Pharmacology of Immunotherapeutic Drugs

Clinton B. Mathias · Jeremy P. McAleer
Doreen E. Szollosi

Pharmacology of Immunotherapeutic Drugs

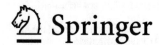
Springer

Clinton B. Mathias
Department of Pharmaceutical
and Administrative Sciences
College of Pharmacy and Health Sciences
Western New England University
Springfield, MA, USA

Jeremy P. McAleer
Pharmaceutical Science and Research
School of Pharmacy
Marshall University
Huntington, WV, USA

Doreen E. Szollosi
Department of Pharmaceutical Sciences
School of Pharmacy and Physician
Assistant Studies
University of Saint Joseph
Hartford, CT, USA

ISBN 978-3-030-19924-1   ISBN 978-3-030-19922-7   (eBook)
https://doi.org/10.1007/978-3-030-19922-7

This Springer imprint is published by the registered company Springer Nature Switzerland AG
The registered company address is: Gewerbestrasse 11, 6330 Cham, Switzerland

Preface

The human immune system is an intricate network of cells and molecules that is critical for our survival and protects our bodies from damage by pathogens, toxins, and other foreign substances. Protection from infection and other injuries prolongs the life of individuals and contributes to their overall health. In contrast, dysregulated immune responses that attack self-antigens or react to harmless substances cause damage to host tissues and induce the development of disease.

Work done by immunologists over the last few decades has revealed a remarkable complexity underlying the mechanisms by which the immune system protects us from infectious organisms while simultaneously avoiding collateral tissue damage. These studies suggest new and hitherto unappreciated roles for many immune cells and molecules in both host protection and disease development, providing novel insights into the mechanisms by which immune cells modulate physiological functions. Chronic inflammation is now known to be causative or a co-culprit in a number of conditions not typically associated with inflammation, including cardiovascular insults (atherosclerosis, coronary artery disease), neurological diseases (Alzheimer's disease, multiple sclerosis), type 2 diabetes, and cancer.

These insights and developments have led to the investigation of a number of immune system components as drug targets for therapeutic purposes. Over the years, this has resulted in the approval by the Food and Drug Administration of several immune-modulating drugs for the treatment of diverse diseases ranging from asthma to cancer. These treatments include general immunosuppressants and antiproliferative agents as well as targeted therapies aimed at modulating specific components of the immune system. This latter category includes various biologics, such as monoclonal antibodies, small molecules, and recombinant cytokines. The immunological principles underlying the activity of these drugs as well as their mechanisms of action is increasingly becoming an important component of health sciences education, including professions such as medicine, pharmacy, and nursing.

We wrote *The Pharmacology of Immunotherapeutic Drugs* in order to bridge the gap between basic science and medical education related to disorders of the immune system. While most pathophysiology and pharmacology textbooks aimed at health science students focus on disease pathogenesis and treatments, there is a dearth of textbooks that are devoted to the immunological mechanisms of disease development and their therapeutic treatment. This is important considering the multitude of immunotherapeutic drugs that have been recently approved for the treatment of a wide variety of diseases. Our book is intended to be a reference for both basic immunologists and clinicians, including medical doctors, pharmacists, and nurses, with the goal of enhancing our understanding of the complexity of the interactions between the immune system and disease. We are not only authors but also teachers, scientists, and lifelong students of immunology who desire to share our passion for immunology with others in the health sciences.

The book opens with a general overview of the immune system, examining the link between inflammation and the onset of disease and providing a synopsis of various pharmacological targets in the context of immunotherapy. While we do cover the basic principles and concepts involved in immunology wherever applicable, it is presupposed that the student will have had prior instruction in basic immunology. A unique feature of this chapter is the inclusion of a comprehensive table listing the various classes and types of immunotherapeutic drugs that are currently approved for the treatment of diseases. Another highlight is a table containing a list of all currently known cytokines and their roles in immune development and function. Lastly, the suggested reading list at the end of Chap. 1 highlights major discoveries in the field of immunology during the last two centuries that have advanced our current understanding of immunology and medicine.

In Chaps. 2 and 3, we build on the preliminary concepts introduced in Chap. 1 and discuss the principles of both innate and adaptive immune processes and their therapeutic modulation. Following this in Chaps. 4, 5, and 6, we focus on inflammatory diseases affecting the major organ systems, such as the respiratory system, the skin, and the gastrointestinal system, and discuss the immunopharmacology of drugs used in their treatment. Similarly, in Chaps. 7 and 8, we cover the basic principles and immune mechanisms involved in autoimmunity and transplantation and discuss the roles of various immunotherapeutic drugs. Lastly, in Chaps. 9 and 10, we discuss the role of immunomodulatory agents in fighting infectious diseases and cancers.

Our book is structured to easily navigate through drug information related to the diseases. Each chapter begins with a table summarizing the drugs discussed in the chapter and their classification. This is followed by a summary of the role of the immune system in health and disease and mechanistic information on how the medications work to treat each disease. In order to provide a historical perspective on drug development, including serendipitous discoveries, trials, and tribulations, "From Bench to Bedside" sections are included at the end of each chapter. Finally, several clinical applications are highlighted in case studies and practice questions that have been added to the chapters.

The development of this textbook has been a long process, and we are grateful to everyone who has played a role in seeing it through completion. We are especially grateful to our family members, who encouraged and supported us in this endeavor throughout the last 2 years. We are also thankful to our colleagues and co-workers, many of whom were willing to review material and provide suggestions and ideas. We are particularly thankful for our coauthors who contributed to chapter material, including Chaps. 7, 9, and 10. A number of students and fellows were willing to read the chapters and make figures and tables. We are grateful for their assistance. We are also thankful to our colleagues who provided materials for case studies, bench to bedside, and practice questions. Lastly, we are thankful to our editors at Springer, who have provided guidance and direction throughout the process.

Immunology is an important subject, not only for the basic science researchers but also for the clinicians. We hope our book helps to illuminate the therapeutic principles behind immunomodulatory drugs for individuals working in health-care fields across several disciplines.

Springfield, MA, USA   Clinton B. Mathias
Huntington, WV, USA   Jeremy P. McAleer
Hartford, CT, USA   Doreen E. Szollosi

Acknowledgments

Contributions to the Drug Table, Glossary, and Answer Key

Victoria Lucero, PharmD
Hector Garcia, PharmD
Yamilia Garcia, PharmD
Ana Gomes, PharmD
Ernest Agyemang, PharmD
Christina Petrelis, PharmD
Zara Saqab, PharmD
Heather DeMar

The authors would like to thank the following reviewers for their thoughtful feedback:

Mohammed Manzoor, PharmD
Alexander Levine, PharmD, BCPS
Swetha Rudraiah, PhD
Junjiang Sun, MD
A.R.M. Ruhul Amin, PhD
Thomas Wadzinski, MD, PhD
Morgan Reynolds, PharmD, CDE
James Knittel, PhD
Diptiman Bose, PhD

Contents

Contributors

Sunna Ahmad, Pharm.D. School of Pharmacy and Physician Assistant Studies, University of Saint Joseph, Hartford, CT, USA

A. R. M. Ruhul Amin, Ph.D. School of Pharmacy, Marshall University, Huntington, WV, USA

Kaitlin Armstrong, Pharm.D. candidate College of Pharmacy and Health Sciences, Western New England University, Springfield, MA, USA

Charles Babcock, Pharm.D., C.D.E., B.C.A.C.P. School of Pharmacy, Marshall University, Huntington, WV, USA

Ngumbah Chumbow, Pharm.D. School of Pharmacy and Physician Assistant Studies, University of Saint Joseph, Hartford, CT, USA

Elizabeth Cohen, Pharm.D., B.C.P.S. Yale New Haven Hospital, New Haven, CT, USA

Daniella D'Aquino, Pharm.D. School of Pharmacy and Physician Assistant Studies, University of Saint Joseph, Hartford, CT, USA

Jennifer Donato, Pharm.D. St. Vincent's Medical Center, Bridgeport, CT, USA

Kirsten Hokeness, Ph.D. Bryant University, Smithfield, RI, USA

Shannon R. M. Kinney, Ph.D. College of Pharmacy and Health Sciences, Western New England University, Springfield, MA, USA

Dylan Krajewski, B.S. College of Pharmacy and Health Sciences, Western New England University, Springfield, MA, USA

Andrea L. Leschak, Pharm.D., B.C.G.P. School of Pharmacy and Physician Assistant Studies, University of Saint Joseph, Hartford, CT, USA

Victoria Lucero, Pharm.D. Yale New Haven Hospital, New Haven, CT, USA

Mohammed K. Manzoor, Pharm.D. School of Pharmacy and Physician Assistant Studies, University of Saint Joseph, Hartford, CT, USA

Michele Riccardi, Pharm.D., B.C.P.S. School of Pharmacy and Physician Assistant Studies, University of Saint Joseph, Hartford, CT, USA

Jeffrey Rovatti, Pharm.D. College of Pharmacy and Health Sciences, Western New England University, Springfield, MA, USA

About the Authors

Clinton B. Mathias received his PhD in Biomedical Sciences with a concentration in Immunology from the University of Connecticut, where he studied the role of innate immune cells in the modulation of allergic asthma. His postdoctoral work at Boston Children's Hospital and Harvard Medical School focused on elucidating mechanisms regulating mast cell homeostasis and function in models of IgE-dependent asthma and food allergy. He is a founding faculty member of the Western New England University College of Pharmacy, where he teaches immunology, infectious diseases, and pharmacology of immunotherapeutic drugs. His research interests are aimed at examining the genetic and environmental factors that govern mast cell responses during allergic inflammation.

Jeremy P. McAleer received his PhD in Biomedical Science from the University of Connecticut where he studied the adjuvant effects of lipopolysaccharide on T cells. His postdoctoral work at Louisiana State University and the University of Pittsburgh focused on the regulation of pulmonary T-cell immunity by commensal microbiota. In 2014, he joined the faculty at Marshall University School of Pharmacy in Huntington, WV, where he teaches immunology and pharmacology and conducts research on the regulation of T-cell immunity by environmental factors.

Doreen E. Szollosi received her PhD in Pathobiology from Brown University where she studied immunosuppression and lymphocyte apoptosis in a mouse model of polymicrobial sepsis at Rhode Island Hospital in Providence. She is a founding faculty member of the University of Saint Joseph School of Pharmacy in Hartford, CT, where she enjoys teaching pharmacy students about the pharmacology of antimicrobials as well as drugs that affect the immune system. Her current research interests include studying the mechanisms of novel anti-inflammatory agents with dual pro-inflammatory cytokine and chemokine suppressive effects.

Overview of the Immune System and Its Pharmacological Targets

1

Clinton B. Mathias

Learning Objectives

1. Describe the process of hematopoiesis and the various types of hematopoietic cells.
2. Describe the processes involved in the education and shaping of immune cells.
3. Describe the role of cell surface receptors and cytokines during immune responses and explain their importance in cell-to-cell communication.
4. Compare and contrast innate and adaptive immune responses in terms of cell types, humoral factors, magnitude, and kinetics.
5. Explain the contribution of immune cells and their mediators to the development of primary and secondary immune responses.
6. Discuss the role of primary and secondary lymphoid organs in the development and activation of immune cells.
7. Describe the various classes and types of immunotherapeutic drugs and discuss their mechanism of action.
8. Describe adverse reactions that can occur with the use of immunotherapeutic drugs.
9. Explain the development of hypersensitivity reactions to immunological drugs.

Clinton B. Mathias (✉)
Department of Pharmaceutical and Administrative Sciences, College of Pharmacy and Health Sciences, Western New England University, Springfield, MA, USA
e-mail: clinton.mathias@wne.edu

Introduction

Since ancient times, humans across many cultures have recognized the vital role that **inflammation** plays in health and disease. The Jews considered blood to be the most sacred of all organs, possessing the life of an animal. Similarly, ancient Egyptians distinguished between good and bad wounds on the basis of the presence or absence of signs of inflammation, while the Hindus in India developed an early system of medicine to treat various inflammatory illnesses. In 460 B.C., the Greek physician Hippocrates first introduced terms such as *edema* and categorized illnesses as acute or chronic. He is also credited with further developing the concept of inflammation and correlating its presence with the resolution and healing of diseases. Based on the Hippocratic canon, the Roman writer Aulus Cornelius Celsus in the first century A.D. accurately described inflammation as consisting of four main characteristics: redness (*rubor*), warmth (*calor*), pain (*dolor*), and swelling (*tumor*). This description of inflammation has stuck with us through the centuries and modern medicine considers the development of inflammation to be critical in the battle against infection and disease.

The nineteenth and twentieth centuries significantly advanced our understanding of how inflammation affects health and disease. The advent of the compound microscope finally

© Springer Nature Switzerland AG 2020
C. B. Mathias et al., *Pharmacology of Immunotherapeutic Drugs*,
https://doi.org/10.1007/978-3-030-19922-7_1

allowed scientists to study the various components of blood, leading to the discovery and characterization of many hematopoietic cell types. Other scientists also discovered tiny organisms called 'microbes' that were ubiquitous throughout nature and hypothesized to cause the development of disease. This was followed by an elegant series of experimental studies by the scientists Robert Koch and Louis Pasteur, who formally established the role of microbes in causing infectious diseases, thus paving the way for understanding the functions of blood cells such as macrophages and mast cells in fighting disease. By the mid-twentieth century, several new advances in immunology had been made including the discovery of **antibodies**, **B cells**, and **T cells**, and their critical role in fighting infectious organisms. Then in 1957, Frank Burnet proposed the **clonal selection theory**, providing an explanation for how immune cells respond to specific infectious antigens, and serving as the basis for our understanding of adaptive immunity. Collectively, these and many other findings had firmly entrenched in the minds of immunologists that inflammation is the body's response to infection. Indeed, as the well-respected immunologist Charles Janeway famously described it several years later, "the immune system evolved to discriminate infectious nonself from noninfectious self" Immunol Today. 1992 Jan;13(1):11–6.

In recent years, work done by immunologists, has led to the discovery and identification of a number of other cell types, receptors, and soluble mediators called **cytokines** (a list of cytokines, their receptors and functions is provided in Table 1.1) that have shaped our current understanding of immunity and how inflammation works. These discoveries have painted a rather complex picture of inflammation that cannot be described solely in terms of the host response to infection or the cardinal characteristics of inflammation first described by Celsus. Indeed, recent studies suggest a far more complicated interplay between various players in regulating the development of inflammation. These include the hematopoietic cells of the immune system, genetic polymorphisms, epigenetic factors, microbes, and several other environmental factors that have the ability to promote or inhibit the development of inflammation. Furthermore, it has now become apparent that inflammation is not simply the body's response to infection, but can also develop towards a host of other antigenic substances including innocuous allergens, food particles, toxic gases, environmental pollutants, and any substance with the potential to cause injury or damage to the host. Lastly, it is now well-established that while the immune system plays a vital role in conferring protection from foreign agents, it is also responsible for the induction of unmitigated inflammatory responses against normal cellular components, leading to chronic inflammatory diseases and autoimmunity. In fact, the persistence of chronic inflammation underlying many different diseases has led to the suggestion that 'inflammation' may be the key to unraveling the unified theory of disease. In support, chronic inflammation is now known to be causative or a co-culprit in a number of conditions not typically associated with inflammation including cardiovascular insults (atherosclerosis, coronary artery disease), neurological diseases (Alzheimer's disease, multiple sclerosis), type 2 diabetes, and cancer.

In this book, we examine the effects of inflammation in the pathogenesis of various diseases and explore the functions of currently approved immunotherapeutic drugs used in their treatment. Specific emphasis will be placed on the roles of immune cells, membrane-bound receptors, and soluble mediators in propagating or preventing a disease and their consideration as established or putative targets for immunotherapy. In the next few sections, a brief synopsis of the immune system including its development and function is provided. This is followed by an overview of the various classes and types of drugs used in immunotherapy. The principles underlying innate and adaptive immune responses as well as therapeutic modulation of the immune system is described in detail in subsequent chapters.

Table 1.1 List of cytokines involved in immune responses

Cytokine/chemokine	Receptor	Produced by	Functions
IL-1α and IL-1β	IL-1R type 1 and type 2	Macrophages, lymohocytes, neutrophils, keratinocytes, fibroblasts, other cells	Proinflammatory cytokine; can act as pyrogen; involved in T_H17 differentiation
IL-1Ra	IL-1R type 1 and type 2	Macrophages, endothelial cells, epithelial cells, neutrophils, keratinocytes, fibroblasts, other cells	Competitive inhibitor of IL-1
IL-2	IL-2R	Activated T cells, DCs, NK cells, NKT cells, mast cells, innate lymphoid cells (ILCs)	Proliferation of T, B, NK cells and ILCs
IL-3	IL-3R	T cells, mast cells, eosinophils, macrophages, NK cells, stromal cells, other cells	Hematopoiesis; growth factor for mast cells, basophils, eosinophils, DCs
IL-4	IL-4R type I and type II	T_H2 cells, basophils, mast cells, eosinophils, NKT cells, γδ T cells	T_H2 differentiation; B cell activation; IgE class switching; upregulation of MHC II; upregulation of CD23 (low affinity receptor for IgE) and IL-4R
IL-5	IL-5R	T_H2 cells, activated eosinophils, mast cells, NK cells, NKT cells, ILC2 cells	Eosinophil differentiation, migration, activation, function, and survival; wound healing
IL-6	IL-6R (soluble IL-6R and gp130)	Endothelial cells, fibroblasts, monocytes, macrophages, T cells, B cells, granulocytes, mast cells, keratinocytes, other cells	Acute phase response; T-cell differentiation, activation, and survival; B-cell differentiation and production of antibodies; leukocyte trafficking and activation; osteoclastogenesis; synovial fibroblast proliferation and cartilage degradation; other functions
IL-7	IL-7R and soluble IL-7R	Monocytes, macrophages, DCs, epithelial cells, B cells, stromal cells	B and T cell development; T cell survival; development and maintenance of ILCs; other functions
IL-8 (CXCL8)	CXCR1 and CXCR2	Monocytes, macrophages, neutrophils, lymphocytes, epithelial cells, keratinocytes, smooth muscle cells, other cells	Chemotactic factor for neutrophils, NK cells, T cells, basophils, eosinophils; angiogenesis
IL-9	IL-9R	T_H2 cells, T_H9 cells, T_H17 cells, mast cells, ILC2s, T_{reg} cells	Proliferation of T cells and mast cells; IgE production; mucus production
IL-10	IL-10R1/ IL-10R2 complex	T_H2 cells, T_{reg} cells, T_H1 cells, macrophages, DCs, B cells, mast cells, other cells	Suppression of DC and T cell function; stimulation of mast cells, NK cells, and B cells
IL-11	IL-11Rα and gp130	Bone marrow stromal cells, fibroblasts, epithelial cells, osteoblasts, other cells	Hematopoietic growth factor for erythroid and myeloid lineages; bone remodeling and stimulation of osteoclasts; epithelial cell repair
IL-12	IL-12Rβ1 and IL-12Rβ2	Macrophages, neutrophils, DCs, B cells, other cells	Development and maintenance of T_H1 cells; NK cell activation; DC maturation; cytotoxic responses

(continued)

Table 1.1 (continued)

Cytokine/chemokine	Receptor	Produced by	Functions
IL-13	IL-13R type I (IL-13Rα1 and IL-4Rα) and type II (IL-13Rα2)	T_H2 cells, mast cells, basophils, eosinophils, NKT cells, ILC2 cells	IgE class-switching; mucus secretion; epithelial cell turnover; MHC II upregulation; smooth muscle hyperreactivity; defense against parasites
IL-14 (alpha-taxilin)	IL-14R	T cells, T cell lymphomas	Proliferation of activated and cancerous B cells
IL-15	IL-15R	Monocytes, macrophages, DCs, CD4 T cells, stromal cells, keratinocytes, other cells	NK cell proliferation and activation; differentiation of γδ T cells; development and maintenance of NK, NKT, and memory CD8 T cells; suppression of CD4 T cells; prevention of eosinophil apoptosis
IL-16 (pro-IL-16)	CD4	Epithelial cells, fibroblasts, T cells, eosinophils, mast cells, DCs	Chemotactic factor for CD4 and CD8 T cells, mast cells, eosinophils, monocytes
IL-17A and IL-17F	IL-17RA	T_H17 cells, CD8 T cells, γδ T cells, NK cells, NKT cells, neutrophils, ILCs	Neutrophil recruitment and activation; promotion of inflammation
IL-17B, IL-17C, IL-17D	IL-17RB; IL-17RA-E; IL-17RD or SEF[a] or IL-17RLM	IL-17B: neuronal cells; IL-17C: epithelial cells; IL-17D: resting B and T cells, skeletal cells, heart, lung, brain, pancreatic cells	Induction of antimicrobial peptides, cytokines, chemokines, metalloproteinases; IL-17B: chondrogenesis and osteogenesis; IL-17C: intestinal barrier modulation; IL-17D: suppression of myeloid progenitor cells
IL-18	IL-18R	Macrophages, DCs, epithelial cells, keratinocytes, osteoblasts, other cells	Promotion of NK cell cytotoxicity; production of IFN-γ in the presence of IL-12
IL-19	IL-20R1/ IL-20R2	Monocytes, B cells, keratinocytes, epithelial cells, other cells	Enhancement of T_H2 cytokine production in keratinocytes; increase IL-6 and TNF-α from monocytes
IL-20	IL-20R1/ IL-20R2 and IL-22R1/ IL-20R2	Monocytes, epithelial cells, keratinocytes	Autocrine regulator of keratinocytes
IL-21	IL-21R	T_H9 cells, T_H17 cells, NKT cells	B cell proliferation and survival; NKT cell proliferation; T cell growth
IL-22	IL-22R	Activated T_H17 cells, T_H22 cells, NK cells, NKT cells, ILCs	Induction of antimicrobial peptides from keratinocytes; keratinocyte repair and healing; tissue reorganization
IL-23	IL-23R	Macrophages and DCs in peripheral tissues	T_H17 proliferation and maintenance; promotion of IL-17 production; NK cell activation; regulation of antibody production
IL-24	IL-20R1/ IL-20R2 and IL-22R1/ IL-20R2	Melanocytes, T cells, keratinocytes, other cells	Tumor suppression

(continued)

Table 1.1 (continued)

Cytokine/chemokine	Receptor	Produced by	Functions
IL-25 (IL-17E)	IL-17RA and IL-17RB	T_H2 cells, mast cells, eosinophils, basophils, epithelial cells	Alarmin cytokine; Induction of T_H2 responses; production of IgE, IL-4, IL-5, IL-13; inhibition of T_H1 and T_H17 responses
IL-26	IL-10R2 chain and IL-20R1 chain	Activated T_H17 cells, NK cells, memory T cells	Regulation of epithelial cells
IL-27	IL-27Rα and gp130	Activated macrophages, DCs, and epithelial cells	Control of differentiation of helper T cell subsets; T_H1 differentiation; induction of T-bet; inhibition of T_H17 responses; upregulation of IL-10
IL-28A/B/IL-29	IL-28R1/ IL-10R2	DCs and other nucleated cells in response to viral infections	Induction of T_H1 and T_{reg} responses; induction of tolerogenic DCs
IL-30 (p28 subunit of IL-27)			Prevention and treatment of cytokine-induced liver injury
IL-31	IL-31RA/ OSMRβ[a]	T_H2 cells, CD8 T cells, macrophages, DCs, keratinocytes, mast cells, other cells	Induction of chemokines from eosinophils and keratinocytes; itching during atopic dermatitis
IL-32	Unknown	Monocytes, macrophages, activated NK cells, activated T cells, epithelial cells	Induction of IL-6, CXCL8, TNF-α in macrophages and other cells; prevention of eosinophil apoptosis
IL-33	ST2	Epithelial cells, endothelial cells, necrotic cells, fibroblasts, stromal cells	Alarmin cytokine; induction of T_H2, mast cell, eosinophil, and ILC2 responses
IL-34	Colony stimulating factor (CSF)-1 receptor	Spleen, heart, brain, liver, kidney, thymus, testes, ovary, small intestine, prostate, colon	Regulation of myeloid lineage and microglial proliferation
IL-35	IL-12Rβ2/ gp130; IL-12Rβ2/ IL-12Rβ2; gp130/gp130	T_{reg} cells, monocytes, epithelial cells, endothelial cells, smooth muscle cells	T_{reg} proliferation; increased IL-10 production; inhibition of effector T cell function
IL-36	IL-36Ra	Endothelial cells, macrophages	Promotion of keratinocyte, DC, and T cell responses to tissue injury or infection
IL-37	IL-18Rα and IL-18BP	Monocytes, tonsil plasma cells, breast carcinoma, lung carcinoma, colon carcinoma, melanoma	Inhibition of IL-18 activity; inhibition of DCs and NK cell activity
IL-38	IL-1R1 with low affinity, IL-36R	Basal epithelia of skin, spleen, fetal liver, placenta, thymus, proliferating B cells of the tonsils	Inhibition of T_H17 responses; inhibition of IL-36
B-cell activating factor (BAFF) or B Lymphocyte Stimulator (BLyS)	TACI,[a] BCMA,[a] BAFF-R	Monocytes, dendritic cells, follicular dendritic cells, bone marrow stromal cells	B cell activation and maturation
Granulocyte colony-stimulating factor (G-CSF or CSF3)	G-CSF receptor	Bone marrow cells, endothelial cells, macrophages, other immune cells	Hematopoiesis; stimulates HSCs to produce neutrophils

(continued)

Table 1.1 (continued)

Cytokine/chemokine	Receptor	Produced by	Functions
Granulocyte-macrophage colony-stimulating factor (GM-CSF or CSF2)	GM-CSF receptor	Macrophages, mast cells, T cells, NK cells, endothelial cells, fibroblasts	Hematopoiesis; stimulates HSCs to produce granulocytes and myeloid cells
IFN-α and IFN-β	IFNAR	All nucleated cells in response to viral infections; plasmacytoid DCs	Antiviral response; interferon response; activation of NK cells; stimulation of DCs; stimulation of ADCC; apoptosis of tumor cells
IFN-γ	IFNGR1/ IFNGR2	T_H1 cells, CD8 T cells, NK cells, NKT cells, macrophages, B cells	Antiviral response; cytotoxic activity; upregulation of MHC II; enhancement of immunoproteasome
Macrophage colony-stimulating factor (M-CSF)	M-CSF receptor	Bone marrow cells, fibroblasts	Acts on HSCs to promote myeloid lineage
Thymic stromal lymphopoietin (TSLP)	CRLF2[a] and IL-7Rα chain	Fibroblasts, epithelial cells, stromal cells	Stimulates DCs and T_H2 responses
Transforming growth factor (TGF)-β	TβR I and TβR II	Epithelial cells, fibroblasts, macrophages, eosinophils, T cells, T_{reg} cells, other cells	Immune tolerance; induction of T_{reg} cells; decreased growth of immune precursors; mesenchymal cell transition; development of cardiac system and bone formation
Tumor Necrosis Factor (TNF)-α	TNFR1 and TNFR2	Macrophages, monocytes, DCs, T cells, mast cells, NK cells, NKT cells, fibroblasts, endothelial cells, other cells	Proinflammatory cytokine; vasodilation; vascular permeability; upregulation of adhesion molecules on endothelial cells; tumorigenesis
TNF-β or Lymphotoxin (LT)-α and LT-β	LT-β receptors	Lymphocytes	Formation of secondary lymphoid organs; anti-proliferative activity; destruction of tumor cell lines; innate immune regulation; pro-carcinogenic activity when upregulated

Adapted and modified from Akdis et. al. Interleukins (from IL-1 to IL-38), interferons, transforming growth factor β, and TNF-α: Receptors, functions, and roles in disease. J Allergy Clin Immunol 2016;138:984–1010

[a]BCMA B-cell maturation antigen, CRLF2 cytokine receptor-like factor 2, OSMRβ oncostatin M specific receptor subunit beta, SEF similar expression to fibroblast growth factor genes, TACI transmembrane activator and calcium modulator and cyclophilin ligand interactor

Overview of the Immune Response

The primary purpose of the immune system is to defend the host against infectious organisms that may compromise the integrity of the host, leading to cellular damage and possible death of the host. Immune responses against pathogens can be compartmentalized into five stages: pathogen detection, acute inflammation, antigen presenta-tion, adaptive immunity, and pathogen destruction (Fig. 1.1). As discussed throughout this book, various cell types are involved at each stage, with their function regulated by cell-to-cell interactions, surface receptors, and cytokines. Many of these receptors and cytokines (which include various **interleukins**) are therapeutic targets for patients with inflammatory diseases.

Infection with a pathogenic organism can lead to three possible outcomes: elimination of the

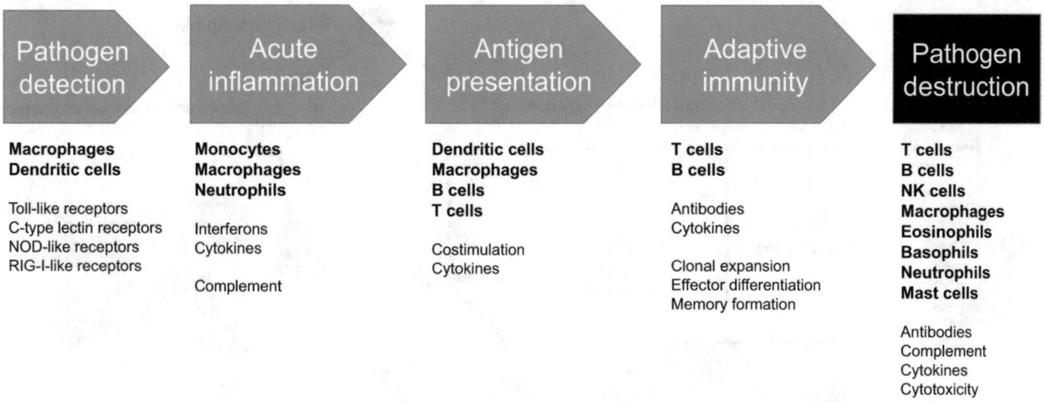

Pathogen detection	Acute inflammation	Antigen presentation	Adaptive immunity	Pathogen destruction
Macrophages **Dendritic cells** Toll-like receptors C-type lectin receptors NOD-like receptors RIG-I-like receptors	**Monocytes** **Macrophages** **Neutrophils** Interferons Cytokines Complement	**Dendritic cells** **Macrophages** **B cells** **T cells** Costimulation Cytokines	**T cells** **B cells** Antibodies Cytokines Clonal expansion Effector differentiation Memory formation	**T cells** **B cells** **NK cells** **Macrophages** **Eosinophils** **Basophils** **Neutrophils** **Mast cells** Antibodies Complement Cytokines Cytotoxicity

Fig. 1.1 Immune responses against pathogenic microorganisms occur in five stages, culminating in pathogen destruction. Examples of cell types, receptor interactions and/or immune checkpoints are indicated for each stage (figure contributed by Jeremy P. McAleer)

organism by the immune system, chronic infection that is held in check by the immune system, or death of the host due to a failure of the immune system to eliminate the pathogen. Most infections are successfully eliminated by the immune system, resulting in tissue healing and cellular memory of the infectious pathogen. A small number of pathogens may cause chronic infections that are not cleared, leading to latency of the infectious organism within the host and subsequent periods of reactivation by environmental or other stimuli. Although these infections are not completely eradicated, they are usually held in check by the immune system for long periods of time, until the immune system is either compromised or completely damaged. In the absence of treatment to restore the immune system or control the infection, this usually results in death of the host.

The immune system is also critical for human survival. In the absence of a functional immune system, the host is unable to protect itself against common environmental microorganisms, ultimately succumbing to various infections that often result in death. Severe cases of this are observed in patients born with primary immunodeficiencies, as exemplified by **Severe combined immune deficiency (SCID).** In this primary immunodeficiency, patients are unable to produce the T and B cells of the adaptive immune system, and survival is not possible, unless therapy is initiated with **hematopoietic stem cell**

transplantation (bone marrow transplantation) to restore the immune system.

In addition to initiating and propagating immune responses, the cells of the immune system play important roles in several other organ systems. Various resident and migrating populations of immune cells such as macrophages and mast cells are present in almost every organ of the body, where they contribute to the integrity of tissues and participate in maintaining organelle function.

Hematopoiesis and Cells of the Immune System

The cells of the immune system are derived and transported via blood, and hence are referred to as hematopoietic cells. The process of formation of blood cells is termed as **hematopoiesis**. All the populations of blood cells are derived from common progenitors termed **hematopoietic stem cells (HSCs)**. These cells are present throughout the adult bone marrow and are long-lasting and self-renewing. They divide in the presence of growth factors and other instructions from stromal cells into several types of progenitor populations, eventually leading to the generation of distinct lineages of red and white blood cells. Thus, HSCs are also said to be pluripotent with the ability to differentiate into many different cell types.

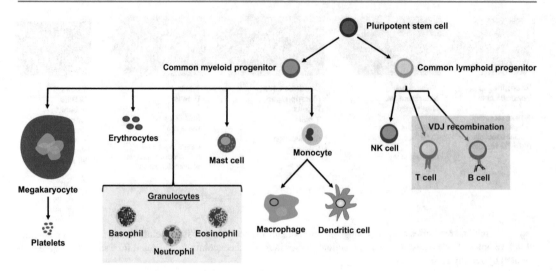

Fig. 1.2 The development of immune cells through hematopoiesis. Pluripotent stem cells are self-renewing and give rise to daughter progeny with a more limited developmental potential. Hematopoiesis occurs in the bone marrow and is guided by growth factors and cell to cell interactions. The common myeloid progenitor gives rise to several innate immune cell types including granulocytes, mast cells, and monocytes. The common lymphoid progenitor gives rise to lymphocytes (T cells, B cells, NK cells) (figure contributed by Jeremy P. McAleer)

In the developing embryo, hematopoiesis begins in the yolk sac. This later shifts to the fetal liver and then the spleen during the third to seventh months of fetal life. During the fourth to fifth months, hematopoiesis is initiated in the fetal bone marrow, and this continues throughout the life of the host. In adults, the major sites of hematopoiesis are the skull, sternum, vertebral column, femurs, pelvis, and ribs.

Hematopoietic cells are divided into two major categories: red blood cells or **erythrocytes** and white blood cells or **leukocytes** (Fig. 1.2). Immune cells are classically referred to as white blood cells, although erythrocytes also participate in the immune response. Two distinct lineages of leukocytes are derived from hematopoiesis: the **myeloid** lineage, which gives rise to **granulocytes**, **monocytes**, **macrophages**, **dendritic cells**, and **mast cells**; and the **lymphoid** lineage which gives rise to **natural killer (NK) cells**, B cells, and various populations of T cells.

Red blood cells and megakaryocytes (which give rise to platelets) are derived from the erythroid progenitor, which is derived from a common myeloid precursor. The primary purpose of erythrocytes is to transport oxygen throughout blood. However, they also participate in the removal of immune complexes containing antibodies bound to their target proteins. Platelets maintain the integrity of blood vessels and initiate and maintain clotting reactions to promote wound healing and prevent blood loss.

The Myeloid Lineage

The myeloid progenitor gives rise to three major cell types: granulocytes, monocyte-derived cells, and mast cells. The granulocytes consist of three major populations of cells: **neutrophils**, **eosinophils**, and **basophils**. They are characterized by the presence of cytoplasmic granules, which house a number of toxic mediators and enzymes that are involved in immune reactions. In addition, they possess many irregular, multi-lobed nuclei, leading to the use of the term **polymorphonuclear (PMN) leukocytes** to describe them.

Neutrophils Are Rapidly Mobilized to Tissues During an Infection

Neutrophils are the most abundant leukocyte present in blood, accounting for up to 70% of the total leukocyte population. Their granules do not stain with acidic or basic dyes, forming the basis for the nomenclature *neutro*phils. Neutrophils are highly specialized cells that are adept in the capture, phagocytosis, and killing of infectious organisms. In addition, they also secrete a number of mediators that enhance inflammation. Neutrophils act as first responders during infections and are rapidly mobilized from the blood to sites of infection. Here, they help initiate and coordinate the capture and killing of microorganisms that have entered the tissue, thriving in the anaerobic conditions present in damaged tissues. Despite their intense activity, neutrophils are short-lived cells that die after their granular contents have been released, resulting in the formation of pus.

Eosinophils and Basophils Protect the Host from Parasitic Infections

Eosinophils derive their name from the pink staining of their granules when stained with the acidic dye eosin. The major function of eosinophils is to initiate defense against parasitic organisms such as helminth worms. These effects are primarily mediated in concert with parasite-specific **IgE antibodies** produced by the B cells of the adaptive immune system. Eosinophils are generated in the bone marrow under the control of stromal cells and several growth factors, including the interleukins **(IL)-3** and **IL-5**. During a parasitic infection, these cytokines, as well as chemokines such as **eotaxin** produced by T cells, induce their migration to tissues, where they promote their differentiation and survival. Once they reach the site of parasitic infection, eosinophils upregulate the high affinity receptor for IgE antibodies, **FcεRI**, and mediate antigen-induced inflammatory reactions resulting in degranulation and the release of toxic mediators such as major basic protein and eosinophil peroxidases which destroy the parasitic organism. In addition to their role in anti-parasitic responses, eosinophils are a major contributor to the development of allergic disease.

Basophils stain with the basic dye hematoxylin. They are a rare granulocyte population that like eosinophils and mast cells have been implicated in IgE-mediated reactions, but have recently been found to also contribute to other types of immune responses. Basophils are mostly present in circulation, where they constitutively express the IgE receptor, FcεRI, and participate in the development of anti-parasitic and allergic responses. Like mast cells and eosinophils, they also depend on growth factors such as IL-3 and **granulocyte-macrophage colony stimulating factor (GM-CSF)** for their differentiation and survival. They are prolific producers of the cytokine **IL-4**, and have been hypothesized to provide the initial source of IL-4 that is required for the differentiation and activation of **helper CD4 T cells** of the T_H2 phenotype. In addition, they have been found to express ligands for costimulatory molecules that activate T cells and have been postulated to act as antigen-presenting cells under some conditions.

Monocytes, Macrophages, and Dendritic Cells Capture and Destroy Pathogens and Alert the Immune System

The second group of myeloid cells consists of monocytes, macrophages, and dendritic cells. Monocytes are a distinct group of cells with indented nuclei that are present throughout the circulation. From the blood, monocytes migrate to tissues where they mature into macrophages or dendritic cells under the control of growth factors such as GM-CSF and IL-4. Macrophages are long-lasting cells that are present in all bodily tissues. Here, they not only perform functions that are unique to the tissue such as the capture of antigens by skin-resident cells or the maintenance of bone homeostasis and integrity by bone-resident **osteoclasts**, but are also involved in the initiation and propagation of immune responses. A primary immune function of macrophages in tissues is to act as sentinel cells that sense and alert the immune system to the presence of infection or danger. Macrophages are well-equipped to do this by virtue of possessing a number of receptors that are adept at both capturing pathogens and initiating an inflammatory signal transduction cascade. Pathogen capture is mediated by various receptors on the surface of macrophages including C-type

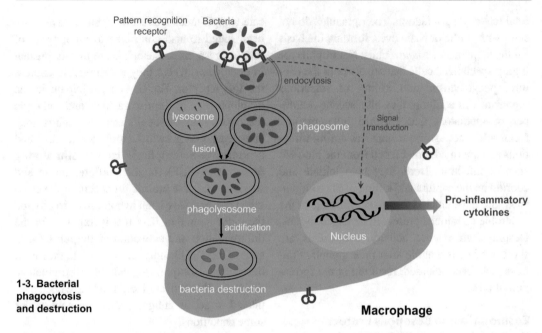

1-3. Bacterial phagocytosis and destruction

Fig. 1.3 Bacterial phagocytosis and destruction. Macrophages detect microbes including bacteria through pattern recognition receptors. This elicits receptor-mediated endocytosis as well as a signal transduction pathway leading to the expression of pro-inflammatory cytokines. Fusion of the phagosome with a lysosome results in acidification within the intracellular compartment and bacterial destruction (figure contributed by Jeremy P. McAleer)

lectin receptors (such as dectins and mannose binding receptors) as well as scavenger receptors. This is subsequently followed by the initiation of **phagocytosis** or receptor-mediated **endocytosis** (Fig. 1.3). This involves pathogen transport via a vesicular pathway that comprises of a series of vesicles that terminate in the cellular phagosome. Here, changes in cellular pH induce the fusion of the phagosome with the lysosome, giving rise to the phagolysosome, where the pathogen is destroyed and degraded. Pathogenic peptides derived from this process may be subsequently used as antigens to induce the activation of T cells during adaptive immune responses.

In addition to receptors for antigen capture, macrophages also express receptors that initiate signal transduction pathways. A vast majority of these belong to the **Toll-like receptor (TLR) family**, which may be expressed either on the plasma membrane or intracellularly. Examples include the TLR4 homodimer, which binds to **lipopolysaccharide**, an endotoxin found in the

cell wall of gram-negative bacteria. Similarly, TLR5 binds bacterial flagellin, while TLR3 binds viral nucleic acids. Binding of ligands by TLRs results in the induction of signaling cascades that culminate in the activation of various transcription factors including **nuclear factor of kappa B (NF-κB)**, a potent transcription factor involved in the activation of a number of immune cytokine genes such as **IL-2**, **TNF-α**, **IL-1**, and **IL-6**.

Dendritic cells also derive from the monocyte lineage and perform similar functions as macrophages in various tissues. In addition, they are equipped with the unique ability to induce the activation of naïve T cells in secondary lymphoid organs, serving as a link between the innate and adaptive immune responses. Once they have captured antigens in peripheral tissues such as the skin, dendritic cells migrate to secondary lymphoid organs such as the draining lymph nodes, where they activate naïve T cells and induce their differentiation into various sub-types.

Mast Cells Protect Against Parasites and Also Promote Inflammation

The third category of myeloid cells, mast cells, are present throughout vascularized tissues, where they sense the presence of pathogens and initiate immune responses. Like eosinophils and basophils, they also possess large numbers of granules containing preformed mediators such as histamine, which are released upon activation and degranulation. Mast cells also constitutively express the IgE receptor, FcεRI, and participate in IgE-mediated anti-parasitic and allergic responses. However, they are highly versatile cells that are also implicated in many other types of immune reactions, and express several other receptors including the TLRs and complement receptors.

The Lymphoid Lineage

The lymphoid lineage of cells gives rise to NK cells, T cells, and B cells. NK cells are a heterogeneous group of innate lymphocytes that express several receptors that are involved in recognizing and attacking tumors or virus-infected cells. NK cells also produce a variety of cytokines that can modulate the function of other cell types such as dendritic cells, macrophages, and T cells.

T cells are the main drivers of the adaptive immune response. They are derived from lymphoid progenitors in the bone marrow, following which they travel to the thymus, where they complete their development and maturation. In the thymus, T cells are educated to recognize the difference between host and foreign antigens under the control of thymic epithelial cells, macrophages, and dendritic cells. T cells derived their name due to their maturation in the thymus gland. Following maturation, naïve T cells exit the thymus and enter circulation, where they are poised to interact with antigens presented by antigen presenting cells such as dendritic cells. Two major types of T cells have been described: **CD4 T cells**, which consist of **helper T cells** and **regulatory T cells** (T_{reg}), and **CD8 T cells**, also referred to as **cytotoxic T cells**.

Helper T cells can be differentiated into many diverse sub-types including the $T_H1, T_H2, T_H9, T_H17, T_H22$, and T_{FH} subsets depending on their phenotype. The differentiation of helper T cells is coordinated by both antigen presenting cells and other innate cell types through the release of distinct cytokines which promote their differentiation. Each type of helper T cell is associated with the expression and activation of transcription factors unique to that particular cell type. Helper T cells are critical to the immune system and perform diverse functions including the coordination of immune responses against intracellular and extracellular bacteria, viruses, parasites, and fungi. The depletion of helper T cells leads to severely compromised immune functions and death, as occurs during the development of **Acquired Immune Deficiency Syndrome (AIDS)**. Regulatory T cells play an important role in regulating or suppressing other cells in the immune system. They suppress unwanted responses to self or foreign antigens and prevent the development of autoimmunity.

In contrast, CD8 T cells are uniquely equipped to mediate adaptive immunity to viral infections. They kill virally-infected cells and may also enhance immune responses to other pathogens. Additionally, these cytotoxic T cells are the adaptive immune system's primary defense against tumors and the development of cancer.

B cells also arise from lymphoid progenitors in the bone marrow and complete their maturation and development there. The origin of their name comes from where they were first discovered, the Bursa of Fabricius, a specialized hematopoietic organ which is only found in birds. The primary function of B cells is the production and secretion of various immunoglobulins or antibody isotypes. Upon maturation, B cells express the **IgM** antibody, which is the first antibody isotype produced during immune responses. Under the direction of T cells, B cells can be further activated to produce various other antibody isotypes such as **IgG, IgA**, and **IgE**.

The Education and Shaping of Immune Cells

Regulation of Immune Cells by Commensal Microbiota

Immune cells are conditioned by their microenvironment. Signals received during infection or other types of host injury have the potential to modulate the functions of immune cells, leading to their activation or suppression. Similarly, several environmental factors have also been shown to modulate the development of immune responses. The host microbiota in particular has an enormous influence on the immune system. During fetal development, fetal cells have no interactions with microorganisms as a result of protection provided by maternal IgG antibodies and the mother's immune cells. This vastly changes as soon as a newborn is exposed to environmental bacteria. Upon birth, each individual is colonized by a host of **commensal** microorganisms, which constitute the normal microflora of the host. These bacteria reside in various mucosal tissues including the gastrointestinal tract, oral cavity, vagina, and skin. Here, they are in constant interaction with immune cells and modulate their activity and function, providing the necessary experience that is required for fighting infections. As such, the immune cells in mucosal tissues remain ever-ready to prevent the development of infection, actively monitoring the microbial population and preventing infection by opportunistic pathogens. This sentinel activity is performed in a manner that minimizes host cellular damage and prevents the development of chronic inflammation.

Commensal microorganisms perform many functions including aiding in digestion, providing metabolites and cofactors for cells, preventing the growth of opportunistic pathogens, and shaping the immune system. The interactions of immune cells with the commensal microflora play a pivotal role in providing the education and experience that is needed for future defense against infections with pathogenic organisms. Exposure to infections, especially during early life, can further modulate the development of the immune system, ensuring that immune cells develop in a healthy fashion that is geared towards host defense and not the development of unnecessary responses. For example, exposure to intracellular bacteria such as mycobacteria in early life may help to prevent a T_H2 bias of the immune system, while exposure to helminth worms is thought to reduce IgE-mediated allergic sensitization.

The diversity and composition of the commensal population is determined by a host of factors including exposure to dietary components and competing species of bacteria. When changes in the microbial composition occur, either due to illness, a change in diet, or treatment with antibiotics, further modulation of the immune system may also occur. In elderly or immunocompromised patients, antibiotic treatment can disrupt the normal microbial composition and allow for the growth of opportunistic pathogens such as *Clostridium difficile*, which are normally held in check by the immune system and by competing bacteria such as enterobacteria.

T and B Cell Education in Primary Lymphoid Organs

Adaptive immune cells gain specific experience in **primary lymphoid organs** such as the **thymus** and **bone marrow,** where they develop and mature. In the thymus, T cells are taught to differentiate between 'self' and 'non-self' antigens. Under the careful coordination of thymic epithelial cells and dendritic cells, they learn to tolerate self-tissues and mediate immune responses against foreign antigens. This selection process ensures that naïve T cells will only be activated against non-self antigens that are presented by host antigen presenting cells, thereby preventing the development of autoimmunity. Immature T cells which have the potential to recognize self-antigens are eliminated and undergo death by apoptosis. In a similar manner, B cells also undergo selection processes in the bone marrow and secondary lymphoid organs. These processes ensure that self-reactive B cells with the potential to bind autoantigens are eliminated from the immune repertoire and only those that can react against non-self antigens are retained. Further selection processes in secondary lymphoid organs such as the lymph node ensure the differentiation and survival of mature B cells that have the potential to react with high affinity against specific antigens and make effective antibodies of various isotypes. Once mature naïve B and T cells enter the circulation, they are held in check by a number of regulatory processes, which are aimed at further preventing the development of autoimmunity.

Upon activation, all immune cells are programmed to differentiate into activated effector cells. Depending on the particular type of injury or antigenic trigger, effector cells mediate the active immune response to pathogens or other foreign agents, inducing the development of inflammation and destroying the foreign organism. The functions of effector cells are further conditioned by the release and activity of various cytokines, which modulate the behavior of the particular immune cell. Various types of effector cells exist depending on the type of cell and the particular immune response. In addition to giving rise to effector cells, adaptive immune cells also differentiate into memory cells. These are long-lasting cells that

remember the particular antigenic exposure and are readily stimulated on antigenic re-exposure resulting in a rapid and potent immune response against the specific antigen.

The Innate Immune Response

The vast majority of infectious organisms are rapidly eliminated by the immune system soon after exposure without causing significant host damage and/or the induction of clinical symptoms. This response is mediated by a combination of both ubiquitously present anti-microbial proteins and molecules as well as the microbicidal activity of cells such as neutrophils and macrophages. This type of response is termed as the **innate immune response**, since it can be mobilized as soon as infection occurs, does not recognize specific antigens, and does not require a prolonged induction phase as in the case of T and B cells (Fig. 1.4).

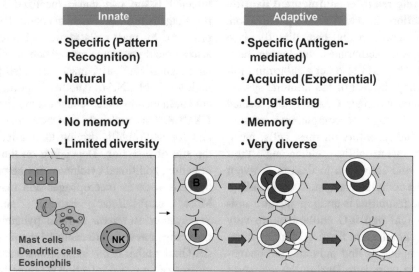

Fig. 1.4 Distinguishing characteristics of the innate and adaptive immune systems. Both innate and adaptive immune cells evolved to recognize foreign antigens. However, they differ with respect to their specificity and capacity to mediate long-lasting immune responses. Innate cells express a variety of receptors for the recognition of pathogen-associated molecular patterns. In contrast, adaptive cells are equipped with the unique ability to recognize distinct antigens by virtue of a single specific surface receptor. The effects of activated innate cells occur immediately. However, adaptive cells must go through a process of clonal selection and clonal expansion prior to activation. Activated adaptive cells can differentiate into effector and memory populations that mediate a tailored and life-long response to antigens

Pre-formed Molecules Provide an Immediate Defense Against Infectious Agents

A number of molecules present in blood and tissues possess anti-microbial activity. These include protease inhibitors such as α2-macroglobulins in the blood, acids in various tissues, lysozyme which degrades peptidoglycan, and **defensins** which are anti-microbial peptides. In addition to these, a unique family of serine proteases play a critical role in the elimination of pathogens and the facilitation of immune responses. These heat-labile proteins, which act on each other during the immune response, are collectively referred to as the **complement system**. The molecules of the complement system are constitutively produced by the liver. Upon antigenic exposure, whether due to changes in the physiological environment or the engagement of receptors, the complement pathway is activated. This results in the activation of key complement molecules such as **C3b**, the primary function of which is to tag pathogens for destruction and facilitate complement-initiated phagocytosis. This is referred to as **complement fixation** or **opsonization**. In addition to opsonization, complement components can directly lyse pathogenic cell membranes, mediating their destruction. They can also act as alarmin molecules, alerting the rest of the immune system to the presence of danger. **C3a** and **C5a**, formed during the cleavage of complement components can bind receptors on mast cells, basophils, and neutrophils, enhancing their recruitment and activation in tissues. A major trigger of the complement system during adaptive immune responses is antigen-specific antibody. Both IgM and IgG antibodies are very effective at complement fixation, binding complement components and inducing the phagocytosis of the pathogen. During the course of inflammation, large numbers of antigen-antibody immune complexes can be formed. Binding of these to the complement component C3b can facilitate the removal of **immune complexes** by erythrocytes which express receptors for C3b.

The Initial Response to Infection

In addition to immunity mediated by the complement system and other molecules, a number of leukocytes play key roles in the initial response to infection. Depending on the type and the site of infection, distinct immunological pathways are activated aimed at terminating the infection.

Early on, cells such as macrophages play a critical role in limiting the numbers of pathogens and alerting other immune cells. Damage to cells of the connective tissue such as a wound, burn, trauma, bite, or other type of injury to the skin induces the rapid activation of macrophages, which perform phagocytosis and release proinflammatory cytokines (Fig. 1.5). Of these, the cytokine, TNF-α, is a potent vasodilator, causing blood vessels to expand and inducing vascular permeability. As a result, endothelial cells lining blood vessels become leaky, allowing the exit of blood constituents including cells and other molecules. TNF-α also upregulates the expression of adhesion molecules on blood vessels, facilitating the migration of neutrophils and other cells that express corresponding ligands to tissues. The arrival of cells and other molecules to the infected tissue can cause localized swelling, resulting in the development of edema. Histamine produced by mast cells at sites of infection is also a potent vasoactivator and can act in a similar manner. Similarly, mast cells also produce high levels of TNF-α. Another important molecule produced by macrophages is the chemokine **CXCL8**. This molecule acts as a chemoattractant for neutrophils, driving their migration to the site of infection. Depending on the type of infection, additional cytokines may be produced by cells such as macrophages and mast cells. Most extracellular bacteria such as *Staphylococcus aureus* or other **pyogenic (pus-inducing) bacteria** are captured *via* phagocytosis. On the other hand, intracellular bacteria and viruses often cause infection by directly infecting the macrophages. Macrophages can also phagocytose other cells that have been infected by the pathogen. In response to viral infections, macrophages make the cytokine IL-12, which can serve to coactivate both dendritic cells and natural killer cells to the pathogen.

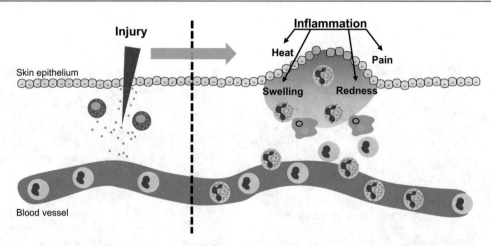

Fig. 1.5 Hallmarks of Inflammation. Injury to a body tissue such as the skin results in the immediate production of cytokines by epithelial cells, which serve to recruit neutrophils and other inflammatory cells from the blood. Release of TNF-α and other cytokines by tissue macrophages make blood vessels permeable, enhancing the migration of leukocytes to the injured area. The dilation of blood vessels and increased leukocyte infiltration at the injured site contributes to the redness, heat, and swelling associated with inflammation. The increase in edema causes pinching of the nerves attached to blood vessels, resulting in the induction of pain (figure contributed by Jeremy P. McAleer)

The Development of Inflammation Gives Rise to the Acute Phase Response

Signaling cascades induced by the engagement of pattern recognition receptors including TLRs on macrophages further enhance inflammation by inducing the activation of transcription factors such as NF-κB and the production of cytokines such as IL-1β and IL-6. Along with TNF-α, IL-1β and IL-6 are considered to be some of the most prominent proinflammatory cytokines produced during the innate immune response. Together, the three cytokines exert both localized and systemic effects to enhance the inflammatory response. IL-1β like TNF-α also acts on endothelial cells and promotes vasodilation. IL-6, and to a lesser effect IL-1β and TNF-α, promotes the **acute phase response**. This refers to a dynamic change in the profile of dozens of serum proteins that are secreted by hepatocytes in the liver. The concentrations of these proteins changes significantly, with proteins such as albumin (which is the most abundant plasma protein) decreasing while those of others such as **C-reactive protein (CRP)** and serum amyloid A increasing over a hundred-fold. The latter are referred to as acute phase proteins and their levels can be directly correlated to the intensity of inflammation. One of these, CRP, is also a trigger of the classical pathway of complement activation.

IL-1β, IL-6, and TNF-α also exert systemic effects. One of these effects includes actions on the temperature control sites of the hypothalamus as well as on fat and muscle cells, with the net effect of altering energy mobilization and raising the body temperature. These cytokines are therefore also referred to as pyrogens. The raised body temperature not only inhibits the growth of pathogens, but also enhances the effects of adaptive immunity.

Macrophages and Neutrophils Destroy Pathogenic Bacteria via Phagocytosis

Phagocytosis of extracellular bacteria by macrophages induces the release of CXCL8 and the eventual recruitment of neutrophils to the infected site. Neutrophils act as first responders and are extremely effective at killing and destroying extracellular bacteria. The responding neutrophils secrete a battery of toxic mediators and degradative enzymes stored in their granules which are extremely destructive to pathogens. The process of pathogen destruction begins with phagocytosis, subsequent to which pathogens are subjected to granule contents of many different types (Fig. 1.6).

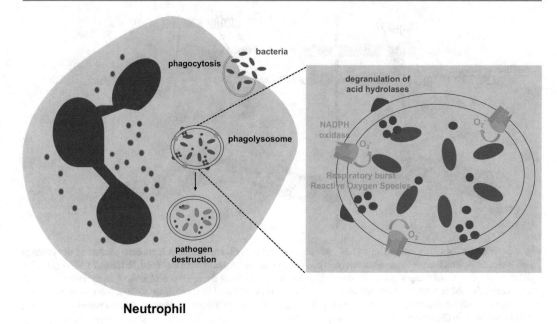

Neutrophil

Fig. 1.6 Neutrophil microbicidal functions. Bacterial endocytosis in neutrophils results in activation of the NADPH oxidase, leading to the production of reactive oxygen species in phagolysosomes and ultimately resulting in bacterial cell death (figure contributed by Jeremy P. McAleer)

One hallmark of pathogen destruction by neutrophils is the induction of the respiratory burst. This involves the activity of enzymes such as NADPH oxidase which raises the pH in the cell and induces the release of a number of toxic oxides and superoxides. These reactive oxygen species enhance the activity of several degradative enzymes and antimicrobial peptides, which cause the death of the pathogen. Eventually the pathogen is completely degraded in the phagolysosome by the action of acid hydrolases. Once the pathogen is destroyed, the neutrophil is spent and also dies. The accumulation of dead neutrophils leads to the formation of pus.

Innate Immunity to Viruses Is Mediated by Natural Killer Cells

In contrast to bacterial infections, infection of cells with viruses induces the recruitment and activation of natural killer cells. Macrophages release **IL-12**, which together with TNF-α, has the ability to activate natural killer cells. However, the most potent activators of NK cells are **type I interferons** which are produced by all cells when infected with viruses, and produced prodigiously by epithelial cells and **plasmacytoid dendritic cells**. The latter, which are different from conventional dendritic cells, are also referred to as **interferon producing cells,** since they can produce a thousand times more type I interferon compared with epithelial cells.

The two main types of type I interferons are **IFN-α** and **IFN-β**. These are produced as soon as a cell is infected and promote what is termed as the **interferon response**. The net effect of the interferon response is to enhance viral resistance in infected cells, upregulate the expression of ligands that bind receptors on NK cells, and promote the activation of NK cells.

NK cells are potent killers of virally-infected cells. They are large granular lymphocytes which circulate throughout blood in a partially active state, where they are prevented from attacking the body's cells via a delicate balance of engagement of activating and inhibitory receptors present on the NK cell surface. These receptors are stochastically expressed on the surface of NK cells, and different NK cell subsets express different combinations of receptors. Under normal conditions, inhibitory receptors on NK cells bind **major**

histocompatibility class (MHC) I molecules which are expressed on every nucleated cell in the body. This signals the NK cell to not engage its activating receptors and prevents killing of uninfected cells. On the other hand, virally-infected cells downregulate MHC I and upregulate ligands for activating receptors on NK cells. These include **stress proteins** such as MHC Class I related polypeptide sequences A and B (**MIC-A** and **MIC-B**), as well as Rae 1. This alters the delicate balance of receptor engagement on NK cells and triggers their activation. Once activated, NK cells are induced to kill the virally infected cells, through a dedicated program of apoptosis mediated by perforin, granzymes, and caspases. In addition to killing, NK cells also produce a host of cytokines which have deleterious effects on infected cells as well as activate other immune cells. One of these is a potent cytokine called **IFN-γ**, which not only exerts anti-viral effects, but also promotes the degradation of the pathogen in antigen presenting cells, and enhances their ability to stimulate the activation of T cells. Depending on the type of response, other cytokines are also produced by specific subsets of NK cells, mimicking the types of cytokines produced by T cell subsets during the adaptive immune response.

Dendritic Cells Initiate the Development of Adaptive Immune Responses

While the major effect of cells such as macrophages, neutrophils, and NK cells is to terminate the pathogen at the site of infection and amplify the effects of the innate immune response, another innate immune cell serves a dual purpose, which is to initiate the activation of the adaptive immune response.

Like macrophages, dendritic cells (DCs) at sites of infection also conduct phagocytosis and release proinflammatory cytokines. However, their major function in immunity is to initiate the activation of naïve or uncommitted T cells to the particular pathogen. Immature DC at sites of infection phagocytose the pathogen and degrade it in either the proteasome or the phagolysosome depending on the type of infection. This results in the production of a number of peptides which may serve as antigenic triggers to activate naïve T cells. Loaded with this cargo of peptides, immature DC travel from infected sites to the draining lymph nodes or the spleen, where they encounter circulating naïve T cells that are moving through the organs. In the process of migration, DCs undergo a change in phenotype, acquiring and upregulating ligands that enhance their ability to activate a naïve T cell. Upon reaching the **lymph node** or **spleen**, the DC is now said to be a mature DC that is capable of initiating T cell activation.

The Adaptive Immune Response

While the primary purpose of the innate immune response is to limit the spread of the infection as much as possible while also paving the way for the adaptive immune response, the goal of the adaptive immune response is to mount a specific, targeted response that completely destroys the pathogen and ensures that the host is never again subjected to infection with the same pathogen (Fig. 1.7).

Principles of the Adaptive Immune Response

The adaptive immune response is mediated by T cells, B cells, and their various mediators such as cytokines and antibodies. The first time an adaptive immune response is mounted against a specific pathogen, it is called the **primary immune response**. Subsequent responses are termed as **secondary responses**. The secondary response is mediated by **memory** T cells and B cells which have formed a memory of the pathogen through the first encounter. The memory response is of much greater magnitude than the primary response, often resulting in termination of the infection without the development of any clinical symptoms.

The development of the adaptive response hinges on the principle of clonal selection and the expansion of T cells and B cells to the specific pathogen. Unlike innate cells, these cell types do not simply recognize the presence of patterns on pathogen surfaces. Rather, every single activated T or B cell is committed to the recognition of a unique **antigen** or **epitope** that is

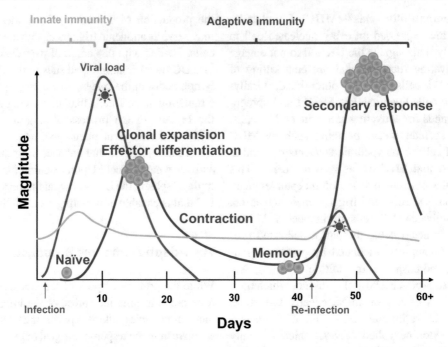

Fig. 1.7 Kinetics of anti-viral immune responses. This diagram outlines the time course of a virus infection and the relative magnitude of subsequent immune responses. Once viruses breach epithelial barriers, there is an incubation period in which symptoms from the infection have not yet occurred. During the next few days, viruses will undergo replication in host cells and begin to infect neighboring cells. The peak of viral replication may occur 7–10 days following initial exposure (red line), with levels declining over the next week or so, until the infection is cleared. The innate immune system is the first line of defense and includes macrophages, neutrophils, dendritic cells, NK cells and complement. The innate immune system can respond within hours following infections to initiate a type I interferon response. While this is important for controlling pathogen load, the magnitude of the innate response is not sufficient to clear the infection (green line). Adaptive immune responses take about a week to develop because they depend on the outgrowth of a single antigen-specific lymphocyte (T cell, B cell; blue line). Lymphocytes that have not yet encountered their antigen in lymph nodes are referred to as naïve. Following their activation by virus antigens, lymphocytes undergo a phase of clonal expansion in which one cell proliferates several times to become a population of thousands of lymphocytes that all recognize the same antigen. Clonal expansion is linked to their effector differentiation, in which lymphocytes acquire the ability to inhibit viral replication and/or dissemination, as described in Chap. 3. Therefore, clonal expansion coincides with the initial decrease observed in viral loads. Following expansion, there is a contraction phase in which most of the effector lymphocytes undergo apoptosis. A small population of memory cells persists, capable of mounting a rapid response to a second infection with the same virus. Memory cells live for several years within the individual (figure contributed by Jeremy P. McAleer)

derived from the pathogen. Recognition of this antigen allows the T or B cell to recognize the entire pathogen and mount a targeted response. The only antigens recognized by T cells are peptides that have been derived from degradation of a pathogen in an antigen presenting cell. In contrast, B cells recognize all sorts of antigens including peptides, glycoproteins, polysaccharides, and other types of pathogen components. Clonal selection refers to the process by which naïve T cells or B cells are selected to become

specific to the particular pathogen. Once a naïve cell is activated to the specific antigen, it then divides into hundreds of similarly activated clones which now act against the pathogen and mediate its destruction.

The Lymphatic System

The first step in the initiation of the adaptive immune response is the antigen-specific activation of a naïve T cell to the offending pathogen. **Naïve** T cells along with naïve B cells circulate throughout lymphoid organs, carried by a complex network of vessels connecting the blood and lymphatic system. The lymphatic system consists of an anastomosing network of lymphatic vessels which originate in connective tissues and collect the extracellular plasma or fluid that leaks out of blood vessels, returning it to the heart. This fluid is called the **lymph** and consists of a number of leukocytes which traverse throughout the lymphatic system, making regular stops at lymph nodes situated at intervening junctions in the lymphatics. At any given time, lymphocytes represent the largest population of leukocytes in the lymph, although they are only a fraction of the total lymphocyte population in the body. The vast majority of lymphocytes are present in the lymphoid organs which serve various areas of the body. Of these, the thymus and bone marrow are referred to as primary or central lymphoid organs since this is where T and B cells develop and mature.

Activation of naïve lymphocytes typically occurs in the secondary or peripheral lymphoid organs, of which the lymph nodes and the spleen are the most prominent (Fig. 1.8). The lymph nodes collect the fluid draining from an infected site such as the skin or the respiratory tract and serve as an ideal location for the encounter between pathogen and naïve T and B cells. Similarly, the spleen acts as a reservoir for the filtration of blood, removing any damaged or senescent red blood cells. It is therefore uniquely poised to handle the activation of lymphocytes to blood-borne pathogens that directly enter the blood stream or eventually reach the blood. Several other organs can also act as secondary lymphoid organs including the tonsils, adenoids, Peyer's patches, and appendix. In addition, less organized lymphoid tissues referred to as tertiary lymphoid organs are present throughout the respiratory, gastrointestinal and urogenital tracts.

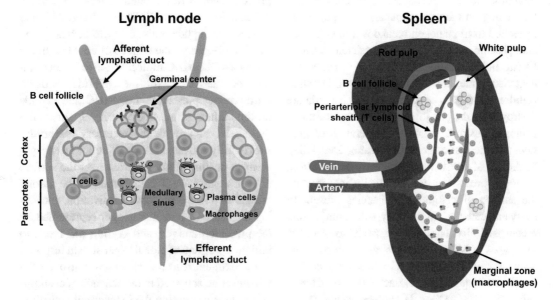

Fig. 1.8 Secondary lymphoid organs. Adaptive immune responses against microorganisms are initiated in lymph nodes and the spleen. These tissues contain organized regions that facilitate interactions between dendritic cells, T cells and B cells, promoting lymphocyte activation against antigens collected in peripheral tissues. In lymph nodes, the paracortical region is populated by T cells, while the outer cortex contains B cells, including germinal centers of activated B cells undergoing clonal expansion. The inner medulla of lymph nodes contains antibody-producing plasma cells and macrophages. Fluid enters lymph nodes through afferent lymphatic vessels, exits through efferent ducts, and ultimately drains into the thoracic duct where it enters the bloodstream. The spleen filters blood and has organized regions termed red pulp and white pulp. The red pulp is a site of red blood cell disposal, while the white pulp contains immune cells. Immune functions of the spleen are similar to that of lymph nodes, with the primary difference being that the spleen collects cells and antigens from blood rather than lymph fluid (figure contributed by Jeremy P. McAleer)

The Activation of Naïve Lymphocytes Occurs in Secondary Lymphoid Organs

In the absence of infection or other immune triggers, naïve lymphocytes constantly traverse the lymphatic system, surveying the lymph nodes for the presence of antigen. Antigen is detected by lymphocytes via a single unique receptor expressed on the surface of T cells and B cells. In T cells, this receptor is simply referred to as the T cell receptor or **TCR**. On B cells, the B cell receptor or **BCR** is the **immunoglobulin** molecule. Every T or B cell will only express one type of receptor, which is constrained by the specific antigen to which it binds, thus ensuring that activated T and B cells will only recognize the specific antigen to which it is activated.

Activation of lymphocytes is initiated in the secondary lymphoid organ. Once an infection has ensued, immature dendritic cells at the site of infection capture the offending pathogen and begin the process of pathogen destruction and migration to the secondary lymphoid organ. Depending on the type of pathogen, peptides are generated from pathogen breakdown in either the endoplasmic reticulum or the vesicular system. **Intracellular pathogens** such as viruses are degraded in the immunoproteasome, while **extracellular pathogens** such as pyogenic bacteria are destroyed in the phagolysosome. The process of pathogen destruction and the generation of peptides is termed as **antigenic processing**. Depending on the site of destruction, peptides generated from pathogen breakdown are eventually loaded onto the surface of ubiquitous molecules present in every nucleated cell of the body, called **major histocompatibility complex** or MHC molecules. Two types of MHC molecules are involved in the activation of T cells: MHC Class I molecules, which are required for the activation of CD8 T cells and **MHC Class II molecules** which are required for the activation of CD4 T cells. As the immature DC migrates toward the secondary lymphoid organ such as a lymph node, it begins to downregulate receptors for antigen capture and upregulate receptors that enhance activation of T cells. Of these, the upregulation of MHC molecules loaded with peptides is paramount for T cell activation to occur. In addition, a number of other receptors for ligands on naïve T cells are also highly expressed. The primary purpose of these is to costimulate the naïve T cell to the specific antigen on MHC molecules. Once the mature DC reaches the lymph node, it is now ready to make contact with a naïve T cell.

The Activation and Differentiation of T Lymphocytes Requires Costimulation and Direction from Cytokines

Three steps are involved in the activation of naïve T cells. First, the TCR on naïve T cells makes contact with the peptide antigen on the surface of MHC molecules on the antigen presenting cell. This is an essential first step which commits the naïve T cell to the specific antigen and provides specific identifying information regarding the nature of the pathogen. It can only effectively be carried out by professional **antigen presenting cells** (APCs) such as dendritic cells, macrophages, and B cells and is referred to as **antigen presentation**. A fundamental criterion of antigen presentation is that the TCR on a T cell will only engage the peptide antigen in the context of an MHC molecule on the surface of an APC. In the absence of the MHC molecule, naïve T cells cannot be activated to the peptide antigen. Furthermore, presentation of MHC and peptide on the surface of an APC is critical, since only these cells can provide the necessary **costimulation** to fully activate the naïve T cell. The engagement of costimulatory molecules on the surface of APCs and naïve T cells serves as the second critical step in the process of activation, conveying the sense of potential danger represented by the presented antigen, and gearing the T cell to initiate a program of clonal expansion in response to the antigen. It also ensures that naïve T cells will never be activated in the absence of costimulation, thus preventing the inadvertent activation of T cells to self-antigens expressed by other cells of the body. The most important costimulatory interaction for the activation of naïve T cells occurs between **CD28** on T cells and **B7 family** molecules such as **CD80** or **CD86** expressed on the surface of APCs. In addition, interactions between other costimulatory molecules play a role in the activation of effector or memory

T cells. These include OX40 (CD134) and OX40 ligand (CD252) as well as ICOS (inducible costimulator on T cells) and ICOS ligand. Engagement of the TCR and costimulatory molecules is facilitated by a tight zone of contact called the **immunological synapse** that is established between the APC and T cell. This allows the binding of a number of other receptors that strengthen the interaction between these molecules. The provision of costimulation initiates a signaling cascade that culminates in the activation of the transcription factor **nuclear factor of activated T cells (NFAT)**, which activates the gene for the cytokine IL-2. In the presence of IL-2, the activated T cell is now stimulated to divide and expand, thus completing the third step involved in T cell activation.

Depending on the type of MHC molecule presenting the antigen, activation results in the initiation of either a cytotoxic or helper T cell response. MHC I molecules present to CD8 T cells initiating a cytotoxic response to viral and tumor antigens. MHC II molecules present to CD4 T cells initiating a helper T cell response to bacterial, viral, fungal, parasitic, and other antigens. The helper T cell response is further delineated by the type of helper T cell activated. In general, T_H1 cells are activated to intracellular bacteria, T_H2 cells to parasitic antigens, and T_H17 cells to extracellular bacteria and fungi. However, in addition to their specified roles in host defense, these subsets exhibit a great degree of versatility and may be induced to perform overlapping and complementary functions depending on the type of antigenic stimulus and the cytokine microenvironment. Additional T helper subsets include follicular helper T cells (T_{FH}) which play a critical role in the secondary lymphoid organs in initiating the activation of naïve B cells. Regulatory T cells (T_{regs}), another type of CD4 T cell, suppress inflammatory responses once the infection is terminated.

Activation of Naïve B Cells

The second step in the development of the adaptive immune response is the activation of naïve B cells to the respective antigen. The recognition of antigen by B cells occurs via the immunoglobulin receptor expressed on its surface. The initial process of recognition involves binding via IgM and other coreceptors expressed on the surface of a B cell, resulting in receptor-mediated endocytosis of the pathogen. Unlike T cells, B cells are not constrained by the recognition of a specific peptide antigen and can recognize various types of macromolecules. Further activation of the B cell requires interactions between the antigen-specific B cell and a similarly activated antigen-specific helper T cell in the secondary lymphoid organ. The B cell presents a peptide antigen on the surface of MHC II to the CD4 T cell and costimulation is provided in the form of **CD40** molecules on the B cell which bind to CD40 ligands (**CD40L**) on the responding T cell. This causes the helper T cell to secrete the cytokines IL-4, IL-5, and IL-6, which stimulate the differentiation and division of B cells into effector, memory, and antibody-producing **plasma B cells**. Helper T cell cytokines also cause B cells to go through a program of antibody refinement, wherein B cells are induced to enhance the quality of their antibodies through repetitive mutations (**somatic hypermutation**), switch their antibody isotype to IgG, IgA or IgE (**isotype switching**), and increase the affinity of their antibodies to the antigen (**affinity maturation**). This ensures that activation results in the production of high affinity antibodies that are aimed at completely destroying the pathogen and terminating the infection. This is accomplished via three distinct mechanisms: **neutralization**, **opsonization**, and **antibody-dependent cellular cytotoxicity (ADCC)**.

Antibodies Are the Highly Specialized Weapons of Adaptive Immunity

Neutralization involves binding of antibodies to the respective antigen or pathogen, prior to cellular entry, thus preventing it from infecting or damaging the cell (Fig. 1.9). An example of neutralization is the binding of antibodies to bacterial toxins preventing their attachment and entry into a target cell. In opsonization, antigen-binding antibodies initiate phagocyte-mediated destruction by binding to antibody or complement receptors on the surfaces of macrophages, dendritic cells, or neutrophils. Lastly, ADCC is mediated by immune

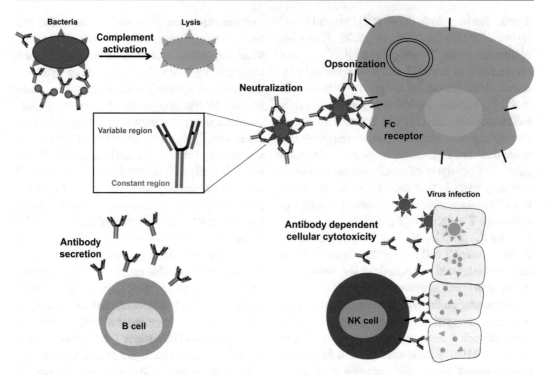

Fig. 1.9 Role of antibodies in host defense. Antibodies produced by B cells have a variable region for antigen binding and constant region that determines antibody function. Antibodies can neutralize pathogens or toxins by preventing their attachment to host cell surfaces. Antibodies attached to bacteria can activate the classical complement pathway, leading to lysis. Macrophages and NK cells, among other cell types, express Fc receptors that recognize constant regions of antibodies. This facilitates the uptake of antibody-coated pathogens by macrophages (opsonization) and the attack of virus-infected cells by NK cells (antibody-dependent cellular cytotoxicity) (figure contributed by Jeremy P. McAleer)

complexes of antigen and IgG molecules bound to IgG receptors on NK cells, triggering their activation and cytotoxic activity. Depending on the type of antigen, different types of antibodies are produced. IgM is the first antibody to be produced during an adaptive response. It is secreted as a pentamer and is very effective at complement activation. However, because of its large size, it is unable to enter many tissues. IgG is the most abundant antibody isotype present in circulation. It is very effective at neutralization, opsonization, and complement activation. Dimeric IgA is the most abundant antibody produced at mucosal surfaces and plays a critical role in mucosal immunity. Lastly, high levels of IgE are produced during infection with parasites such as helminth worms.

The production of high quality antibodies aimed at terminating the infection represents the peak of the adaptive immune response and typically occurs approximately 1 week after the onset

of infection. At this time, elevated numbers of antibodies may be found in the sera of infected individuals. Depending on the type of dominating helper T cell response, some types of antibodies may predominate over others. For example, IgG1 and IgE antibodies are typically by-products of a T_H2-type response, whereas in T_H1-mediated responses, IgG2a antibodies predominate.

As the immune response progresses, the quality of antibodies continues to improve. This is a result of numerous changes in the antigen-binding portion or variable region of the antibody molecule, and its primary purpose is to increase the overall binding and effectiveness of the antibody. One process called somatic hypermutation involves the generation of successive mutations in the complementarity determining regions (CDR)s of the antigen-binding site. The purpose of this mutation is to increase the binding of the antibody for the antigen. Similarly, transcriptional changes in IgM molecules result in switching of the IgM isotype of antibody to either the IgG, IgA, or IgE isotype. Lastly, processes such as affinity maturation increase the individual affinity of the antibody molecule and contribute to the strength or avidity of the overall binding. As such, successive exposures with the antigen exponentially increase the overall number and quality of the antibodies produced.

The Successful Outcome of the Adaptive Immune Response Results in Termination of the Infection

The combined actions of antibodies as well as effector T and B cells serves to eventually clear the infection from the patient. This changes the dynamics of the infection from one in which the pathogen predominates to one controlled by the immune system. As the numbers and effects of the pathogens subside, a dramatic improvement in the patient's condition occurs and the patient begins to experience relief from infection-associated symptoms. Control of the infection is also accompanied by the induction of several populations of regulatory cells, whose purpose is to aid in the resolution of inflammation, prevent inadvertent responses, and spur on the process of healing. Of these, CD4-positive regulatory T cells play a pivotal role in the suppression of unwanted T cell responses and the resolution of inflammation. Similarly, as the populations of effector T cells and B cells dwindle, subsets of antigen-specific memory T and B cell populations continue to persist and clones of these cells are retained interminably, poised to encounter a repeated strike by the same pathogen. When such a strike does occur, these cells are readily activated, mounting a rapid, potent memory T or B cell response that completely eliminates the pathogen before it has had a chance to initiate the process of infection.

Pharmacological Approaches to Treating Inflammation

Although the singular purpose of inflammation is to target and eliminate a perceived threat such as a pathogen, injury, or danger to the host, at the height of inflammation, most individuals are left feeling utterly feeble and helpless. In the midst of a high fever, patients often experience weakness, lethargy, fatigue and other symptoms that are geared toward encouraging the patient to rest so that the body's resources and energy may be expended toward the goal of eliminating the infection. This is also accompanied by other symptoms such as chills, muscle weakness, shivering, and organ-associated symptoms that contribute to the deterioration of the patient's health and overall malaise. In the presence of chronic inflammation, inflammation often continues to persist at a subclinical level, and contributes to fibromyalgia, pain, and decline in health of the patient. As such, a number of drugs have been developed with the aim of subduing inflammation or reducing some of the symptoms associated with it, without sacrificing the overall effectiveness of the immune response.

Drugs such as non-steroidal anti-inflammatory drugs (NSAIDs) including aspirin, ibuprofen, and naproxen have been used for quite some time to bring about an overall reduction in pains and aches all over the body. These drugs act by typically targeting intermediaries in the inflammatory pathways such as enzymes that act on nerve cells and induce pain. Similarly, other drug classes such as **corticosteroids** mediate an overall suppression of the immune response, resulting in attenuation of inflammation-associated pain and pathology. More recently, advances in basic science research have resulted in fundamental breakthroughs regarding our understanding of the immunologic basis of many diseases, elucidating several new and selective targets for therapeutic purposes. These include among others cytokines, chemokines and their receptors, signaling molecules, mediators involved in leukocyte trafficking, and cellular targets such as activated T and B cells. Similarly, a number of drugs that can stimulate the immune response have also been developed for some diseases. A short description of the different types of drugs is provided below. Table 1.2 summarizes the present list of immunotherapeutic drugs approved by the Food and Drug Administration (FDA) for the treatment of many diseases.

Table 1.2 Currently available drugs used in the treatment or modulation of inflammation (table contributed by Doreen E. Szollosi, Jeremy P. McAleer and Clinton B. Mathias)

Drug	Target/action	Chapter(s)
Abatacept (Orencia®)	CTLA-4 fusion protein, Selective T-Cell Costimulation inhibitor	3, 7
Adalimumab (Humira®)	Anti-TNF-α monoclonal antibody	2, 5–7
Aldesleukin (Proleukin®)	Recombinant Interleukin-2	3, 10
Alefacept (Amevive®)	CD2 inhibitor, discontinued	5
Alemtuzumab (Lemtrada®)	Anti-CD52 monoclonal antibody, leukocyte depletion	7, 8
Anakinra (Kineret®)	IL-1 receptor antagonist	2, 7
Antithymocyte globulin (Thymoglobulin®)	Polyclonal rabbit anti-thymocyte globulin	7, 8
Apremilast (Otezla®)	Phosphodiesterase (PDE) 4 inhibitor	5
Atezolizumab (Tecentriq®)	Anti-PD-L1 monoclonal antibody, checkpoint inhibitor	3, 10
Avelumab (Bavencio®)	Anti-PD-L1 monoclonal antibody, checkpoint inhibitor	10
Axicabtagene ciloleucel (Yescarta™)	CAR-T cell therapy	10
Azathioprine (Imuran®, Azasan®)	Purine analog, anti-proliferative agent	5–8
Balsalazide (Colazal®)	5-aminosalicylate, anti-inflammatory	6
Baricitinib (Olumiant®)	Janus kinases (JAK) inhibitor	7
Basiliximab (Simulect®)	Anti-IL-2 receptor monoclonal antibody	3, 7, 8
Belatacept (Nulojix®)	CTLA-4 fusion protein, Selective T cell costimulation inhibitor	3, 8
Belimumab (Benlysta®)	Anti-B lymphocyte stimulator (BLyS; BAFF) monoclonal antibody	3, 7
Benralizumab (Fasenra®)	Anti-IL-5R monoclonal antibody	3, 4
Bevacizumab (Avastin®)	Anti-VEGF monoclonal antibody	10
Blinatumomab (Blincyto®)	Anti-CD19/CD3 monoclonal diabody	10
Brentuximab vedotin (Adcetris®)	Anti-CD30 monoclonal antibody conjugated to an antineoplastic agent	10
Brodalumab (Siliq™)	Anti-IL-17 receptor monoclonal antibody	3, 5, 7
Budesonide (Entocort)	Glucocorticoid receptor activation, anti-inflammatory	4, 6
Canakinumab (Ilaris®)	IL-1 receptor antagonist	2, 7
Certolizumab pegol (Cimzia®)	Anti-TNF-α antibody fragment	2, 5, 7
Cetuximab (Erbitux®)	Anti-EGFR monoclonal antibody	10
Cromolyn sodium	Inhibitor of mast cell degranulation	4
Cyclophosphamide (Cytoxan®, Procytox®)	Alkylating agent of the nitrogen mustard type	7, 8
Cyclosporine (Neoral®, Sandimmune®)	Calcineurin Inhibitor	3, 5–8
Daclizumab (Zenapax®, Zinbryta®)	Anti-IL-2 receptor monoclonal antibody, both brands discontinued	3, 8
Daratumumab (Darzalex®)	Anti-CD38 monoclonal antibody	10
Darbepoetin (Aranesp®)	Erythropoietin (long-acting)	10
Denosumab (Xgeva®, Prolia®)	Anti-RANKL monoclonal antibody	10
Dimethyl fumarate (Tecfidera®)	Immunomodulatory	7
DTaP vaccine (Daptacel®, Infanrix®)	Inactivated vaccine, diphtheria, tetanus, acellular pertussis	9
Dupilumab (Dupixent®)	Anti-IL-4Rα monoclonal antibody	3–5
Durvalumab (Imfinzi®)	Anti-PD-L1 monoclonal antibody	10
Elotuzumab (Empliciti)	SLAMF7-directed immunostimulatory antibody	10
Eltrombopag (Promacta®)	Thrombopoietin receptor agonist	10
Epoetin (Epogen®, Procrit®)	Erythropoietin	10
Etanercept (Enbrel®)	Anti-TNF-α fusion protein	2, 5–8
Everolimus (Afinitor®)	mTOR inhibitor, anti-proliferative agent	8
Filgrastim (Neupogen®)	G-CSF	10
Fingolomod (Gilenya®)	Immunomodulatory	7

(continued)

Table 1.2 (continued)

Drug	Target/action	Chapter(s)
Fluticasone	Glucocorticoid	4, 7
Glatiramer acetate (Copaxone®)	Immunomodulatory	7
Golimumab (Simponi®)	Anti-TNF-α monoclonal antibody	2, 5–7
Guselkumab (Tremfya®)	Anti-IL-23 monoclonal antibody	5, 7
Hepatitis A vaccine (Havrix®)	Inactivated (Viral) Vaccine	9
Hepatitis B vaccine (Recombivax Hb®, Engerix-b®, Heplisav-B®)	Inactivated (Viral) Vaccine	9
Hepatitis A, Hepatitis B combo vaccine (Twinrix®)	Inactivated (Viral) Vaccine	9
Herpes zoster vaccines (Zostavax®, Shingrix®)	Live attenuated vaccine (Zostavax®)	9
	Recombinant (Shingrix®)	
HPV vaccine (Gardasil-9®)	Inactivated (viral) vaccine	9
Hydrocortisone	Glucocorticoid	4, 5, 7
Hydroxychloroquine (Plaquenil®)	Anti-protozoan Agent + Anti-rheumatic (immunosuppressant, exact mechanism unknown)	7
Ibritumomab tiuxetan (Zevalin®)	Anti-CD20 monoclonal antibody + radioimmunotherapy	10
Imiquimod (Aldara®, Zyclara®)	TLR7 agonist	10
Infliximab (Remicade®)	Anti-TNF-α monoclonal antibody	2, 5–7
Influenza vaccines (various brands)	Inactivated influenza virus vaccine	9
	Live attenuated influenza vaccine, or	
	Recombinant influenza vaccine	
Interferon alfa-2b (Intron A®)	Interferon	6, 10
Interferon beta-1a (Avonex®, Rebif®) pegylated (Plegridy®)	Type 1 Interferon	2, 6, 7
Interferon beta-1b (Betaseron®)	Type 1 Interferon	6, 7
Interferon gamma-1b (Actimmune®)	Type 2 Interferon	7
Intravenous immune globulin, IVIG (Gammagard®), SCIG (Vivaglobin®)	Polyclonal IgG Immune Globulin, for antibody reconstitution or suppressing hyperacute organ rejection	6–8
Ipilimumab (Yervoy®)	CTLA-4 antagonist	10
Ixekizumab (Taltz®)	Anti-IL-17 monoclonal antibody	3, 5, 7
Leflunomide (Arava®)	Pyrimidine synthesis inhibitor	7
Lenalidomide (Revlimid®)	IMiDᵃ/immunomodulator	10
MMR/MMRV vaccines	Live attenuated vaccines for measles, mumps, and rubella. MMRV includes varicella	9
Meningococcal vaccines	Conjugate, polysaccharide, or protein vaccine	9
Mepolizumab (Nucala®)	Anti-IL-5 monoclonal antibody	3, 4
6-Mercaptopurine	Purine analog, anti-proliferative agent	5, 6
Mesalamine (Asacol®, Canasa®, Lialda®, Pentasa®, Rowasa®)	5-aminosalicylate, anti-inflammatory	6
Methotrexate (Rheumatrex®)	Purine and pyrimidine synthesis inhibitor, anti-proliferative agent	5–7
Methoxy polyethylene glycol-epoetin beta (Mircera®)	Erythropoietin (long acting)	10
Methylprednisone	Glucocorticoid	4, 5, 7
Mitoxantrone (Novantrone®)	Immunomodulatory	7
Moxetumomab pasudotox (Lumoxiti®)	Anti-CD22 monoclonal antibody	10
Muromonab (Orthoclone OKT3®)	Anti-CD3 monoclonal antibody, discontinued	3, 8
Mycophenolate mofetil (CellCept®)	Inhibitor of inosine-5′-monophosphate dehydrogenase, anti-proliferative agent	7, 8

(continued)

Table 1.2 (continued)

Drug	Target/action	Chapter(s)
Natalizumab (Tysabri®)	Anti-$\alpha_4\beta_1$ integrin monoclonal antibody	2, 6, 7
Necitumumab (Portrazza®)	Anti-EGFR monoclonal antibody	10
Nivolumab (Opdivo®)	Anti-PD1 monoclonal antibody, checkpoint inhibitor	3, 10
Obinutuzumab (Gazyva®)	Anti-CD20 monoclonal antibody	3, 10
Ocrelizumab (Ocrevus®)	Anti-CD20 monoclonal antibody	3, 7
Ofatumumab (Arzerra®)	Anti-CD20 monoclonal antibody, B cell death	3, 10
Olsalazine (Dipentum)	5-aminosalicylate, anti-inflammatory	6
Omalizumab (Xolair®)	Anti-IgE monoclonal antibody	4
Oprelvekin (Neumega®)	Recombinant IL-11	10
Palivizumab (Synagis®)	Respiratory syncytial virus monoclonal antibody	1
Panitumumab (Vectibix®)	Anti-EGFR monoclonal antibody	10
PCV (Prevnar 13®)	Pneumococcal conjugate vaccine	9
Pegfilgrastim (Neulasta®)	Pegylated G-CSF	10
Peginterferon alfa-2a, 2b (Pegasys®, Pegintron®, Sylatron®)	Covalent conjugate of recombinant alfa-2a, 2b interferon	2, 10
Pembrolizumab (Keytruda®)	Anti-PD-1 monoclonal antibody, checkpoint inhibitor	3, 10
Pentostatin (Nipent®)	Adenosine deaminase inhibitor, anti-proliferative agent	8
Pertuzumab (Perjeta®)	Anti-HER2 monoclonal antibody	10
Pimecrolimus (Elidel®)	Calcineurin inhibitor	5, 6
Pomalidomide (Pomalyst®)	IMiD[a]/Immunomodulatory	10
PPSV23 (Pneumovax 23®)	Pneumococcal polysaccharide vaccine	9
Prednisone/prednisolone	Glucocorticoid/anti-inflammatory	4–7
Ramucirumab (Cyramza®)	Anti-VEGFR1 monoclonal antibody	10
Rh$_o$(D) Immune Globulin (Rhogam®)	Anti-D (Rho) immunoglobulin, prevents maternal sensitization against fetal Rho(D) antigens	3, 8
Reslizumab (Cinqair®)	Anti-IL-5 monoclonal antibody	3, 4
Rilonacept (Arcalyst®)	IL-1 receptor inhibitor	2, 7
Rituximab (Rituxan®)	Anti-CD20 monoclonal antibody	3, 7, 8, 10
Romiplostim (Nplate®)	Thrombopoietin analog	10
Sargramostim (Leukine®)	GM-CSF	10
Sarilumab (Kevzara®)	Anti-IL-6 receptor monoclonal antibody	7
Secukinumab (Cosentyx®)	Anti-IL-17A monoclonal antibody	3, 5, 7
Siltuximab (Sylvant®)	Anti-IL-6 monoclonal antibody	2, 7
Sipuleucel-T (Provenge®)	Dendritic cell-based prostate cancer vaccine	10
Sirolimus (Rapamune®)	mTOR kinase inhibitor, anti-proliferative	3, 8
Sulfasalazine (Azulfidine®, Sulfazine®)	5-Aminosalicylic Acid Derivative, anti-inflammatory	6, 7
Tacrolimus (Prograf®, Protopic®)	Calcineurin Inhibitor	3, 5–8
Talimogene laherparepvec (Imlygic®)	Modified *Herpes simplex virus-1* therapy	10
Tdap (Boostrix,® Adacel®)	Toxoid, acellular pertussis vaccine	9
Teriflunomide (Aubagio®)	Immunomodulatory	7
Thalidomide (Thalomid®)	IMiD[a]/Immunomodulatory	6, 10
Tildrakizumab (Ilumya®)	Anti-IL-23 monoclonal antibody	5, 7
Tisagenlecleucel (Kymriah®)	CAR-T cell therapy	10
Tocilizumab (Actemra®)	Anti-IL-6 receptor monoclonal antibody	2, 7, 8
Tofacitinib (Xeljanz®)	Janus kinases (JAK) inhibitor	7
Trastuzumab (Herceptin®)	Anti-HER2 monoclonal antibody	10
Ustekinumab (Stelara®)	Anti-IL-12/IL-23p40 monoclonal antibody	2, 5, 7
Varicella zoster (Varivax®)	Live attenuated varicella zoster virus vaccine	9
Vedolizumab (Entyvio®)	Anti-$\alpha_4\beta_7$ integrin monoclonal antibody, inhibits leukocyte migration	2, 6, 7

[a]*IMiD* immune modulatory imide drug

Inhibitors of Inflammation

Glucocorticoids

Glucocorticoids (corticosteroids) have remained the mainstay of immunotherapy for several decades and are widely prescribed for the treatment of many chronic inflammatory diseases such as asthma and rheumatoid arthritis. They work by inducing a general suppression of the immune system and thereby preventing inflammation-associated pathology. The mechanism of action of glucocorticoids is described in detail in Chaps. 4 and 6. Since glucocorticoids are broadly effective, long-term treatment with systemic corticosteroids is not recommended and is associated with several adverse effects including susceptibility to infections and the development of cancer. However, the use of selective formulations such as inhaled corticosteroids for chronic asthma have proven to be extremely beneficial and effective in the treatment of inflammatory conditions.

Anti-histamines (Histamine Receptor Antagonists)

These are widely available over the counter and used in the symptomatic treatment of diverse conditions including allergies, acidity, sleeplessness and anxiety. They include both competitive inhibitors of histamine as well as inverse agonists of histamine receptors and work primarily by targeting histamine produced by cells such as mast cells, preventing its binding to one of four types of histamine receptors. Induction of histamine signaling can result in the development of vasodilation, vascular permeability and smooth muscle constriction, resulting in symptoms such as coughing, sneezing or itching. Thus, anti-histamines provide a temporary resolution of these symptoms by curtailing histamine-induced effects. The mechanism of action of anti-histamines is described in Chap. 4.

Anti-eicosanoids

Derivatives of the arachidonic acid pathway such as **prostaglandins** and **leukotrienes** play a vital role in inflammation, inducing a variety of physiological responses such as vasodilation, vascular permeability, smooth muscle reactivity, recruitment of immune cells, thrombosis and gastrointestinal secretion. These derivatives along with other arachidonate metabolites such as thromboxane A_2, lipoxins, and hepoxilins are collectively referred to as eicosanoids. In addition to the above effects, eicosanoids such as prostaglandins contribute to the development of inflammation by inducing both pyrogenic and neurological effects such as fever and pain. A number of widely available agents have been developed to target the effects of both prostaglandins and leukotrienes. These include inhibitors of the enzymes that are necessary for their derivation from arachidonic acid as well as specific leukotriene receptor antagonists. Prostaglandins are synthesized via the cyclooxygenase (COX) pathway of arachidonic acid metabolism, whereas leukotrienes are derived via the 5-lipoxygenase pathway. Both COX 1 and COX2 inhibitors as well as selective COX2 inhibitors are widely available as over-the-counter agents. These include several NSAIDs such as aspirin, ibuprofen, acetaminophen and COX2 inhibitors such as celecoxib (Celebrex®). The NSAIDS and COX2 inhibitors are not discussed further in this book. Inhibitors of leukotriene synthesis and function are also available and are commonly prescribed for the treatment of chronic inflammatory diseases such as asthma. The mechanism of action of leukotriene antagonists is described in detail in Chap. 4.

Calcineurin Inhibitors (Specific Inhibitors of T Cell Function)

The **calcineurin inhibitors cyclosporine** and **tacrolimus** revolutionized the treatment of solid organ and hematopoietic stem cell or bone marrow transplantation. In fact, the advent of cyclosporine in the therapeutics of transplantation is referred to as the cyclosporine era of transplantation. Both cyclosporine and tacrolimus act by suppressing the proliferation of T cells via the inhibition of NFAT activation and the blockade of IL-2 release. Cyclosporine is a peptide antibiotic that binds to cyclophilin, a member of a class of intracellular proteins termed as immunophilins. The cyclosporine-cyclophilin complex then inhibits the phosphatase calcineurin, which is required for the activation of the T cell specific transcription factor NFAT (nuclear factor of activated T cells). Tacrolimus (FK 506), a macrolide antibiotic, produced by *Streptomyces tsukubaensis*, acts in a similar manner by binding to the immunophilin, FK binding protein. Calcineurin inhibitors are widely used in solid organ and hematopoietic stem cell transplantation and along with glucocorticoids remain the mainstay of therapy. Topical calcineurin inhibitors are also used in the treatment of dermatologic diseases such as atopic dermatitis and psoriasis. The mechanism of action of calcineurin inhibitors is described in Chaps. 5, 7, and 8.

Inhibitors of Proliferation

Sirolimus (Rapamycin) and Everolimus
These drugs also inhibit T cell activation and block the release of IL-2 and other T cell-derived cytokines. Although, like the calcineurin inhibitors, they also complex with an immunophilin, FK506-binding protein 12, their mechanism of action is dependent on the inhibition of the protein kinase, mTOR (molecular target of rapamycin), which is essential for cell growth, proliferation, and metabolism. Both these drugs are mainly used in transplantation therapy.

Mycophenolate Mofetil (MMF)
MMF is semisynthetic derivative of mycophenolic acid (MPA), which is produced by the mold *Penicillium glaucus*. It is a pro-drug that is converted to its active metabolite MPA *in vivo*, which selectively and reversibly inhibits inosine monophosphate dehydrogenase, an enzyme required for the synthesis of guanine nucleotides in T and B cells. The inosine monophosphate dehydrogenase-dependent *de novo* pathway of guanine synthesis is essential for T and B cell proliferation and function, due to the absence of alternative salvage pathways which exist in other cell types. As a result, inhibition of this enzyme by MPA leads to the suppression of T and B cell proliferation and function. MMF is mainly used in transplantation therapy, but is also being considered for therapeutic

purposes in rheumatoid arthritis, inflammatory bowel disease, and lupus nephritis.In addition, it is also commonly prescribed off-label for the treatment of systemic lupus erythematosus.

Azathioprine
Azathioprine is a cytotoxic drug that is mainly used for the treatment of solid-organ transplantation. It is a pro-drug that is converted in vivo to 6-mercaptopurine, which is subsequently converted to other derivatives that inhibit *de novo* purine synthesis. This results in the death of stimulated lymphocytes, dampening the induction of T and B cell mediated immunity. Due to its cytotoxic effects, the major toxicity associated with azathioprine is bone marrow suppression resulting in leukopenia, thrombocytopenia, and/or anemia. It is used for the maintenance of renal allografts, and also sometimes in the treatment of rheumatoid arthritis, Crohn's disease, and acute glomerulonephritis associated with systemic lupus erythematosus.

Other Anti-proliferative Drugs
Other anti-proliferative and cytotoxic drugs include **thalidomide**, which inhibits angiogenesis, has anti-inflammatory effects, and is used in the treatment of multiple myeloma and other cancers; **cyclophosphamide**, a cytotoxic agent, which destroys immune cells by alkylating resting and proliferating cells and is used in the treatment of some autoimmune disorders; and pyrimidine synthesis inhibitors such as **leflunomide** and **teriflunomide**, which inhibit the mitochondrial enzyme dihydroorotate dehydrogenase required for pyrimidine synthesis and immune cell function, and are used in the treatment of rheumatoid arthritis and relapsing-remitting multiple sclerosis. In addition, other cytotoxic drugs such as **methotrexate** are also commonly used for various therapeutic purposes.

Biologics

Over the last few decades, revolutionary advances in the understanding of the immunological basis of diseases and molecular and cell biology techniques, have resulted in the development of several new biologics that specifically target components of immune-mediated pathways such as immune cells, cytokines, cell signaling molecules, and various receptors and their associated ligands. These classes of drugs include monoclonal antibodies, small molecule inhibitors, fusion proteins, and various receptor antagonists.

Monoclonal Antibodies

Since the advent of recombinant DNA technology, various monoclonal antibodies are now therapeutically used for the treatment of a number of diseases. Based on whether they incorporate the variable and/or **complementarity-determining regions (CDRs)** of mouse antibodies, they are referred to as **chimeric** (composed of mouse variable chains), **humanized** (composed of mouse CDR sequences), or **fully human** (consisting of no mouse chains or sequences). The first monoclonal antibodies were produced using **hybridomas** derived from myeloma cell lines, although they are now frequently produced commercially using recombinant DNA technology. The different classes of therapeutic monoclonal antibodies are described more extensively in Chap. 3. Examples of prototypic antibodies belonging to the different classes include **rituximab (Rituxan®)**, a chimeric anti-CD20 antibody used in the treatment of non-Hodgkin's lymphoma, **omalizumab (Xolair®)**, a humanized anti-IgE antibody used in the treatment of asthma, and **adalimumab (Humira®)**, a fully human anti-TNFα antibody used in the treatment of rheumatoid arthritis.

In addition to treatment of inflammatory diseases, a number of monoclonal antibodies targeting various cell surface molecules and pathways have also been developed for the treatment of diverse types of cancers. These include inhibitors of angiogenesis, proliferation, and cell signaling. Examples include **alemtuzumab**, an anti-CD52 antibody that depletes B and T cells and is used for the treatment of B-cell chronic lymphocytic leukemia, **bevacizumab**, which inhibits vascular endothelial growth factor (VEGF) and blocks angiogenesis in tumors, and **trastuzumab**, which blocks the extracellular domain of HER-2/*neu* in

breast cancer patients and prevents signaling in HER-2/*neu*-positive tumors. Several monoclonal antibodies are also used to specifically deliver toxins and radioisotopes to tumor cells.

Similarly, monoclonal antibodies that target infectious organisms have also been approved by the FDA. **Palivizumab (Synagis®)** is a humanized neutralizing IgG antibody that is used to prevent respiratory syncytial virus (RSV) infections in children at increased risk of severe disease. This includes children who were born prematurely and are under 6 months of age, and children who may be at high risk of RSV infection due to bronchopulmonary dysplasia or congenital heart disease. The drug is given once a month during RSV season and provides protection by binding an epitope in the F protein subunit of RSV. This results in the inhibition of viral fusion and the prevention of syncytia within the lungs, which are necessary for the intercellular spread of the virus.

T Cell Checkpoint Inhibitors

More recently, a number of T cell specific inhibitors have been developed that selectively inhibit or enhance the activation of T cells for the treatment of non-immune cell cancers. Checkpoint inhibitors such as **anti-PD1 (pembrolizumab** and **nivolumab)** and **anti-CTLA-4 (ipilimumab)** enhance T cell activity against tumors by presumably increasing their costimulatory activity (Figs. 10.2 and 10.3). In contrast, the fusion proteins **abatacept** and **belatacept**, which consist of the extracellular domain of human **CTLA-4** fused with the constant regions of IgG, inhibit the costimulation of T cells and dampen T cell activity. The 2018 Nobel Prize in Physiology or Medicine was awarded to Drs. James P. Allison and Tasuko Honjo for their work on T cell checkpoint inhibitors. In addition to the drugs mentioned above, several others have been approved by the FDA for the treatment of various cancers and inflammatory diseases, and others are currently in development.

Cytokine Inhibitors

Insights into immune signaling mechanisms and the cross-talk between various immune cells have led to the development of several drugs that block cytokine function by inhibiting their binding, signaling, or activity. The first cytokine antagonists to be developed included both monoclonal antibodies and fusion proteins targeting the pro-inflammatory cytokine, TNF-α. These include **infliximab**, **etanercept**, and **certolizumab pegol**. More recently, a number of other cytokine antagonists have been developed targeting various cytokines including IL-1, IL-2, IL-5, IL-6, IL-12 and IL-23, and IL-17. In addition, inhibitors that target the JAK-STAT pathway of cytokine signaling have also been approved by the FDA and others are currently in development. It is also anticipated that several new drugs targeting various cytokines and their signaling pathways will be approved by the FDA in the near future. Presently FDA-approved drugs targeting various cytokines are described throughout this textbook.

Immune Cell Recruitment Inhibitors

The migration of immune cells to various organs is a critical component of inflammatory reactions during chronic inflammatory diseases. As such, a number of drugs have been developed that inhibit the expression or function of adhesion molecules on leukocytes or blood vessels and prevent the migration of effector cells to target tissues. Examples of these drugs include the integrin inhibitors **natalizumab** and **vedolizumab** used in the treatment of multiple sclerosis and Crohn's diseases as well as leukocyte function-associated antigen-1 (LFA-1) inhibitors such as **efalizumab**, which was previously used for the treatment of Crohn's disease, but was subsequently withdrawn.

Immunomodulatory Drugs

Recombinant Cytokines

Interferons

Interferons have been used for therapeutic purposes since as early as the 1980s. While initially studied mainly in the context of anti-viral responses, increasing evidence suggests that they have a number of immunomodulatory effects. These include the enhancement of antigen presentation, phagocytosis, upregulation of MHC Class I and II, and the induction of the immunoproteasome. They are also potent inducers of the antiviral cytotoxic response by both NK cells and cytotoxic T cells. The two main types of interferon that have been extensively studied in humans are both used for immunotherapeutic purposes. These include the type I interferons IFN-α and IFN-β as well as the type II interferon, IFN-γ. The type I interferons are produced by cells such as epithelial cells and plasmacytoid dendritic cells soon after infection and both activate NK cells as well as increase the intensity of anti-viral resistance through a series of molecular and cellular events, which are collectively termed as the interferon response. IFN-γ is produced by both activated NK cells and T cells (T_H1 and CD8 T cells) and further contributes to the antiviral response by inhibiting viral replication and activating various immune cells such as phagocytes. A number of interferon drugs comprising of all three types have been developed for the treatment of several diseases. While their mechanism of action is not always clear, they are therapeutically effective.

IFN-α is used for the treatment of a variety of cancers. These include hairy cell leukemia, malignant melanoma, follicular lymphoma, and Kaposi's sarcoma (seen in patients with AIDS). It is also used for the treatment of chronic hepatitis B and until recently, was also commonly used in conjunction with ribavirin for the treatment of chronic hepatitis C. IFN-β is currently FDA-approved for the treatment of relapsing multiple sclerosis and is used to reduce the frequency of clinical exacerbations. IFN-γ is currently used to reduce the frequency and severity of infections associated with chronic granulomatous disease, which is an immune deficiency resulting in defective phagocytic function due to the absence of NADPH oxidase activity.

Adverse effects associated with interferon therapy include flu-like symptoms such as fever, chills and headaches, gastrointestinal reactions, rash, myalgia, and injection site reactions.

Interleukin-2

IL-2 is a cytokine that is critical for the proliferation and division of T cells and induces their function and activity. Human recombinant IL-2 (**aldesleukin** or **Proleukin**®) is used for the treatment of metastatic renal cell carcinoma and melanoma. It stimulates lymphocytes and enhances their activity against the tumor. Adverse effects include flu-like symptoms as well as a serious but uncommon cardiovascular toxicity resulting from capillary leak syndrome.

Immunization

Immunization used in the prevention of various diseases can be classified as active or passive. **Active immunization** involves the induction of systemic immune responses to specific antigens, and often results in the acquisition of life-long immunity. The most commonly utilized application of active immunization has been the **vaccination** of a population against prevalent infectious pathogens. A number of vaccines described in Chap. 9 are currently in use against a wide variety of bacterial and viral infections. These include diphtheria, pertussis, tetanus, measles, mumps, polio, meningitis (bacterial and viral), chicken pox, shingles, rota viruses, influenza, and human papilloma virus, among others. In addition to protection from infectious organisms, therapeutic vaccines have also been developed or are being considered for other types of diseases. This includes cancer vaccines that utilize various types of cancer antigens (as described in Chap. 10) and vaccines to prevent the development of allergic disorders (as described in Chap. 4).

Passive immunization has also been used for the treatment of diseases and historically has included the transfer of antibodies from both animals and humans to patients. The passive transfer of antibodies is indicated when individuals are unable to make antibodies due to a congenital or acquired deficiency, when exposed to lethal doses of an infectious or toxic agent such as venoms and there is no time for the development of adaptive immunity, or when a particular disease can be ameliorated with the passive transfer of antibodies. Depending on the disease, both non-specific and highly-specific immunoglobulins may be used. Protection typically lasts for 1–3 months, by which time many immune-competent individuals should be able to generate adaptive immune responses. Specific immunoglobulin preparations are available for several diseases including rabies, tetanus, botulism, and respiratory syncytial virus. **Rho(D)** is a specific IgG preparation given to Rh-negative pregnant women for the prophylaxis of hemolytic disease of the newborn in the developing fetus.

Intravenous Immunoglobulin (IVIG)

Non-specific immune globulin is derived from the pooled plasma of thousands of adults and is used for the treatment of a variety of diseases. It mainly consists of IgG molecules and its initial application was primarily for the treatment of antibody deficiencies such as **agammaglobulinemia**. However, more recently, it has been considered for the treatment of several autoimmune diseases, both FDA-approved and off-label. The effects of IVIG are thought to be mediated through a combination of factors. This includes the saturation of both activating and inhibitory **Fc receptor**s for IgG as well as the **FcRn receptor** which enhances the half-life of IgG in serum. This prevents autoantibodies from engaging Fc receptors and inducing phagocytosis. The pooled preparation is also thought to contain anti-idiotypic antibodies, *i.e.* antibodies that bind to other antibodies such as the autoantibodies that exist within the patient. In addition, they may also contain helpful antibodies against B cell proliferation and survival factors, thus shutting down the production of autoantibodies. Lastly, they are thought to downregulate antigen presentation and complement activation.

Allergen Immunotherapy

Allergen immunotherapy or allergen desensitization is an immunotherapeutic procedure that has existed since the early 1900s. It is mostly used in the treatment of allergic diseases with the aim of shifting the immunologic response from a pathologic IgE-dominated response to a protective IgG4-dominant response. The induction of the tolerogenic response is thought to be dependent on the production of immunoregulatory cytokines such as IL-10.

The Adverse Effects Associated with Immunotherapy

As in the case of any type of pharmacological treatment, there exists the potential for the development of both minor and serious, or even life-threatening adverse effects. The development of adverse effects is often correlated with the dose, duration, and route of therapy, but other factors also play a role such as age, gender, and the immune status of the patient. Short-term treatment often results in minimal side effects, which are reversible after the end of treatment. However, long-term treatment may be associated with longer-lasting adverse effects. The immune specificity of the drug is also an important factor. For example, short term treatment with the glucocorticoid, oral prednisone, may result in weight gain, insomnia, fluid retention, and mood changes. However, long-term treatment is associated with osteoporosis, hypertension, weight gain, glaucoma, diabetes, muscle weakness and Cushing syndrome. In contrast, the major effect associated with long-term treatment with calcineurin inhibitors is the development of irreversible nephrotoxicity and impaired renal function. The route of treatment is also an important factor. For example, topical treatment with calcineurin inhibitors is associated with limited toxicities such as the development of rashes associated with herpes simplex virus infections. Similarly, one adverse effect of inhaled corticosteroids is the potential for development of oral candidiasis.

Inhibition of specific types of immune cells or their mediators such as cytokines is often associated with adverse effects relative to the functions of the specific target. For example, inhibition of TNF-α may result in the activation of latent tuberculosis, while the inhibition of IL-17 may result in the occurrence of upper respiratory tract infections or fungal infections. Similarly, enhancement of T cell costimulation for cancer treatment may be associated with the risk for developing autoimmunity. Chronic treatment with almost all immunosuppressive drugs is associated with the risk of development of infections. This is further enhanced in the case of transplantation recipients receiving long-term treatment

with a wide variety of immunosuppressive drugs. As such, patients are often advised about the potential for developing infections and closely monitored throughout the duration of therapy. Long-term treatment over several years can also increase the risk of development of cancers such as carcinomas of the skin and genital tract and Kaposi's sarcoma. Transplantation recipients in particular are two to four times more likely to develop these cancers compared to the general population.

Hypersensitivity Reactions to Drugs

Drug hypersensitivities are immune-mediated reactions to drugs. Depending on the type of drug, they may be mediated by IgE or IgG antibodies and often involve the activation of T cells, B cells and phagocytes. Symptoms may range from mild to severe, and may include the development of rash, serum sickness, or in rare cases anaphylaxis.

Many drugs act as haptens that bind to cell-surface molecules, resulting in the formation of immunogenic peptides that stimulate the immune system. For example, in some individuals, penicillin can conjugate with erythrocytes resulting in the production of modified epitopes that stimulate T_H2 cells and induce the production of IgE antibodies. Subsequently treatment with penicillin can induce severe IgE-mediated anaphylactic reactions (**type I hypersensitivity** reactions) that can have fatal consequences. Conversely, the induction of IgG antibodies can trigger the complement-mediated phagocytic destruction of erythrocytes resulting in anemia (**type II hypersensitivity** reactions). Recent findings implicate a single, specific receptor, MrgprX2, on mast cells that is often involved in pseudo-allergic reactions to various drugs.

Some drugs such as large proteins or therapeutic monoclonal antibodies can directly stimulate antibodies resulting in **type III hypersensitivity** reactions and the development of serum sickness. This is often accompanied by fever, chills, rash and vasculitis in the target tissues. The reactions are mediated by immune complexes of the drug with IgG antibodies and subside when the immune complexes are cleared.

Steven-Johnson syndrome/toxic epidermal necrolysis (SJS/TEN) is a severe reaction to some types of drugs that induces skin necrosis and detachment. The mucus membranes of the eyes, mouth, and genitals are often affected. The onset of SJS/TEN is a significant medical emergency and is life-threatening. The first symptoms include fever and flu-like symptoms, which is followed 1–3 days later by various rashes leading to blistering and peeling of the skin, starting with the face and spreading to other areas of the body. The reaction is triggered by certain medications such as **allopurinol**, anti-epileptics, cancer therapies, and antibiotics and often occur 1–3 weeks after therapy. It may also be triggered by infections. People with a weakened immune system, HIV, a family history of SJS/TEN, and certain polymorphisms in HLA-B are particularly at risk. The reaction is thought to be mediated by activated CD8 T cells which cause the blistering and is considered a **type IV hypersensitivity** reaction. Treatment includes supportive therapy and treatment with cyclosporine, IVIG, plasma exchange, and corticosteroids.

Summary

The immune system plays a critical role in host defense and is required for human survival. The cells of the immune system are generated through the process of hematopoiesis in the bone marrow. Innate immune responses are triggered immediately after infection, injury, or other trauma and involve the activity of various cell types including myeloid cells, granulocytes, and mast cells. These cells in coordination with a number of proinflammatory cytokines initiate host defense and alert the immune system. Neutrophils are efficient defenders of the host against bacterial infections, while NK cells are quick to respond to viral infections. Dendritic cells survey the infectious site for pathogens and act as an important link between the innate and adaptive immune responses. Adaptive immune responses are established several days after infection and mediate specific, potent, and long-lasting responses against pathogenic antigens. Helper CD4 T cells drive the adaptive immune response and differentiate into various subsets depending on the specific type of pathogen. Cytotoxic CD8 T cells are activated against viral and tumor antigens. The activation of T cells and their effector function is dependent on dendritic cells, other antigen presenting cells, and cytokines, which regulate their function. B cells are also activated to pathogenic antigens and produce various antibodies, which can destroy the pathogen. When the infection begins to clear, the adaptive immune response wanes, and memory lymphocytes are generated that persist during life and provide protection against future attacks.

Recent advances in immunology research have significantly enhanced our understanding of the immunological basis of many diseases. Immune cells and their mediators are not only involved in host defense against foreign pathogens, but also play a vital role in maintaining homeostatic integrity and participate in reactions that contribute to the development of either immunity or tolerance. Further investigation of the mechanisms involved in these processes have resulted in the elucidation of several new immune-mediated targets for therapeutic purposes, leading to the development of novel drugs that target the immune system. These drugs belong to various classes inducing immunosuppression, inhibiting proliferation of immune cells, and modulating immune activity. The latter category includes several monoclonal antibodies and other biologics that target specific immune cells and molecules. In addition, several types of drugs also stimulate the immune system. These include various vaccines as well as recombinant cytokines that can activate immune activity against specific targets. It is anticipated that in future years, the complexity of the various interactions between immune cells and their mediators will be further uncovered, leading to the development of even more immunotherapeutic drugs.

Practice Questions

1. Provide three examples each of an innate and an adaptive immune cell and list at least one function of each cell type.

2. Provide examples of how microbiota influence the development of the immune response.
3. Describe the cardinal characteristics of inflammation and explain the immunological mechanisms underlying their development.
4. _____ is a cytokine produced by macrophages that causes the dilation of blood vessels and promotes the recruitment of leukocytes to injured tissues.
   (a) TNF-α
   (b) IL-6
   (c) IL-1β
   (d) IL-5
5. _____ is a chemokine produced by macrophages that enhances the recruitment of neutrophils to injured tissues.
   (a) CXCL8
   (b) Eotaxin
   (c) TNF-α
   (d) IL-5
6. Which of the following represent examples of innate cells that are involved in IgE-mediated immune responses to parasites? Select all that apply.
   (a) T$_H$2 cells
   (b) Eosinophils
   (c) Basophils
   (d) Neutrophil
7. The_____ is involved in the phagocytosis-mediated killing of bacterial cells by neutrophils.
   (a) activation of NF-κB
   (b) respiratory burst
   (c) release of cytokines
   (d) induction of costimulation
8. _____ is a growth factor required for the generation of eosinophils in the bone marrow. Select all that apply.
   (a) IL-3
   (b) IL-6
   (c) IL-1β
   (d) IL-5
9. What do you mean by the interferon response? How does it affect the activation of NK cells?
10. Explain how cell surface receptors contribute to the NK cell-mediated killing of virally-infected cells.

11. Explain the process involved in the activation of naïve T cells to a novel antigen.
12. Which of the following molecules is expressed by dendritic cells as they migrate towards draining lymph nodes after capture of an antigen?
   (a) CD80
   (b) MHC I
   (c) IL-6 receptor
   (d) CD28
13. The engagement of _____ molecules is a critical second step in the activation of naïve T cells to an antigen.
   (a) TLR
   (b) adhesion
   (c) costimulatory
   (d) inhibitory
14. Describe the various subsets of helper T cells and give one example of their immunological function.
15. Explain the mechanisms by which antibodies combat infectious organisms.
16. _____ is a costimulatory molecule expressed on B cells required for the induction of isotype switching in antibody molecules.
   (a) CD28
   (b) CD40
   (c) ICOS
   (d) PD-1
17. How does somatic hypermutation contribute to the development of the B cell repertoire?
18. _____ is an example of an eicosanoid produced by mast cells after IgE-mediated activation.
   (a) Histamine
   (b) Leukotriene
   (c) Tryptase
   (d) IL-6
19. Which of the drugs below complexes with FK506BP12 and inhibits the actions of mTOR?
   (a) Tacrolimus
   (b) Everolimus
   (c) Cyclosporine
   (d) Abatacept
20. _____ is a drug that inhibits purine synthesis *via* derivatives of 6-mercaptopurine.

(a) Azathioprine

(b) Methotrexate

(c) Cyclophosphamide

(d) IL-5

21. _____ is an example of a drug that inhibits T cell-mediated responses by inhibiting T cell costimulation.

(a) Abatacept

(b) Ipilimumab

(c) Pembrolizumab

(d) Nivolumab

22. _____ is a chimeric monoclonal antibody used in the treatment non-Hodgkin's lymphoma.

(a) Rituxan

(b) Xolair

(c) Humira

(d) Cosentyx

23. Which of the following are examples of inhibitors of TNF-α? Select all that apply.

(a) Etanercept

(b) Infliximab

(c) Adalimumab

(d) Secukinumab

24. Which of the following is an example of an immunotherapeutic drug used in the treatment of metastatic renal carcinoma?

(a) Rituximab

(b) Aldesleukin

(c) Nivolumab

(d) Alemtuzumab

25. _____ is a receptor on mast cells that is involved in pseudo-allergic reactions to drugs

(a) MrgprX2

(b) FcεRI

(c) TLR

(d) Leukotriene receptor D4

26. _____ is an example of a severe hypersensitivity reaction that can develop in some people who are treated with allopurinol.

(a) Type II hypersensitivity reactions

(b) Anaphylaxis.

(c) Steven Johnson syndrome

(d) Serum sickness

Suggested Reading[1]

Jenner E. An inquiry into the causes and effects of variolae vaccinae: a disease discovered in some Western Counties of England. London: Sampson Low; 1798. p. 75.

Jenner E. Letter addressed to the medical profession generally, relative to vaccination. Lond Med Phys J. 1821;45:277–80.

Pasteur L. Sur les maladies virulentes, et en particulier sur la maladie appelee vulgairement cholera des poules. C R Acad Sci. 1880;90:248–9.

Pasteur LC, Roux E. Compte rendu sommaire des experiences faites a Pouilly-Le-Fort, pres de Melun, sur la vaccination charnonneuse. C R Acad Sci. 1881;92:1378–83.

Koch R. A further communication on a remedy for tuberculosis. Br Med J. 1891;1:125–7.

Koch R. An address on the fight against tuberculosis in the light of the experience that has been gained in the successful combat of other infectious diseases. Br Med J. 1901;2:189–93.

Weil R. Studies in anaphylaxis. XIV. On the relation between precipitin and sensitizin. J Immunol. 1916;1:1–18.

Lurie MB. A correlation between the histological changes and the fate of living tubercule bacilli in the organs of infected rabbits. J Exp Med. 1933;57:31–54.

Gibson T, Medawar PB. The fate of skin homografts in man. J Anat. 1943;77:299–310 294.

Chase MW. The cellular transfer of cutaneous sensitivity to tuberculin. Proc Soc Exp Biol Med. 1945;59:134.

Coombs RR, Mourant AE, Race RR. A new test for the detection of weak and incomplete Rh agglutinins. Br J Exp Pathol. 1945;26:255–66.

Owen RD. Immunogenetic consequences of vascular anastomoses between bovine twins. Science. 1945;102:400–1.

Fagraeus A. Plasma cellular reaction and its relation to the formation of antibodies in vitro. Nature. 1947;159:499.

Fagraeus A. The plasma cellular reaction and its relation to the formation of antibodies in vitro. J Immunol. 1948;58:1–13.

Snell GD. Methods for the study of histocompatibility genes. J Genet. 1948;49:87–108.

Bordley JE, Carey RA, et al. Preliminary observations on the effect of adrenocorticotropic hormone in allergic diseases. Bull Johns Hopkins Hosp. 1949;85:396–8.

Hench PS, Kendall EC, Slocumb CH, Polley HF. Effects of cortisone acetate and pituitary ACTH on rheumatoid

[1]The suggested reading list below was created with the aim of highlighting classic papers in immunology that describe seminal findings in the field of immunology. Many of these discoveries have advanced our current understanding of immunology and medicine and several have resulted in the receipt of the Nobel Prize.

arthritis, rheumatic fever and certain other conditions. Arch Intern Med (Chic). 1950;85:545–666.

Billingham RE, Brent L, Medawar PB. Actively acquired tolerance of foreign cells. Nature. 1953;172:603–6.

Jerne NK. The natural-selection theory of antibody formation. Proc Natl Acad Sci U S A. 1955;41:849–57.

Billingham RE, Brent L, Medawar PB. The antigenic stimulus in transplantation immunity. Nature. 1956;178:514–9.

Isaacs A, Lindenmann J. Virus interference. I. The interferon. Proc R Soc Lond B Biol Sci. 1957;147:258–67.

Isaacs A, Lindenmann J, Valentine RC. Virus interference. II. Some properties of interferon. Proc R Soc Lond B Biol Sci. 1957;147:268–73.

Nossal GJ, Lederberg J. Antibody production by single cells. Nature. 1958;181:1419–20.

Porter RR. Separation and isolation of fractions of rabbit gamma-globulin containing the antibody and antigenic combining sites. Nature. 1958;182:670–1.

Burnet FM. The clonal selection theory of acquired immunity. Cambridge: Cambridge University Press; 1959.

Nowell PC. Phytohemagglutinin: an initiator of mitosis in cultures of normal human leukocytes. Cancer Res. 1960;20:462–6.

Yalow RS, Berson SA. Immunoassay of endogenous plasma insulin in man. J Clin Invest. 1960;39:1157–75.

Dresser DW. Effectiveness of lipid and lipidophilic substances as adjuvants. Nature. 1961;191:1169–71.

Burnet FM. The immunological significance of the thymus: an extension of the clonal selection theory of immunity. Australas Ann Med. 1962;11:79–91.

Dresser DW. Specific inhibition of antibody production. II. Paralysis induced in adult mice by small quantities of protein antigen. Immunology. 1962;5:378–88.

Mackaness GB. Cellular resistance to infection. J Exp Med. 1962;116:381–406.

Mackaness GB. The immunological basis of acquired cellular resistance. J Exp Med. 1964;120:105–20.

Cooper MD, Peterson RD, Good RA. Delineation of the thymic and bursal lymphoid systems in the chicken. Nature. 1965;205:143–6.

Brenner S, Milstein C. Origin of antibody variation. Nature. 1966;211:242–3.

Cooper MD, Raymond DA, Peterson RD, South MA, Good RA. The functions of the thymus system and the bursa system in the chicken. J Exp Med. 1966;123:75–102.

Ishizaka K, Ishizaka T. Physicochemical properties of reaginic antibody. 1. Association of reaginic activity with an immunoglobulin other than gammaA- or gammaG-globulin. J Allergy. 1966a;37:169–85.

Ishizaka K, Ishizaka T. Physicochemical properties of reaginic antibody. 3. Further studies on the reaginic antibody in gamma-A-globulin preparations. J Allergy. 1966b;38:108–19.

Ishizaka K, Ishizaka T, Lee EH. Physiochemical properties of reaginic antibody. II. Characteristic properties of reaginic antibody different from human gamma-A-isohemagglutinin and gamma-D-globulin. J Allergy. 1966a;37:336–49.

Ishizaka K, Ishizaka T, Hornbrook MM. Physico-chemical properties of human reaginic antibody. IV. Presence of a unique immunoglobulin as a carrier of reaginic activity. J Immunol. 1966b;97:75–85.

Ishizaka K, Ishizaka T, Hornbrook MM. Physicochemical properties of reaginic antibody. V. Correlation of reaginic activity wth gamma-E-globulin antibody. J Immunol. 1966c;97:840–53.

Edelman GM, Gally JA. Somatic recombination of duplicated genes: an hypothesis on the origin of antibody diversity. Proc Natl Acad Sci U S A. 1967;57:353–8.

Henney CS, Ishizaka K. An antigenic determinant of human gamma-globulin susceptible to papain digestion. J Immunol. 1967;99:695–702.

Ishizaka K, Ishizaka T. Identification of gamma-E-antibodies as a carrier of reaginic activity. J Immunol. 1967;99:1187–98.

Ishizaka K, Ishizaka T, Menzel AE. Physicochemical properties of reaginic antibody. VI. Effect of heat on gamma-E-, gamma-G- and gamma-A-antibodies in the sera of ragweed sensitive patients. J Immunol. 1967a;99:610–8.

Ishizaka K, Ishizaka T, Terry WD. Antigenic structure of gamma-E-globulin and reaginic antibody. J Immunol. 1967b;99:849–58.

Johansson SG, Bennich H. Immunological studies of an atypical (myeloma) immunoglobulin. Immunology. 1967;13:381–94.

Mintz B, Silvers WK. "Intrinsic" immunological tolerance in allophenic mice. Science. 1967;158:1484–6.

Mishell RI, Dutton RW. Immunization of dissociated spleen cell cultures from normal mice. J Exp Med. 1967;126:423–42.

Edelman GM, et al. The covalent structure of an entire gammaG immunoglobulin molecule. Proc Natl Acad Sci U S A. 1969;63:78–85.

Klinman NR. Antibody with homogeneous antigen binding produced by splenic foci in organ culture. Immunochemistry. 1969;6:757–9.

McDevitt HO, Chinitz A. Genetic control of the antibody response: relationship between immune response and histocompatibility (H-2) type. Science. 1969;163:1207–8.

Raff MC. Two distinct populations of peripheral lymphocytes in mice distinguishable by immunofluorescence. Immunology. 1970;19:637–50.

Wu TT, Kabat EA. An analysis of the sequences of the variable regions of Bence Jones proteins and myeloma light chains and their implications for antibody complementarity. J Exp Med. 1970;132:211–50.

Armstrong JA, D'Arcy Hart P. Response of cultured macrophages to Mycobacterium tuberculosis, with observations on fusion of lysosomes with phagosomes. J Exp Med. 1971;134:713–40.

Craig SW, Cebra JJ. Peyer's patches: an enriched source of precursors for IgA-producing immunocytes in the rabbit. J Exp Med. 1971;134:188–200.

Cudkowicz G, Bennett M. Peculiar immunobiology of bone marrow allografts. I. Graft rejection by irradiated responder mice. J Exp Med. 1971a;134:83–102.

Cudkowicz G, Bennett M. Peculiar immunobiology of bone marrow allografts. II. Rejection of parental grafts by resistant F 1 hybrid mice. J Exp Med. 1971b;134:1513–28.

Engvall E, Perlmann P. Enzyme-linked immunosorbent assay (ELISA). Quantitative assay of immunoglobulin G. Immunochemistry. 1971;8:871–4.

Jerne NK. The somatic generation of immune recognition. Eur J Immunol. 1971;1:1–9.

Mitchison NA. The carrier effect in the secondary response to hapten-protein conjugates. I. Measurement of the effect with transferred cells and objections to the local environment hypothesis. Eur J Immunol. 1971a;1:10–7.

Mitchison NA. The carrier effect in the secondary response to hapten-protein conjugates. II. Cellular cooperation. Eur J Immunol. 1971b;1:18–27.

Sprent J, Miller JF, Mitchell GF. Antigen-induced selective recruitment of circulating lymphocytes. Cell Immunol. 1971;2:171–81.

Klinman NR. The mechanism of antigenic stimulation of primary and secondary clonal precursor cells. J Exp Med. 1972;136:241–60.

Babior BM, Kipnes RS, Curnutte JT. Biological defense mechanisms. The production by leukocytes of superoxide, a potential bactericidal agent. J Clin Invest. 1973;52:741–4.

Cotton RG, Milstein C. Letter: fusion of two immunoglobulin-producing myeloma cells. Nature. 1973;244:42–3.

Steinman RM, Cohn ZA. Identification of a novel cell type in peripheral lymphoid organs of mice. I. Morphology, quantitation, tissue distribution. J Exp Med. 1973;137:1142–62.

Strander H, Cantell K, Carlstrom G, Jakobsson PA. Clinical and laboratory investigations on man: systemic administration of potent interferon to man. J Natl Cancer Inst. 1973;51:733–42.

Bottazzo GF, Florin-Christensen A, Doniach D. Islet-cell antibodies in diabetes mellitus with autoimmune polyendocrine deficiencies. Lancet. 1974;2:1279–83.

Brandtzaeg P. Mucosal and glandular distribution of immunoglobulin components: differential localization of free and bound SC in secretory epithelial cells. J Immunol. 1974;112:1553–9.

MacCuish AC, Irvine WJ, Barnes EW, Duncan LJ. Antibodies to pancreatic islet cells in insulin-dependent diabetics with coexistent autoimmune disease. Lancet. 1974;2:1529–31.

Owen JJ, Cooper MD, Raff MC. In vitro generation of B lymphocytes in mouse foetal liver, a mammalian 'bursa equivalent'. Nature. 1974;249:361–3.

Steinman RM, Cohn ZA. Identification of a novel cell type in peripheral lymphoid organs of mice. II. Functional properties in vitro. J Exp Med. 1974;139:380–97.

Zinkernagel RM, Doherty PC. Restriction of in vitro T cell-mediated cytotoxicity in lymphocytic choriomeningitis within a syngeneic or semiallogeneic system. Nature. 1974;248:701–2.

Bevan MJ. The major histocompatibility complex determines susceptibility to cytotoxic T cells directed against minor histocompatibility antigens. J Exp Med. 1975;142:1349–64.

Cantor H, Boyse EA. Functional subclasses of T-lymphocytes bearing different Ly antigens. I. The generation of functionally distinct T-cell subclasses is a differentiative process independent of antigen. J Exp Med. 1975a;141:1376–89.

Cantor H, Boyse EA. Functional subclasses of T lymphocytes bearing different Ly antigens. II. Cooperation between subclasses of Ly+ cells in the generation of killer activity. J Exp Med. 1975b;141:1390–9.

Kohler G, Milstein C. Continuous cultures of fused cells secreting antibody of predefined specificity. Nature. 1975;256:495–7.

Burnet FM. A modification of Jerne's theory of antibody production using the concept of clonal selection. CA Cancer J Clin. 1976;26:119–21.

Hozumi N, Tonegawa S. Evidence for somatic rearrangement of immunoglobulin genes coding for variable and constant regions. Proc Natl Acad Sci U S A. 1976;73:3628–32.

Solley GO, Gleich GJ, Jordon RE, Schroeter AL. The late phase of the immediate wheal and flare skin reaction. Its dependence upon IgE antibodies. J Clin Invest. 1976;58:408–20.

Robinson JH, Owen JJ. Generation of T-cell function in organ culture of foetal mouse thymus. II. Mixed lymphocyte culture reactivity. Clin Exp Immunol. 1977;27:322–7.

Ruscetti FW, Morgan DA, Gallo RC. Functional and morphologic characterization of human T cells continuously grown in vitro. J Immunol. 1977;119:131–8.

Silverton EW, Navia MA, Davies DR. Three-dimensional structure of an intact human immunoglobulin. Proc Natl Acad Sci U S A. 1977;74:5140–4.

Brack C, Hirama M, Lenhard-Schuller R, Tonegawa S. A complete immunoglobulin gene is created by somatic recombination. Cell. 1978;15:1–14.

Baker PE, Gillis S, Smith KA. Monoclonal cytolytic T-cell lines. J Exp Med. 1979;149:273–8.

Kung P, Goldstein G, Reinherz EL, Schlossman SF. Monoclonal antibodies defining distinctive human T cell surface antigens. Science. 1979;206:347–9.

Murphy RC, Hammarstrom S, Samuelsson B. Leukotriene C: a slow-reacting substance from murine mastocytoma cells. Proc Natl Acad Sci U S A. 1979;76: 4275–9.

Parks DR, Bryan VM, Oi VT, Herzenberg LA. Antigen-specific identification and cloning of hybridomas with a fluorescence-activated cell sorter. Proc Natl Acad Sci U S A. 1979;76:1962–6.

Reinherz EL, Kung PC, Goldstein G, Schlossman SF. Separation of functional subsets of human T cells by a monoclonal antibody. Proc Natl Acad Sci U S A. 1979;76:4061–5.

Silverstein AM. History of immunology. Cell Immunol. 1979a;42:1–2.

Silverstein AM. History of immunology. Cellular versus humoral immunity: determinants and consequences of an epic 19th century battle. Cell Immunol. 1979b;48:208–21.

Davis MM, et al. An immunoglobulin heavy-chain gene is formed by at least two recombinational events. Nature. 1980;283:733–9.

Early P, Huang H, Davis M, Calame K, Hood L. An immunoglobulin heavy chain variable region gene is generated from three segments of DNA: VH, D and JH. Cell. 1980;19:981–92.

Silverstein AM, Bialasiewicz AA. History of immunology. A history of theories of acquired immunity. Cell Immunol. 1980;51:151–67.

Van Wauwe JP, De Mey JR, Goossens JG. OKT3: a monoclonal anti-human T lymphocyte antibody with potent mitogenic properties. J Immunol. 1980;124:2708–13.

Kappler JW, Skidmore B, White J, Marrack P. Antigen-inducible, H-2-restricted, interleukin-2-producing T cell hybridomas. Lack of independent antigen and H-2 recognition. J Exp Med. 1981;153:1198–214.

Silverstein AM, Miller G. History of immunology. The royal experiment on immunity: 1721-1722. Cell Immunol. 1981;61:437–47.

Steiner H, Hultmark D, Engstrom A, Bennich H, Boman HG. Sequence and specificity of two antibacterial proteins involved in insect immunity. Nature. 1981;292:246–8.

Ziegler K, Unanue ER. Identification of a macrophage antigen-processing event required for I-region-restricted antigen presentation to T lymphocytes. J Immunol. 1981;127:1869–75.

Allison JP, McIntyre BW, Bloch D. Tumor-specific antigen of murine T-lymphoma defined with monoclonal antibody. J Immunol. 1982;129:2293–300.

Butcher EC, et al. Surface phenotype of Peyer's patch germinal center cells: implications for the role of germinal centers in B cell differentiation. J Immunol. 1982;129:2698–707.

Howard M, et al. Identification of a T cell-derived b cell growth factor distinct from interleukin 2. J Exp Med. 1982;155:914–23.

Isakson PC, Pure E, Vitetta ES, Krammer PH. T cell-derived B cell differentiation factor(s). Effect on the isotype switch of murine B cells. J Exp Med. 1982;155:734–48.

Silverstein AM. History of immunology. Development of the concept of immunologic specificity, I. Cell Immunol. 1982a;67:396–409.

Silverstein AM. History of immunology: development of the concept of immunologic specificity: II. Cell Immunol. 1982b;71:183–95.

Takahashi N, et al. Structure of human immunoglobulin gamma genes: implications for evolution of a gene family. Cell. 1982;29:671–9.

Turkeltaub PC, Rastogi SC, Baer H, Anderson MC, Norman PS. A standardized quantitative skin-test assay of allergen potency and stability: studies on the allergen dose-response curve and effect of wheal, erythema, and patient selection on assay results. J Allergy Clin Immunol. 1982;70:343–52.

Haskins K, et al. The major histocompatibility complex-restricted antigen receptor on T cells. I. Isolation with a monoclonal antibody. J Exp Med. 1983;157:1149–69.

Kappler J, et al. The major histocompatibility complex-restricted antigen receptor on T cells in mouse and man: identification of constant and variable peptides. Cell. 1983;35:295–302.

Tonegawa S. Somatic generation of antibody diversity. Nature. 1983;302:575–81.

Auron PE, et al. Nucleotide sequence of human monocyte interleukin 1 precursor cDNA. Proc Natl Acad Sci U S A. 1984;81:7907–11.

Gough NM, et al. Molecular cloning of cDNA encoding a murine haematopoietic growth regulator, granulocyte-macrophage colony stimulating factor. Nature. 1984;309:763–7.

Hedrick SM, Cohen DI, Nielsen EA, Davis MM. Isolation of cDNA clones encoding T cell-specific membrane-associated proteins. Nature. 1984;308:149–53.

Marshall BJ, Warren JR. Unidentified curved bacilli in the stomach of patients with gastritis and peptic ulceration. Lancet. 1984;1:1311–5.

McKean D, et al. Generation of antibody diversity in the immune response of BALB/c mice to influenza virus hemagglutinin. Proc Natl Acad Sci U S A. 1984;81:3180–4.

Morrison SL, Johnson MJ, Herzenberg LA, Oi VT. Chimeric human antibody molecules: mouse antigen-binding domains with human constant region domains. Proc Natl Acad Sci U S A. 1984;81:6851–5.

Rock KL, Benacerraf B, Abbas AK. Antigen presentation by hapten-specific B lymphocytes. I. Role of surface immunoglobulin receptors. J Exp Med. 1984;160:1102–13.

Townsend AR, McMichael AJ, Carter NP, Huddleston JA, Brownlee GG. Cytotoxic T cell recognition of the influenza nucleoprotein and hemagglutinin expressed in transfected mouse L cells. Cell. 1984;39:13–25.

Babbitt BP, Allen PM, Matsueda G, Haber E, Unanue ER. Binding of immunogenic peptides to Ia histocompatibility molecules. Nature. 1985;317:359–61.

Beutler B, Milsark IW, Cerami AC. Passive immunization against cachectin/tumor necrosis factor protects mice from lethal effect of endotoxin. Science. 1985;229:869–71.

Jenner E, Pasteur L. [From Jenner to Pasteur or the development of ideas on vaccination]. Bull Acad Natl Med. 1985;169:771–8.

Lanzavecchia A. Antigen-specific interaction between T and B cells. Nature. 1985;314:537–9.

Nakano T, et al. Fate of bone marrow-derived cultured mast cells after intracutaneous, intraperitoneal, and intravenous transfer into genetically mast cell-deficient W/Wv mice. Evidence that cultured mast cells can give rise to both connective tissue type and mucosal mast cells. J Exp Med. 1985;162:1025–43.

Brenner MB, et al. Identification of a putative second T-cell receptor. Nature. 1986;322:145–9.

Clark EA, Ledbetter JA. Activation of human B cells mediated through two distinct cell surface differentiation antigens, Bp35 and Bp50. Proc Natl Acad Sci U S A. 1986;83:4494–8.

Dustin ML, Rothlein R, Bhan AK, Dinarello CA, Springer TA. Induction by IL 1 and interferon-gamma: tissue distribution, biochemistry, and function of a natural adherence molecule (ICAM-1). J Immunol. 1986;137:245–54.

Jones PT, Dear PH, Foote J, Neuberger MS, Winter G. Replacing the complementarity-determining regions in a human antibody with those from a mouse. Nature. 1986;321:522–5.

Karre K, Ljunggren HG, Piontek G, Kiessling R. Selective rejection of H-2-deficient lymphoma variants suggests alternative immune defence strategy. Nature. 1986;319:675–8.

Kehrl JH, et al. Production of transforming growth factor beta by human T lymphocytes and its potential role in the regulation of T cell growth. J Exp Med. 1986;163:1037–50.

Mosmann TR, Cherwinski H, Bond MW, Giedlin MA, Coffman RL. Two types of murine helper T cell clone. I. Definition according to profiles of lymphokine activities and secreted proteins. J Immunol. 1986;136:2348–57.

Rothlein R, Dustin ML, Marlin SD, Springer TA. A human intercellular adhesion molecule (ICAM-1) distinct from LFA-1. J Immunol. 1986;137:1270–4.

Royer-Pokora B, et al. Cloning the gene for an inherited human disorder—chronic granulomatous disease—on the basis of its chromosomal location. Nature. 1986;322:32–8.

Sen R, Baltimore D. Inducibility of kappa immunoglobulin enhancer-binding protein Nf-kappa B by a post-translational mechanism. Cell. 1986a;47:921–8.

Sen R, Baltimore D. Multiple nuclear factors interact with the immunoglobulin enhancer sequences. Cell. 1986b;46:705–16.

Bjorkman PJ, et al. Structure of the human class I histocompatibility antigen, HLA-A2. Nature. 1987a;329:506–12.

Bjorkman PJ, et al. The foreign antigen binding site and T cell recognition regions of class I histocompatibility antigens. Nature. 1987b;329:512–8.

Brunet JF, et al. A new member of the immunoglobulin superfamily—CTLA-4. Nature. 1987;328:267–70.

Cher DJ, Mosmann TR. Two types of murine helper T cell clone. II. Delayed-type hypersensitivity is mediated by TH1 clones. J Immunol. 1987;138:3688–94.

Doyle C, Strominger JL. Interaction between CD4 and class II MHC molecules mediates cell adhesion. Nature. 1987;330:256–9.

Jenkins MK, Schwartz RH. Antigen presentation by chemically modified splenocytes induces antigen-specific T cell unresponsiveness in vitro and in vivo. J Exp Med. 1987;165:302–19.

Kappler JW, Roehm N, Marrack P. T cell tolerance by clonal elimination in the thymus. Cell. 1987;49:273–80.

Orme IM. The kinetics of emergence and loss of mediator T lymphocytes acquired in response to infection with Mycobacterium tuberculosis. J Immunol. 1987;138:293–8.

Snapper CM, Paul WE. Interferon-gamma and B cell stimulatory factor-1 reciprocally regulate Ig isotype production. Science. 1987;236:944–7.

Yoshimura T, Matsushima K, Oppenheim JJ, Leonard EJ. Neutrophil chemotactic factor produced by lipopolysaccharide (LPS)-stimulated human blood mononuclear leukocytes: partial characterization and separation from interleukin 1 (IL 1). J Immunol. 1987a;139:788–93.

Yoshimura T, et al. Purification of a human monocyte-derived neutrophil chemotactic factor that has peptide sequence similarity to other host defense cytokines. Proc Natl Acad Sci U S A. 1987b;84:9233–7.

Bird RE, et al. Single-chain antigen-binding proteins. Science. 1988;242:423–6.

Goodnow CC, et al. Altered immunoglobulin expression and functional silencing of self-reactive B lymphocytes in transgenic mice. Nature. 1988;334:676–82.

Schall TJ, et al. A human T cell-specific molecule is a member of a new gene family. J Immunol. 1988;141:1018–25.

Shaw JP, et al. Identification of a putative regulator of early T cell activation genes. Science. 1988;241:202–5.

Coffman RL, Lebman DA, Shrader B. Transforming growth factor beta specifically enhances IgA production by lipopolysaccharide-stimulated murine B lymphocytes. J Exp Med. 1989;170:1039–44.

Emmel EA, et al. Cyclosporin A specifically inhibits function of nuclear proteins involved in T cell activation. Science. 1989;246:1617–20.

Fiorentino DF, Bond MW, Mosmann TR. Two types of mouse T helper cell. IV. Th2 clones secrete a factor that inhibits cytokine production by Th1 clones. J Exp Med. 1989;170:2081–95.

Janeway CA Jr. Approaching the asymptote? Evolution and revolution in immunology. Cold Spring Harb Symp Quant Biol. 1989;54(Pt 1):1–13.

Lefrancois L, Goodman T. In vivo modulation of cytolytic activity and Thy-1 expression in TCR-gamma delta+ intraepithelial lymphocytes. Science. 1989;243:1716–8.

Porcelli S, et al. Recognition of cluster of differentiation 1 antigens by human CD4-CD8-cytolytic T lymphocytes. Nature. 1989;341:447–50.

Schatz DG, Oettinger MA, Baltimore D. The V(D)J recombination activating gene, RAG-1. Cell. 1989;59:1035–48.

Sonoda E, et al. Transforming growth factor beta induces IgA production and acts additively with interleukin 5 for IgA production. J Exp Med. 1989;170:1415–20.

Townsend A, et al. Association of class I major histocompatibility heavy and light chains induced by viral peptides. Nature. 1989;340:443–8.

Wright AE, Douglas SR, Sanderson JB. An experimental investigation of the role of the blood fluids in connection with phagocytosis. 1903. Rev Infect Dis. 1989;11:827–34.

Conrad DH, Ben-Sasson SZ, Le Gros G, Finkelman FD, Paul WE. Infection with Nippostrongylus brasiliensis or injection of anti-IgD antibodies markedly enhances Fc-receptor-mediated interleukin 4 production by non-B, non-T cells. J Exp Med. 1990;171:1497–508.

Hombach J, Tsubata T, Leclercq L, Stappert H, Reth M. Molecular components of the B-cell antigen receptor complex of the IgM class. Nature. 1990;343:760–2.

Koller BH, Marrack P, Kappler JW, Smithies O. Normal development of mice deficient in beta 2M, MHC class I proteins, and CD8+ T cells. Science. 1990;248:1227–30.

Le Gros G, Ben-Sasson SZ, Seder R, Finkelman FD, Paul WE. Generation of interleukin 4 (IL-4)-producing cells in vivo and in vitro: IL-2 and IL-4 are required for in vitro generation of IL-4-producing cells. J Exp Med. 1990;172:921–9.

Linsley PS, Clark EA, Ledbetter JA. T-cell antigen CD28 mediates adhesion with B cells by interacting with activation antigen B7/BB-1. Proc Natl Acad Sci U S A. 1990;87:5031–5.

Monaco JJ, Cho S, Attaya M. Transport protein genes in the murine MHC: possible implications for antigen processing. Science. 1990;250:1723–6.

Moore KW, et al. Homology of cytokine synthesis inhibitory factor (IL-10) to the Epstein-Barr virus gene BCRFI. Science. 1990;248:1230–4.

Oettinger MA, Schatz DG, Gorka C, Baltimore D. RAG-1 and RAG-2, adjacent genes that synergistically activate V(D)J recombination. Science. 1990;248:1517–23.

Ruddle NH, et al. An antibody to lymphotoxin and tumor necrosis factor prevents transfer of experimental allergic encephalomyelitis. J Exp Med. 1990;172:1193–200.

Zijlstra M, et al. Beta 2-microglobulin deficient mice lack CD4-8+ cytolytic T cells. Nature. 1990;344:742–6.

Falk K, Rotzschke O, Stevanovic S, Jung G, Rammensee HG. Allele-specific motifs revealed by sequencing of self-peptides eluted from MHC molecules. Nature. 1991;351:290–6.

Fiorentino DF, et al. IL-10 acts on the antigen-presenting cell to inhibit cytokine production by Th1 cells. J Immunol. 1991;146:3444–51.

Holmes WE, Lee J, Kuang WJ, Rice GC, Wood WI. Structure and functional expression of a human interleukin-8 receptor. Science. 1991;253:1278–80.

Murphy PM, Tiffany HL. Cloning of complementary DNA encoding a functional human interleukin-8 receptor. Science. 1991;253:1280–3.

Pearce EJ, Caspar P, Grzych JM, Lewis FA, Sher A. Downregulation of Th1 cytokine production accompanies induction of Th2 responses by a parasitic helminth, Schistosoma mansoni. J Exp Med. 1991;173:159–66.

Rudensky A, Preston-Hurlburt P, Hong SC, Barlow A, Janeway CA Jr. Sequence analysis of peptides bound to MHC class II molecules. Nature. 1991;353:622–7.

Todd JA, et al. Genetic analysis of autoimmune type 1 diabetes mellitus in mice. Nature. 1991;351:542–7.

von Behring E, Kitasato S. [The mechanism of diphtheria immunity and tetanus immunity in animals. 1890]. Mol Immunol. 1991;28(1317):1319–20.

Carter RH, Fearon DT. CD19: lowering the threshold for antigen receptor stimulation of B lymphocytes. Science. 1992;256:105–7.

Ishida Y, Agata Y, Shibahara K, Honjo T. Induced expression of PD-1, a novel member of the immunoglobulin gene superfamily, upon programmed cell death. EMBO J. 1992;11:3887–95.

Janeway CA Jr. The immune system evolved to discriminate infectious nonself from noninfectious self. Immunol Today. 1992;13:11–6.

Karlhofer FM, Ribaudo RK, Yokoyama WM. MHC class I alloantigen specificity of Ly-49+ IL-2-activated natural killer cells. Nature. 1992;358:66–70.

Noelle RJ, et al. A 39-kDa protein on activated helper T cells binds CD40 and transduces the signal for cognate activation of B cells. Proc Natl Acad Sci U S A. 1992;89:6550–4.

Schindler C, Shuai K, Prezioso VR, Darnell JE Jr. Interferon-dependent tyrosine phosphorylation of a latent cytoplasmic transcription factor. Science. 1992;257:809–13.

Velazquez L, Fellous M, Stark GR, Pellegrini S. A protein tyrosine kinase in the interferon alpha/beta signaling pathway. Cell. 1992;70:313–22.

Watanabe-Fukunaga R, Brannan CI, Copeland NG, Jenkins NA, Nagata S. Lymphoproliferation disorder in mice explained by defects in Fas antigen that mediates apoptosis. Nature. 1992;356:314–7.

Zychlinsky A, Prevost MC, Sansonetti PJ. Shigella flexneri induces apoptosis in infected macrophages. Nature. 1992;358:167–9.

Brown JH, et al. Three-dimensional structure of the human class II histocompatibility antigen HLA-DR1. Nature. 1993;364:33–9.

Gay D, Saunders T, Camper S, Weigert M. Receptor editing: an approach by autoreactive B cells to escape tolerance. J Exp Med. 1993;177:999–1008.

Heinzel FP, Rerko RM, Hatam F, Locksley RM. IL-2 is necessary for the progression of leishmaniasis in susceptible murine hosts. J Immunol. 1993;150:3924–31.

Hsieh CS, et al. Development of TH1 CD4+ T cells through IL-12 produced by Listeria-induced macrophages. Science. 1993;260:547–9.

Noguchi M, et al. Interleukin-2 receptor gamma chain mutation results in X-linked severe combined immunodeficiency in humans. Cell. 1993;73:147–57.

Shinkai Y, et al. Restoration of T cell development in RAG-2-deficient mice by functional TCR transgenes. Science. 1993;259:822–5.

Tiegs SL, Russell DM, Nemazee D. Receptor editing in self-reactive bone marrow B cells. J Exp Med. 1993;177:1009–20.

De Togni P, et al. Abnormal development of peripheral lymphoid organs in mice deficient in lymphotoxin. Science. 1994;264:703–7.

Hogquist KA, et al. T cell receptor antagonist peptides induce positive selection. Cell. 1994;76:17–27.

Iwashima M, Irving BA, van Oers NS, Chan AC, Weiss A. Sequential interactions of the TCR with two distinct cytoplasmic tyrosine kinases. Science. 1994;263:1136–9.

Jardetzky TS, et al. Three-dimensional structure of a human class II histocompatibility molecule complexed with superantigen. Nature. 1994;368:711–8.

Lau LL, Jamieson BD, Somasundaram T, Ahmed R. Cytotoxic T-cell memory without antigen. Nature. 1994;369:648–52.

Saint-Ruf C, et al. Analysis and expression of a cloned pre-T cell receptor gene. Science. 1994;266:1208–12.

Sallusto F, Lanzavecchia A. Efficient presentation of soluble antigen by cultured human dendritic cells is maintained by granulocyte/macrophage colony-stimulating factor plus interleukin 4 and downregulated by tumor necrosis factor alpha. J Exp Med. 1994;179:1109–18.

Surh CD, Sprent J. T-cell apoptosis detected in situ during positive and negative selection in the thymus. Nature. 1994;372:100–3.

Walunas TL, et al. CTLA-4 can function as a negative regulator of T cell activation. Immunity. 1994;1:405–13.

Krummel MF, Allison JP. CD28 and CTLA-4 have opposing effects on the response of T cells to stimulation. J Exp Med. 1995;182:459–65.

McBlane JF, et al. Cleavage at a V(D)J recombination signal requires only RAG1 and RAG2 proteins and occurs in two steps. Cell. 1995;83:387–95.

Robey E, Allison JP. T-cell activation: integration of signals from the antigen receptor and costimulatory molecules. Immunol Today. 1995;16:306–10.

Sakaguchi S, Sakaguchi N, Asano M, Itoh M, Toda M. Immunologic self-tolerance maintained by activated T cells expressing IL-2 receptor alpha-chains (CD25). Breakdown of a single mechanism of self-tolerance causes various autoimmune diseases. J Immunol. 1995;155:1151–64.

Yao Z, et al. Herpesvirus Saimiri encodes a new cytokine, IL-17, which binds to a novel cytokine receptor. Immunity. 1995;3:811–21.

Feng Y, Broder CC, Kennedy PE, Berger EA. HIV-1 entry cofactor: functional cDNA cloning of a seven-transmembrane, G protein-coupled receptor. Science. 1996;272:872–7.

Garboczi DN, et al. Structure of the complex between human T-cell receptor, viral peptide and HLA-A2. Nature. 1996;384:134–41.

Garcia KC, et al. An alphabeta T cell receptor structure at 2.5 A and its orientation in the TCR-MHC complex. Science. 1996;274:209–19.

Larsen CP, et al. Long-term acceptance of skin and cardiac allografts after blocking CD40 and CD28 pathways. Nature. 1996;381:434–8.

Lemaitre B, Nicolas E, Michaut L, Reichhart JM, Hoffmann JA. The dorsoventral regulatory gene cassette spatzle/Toll/cactus controls the potent antifungal response in Drosophila adults. Cell. 1996;86:973–83.

Medzhitov R, Preston-Hurlburt P, Janeway CA Jr. A human homologue of the Drosophila Toll protein signals activation of adaptive immunity. Nature. 1997;388:394–7.

Muzio M, Ni J, Feng P, Dixit VM. IRAK (Pelle) family member IRAK-2 and MyD88 as proximal mediators of IL-1 signaling. Science. 1997;278:1612–5.

Wesche H, Henzel WJ, Shillinglaw W, Li S, Cao Z. MyD88: an adapter that recruits IRAK to the IL-1 receptor complex. Immunity. 1997;7:837–47.

Zheng W, Flavell RA. The transcription factor GATA-3 is necessary and sufficient for Th2 cytokine gene expression in CD4 T cells. Cell. 1997;89:587–96.

Butz EA, Bevan MJ. Massive expansion of antigen-specific CD8+ T cells during an acute virus infection. Immunity. 1998;8:167–75.

Monks CR, Freiberg BA, Kupfer H, Sciaky N, Kupfer A. Three-dimensional segregation of supramolecular activation clusters in T cells. Nature. 1998;395:82–6.

Murali-Krishna K, et al. Counting antigen-specific CD8 T cells: a reevaluation of bystander activation during viral infection. Immunity. 1998;8:177–87.

Poltorak A, et al. Defective LPS signaling in C3H/HeJ and C57BL/10ScCr mice: mutations in Tlr4 gene. Science. 1998;282:2085–8.

Schellekens GA, de Jong BA, van den Hoogen FH, van de Putte LB, van Venrooij WJ. Citrulline is an essential constituent of antigenic determinants recognized by rheumatoid arthritis-specific autoantibodies. J Clin Invest. 1998;101:273–81.

Bauer S, et al. Activation of NK cells and T cells by NKG2D, a receptor for stress-inducible MICA. Science. 1999;285:727–9.

Dong H, Zhu G, Tamada K, Chen L. B7-H1, a third member of the B7 family, co-stimulates T-cell proliferation and interleukin-10 secretion. Nat Med. 1999;5:1365–9.

Forster R, et al. CCR7 coordinates the primary immune response by establishing functional microenvironments in secondary lymphoid organs. Cell. 1999;99:23–33.

Grakoui A, et al. The immunological synapse: a molecular machine controlling T cell activation. Science. 1999;285:221–7.

Hoshino K, et al. Cutting edge: Toll-like receptor 4 (TLR4)-deficient mice are hyporesponsive to lipopolysaccharide: evidence for TLR4 as the Lps gene product. J Immunol. 1999;162:3749–52.

Nishimura H, Nose M, Hiai H, Minato N, Honjo T. Development of lupus-like autoimmune diseases by disruption of the PD-1 gene encoding an ITIM motif-carrying immunoreceptor. Immunity. 1999;11:141–51.

Nutt SL, Heavey B, Rolink AG, Busslinger M. Commitment to the B-lymphoid lineage depends on the transcription factor Pax5. Nature. 1999;401:556–62.

Sallusto F, Lenig D, Forster R, Lipp M, Lanzavecchia A. Two subsets of memory T lymphocytes with distinct homing potentials and effector functions. Nature. 1999;401:708–12.

Muramatsu M, et al. Class switch recombination and hypermutation require activation-induced cytidine deaminase (AID), a potential RNA editing enzyme. Cell. 2000;102:553–63.

Szabo SJ, et al. A novel transcription factor, T-bet, directs Th1 lineage commitment. Cell. 2000;100:655–69.

Chambers CA, Kuhns MS, Egen JG, Allison JP. CTLA-4-mediated inhibition in regulation of T cell responses: mechanisms and manipulation in tumor immunotherapy. Annu Rev Immunol. 2001;19:565–94.

Girardi M, et al. Regulation of cutaneous malignancy by gammadelta T cells. Science. 2001;294:605–9.

Masopust D, Vezys V, Marzo AL, Lefrancois L. Preferential localization of effector memory cells in nonlymphoid tissue. Science. 2001;291:2413–7.

Shankaran V, et al. IFNgamma and lymphocytes prevent primary tumour development and shape tumour immunogenicity. Nature. 2001;410:1107–11.

Arase H, Mocarski ES, Campbell AE, Hill AB, Lanier LL. Direct recognition of cytomegalovirus by activating and inhibitory NK cell receptors. Science. 2002;296:1323–6.

Fontenot JD, Gavin MA, Rudensky AY. Foxp3 programs the development and function of CD4+CD25+ regulatory T cells. Nat Immunol. 2003;4:330–6.

Hori S, Nomura T, Sakaguchi S. Control of regulatory T cell development by the transcription factor Foxp3. Science. 2003;299:1057–61.

Pentcheva-Hoang T, Egen JG, Wojnoonski K, Allison JP. B7-1 and B7-2 selectively recruit CTLA-4 and CD28 to the immunological synapse. Immunity. 2004;21:401–13.

Silverstein AM. Paul Ehrlich, archives and the history of immunology. Nat Immunol. 2005;6:639.

Khanna KM, McNamara JT, Lefrancois L. In situ imaging of the endogenous CD8 T cell response to infection. Science. 2007;318:116–20.

Kaufmann SH. Immunology's foundation: the 100-year anniversary of the Nobel Prize to Paul Ehrlich and Elie Metchnikoff. Nat Immunol. 2008a;9:705–12.

Kaufmann SH. Paul Ehrlich: founder of chemotherapy. Nat Rev Drug Discov. 2008b;7:373.

Robinson JH, Owen JJ. Pillars article: generation of T-cell function in organ culture of foetal mouse thymus I. Mitogen responsiveness. 1975. J Immunol. 2008;181:7437–44.

Xu Z, Zan H, Pone EJ, Mai T, Casali P. Immunoglobulin class-switch DNA recombination: induction, targeting and beyond. Nat Rev Immunol. 2012;12:517–31.

Cooper MD. The early history of B cells. Nat Rev Immunol. 2015;15:191–7.

Gitlin AD, Nussenzweig MC. Immunology: fifty years of B lymphocytes. Nature. 2015;517:139–41.

Akdis M, et al. Interleukins (from IL-1 to IL-38), interferons, transforming growth factor β, and TNF-α: receptors, functions, and roles in disease. J Allergy Clin Immunol. 2016;138:984–1010.

Modulation of the Innate Immune System

2

Doreen E. Szollosi and Clinton B. Mathias

Learning Objectives

1. Identify the mechanisms by which components of the innate immune system protect the body from infection.
2. Discuss the events involved in the inflammatory response.
3. Identify innate immune receptors and cytokines.
4. Recognize pathogen-associated molecular patterns (PAMPs) and predict how the immune system will recognize them.
5. Recognize the biological structure of the TNF-α inhibitors.
6. Discuss the pharmacology of the TNF-α, IL-1, IL-6, and IL-12 inhibitors, including mechanism of action, clinical uses, and adverse effects.
7. Discuss the pharmacology of the integrin inhibitors, including mechanism of action, clinical uses, and adverse effects.
8. Discuss the pharmacology of interferon therapies including mechanism of action, clinical uses, and adverse effects.

Drugs discussed in this chapter

Drug	Classification
Adalimumab (Humira®)	Anti-TNF-α monoclonal antibody
Anakinra (Kineret®)	Recombinant IL-1R antagonist
Canakinumab (Ilaris®)	Anti-IL-1β antibody
Certolizumab pegol (Cimzia®)	Anti-TNF-α antibody fragment
Etanercept (Enbrel®)	Anti-TNF-α fusion protein
Golimumab (Simponi®)	Anti-TNF-α monoclonal antibody
Infliximab (Remicade®)	Anti-TNF-α monoclonal antibody
Interferon alfa-2a, 2b (Pegasys®, Pegintron®)	Interferon
Interferon beta-1a (Avonex®)	Interferon
Natalizumab (Tysabri®)	Anti-α4β1 integrin monoclonal antibody
Rilonacept (Arcalyst®)	Anti-IL-1 fusion protein
Sarilumab (Kevzara®)	Anti-IL-6 receptor monoclonal antibody
Siltuximab (Sylvant®)	Anti-IL-6 monoclonal antibody
Tocilizumab (Actemra®)	Anti-IL-6 receptor monoclonal antibody
Ustekinumab (Stelara®)	Anti-IL-12/23 monoclonal antibody
Vedolizumab (Entyvio®)	Anti-α4β7 integrin monoclonal antibody

D. E. Szollosi (✉)
Department of Pharmaceutical Sciences, School of Pharmacy and Physician Assistant Studies, University of Saint Joseph, Hartford, CT, USA
e-mail: dszollosi@usj.edu

C. B. Mathias
Department of Pharmaceutical and Administrative Sciences, College of Pharmacy and Health Sciences, Western New England University, Springfield, MA, USA
e-mail: clinton.mathias@wne.edu

© Springer Nature Switzerland AG 2020
C. B. Mathias et al., *Pharmacology of Immunotherapeutic Drugs*,
https://doi.org/10.1007/978-3-030-19922-7_2

Introduction

As the immune system's first defense against foreign invaders, innate immune cells and mediators play important roles in keeping the body free from infection. Because innate immune cells and their receptors are only equipped to recognize molecular patterns of potential pathogens and not specific antigens, their job is said to be non-specific. In some instances, however, the inappropriate response of the innate immune system can play a role in the pathophysiology of conditions in which chronic inflammation contributes to disease symptoms and progression. Here, we will discuss and outline the normal physiological role of the innate immune system and its components, and then highlight these as potential drug targets in disease states in which the immune system may be over-activated (i.e. autoimmunity).

First Barriers to Infection

Non-cellular Defenses

The body's first lines of defense against infection by foreign invaders includes its physical barriers. These barriers include the skin and epithelia of the digestive, respiratory, and urogenital tracts—all areas of the body that are able to have first contact with the outside environment. Some of these barriers are colonized with the body's microbiome, or microorganisms that have a commensalistic relationship with the host, creating a type of microbial antagonism that makes it difficult for disease-causing pathogens to penetrate and cause infection. Infants begin to be colonized with commensal microorganisms at birth. Besides these microbiological barriers, mechanical and chemical barriers also exist to prevent colonization by potential pathogens. Examples of these barriers can be found in Table 2.1.

If a pathogen penetrates any of the physical barriers, plasma proteins in the form of what is called the complement system are an immediate non-cellular defense against bacteria and virus particles. The **complement system** is a cascade of approximately 30 serine proteases that cleave

Table 2.1 Physical barriers at external surfaces

Tissue	Mechanical barriers	Chemical barriers
Skin	Tight junctions between epithelial cells, sweat	Antimicrobial peptides and fatty acids
Lungs	Tight junctions between epithelial cells Tracheal cilia, movement of mucus	Surfactant Antimicrobial peptides
Eyes, Nasopharynx	Tight junctions between epithelial cells Nasal cilia movement, tears	Enzymes in saliva and tears, antimicrobial peptides
Gut	Tight junctions between epithelial cells, movement of fluid	Low pH, antimicrobial enzymes, antimicrobial peptides

subsequent proteases in the pathway, one of the most important being C3, and induce the removal or destruction of pathogens. The net effect of the activities of individual complement proteins in the cascade is to induce either the opsonization or lysis of pathogens and the recruitment of inflammatory cells to infectious sites. The complement cascades are arranged into three different pathways: Alternative, Classical, and Mannose-Binding Lectin (MBL) (Fig. 2.1). The alternative pathway is the first to be activated during initial infection and involves the protease C3 which is made in the liver and released into the blood. When C3 is hydrolyzed, especially near the surface of a pathogen, it becomes subsequently cleaved by an enzyme, C3 convertase into C3a and C3b. C3b is then able to bind covalently to the surface of the pathogen. This creates a positive feedback loop in which the deposition of more C3b results in further cleavage of C3 by C3 convertase, resulting in a coating of the pathogen by C3b. This C3b "coating" is then able to interact with complement receptors on phagocytes, resulting in a more efficient phagocytosis. The process of coating with complement for phagocytosis is known as opsonization.

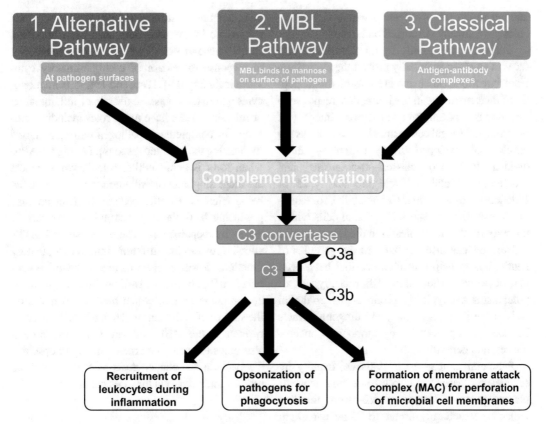

Fig. 2.1 Activation and roles of the three complement pathways. Activation of complement results in recruitment of leukocytes, opsonization of pathogens to promote phagocytosis, and formation of the membrane attack complex to aid is destruction of microbes via perforation of cell membranes

The MBL and classical pathways are activated later during infection, but result in the same effect, which is the deposition of C3b on the surfaces of pathogens. The MBL pathway is initiated when mannose-binding lectin, an acute phase protein produced by the liver during infection, binds mannose residues on the surface of pathogens. This activates the complement cascade via the lectin pathway. Similarly, the classical pathway is activated when C-reactive protein, another acute phase protein, binds phosphorylcholine on pathogen surfaces and triggers complement proteins. It is also activated by antibodies that are produced during the adaptive immune response.

While opsonization is one of the most important effects of complement, products beyond C3b are also integral for pathogen killing. Complement C5 is structurally similar to C3 and can be cleaved

by C5 convertase into C5a and C5b. C5b initiates the forming of the membrane attack complex (MAC) which is composed of C5, C6, C7, and C9 interactions with the bacterial cell membrane. These, in effect, poke holes in the cell membranes of bacterial cells, causing them to lyse and die.

Lastly, while C3b and C5b contribute to important effector mechanisms of complement, the smaller components of C3 and C5 cleavage, C3a and C5a, sometimes referred to as anaphylatoxins for their ability to induce anaphylaxis, can help recruit leukocytes to the site of infection. Specific activities include the degranulation of mast cells and basophils with the consequent release of histamine, and a vasodilating effect on blood vessels that allows for easier passage of leukocytes out of the blood and into the site of infection. C5a in particular can act as a chemoattractant to help neutrophils and monocytes adhere to blood vessel walls and get to the site of infection where C3b molecules have already opsonized pathogens.

Defensins are usually found at mucosal surfaces in an effort to initially protect the epithelium from infection. Defensins are antimicrobial peptides; their main role in the immediate response to infection is to penetrate and disrupt the integrity of bacterial and fungal cell membranes, as well as the envelope of enveloped viruses. Defensins can be divided into two classes—α-defensins and β-defensins 6 and 4 There are six types of α-defensins. α-defensins HD5 and HD6, for example, are secreted by special epithelial cells within the crypts of the small intestine called Paneth cells. α-defensins can also be found in the granules of neutrophils to help kill microbes that have been phagocytosed. The four different types of β-defensins are typically produced by epithelial cells of the skin, respiratory, and urogenital tracts but can also be produced by monocytes, macrophages, and dendritic cells.

Pathogen damage to host tissue, usually by secreted proteases can also initiate the release of plasma proteins known as α2-macroglobulins which are structurally similar to C3 but can aid in the inactivation of microbial proteases by chemically inducing a conformational change. The covalent binding of the α2-macroglobulin to the protease forms a complex that can then be cleared by macrophages which recognize this complex via a receptor present on the surface.

The Acute Phase Response

The innate immune response that occurs soon after the start of an infection and involves the production and systemic release of acute phase proteins by the liver is termed as the acute phase response (APR). This is mediated in response to trauma, infection, or inflammatory stimuli and usually occurs when immediate immune barriers have been breached. **Acute phase proteins (APPs)** are made in the liver in response to release of proinflammatory cytokines including IL-1, IL-6, and TNF-α from monocytes and macrophages at the site of inflammation or infection. APPs have many roles including activation of complement, pathogen elimination, and modulating the immune response. During the APR, when fever is being initiated, leukocyte numbers are increasing, and proinflammatory cytokines are being released, Kupffer cells in the liver are also producing IL-6, the major stimulus for release of APPs by hepatocytes. There are several APPs which provide for different immunomodulatory functions. Positive APPs include **C-reactive protein (CRP)**, fibrinogen, D-dimer protein, and mannose-binding protein which binds to mannose on the surface of pathogens and helps to activate complement in the MBL pathway. C-reactive protein also binds to bacterial surfaces, acting to opsonize the bacteria for phagocytosis as well as activate more complement via the classical pathway.

Innate Immune Cells

The innate immune system is made up of leukocytes that have various overlapping roles in ridding the body of potential pathogens. If the body's primary borders are breached, innate immune cells are one of the next lines of defense (with nonspecific receptors for foreign invaders) to rid the body of the invader. These cells include macrophages, neutrophils, dendritic cells, eosinophils, basophils (Fig. 2.2) mast cells, and NK cells. As will be discussed, these cells release mediators (cytokines and chemokines) that

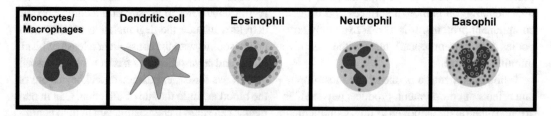

| Monocytes/ Macrophages | Dendritic cell | Eosinophil | Neutrophil | Basophil |

Fig. 2.2 Morphology of cells of the innate immune system

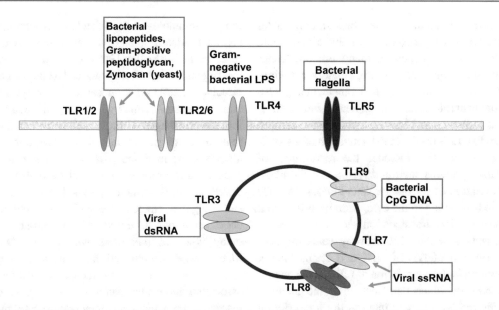

Fig. 2.3 Toll-like receptors and the ligands they recognize. Some TLRs exist on the cell surface while others are internalized

further stimulate the innate response, so the infection is controlled while the adaptive arm of the immune system is mounting a response.

Many innate immune cells use receptors to detect infection. Bacterial components, such as **lipopolysaccharide (LPS)** signal to innate immune cells that an infection is present. LPS is found in the cell walls of Gram-negative bacteria, of which many human pathogens exist. **Toll-like receptors (TLRs)**, of which there are at least ten, recognize a broad spectrum of pathogen components, and are usually found on mast cells, macrophages, and dendritic cells. TLRs are transmembrane proteins consisting of approximately 700–1100 amino acids with extracellular, transmembrane, as well as cytoplasmic domains, with the extracellular portion containing the site for ligand binding. TLRs 1, 2, 4, and 5 are expressed in the cell membrane and usually interact with extracellular components of pathogens. As is the case with LPS (recognized by TLR4), many ligands are from bacterial cell walls and membranes, including lipoteichoic acids and lipoproteins (recognized by TLR 1/2). Bacterial flagellin can be recognized by TLR5. Some TLRs (3, 7, 8, and 9) exist intracellularly

in the endosomes and lysosomes. After a pathogen has been phagocytosed, it will end up in one of these organelles to be broken down. At that point, microbial DNA and RNA are exposed and can be recognized by these internal TLRs. TLRs 3, 7, and 8 are typically responsible for recognizing viral RNA while TLR9 recognizes bacterial DNA. Figure 2.3 illustrates Toll-like receptors and their ligands.

After binding to their ligand, TLRs convert the signal to a response by the cell via a signal transduction pathway. Protein kinases which phosphorylate other proteins to activate them, are also a part of the TLR pathways. Some commonly studied messengers in the TLR pathways include IRAKs (IL-1 receptor-associated kinases) and MAPKs (mitogen-activated protein kinases). Kinases in this pathway are possible drug targets for mitigation of certain conditions in which inflammation contributes to the pathophysiology of the disease. The goal of the TLR pathway is to transcribe genes responsible for production of inflammatory mediators in response to the pathogen that was detected. The mediators, generally cytokines and chemokines, are released by the cell to activate other immune cells to help fight the infection.

The activation of the transcription factor **nuclear factor-kB (NF-kB)** plays a paramount role in the induction of many immune genes including genes for pro-inflammatory cytokines TNF-α, IL-1 and IL-6, and others that play a prominent role in immune responses. Engagement of a TLR such as TLR4 by a pathogenic component like LPS results in the activation of a signaling cascade that includes the recruitment of adapter proteins such as MyD88 and the phosphorylation of various tyrosine kinases. Inactive NF-κB is bound in the cytoplasm by IκB, which prevents its translocation to the nucleus. Activation of the TLR pathway leads to phosphorylation of IκB by IKK or I kappa kinase, resulting in the degradation of IκB and the release of NF-κB, which can now enter the nucleus. Activated NF-κB now induces the transcription of genes for proinflammatory cytokines (Fig. 2.4).

Agranular Leukocytes

Monocytes are large mononuclear cells. This cell type was discovered in the late 1800s by the famed immunologist Ilya Metchnikoff who used starfish to identify phagocytes after injury with a rose thorn. Since the 1960s, classical research has suggested that after spending 1–2 days in the circulation, inflammation causes monocytes to enter the tissues, which where they differentiate into **macrophages**. However, more recent findings have suggested that some macrophages already exist in tissues (tissue-resident macrophages), and probably arose during embryonic development. Both monocytes and macrophages can recognize, phagocytose, and destroy cellular debris, cells that have undergone apoptosis, and many types of pathogens without any help. Macrophages are covered in cell surface receptors, including TLRs, to recognize pathogen associated molecular patterns (PAMPs). Upon recognition of a pathogen, they release cytokines to signal to other cells that there is an infection present. They are also considered to be one of the three types of antigen-presenting cells that can help coordinate the innate and adaptive immune responses.

Fig. 2.4 TLR4 recognizes bacterial LPS. Activation of this signaling pathway results in translocation of the transcription factor NF-kB to the nucleus, leading to transcription of pro-inflammatory cytokines that aid in activation and recruitment of other immune cells to help fight the infection

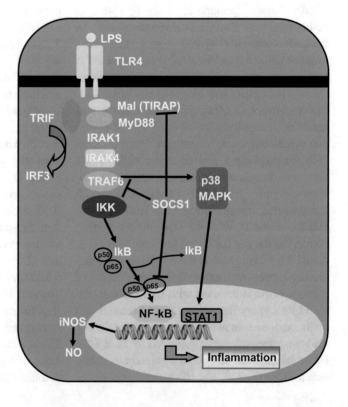

Table 2.2 Macrophage nomenclature based on tissue of residence

Tissue	Macrophage nomenclature
Bone	Osteoclast
Lung	Alveolar macrophage
CNS	Microglial cell
Liver	Kupffer cell
Connective tissue	Histiocytes
Spleen	White pulp, red pulp, marginal-zone, metallophil macrophages

Macrophages are derived from common myeloid progenitors in the bone marrow, where their development is controlled by macrophage colony-stimulating factor (M-CSF) produced by stromal cells. This growth factor drives the differentiation of progenitor cells to become monoblasts, which are committed to the monocyte lineage and eventually differentiate into macrophages in the tissues. Macrophages within tissues (both those derived from monocytes and tissue-resident macrophages) may be referred to by different names (Table 2.2).

On their surfaces, macrophages express several different receptors to help them recognize pathogens or phagocytose pathogens that have been "tagged" by other components of the immune system for removal. These include TLRs but also complement receptors and scavenger receptors whose ligands are diverse microbial proteins. In addition to the recognition of pathogens, TLRs also induce intracellular signaling that leads to macrophage activation. Complement receptors and scavenger receptors help macrophages recognize complexes targeted for phagocytosis. This binding usually results in an irreversible "capture" of the pathogen by the macrophage and results in receptor-mediated endocytosis, or engulfment of the target into a phagosome. The phagosome combines with the lysosome to form a phagolysosome wherein destructive enzymes in the membrane-bound vesicle mediate pathogen killing.

Macrophages may be activated based on stimuli produced by innate immune cells during early tissue damage or infection and thus can have different effects on the resulting physiology of the responding macrophages. Classically activated macrophages become active as a result of the cell-mediated immune response and their major function is the removal of pathogens during infection. These macrophages tend to be primed and activated by IFN-γ produced by innate or adaptive cells during the immune response and release TNF-α for enhanced microbicidal activity. NK cells are a major source of IFN-γ during the innate immune response. During the adaptive immune response, T_H1 cells helps maintain this classically activated macrophage population. Interactions between macrophages and T cells will be explored further in Chap. 3. Upon activation, macrophages release a host of pro-inflammatory cytokines, superoxide, oxygen radicals, and nitric oxide. These mediators serve to destroy the infectious organism and alert the rest of the immune system. Cytokines produced by macrophages include a number of pro-inflammatory cytokines such as IL-1, IL-6, and TNF-α, as well as those that induce that the recruitment of neutrophils (such as CXCL8) and those that activate NK cells (such as IL-12). In addition to IL-1, and IL-6, other cytokines released include IL-23 which aid in the development of IL-17-producing T_H17 cells. These cells induce the activation of neutrophils to extracellular pathogens and are also implicated in autoimmunity. While classically activated macrophages are essential for host defense against infection, their effects must be highly regulated to prevent tissue damage. In the absence of such regulation, they can become highly pathogenic as occurs during certain autoimmune disorders such as inflammatory bowel disease or rheumatoid arthritis.

Other types of macrophages can also play a large role in wound healing and are necessary for tissue repair. In doing so they are activated by both innate and adaptive mediators. An early mediator released by mast cells and basophils is the cytokine IL-4, which is produced in response to tissue injury or even fungal infection. IL-4 is also produced during the adaptive response by T_H2 cells, primarily at mucosal surfaces including the lung and intestines. IL-4 released during these responses (innate or adaptive) results in increased arginase activity in macrophages. Arginine is then converted to another amino acid (ornithine), which is a precursor of collagen and leads to production of extracellular matrix for tissue repair. While the response of wound healing macrophages is not aimed at pathogen removal, there is evidence to suggest that this subset of macrophages may play a role in anti-fungal and antiparasitic responses. Like classically-activated macrophages, a dysregulation of the matrix-building effects of wound healing macrophages may also be responsible for some of the pathological manifestations of autoimmunity.

Lastly, regulatory macrophages have anti-inflammatory activity and can be activated either innate or adaptive immune responses. These macrophages usually produce high levels of IL-10 and downregulate IL-12 and other pro-inflammatory cytokines. Later in the adaptive response, regulatory macrophages suppress the immune response and decrease inflammation.

Dendritic cells (DCs) are also derived from the myeloid lineage and are found at ports of microbial entry such as the skin, the respiratory tract, and the gastrointestinal/genitourinary (GI/GU) tracts. DCs are commonly recognized by their dendrite-like projections and are essential for innate/adaptive immune crosstalk. Myeloid DCs are central to this task, first engulfing the pathogen at the site of infection, then processing its antigens and displaying them on their cell surface for CD4 T cells to "see" on MHC II molecules in the secondary lymph nodes. When DCs themselves are infected by viruses or intracellular bacteria, processed antigens are similarly presented on the surface of MHC I molecules to CD8 T cells. This makes DCs one of the professional antigen-presenting cells (APCs). Antigens that are picked up in the blood may be transported to the spleen, while antigens captured in the respiratory, GI, or reproductive tissues are transported through a draining lymphatic vessel to the closest lymph node. At the sites of infection or antigen capture, these DCs are referred to as immature DCs (iDCs). As they migrate toward the secondary lymphoid organ, they undergo several physiologic changes that make them better equipped for their interaction with naive T cells and are referred to as mature DCs.

Like macrophages, DCs also sense pathogens and undergo activation through TLR-mediated signaling. DCs express all the TLRs except TLR9. The induction of TLR signaling activates the DC and enhances its ability to engulf and process antigen for display on MHC II. It also increases surface expression of CCR7, which is a receptor for the chemokine CCL21 expressed within secondary lymphoid organs. This induces the migration of DCs to the secondary lymphoid organ, where they can prepare to interact with naïve T cells. Specific DC/T cell interactions will be elaborated on in Chap. 3.

Granular Leukocytes

Neutrophils are one of the major pathogen-fighting leukocytes recruited to the site of infection. They have a short lifespan of approximately 8–12 h in the circulation and 1–2 days in the tissue. They are formed in the bone marrow in response to GM-CSF and are generally found circulating in the bloodstream until they are called to a site of infection. Neutrophils account for 50–70% of circulating leukocytes, and as such much of the bone marrow is dedicated to their development. Neutrophil count is normally defined as Absolute Neutrophil Count (ANC) which is the portion of the total white blood cell count that is made up of neutrophils. It is defined as:

$$\frac{[\% \text{ of mature neutrophils} + \% \text{ of almost mature neutrophils (bands)}] \times \text{total WBC count}}{100}$$

A normal ANC is approximately 1500–8000/mm³. A level less than 1000 is referred to as neutropenia. A higher than normal level is considered neutrophilia, which is most often indicative of infection, but can also occur as a result of any type of acute inflammation.

Two hematopoietic growth factors that are essential for neutrophil function are granulocyte colony stimulating factor (G-CSF) and granulocyte-macrophage colony stimulating factor (GM-CSF). G-CSF is a glycoprotein which acts on granulocyte precursors in the bone marrow to produce differentiated granulocytes and release them into the bloodstream. G-CSF can also enhance neutrophil function and stimulate the release of proinflammatory cytokines by neutrophils such as TNF-α. In contrast, GM-CSF can recruit and enhance the functions of both neutrophils and monocytes. Due to their ability to mobilize circulating neutrophils, these factors are often used therapeutically in immunosuppressed patients, most notably those who are neutropenic from undergoing chemotherapy.

To get to the site of infection, neutrophils must squeeze themselves out of the bloodstream, a process called diapedesis. The small cytokine/chemokine, CXCL8 (IL-8) is a potent chemoattractant molecule that helps call neutrophils from the circulation, through the tissue, and to the site of inflammation or injury. CXCL8 is a chemokine which binds to chemokine receptors CXCR1 and CXCR2, both of which are expressed on neutrophils. These receptors may also be expressed on epithelial and endothelial cells, as well as fibroblasts and neurons, but one of the main roles of CXCL8 is neutrophil recruitment.

Neutrophils are activated by LPS, TNF, chemokines, and growth factors. Once they reach the sites of infection, the vast repertoire of pattern recognition receptors expressed by neutrophils allow them to recognize various types of microbes and phagocytose opsonized pathogens. C-type lectin receptors like Dectin-1 recognize fungal β-glucan. The cytosolic microbial sensors NOD1 and NOD2 can recognize peptidoglycan molecules of Gram-negative and Gram-positive bacteria, respectively. Lastly, neutrophils also express a wide array of Toll-like receptors, including TLRs 1, 2, 4, 5, 6, 8, and 10 and complement receptors.

At the site of infection, neutrophils help macrophages in cleaning up the infection by recognizing, phagocytosing, and killing pathogens. The destruction of pathogens by neutrophils occurs within the phagolysosome. This internal microbial killing is aided by hydrogen peroxide, as well as several enzymes and antimicrobial peptides, which kill the ingested bacteria. When pathogens are engulfed into the phagosome, the activity of enzymes such as NADPH oxidase produces superoxide radicals that are rapidly converted to hydrogen peroxide. This raises the pH of the phagosome to 7.8–8.0, activating antimicrobial peptides and other enzymes that attack the engulfed pathogen. After about 10–15 min, the pH of the phagosome returns to 7.0, inducing the formation of the phagolysosome. Here the pathogen is completely degraded by acid hydrolases. The release of hydrogen peroxide and other superoxide radicals is referred to as the respiratory burst and has the potential to harm neighboring cells. Enzymes that inactive these molecules such as catalase are also produced during the respiratory burst and limit the damage to host cells.

The successful destruction of the pathogen through the release of granular contents results in the death of the neutrophil and its phagocytosis by nearby macrophages. In addition to the above-mentioned method of pathogen destruction, neutrophils can also kill pathogens during the process of dying themselves. This process called netosis produces neutrophil extracellular traps (NETs) which consists of nuclear contents, defensins, and other proteins that can trap and destroy pathogens.

Basophils and Mast cells Basophils, like the other leukocytes, are produced in the bone marrow and circulate in the peripheral blood. During a parasitic infection, they can be recruited to tissues, where they can be activated to release granular contents and various cytokines. Basophils make up less than approximately 1–2% of circulating leukocytes. They have a bilobed nucleus and contain many large cytoplasmic granules. These contain several preformed mediators including heparin and the vasodilator histamine. Basophils share many similarities and functional characteristics with their tissue-resident counterparts, the mast cells. They are the only circulating leukocytes that contain histamine, which is rapidly released when they are activated. In addition, they also release a number of cytokines including IL-4, IL-13 and GM-CSF and synthesize lipid mediators including the prostaglandins and leukotrienes as well as platelet activating factor. They also express receptors for various cytokines and chemokines, and Fc receptors for antibodies such as IgE.

In contrast to basophils, mast cells are tissue-resident immune cells that have a sentinel role in immune function and protect the host from parasitic infections; their precursors come from the bone marrow and circulate in the blood until they *home* to the tissues to mature, usually the blood vessels or epithelial surfaces. Mast cells are approximately 20 μm in diameter and contain an abundance of cytoplasmic granules compared to basophils. These contain a number of mediators including histamine, tryptases, heparin, and TNF-α among others. When activated, mast cells are also induced to release numerous cytokines and synthesize lipid mediators such as leukotrienes and prostaglandins.

Both mast cells and basophils constitutively express the high affinity receptor for IgE antibodies, FcεRI. During a parasitic infection, large amounts of parasite-specific IgE are made which bind the receptor on mast cells and basophils. When parasitic antigens bind these IgE molecules, they induce aggregation of the receptor, which induces degranulation of the mast cells and a FcεRI-mediated signaling cascade. This results in the release of preformed mediators such as TNFα, histamine, and proteoglycans and the *de novo* synthesis of cytokines, lipid mediators, and platelet activating factor. In addition to IgE-mediated activation, mast cells and basophils can also be activated via other means including TLRs. The binding of TLR3 on mast cells by dsRNA induces the release of IFN-γ.

Both mast cells and basophils are pathologic during the development of allergic reactions, including allergic rhinitis, urticaria, asthma, and anaphylaxis. Mast cells can also contribute to other conditions such as rheumatoid arthritis, osteoporosis, and cancers.

Eosinophils Like mast cells and basophils, eosinophils are also involved in host defense against parasitic worm infections. They are also involved in the pathogenesis of conditions such as allergic asthma. Eosinophils have a bilobed nucleus and release two main types of granules—specific granules and primary granules. The specific granules contain major basic protein,

eosinophil peroxidase, eosinophil cationic protein, and eosinophil-derived neurotoxin.

The development of eosinophils is mediated by cytokines such as IL-5, IL-3, and GM-CSF. IL-5 released at the site of helminth infection promotes the generation and differentiation of eosinophils from bone marrow progenitors, after which they enter the circulation and home to the tissues. Many eosinophils that are located in the tissues exist in the gastrointestinal tract mucosal surfaces during homeostasis, and at T_H2-dominated sites of inflammation where IL-4 and IL-13 are released. Here, the upregulation of eotaxin and cell adhesion molecules by various immune cells induces the recruitment of eosinophils. On their surfaces, eosinophils express Fc receptors for antibodies including IgE, IgA, and IgG. The receptor for IgE is induced during infection. Eosinophils also express other receptors including complement receptors, cytokine receptors, and chemokine receptors. They also express adhesion molecules, leukotriene and prostaglandin receptors, and TLRs 7 and 8. Upon activation by the cross-linking of Fc receptors, eosinophils release pro-inflammatory mediators including granule-stored cationic proteins, newly-synthesized eicosanoids, and cytokines. While a normal level of eosinophils in the peripheral blood is up to $500/mm^3$, an elevated level (eosinophilia) may indicate atopic asthma (usually mild eosinophilia in blood), a drug reaction, or helminth infection. With atopic asthma, eosinophilia is more likely to be found in nasal secretions, sputum, or the bronchoalveolar lavage (BAL).

Natural Killer (NK) cells play a prominent role in the initiation and maintenance of antiviral immunity. They are also extremely effective against cancerous cells. Under the microscope, NK cells look like T and B cells, deriving from the common lymphoid progenitor and the lymphoid lineage. They are a highly diverse cell type consisting of heterogeneous subsets that can carry out cytotoxic function or release inflammatory cytokines. In humans they are identified on the basis of the adhesion molecule CD56, as well as other NK cell markers. Similarly, in mice they can be identified using markers such as NK1.1

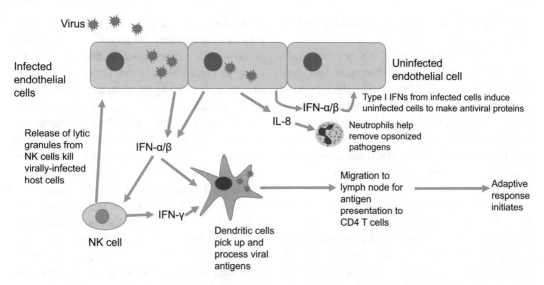

Virus

Infected endothelial cells

Uninfected endothelial cell

IFN-α/β

Type I IFNs from infected cells induce uninfected cells to make antiviral proteins

IL-8

Neutrophils help remove opsonized pathogens

Release of lytic granules from NK cells kill virally-infected host cells

IFN-α/β

Migration to lymph node for antigen presentation to CD4 T cells

Adaptive response initiates

IFN-γ

NK cell

Dendritic cells pick up and process viral antigens

Fig. 2.5 Antiviral immunity and the roles of NK cells. Host cells infected with a virus begin releasing Type I IFNs (IFN-αβ) which signal to neighboring uninfected cells to begin making antiviral proteins. Type I IFNs also activate NK cells to release lytic granules which will kill virally-infected cells. This also stimulates NK cells to release IFN-γ to initiate the adaptive response by promoting DC processing of viral antigen for presentation to CD4 T cells

and DX5. These populations can be further divided into those that perform cytotoxic activity (CD56 dim) and those that release cytokines (CD56 bright). They are distinguished from T cells and other invariant T cells such as NKT cells based on the absence of CD3.

NK cells play a vital role in the induction of immune responses to viruses and tumors. Their activation and cytotoxic functions are governed by an intricate balance between the functions of various surface receptors that promote either activation or inhibition of cell function. These receptors are stochastically expressed on various cell subsets and include inhibitory receptors such as the lectin CD94-NKG2 and KIR receptors and activating receptors such as NKG2D. The inhibitory receptors bind HLA-E molecules on the surface of endogenous cells which prevents the activation of NK cells. Infection or other inflammatory conditions can induce loss of MHC class I and induction of stress proteins such as MICA and MICB. This results in disengagement of the inhibitory MHC I receptor and engagement of activating receptors such as NKG2D with its ligand (MICA/B), inducing activation and NK cell-mediated cytotoxicity.

Activation of NK cells can occur in response to several stimuli, predominantly the release of type I interferons by infected cells (Fig. 2.5). Soon after viral entry, both infected cells and neighboring epithelial cells produce large amounts of IFN-α and IFN-β. In addition, plasmacytoid dendritic cells, also called interferon producing cells, are potent producers of type I interferons. The release of type I interferons results in the induction of the interferon response, leading to resistance to viral infection and the activation of NK cells. This results in the killing of infected cells by activated NK cells. In addition to type I interferons, NK cells can also be activated via cross-talk with macrophages and DCs. These cells produce cytokines such as IL-12 and IL-15, which can promote their activation and function.

Activated NK cells produce large amounts of IFN-γ. This cytokine not only has the ability to promote anti-viral effects, but also has other effects on the immune system such as the activation of the immunoproteasome and the upregulation of MHC II on APCs. In addition, NK cells are known to produce other cytokines including TNF-α and type II cytokines such as IL-13 and IL-5.

The cytotoxic functions of NK cells are mediated via the induction of caspases and programmed cell death. They involve the release of perforin and granzymes from granular contents. While perforin and other proteins such as granulysin poke holes into the target cell membrane, granzymes initiate proteolytic cleavage reactions resulting in the induction of apoptosis and death of the infected cell.

NK cells can also be activated to perform antibody dependent cellular cytotoxicity or ADCC. This occurs when antigen-specific IgG antibodies engage the FcγRIII or CD16 receptor on NK cells, inducing their activation. Activated NK cells then kill target cells expressing the antigen. ADCC is a common mechanism of action of many therapeutic drugs such as rituximab.

Inflammation

Inflammation is the characteristic response to infection (non-self) or the presence of danger. The process of immunity begins when normal host defenses are breached and when the immune system senses a threat to the host. This can occur as a result of pathogen sensing by TLRs or the production of alarmin cytokines by epithelial and other sentinel cells indicating the presence of injury or danger. The type of immune response that is initiated ultimately depends on the type of pathogen and the offended target tissue. Various strategies are employed by the immune system depending on whether the pathogen is extracellular or intracellular, or depending on the type of injury or danger to tissue. The initial response is targeted towards the presence of molecular patterns such as LPS, while the latter adaptive response is more specific and antigenic in nature. Extracellular offenders include extracellular bacteria, some fungi, virions in the extracellular space and allergens. Intracellular offenders include viruses, intracellular bacteria and some parasites.

A ubiquitous initial response to the entry of extracellular bacteria is the induction of the complement system. As described earlier, this complex system involves the activation of a number of heat-labile serine proteases that are constitutively produced by the liver. These are classified as C1-C9, depending on when they were discovered and the functions they perform. Several complement proteins can be further cleaved into smaller components by enzymes referred to as convertases. The most important complement component is C3. This protein is normally present in the inactive state, but in the presence of infection or on engagement of complement components by ligands such as mannose-binding protein, C-reactive protein (CRP) or antibody, it can be hydrolyzed or cleaved into a larger C3b molecule and a smaller C3a molecule. C3b tags the extracellular pathogen, initiating the process of complement fixation. In the case of some bacteria such as *Neisseria*, the deposition of C3b on the bacterial surface can lead to further events in the complement cascade, resulting in the cleavage of C5 and the formation of the **membrane attack complex (MAC)**, which perforates pathogen cell membranes and induces their lysis. Pathogen-bound C3b itself is detected by complement receptors on cells such as macrophages, resulting in the induction of phagocytosis. Other complement components, such as C3a and C5a induce the recruitment of neutrophils and induce mast cell and basophil activation. Thus, activation of complement has the net effect of inducing phagocyte recruitment, opsonizing macrophages and neutrophils for phagocytosis, and lysing bacterial cell membranes. All of these result in death of the pathogen.

In addition to complement activation, several other non-specific mechanisms may also contribute to innate defense including the production of antimicrobial peptides such as defensins, the activation of the kinin system and the production of α-macroglobulins.

The induction of infection or the presence of injury also results in the secretion of a number of cytokines and immune mediators by injured cells. Depending on the type of injury or infection, cells such as epithelial cells can release a vast number of mediators including cytokines such as TNF-α, IL-33, IL-25, thymic stromal lymphopoietin

(TSLP) and type I interferons, various chemokines, and antimicrobial peptides. This has the net effect of recruiting and activating various innate cells such as macrophages, dendritic cells, innate lymphoid cells, mast cells, and NK cells.

Pathogen sensing by macrophages using either scavenger receptors or the TLRs results in the activation of NF-κB, and the induction of genes for various cytokines. Some of the first cytokines to be produced by macrophages are the proinflammatory cytokines TNF-α, IL-1 and IL-6. TNF-α is a potent cytokine that has pleiotropic effects on the immune system. It induces vasodilation increasing the flow of blood within blood vessels and causes vascular permeability, allowing cells and molecules to leak out of blood vessels. It also promotes the expression of adhesion molecules on blood vessels to enable leukocyte migration. Mast cells in tissues can also be activated resulting in the production of histamine which can also contribute to vasodilation.

IL-1 and IL-6 are pyrogenic and raise the body temperature, making it difficult for pathogens to survive. IL-6 also acts on hepatic cells inducing the acute phase response, by leading to the increased production of the acute phase proteins MBP and CRP. These acute phase proteins further act to activate the lectin and the classical pathways of the complement cascade.

In addition to these cytokines, macrophages also produce the chemokine CXCL8, which is a chemotactic migratory factor for neutrophils, drawing in neutrophils from blood vessels. Neutrophils act as first responders, quickly phagocytosing bacteria and producing cytokines. The phagocytic response is dependent on the release of several antibacterial substances in neutrophil granules and the induction of a respiratory burst, resulting in the release of superoxides that damage the bacteria. Eventually, acid hydrolases within the neutrophil granules completely digest the bacteria, leading to death of the neutrophil and the formation of pus.

Similarly, when infection occurs due to intracellular pathogens such as intracellular bacteria or viral infection, macrophages can produce additional cytokines such as IL-12. The concomitant production of type I interferons by virally infected cells has the net effect of activating NK cells and inducing their recruitment to the infected tissue.

The series of physiologic events give rise to the four main hallmarks of inflammation described since ancient times which include redness (rubor), pain (dolor), heat (calor), and swelling (tumor). Vasodilation results in increased blood volume contributing to redness; vascular permeability leads to leakage of blood vessel constituents such as cells and molecules into tissues resulting in swelling or edema; the swelling has the effect of pinching on associated nerves resulting in pain; and the cumulative effects of vasodilation and cytokine function make the inflamed area warm to touch.

Innate Immune Deficiencies

Genetic mutations leading to dysfunction in one or more components in the innate immune system can often manifest in an immunodeficiency disorder characterized by frequent and recurrent infections. Some of these disorders are outlined in Table 2.3.

Therapeutic Inhibitors Which Target the Innate Immune Response

Phagocyte recruitment

Targeting **cell adhesion molecules (CAMs)** to reduce leukocyte recruitment may be an effective method of reducing inflammation in certain disease states in which leukocyte migration contributes to inflammation. CAMs allow cells to bind and interact with their extracellular environment, including other cells. Certain CAMs allow leukocytes to migrate out of general circulation, "roll" along the surface of blood vessels, and permeate through tissue to reach tissues where they contribute to inflammation and injury (Fig. 2.6). Leukocytes expressing a specific CAM, **α₄β₇ integrin**, have been implicated in the

Table 2.3 Primary immunodeficiencies affecting the innate immune system

Disease	Deficiency	Mutation	Clinical manifestations
Chronic granulomatous disease	Phagocytes unable to produce reactive oxygen species for intracellular killing of microorganisms	Mutation in phagocyte oxidase enzyme (cytochrome b558)	Formation of granulomas, recurrent infections including pneumonia, skin abscesses
NK cell deficiency	Classic—absence of NK cells within peripheral blood lymphocytes Functional—NK cells are present but dysfunctional	Classic—mutations in GATA2, MCM4 Functional—mutation in CD16	Susceptibility to viruses such as VZV, EBV, HSV, HPV, and CMV
Leukocyte adhesion deficiency (LAD)	LAD1—deficient β2 integrin expression resulting in defective leukocyte adhesion LAD2—deficient expression of ligands for E- and P-selectins, decreasing leukocyte migration into tissues LAD3—defective adhesive function of integrins on leukocytes and platelets	LAD1—mutation in β chain of β2 integrin LAD2—mutation in sialyl-Lewis X component of selectin ligands LAD3—mutation in Kindlin 3 protein needed for integrin activation	LAD1—recurrent bacterial and fungal skin infections, gingivitis, periodontitis, slow wound healing LAD2—recurrent bacterial infections, pneumonia, otitis media, cellulitis, periodontitis LAD3—recurrent bacterial and fungal infections, increased bleeding tendency
Complement deficiency	C3—defective complement cascade activation C2,C4—defective activation of classical pathway, inability to clear immune complexes	C3 gene mutation C2 or C4 gene mutation	C3—recurrent bacterial infections (particularly gram-negative), sinusitis, tonsillitis, otitis media C2,C4—increased risk of infection, pneumonia, meningitis, sepsis Deficiency in complement may also lead to a lupus-like conditions due to inability to clear immune complexes
Chédiak-Higashi syndrome	Defective phagolysosome formation in neutrophils, macrophages, and dendritic cells. Defective NK cell granules	Mutation in lysosomal trafficking regulatory protein (CHS1)	Susceptibility to infection, particularly by Staphylococci and Streptococci. Associated with oculocutaneous albinism

pathogenesis of inflammatory bowel diseases such as ulcerative colitis and Crohn's disease. Cells expressing $\alpha_4\beta_7$ integrin have been shown to exhibit preferential binding to endothelial surfaces of the GI tract.

Vedolizumab (Entyvio®) is a relatively new antibody that targets the $\alpha_4\beta_7$ integrin. It inhibits leukocyte binding to the GI tract, significantly decreases the symptoms of inflammatory bowel disease (IBD) and is approved for adult ulcerative colitis and Crohn's disease. Adverse effects of vedolizumab include infusion-related reactions, nasopharyngitis, headache, arthralgia, and upper respiratory tract infection.

Natalizumab (Tysabri®) is another humanized monoclonal antibody with a similar mechanism of action in that it is an $\alpha_4\beta_1$ integrin inhibitor used for Crohn's disease and multiple sclerosis. The most common adverse effects include headache, pain in the arms and legs, abdominal pain, fatigue, joint pain, vaginitis, urinary tract infection, and lung infection. Taking natalizumab increases a patient's risk of developing a rare but severe brain infection called progressive multifocal leukencephalopathy (PML). The risk increases with long-term use (greater than 2 years), infection with John Cunningham (JC) virus, or taking other immunosuppressant drugs before beginning natalizumab. Patients should be tested periodically for JC virus, and because of the PML risk, natalizumab is only distributed through the TOUCH®

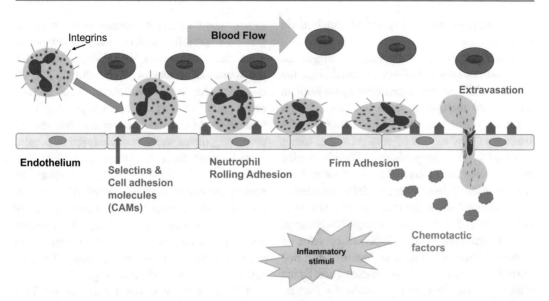

Fig. 2.6 Leukocyte recruitment to the site of inflammation is initiated by stimuli at the site of infection, i.e. cytokines and chemotactic factors. Neighboring endothelial cells begin expressing selections and adhesion molecules which bind to integrins on the surface of neutrophils, causing them to slow down and "stick" to the CAM-expressing endothelial cells. As neutrophils "roll" they adhere to the endothelium more firmly and extravasate out of the blood vessel into the inflamed tissue where they sense chemokines and other inflammatory mediators

prescribing program to help patients understand the risk of PML and if necessary, diagnose it earlier if it occurs.

Table 2.4 Cytokine families

Hematopoietin family	TNF family	IFN family
EPO, IL-2, IL-3, IL-4, IL-6, G-CSF, GM-CSF	TNF-α, TNF-β, FasL	IFN-α, IFN-β, IFN-γ

Pro-inflammatory Cytokines

While it is important to understand the pivotal roles innate immune cells play in the immune response, it is also important to know that many of their activities are mediated by cell to cell communication through cytokines. Thus, cytokines represent an important therapeutic target in several inflammatory diseases, in which in the case of inappropriate inflammation, one can intervene with pharmacotherapy in an effort to "turn off" or suppress intercellular crosstalk to reduce symptoms.

Cytokines are small proteins that are released in response to a stimulus and induce responses by binding to their specific receptor. There are three main families of cytokines, the larger families being the Hematopoietin and TNF families, as well as the smaller IFN family (Table 2.4).

The three main pyrogenic (fever-inducing) cytokines are **IL-1, TNF-α,** and **IL-6**. Acting on the hypothalamus to increase the temperature of the body, fever allows for decreased viral and bacterial replication, increased antigen processing, and a more efficient adaptive immune response. The effects of these pyrogenic cytokines are outlined in Fig. 2.7.

TNF Inhibition

Tumor Necrosis Factor-α (TNF-α) was first described in 1975 by the laboratory of Dr. Lloyd Old at the Sloan Kettering Memorial Cancer Center in New York. Dr. Old's team observed that a cytotoxic factor produced during infection with endotoxins could cause the necrosis of tumors. Previously in 1968 Gale Granger from the University of California and Nancy Ruddle from Yale University had described another TNF family member, which they called lymphotoxin (TNF-β).

The hypothesis that infections can trigger the regression of tumors had been around since the late nineteenth century, when the surgeon William Coley used therapeutic dead bacteria (Coley's toxins) to treat sarcomas. This treatment was based on a few reports of erysipelas and tumor regression. Not surprisingly, Coley's toxins induced fever and chills and patients but without true infection. Subsequently, in 1943, scientists at the National Cancer Institute isolated lipopolysaccharide (LPS) from Gram-negative bacteria, and in turn used it to induce the necrosis of tumors. Subsequent research demonstrated that animals injected with LPS produced mediators which they considered to be anti-tumor factors, and accordingly named these mediators "tumor necrosis factor."

Macrophages are the main cell type that can secrete TNF, but it can also be produced by neutrophils, NK cells, mast cells, eosinophils, and CD4 T cells. TNF-α is an endogenous pyrogen, meaning it acts on the hypothalamus to induce fever to slow down pathogen replication in the body. It can also induce apoptosis through death receptor TNFR1. As a signal transducer, TNF activates MAPK pathways which can result in cellular differentiation and proliferation, as well

as activates transcription factor NF-κB which is generally proinflammatory and anti-apoptotic. Thus, the activation of NF-κB often masks the pro-apoptotic effects of TNF through TNFR1 signaling. As a chemoattractant, TNF recruits neutrophils not only by encouraging the bone marrow to release new neutrophils, but also by promoting the expression of adhesion molecules on the endothelium, and acting as a direct chemoattractant. In the liver, it can stimulate the acute phase response and the release of C-reactive protein and complement for opsonization of bacteria. In macrophages, it helps to stimulate phagocytosis and PGE2. In other tissues, it can promote insulin resistance. Its many effects on various tissues are outlined in Fig. 2.7.

TNF-α can exist in two forms: soluble TNF and transmembrane TNF, with macrophages being the biggest producers. Two receptors exist which have different outcomes upon receptor ligation. TNF receptor 1 (TNFR1) is widely expressed on most cell types (with the exception of erythrocytes) and as mentioned, plays a role in apoptosis and induction of acute inflammation. It binds both soluble and transmembrane TNF. With regard to TNFR2, several studies have suggested that signaling through the TNFR2 mediates cell survival. TNF-α plays a variety of roles in the immune response. It has been reported in humans

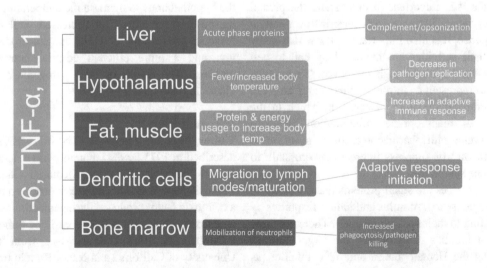

Fig. 2.7 Effects of pyrogenic cytokines IL-1, IL-6, and TNF-α on tissues

that after immune encounter with Gram-negative LPS, TNF becomes elevated in the blood 60–90 min later, and is associated with fever and flu-like symptoms including chills and myalgia. TNF-β is very similar to TNF-α in the response it elicits, binds to the same receptor, and has 30% homology. The main difference is that TNFβ is produced primarily by T cells and is thus often referred to as lymphotoxin.

The first TNF inhibitor biologic drugs were approved by the FDA in 1998 for rheumatoid arthritis (RA) and Crohn's disease. Most of the TNF inhibitors are monoclonal antibodies (except for the etanercept fusion protein) and have indications for gastroenterological, rheumatological, and dermatological conditions (Table 2.5). Nomenclature of monoclonal antibodies will be further described in Chap. 3.

Etanercept (Enbrel®) is a fusion protein (not an antibody) that binds to TNF in both its alpha and beta forms. TNFβ is also known as lymphotoxin-alpha (LT-α). Etanercept is indicated for the treatment of RA, polyarticular juvenile idiopathic arthritis (JIA), plaque psoriasis, psoriatic arthritis, and ankylosing spondylitis. Etanercept is given as a subcutaneous injection.

Infliximab (Remicade®) is a human-mouse chimeric IgG monoclonal antibody with Human Fc region and murine variable regions. Due to this, it is generally considered to be more immunogenic than the other anti-TNF biologics. It can neutralize all forms of TNF-α (including extracellular, transmembrane, and receptor-bound TNF). Infliximab has several indications including Crohn's disease, ulcerative colitis, RA, psoriatic arthritis, ankylosing spondylitis, and plaque psoriasis. Unlike the other TNF inhibitors, infliximab is usually given in the form of IV infusion.

Adalimumab (Humira®) gets its name from being a "Human Monoclonal Antibody in Rheumatoid Arthritis". Thus, is a fully human IgG antibody targeting TNF. Besides its indication for RA, adalimumab is also used to treat juvenile idiopathic arthritis, psoriatic arthritis, ankylosing spondylitis, Crohn's disease, ulcerative colitis, plaque psoriasis, hidradenitis suppurativa, and uveitis. Adalimumab is given as a subcutaneous injection.

Certolizumab pegol (Cimzia®) is a pegylated Fab fragment of a humanized anti-TNF monoclonal antibody and is indicated for moderate to severe RA, psoriatic arthritis, active ankylosing spondylitis, and Crohn's disease. Unlike the other anti-TNF biologics, certolizumab does not have an Fc region. Its pegylation on the Fab fragment, however, increases its bioavailability, extends its half-life, and decreases its dosing frequency. Certolizumab is given as a subcutaneous injection.

Golimumab (Simponi®), like adalimumab is a fully human monoclonal antibody used for

Table 2.5 Clinical uses of approved TNF-inhibitors

	Etanercept	Infliximab	Adalimumab	Certolizumab	Golimumab
Gastroenterology					
Crohn's disease		✓	✓	✓	
Ulcerative colitis		✓	✓		✓
Rheumatology					
Rheumatoid arthritis	✓	✓	✓	✓	✓
Psoriatic arthritis	✓	✓	✓	✓	✓
Ankylosing spondylitis	✓	✓	✓	✓	✓
Juvenile idiopathic arthritis	✓		✓		
Dermatology					
Plaque psoriasis	✓	✓	✓		
Hidradenitis suppurativa			✓		
Opthamology					
Uveitis			✓		

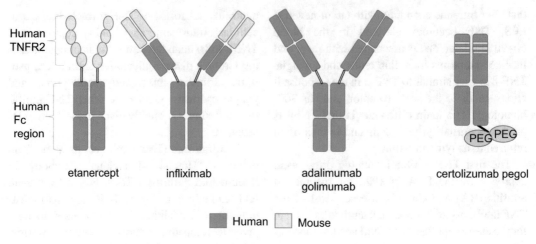

Fig. 2.8 Antibody structures of current TNF-α inhibitors

moderate to severe RA, psoriatic arthritis, active ankylosing spondylitis, and moderate to severe ulcerative colitis. Like most of the other TNF inhibitors, golimumab is also given as a subcutaneous injection. Another form of golimumab, **Simponi Aria®** is given via IV infusion.

The structures of the TNF inhibitors can be compared in Fig. 2.8.

There are, however, several potential problems with TNF inhibitors, depending on the patient. One of the most common is increased risk of infection, particularly from intracellular pathogens. This is why the TNF inhibitors should not be started without first completing a tuberculin skin test to rule out latent tuberculosis. Increased risk of malignancy is also present while on one of these drugs. Other possible adverse events include hypersensitivity reactions, worsening of congestive heart failure or new onset of CHF, Hepatitis B reactivation, neurological reactions, and pancytopenia or anemia. Other possible issues with the TNF inhibitors include:

- Primary non-response in approximately 25–50% of patients
- Loss of response in some patients
- Incomplete pain relief despite an indicated decrease in inflammation
- Incomplete clinical response
- High cost

IL-1 Inhibition

The **interleukin-1 (IL-1)** family is a group of pro-inflammatory cytokines involved in the pathogenesis of many inflammatory diseases. Thus, the IL-1 family represents a potential therapeutic target. There are three forms of IL-1 that are known to exist: IL-1α, IL-1β, and IL-1Ra. IL-1 receptor antagonist (IL-1Ra) is a natural antagonist for IL-1 and can be produced synthetically to be used as a therapy. One of these is **anakinra (Kineret®)** which is a recombinant IL-1 receptor antagonist that competitively inhibits IL-1, specifically IL-1α and IL-1β, and is used for the treatment of RA in patients who have failed one or more disease modifying antirheumatic drugs (DMARDs). It is also approved for the treatment of Neonatal Onset Multisystem Inflammatory Disease (NOMID), a type of Cryopyrin Associated Periodic Syndromes (CAPS). RA patients who take anakinra experience a delayed progression of their physical symptoms, and those with NOMID experience improvement in symptoms and reduction in SAA and CRP levels.

Like TNF-α, IL-1β is an endogenous pyrogen and is mainly released by monocytes and macrophages, but also NK cells, dendritic cells, and epithelial cells early in the immune response. As mentioned earlier, the release of IL-1β and other endogenous pyrogens stimulates the release of APPs from the liver and acts on the hypothalamus to induce fever. It can also act as as a chemoattractant for granulocytes, and in mast cells it can induce histamine release, contributing to inflammation at the site of inflammation.

Some biologics have been designed to target IL-1 itself. **Rilonacept (Arcalyst®)** is a dimeric fusion protein that binds to and inhibits the actions of IL-1β and is approved for the treatment of CAPS, a group of rare, inherited autoinflammatory diseases in which IL-1β is overproduced. IL-1β is a highly pro-inflammatory member of the IL-1 family. Rilonacept decreases the severity of symptoms associated with CAPS, and the levels of Serum Amyloid A (SAA) and C-Reactive Protein (CRP) which are indicators of inflammation that are generally elevated in patients with CAPS. **Canakinumab (Ilaris®)** is another IL-1β inhibitor and is used to treat Systemic Juvenile Idiopathic Arthritis (SJIA), and a number of Periodic Fever Syndromes. Periodic Fever Syndrome is a group of autoinflammatory diseases characterized by cyclical fevers, which includes CAPS. Canakinumab is a human monoclonal IL-1β antibody that binds to and neutralizes IL-1β, which is overproduced in Periodic Fever Syndromes and SJIA. It also decreases CRP and SAA levels and improves symptoms of both of these conditions. In addition to increased risk of infection, the IL-1 inhibitors seem to be generally well-tolerated with the most common adverse effect being injection site reaction.

IL-6 Inhibition

As with TNF and IL-1, **IL-6** is also an endogenous pyrogen and a pleiotropic cytokine with roles that can include both pro- and anti-inflammatory. As a pyrogen it acts on the nervous system to induce fever, as well as the liver to release acute phase proteins. Because IL-6 which is released by T cells and macrophages in response to infection and trauma also plays an important role in inflammation, studies have demonstrated that anti-IL-6 treatments, particularly in RA, are also efficacious. IL-6 transmits its pro-inflammatory signal through a soluble IL-6 receptor and a transmembrane protein called gp130 (CD130) which is ubiquitously expressed

in all cells. When IL-6 binds to its receptor, gp130 dimerizes, leading to activation of JAK family kinases. This is known as trans signaling. These kinases will phosphorylate and activate STAT transcription factors, leading to the transcription of several more cytokines. This can lead to recruitment of monocytes to the site of inflammation, increased adhesion molecule expression on endothelial cells, as well as promotion of T_H17 cells. The anti-inflammatory effects of IL-6 tend to occur through classical signaling at the IL-6 receptor, which is only expressed on macrophages, neutrophils, hepatocytes, and some T-lymphocytes. It is thought that this type of signaling inhibits endothelial cell apoptosis and promotes intestinal epithelial cell proliferation.

Tocilizumab (Actemra®) is a humanized anti-IL-6 monoclonal antibody that exerts its effects via inhibition of the IL-6 receptor (Fig. 2.9), which can be both membrane-bound and soluble. Tocilizumab is currently used for the treatment of severe RA.

Sarilumab (Kevzara®) is a recently approved human monoclonal antibody targeting the IL-6 receptor. Like tocilizumab, sarilumab was also approved for treatment of RA.

Siltuximab (Sylvant®) is a chimeric monoclonal antibody that binds to IL-6 itself (Fig. 2.9) and is currently approved for the treatment of Multicentric Castleman's disease, a rare group of lymphoproliferative disorders characterized by excessive release of proinflammatory cytokines including IL-6. Siltuximab has shown some ability to promote tumor cell apoptosis and may be recommended as a cancer treatment.

The main adverse effects associated with the IL-6 inhibitors include increased risk of infection, increase in liver enzymes, neutropenia, infusion-related reactions, and perforation in the stomach or intestines. Several other IL-6 inhibitors, including olokizumab, and clazakizumab are currently undergoing clinical trials for RA and renal transplant rejection, respectively.

IL-12/IL-23 Inhibition

IL-12 is a heterodimeric cytokine known as p70 (made up of p35 and p40 subunits) produced mainly by antigen presenting cells, (B cells,

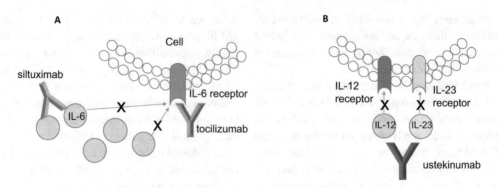

Fig. 2.9 Mechanisms of action of IL-6 and IL-12/23 monoclonal antibodies. (**a**) While tocilizumab binds to IL-6 receptor, siltuximab is able to bind to circulating IL-6. Both prevent IL-6 from binding to its receptor, thereby suppressing its anti-inflammatory effect. (**b**) Ustekinumab binds to the p40 subunit found on both IL-12 and IL-23, preventing both from binding to their receptors

macrophages, and dendritic cells) usually in response to TLR recognition of intracellular pathogens. While IL-12 may induce production of other cytokines, including IFN-γ and TNF-α from NK cells and T cells, it can also act to enhance the activity of these cells as well as act as a growth factor. Early in infection, IL-12 aids in activating phagocytes. Later in the immune response, IL-12 acts to bridge the innate response to the antigen-specific adaptive response, specifically enhancing the cytotoxic activities of NK and CD8 T cells. To promote adaptive immunity, IL-12 induces IFN-γ in favor of T_H1 cell differentiation as well as cytotoxic T cell generation. IL-12 is also thought to be anti-angiogenic in that it upregulates the chemokine CXCL10 which inhibits new blood vessel formation in tumors. Because it activates CD8 T cells, it may also enhance CD8 T cell-induced apoptosis of certain tumor cells. Thus, IL-12 may have an important anticancer role. A related cytokine, **IL-23** is similar to IL-12 in that it also uses the IL-12 p40 subunit in its signaling. Like IL-12, IL-23 also induces IFN-γ and activates T cells. IL-23 may also act to enhance IL-10 release and synthesis of IL-17.

Ustekinumab (Stelara®) is an anti-IL-12 monoclonal antibody approved for the treatment of psoriatic arthritis. Ustekinumab is a human antibody which binds to the p40 subunit of cytokines IL-12 and IL-23, preventing them from

binding to their receptors (Fig. 2.9). The most common adverse effects include injection site reactions, cold symptoms, headache, fatigue, skin rash, and itching.

Type I Interferons

Interferons (IFN) play a role in antiviral immunity. For example, once a cell is infected with a virus, it begins releasing IFNs-α and -β. Since viruses are intracellular pathogens, they are recognized by several different internalized pattern recognition receptors (PRRs) including TLR9 which recognizes viral DNA, as well as TLR3, 7, and 8 which recognize various types of viral RNA. Activation of these receptors with their viral ligands initiates a downstream signaling cascade that results in the transcription of type I IFN genes. IFNs-α and -β released by the infected cell bind to IFN receptor on infected and nearby uninfected cells, resulting in JAK-STAT signaling. STATs will then activate transcription of several genes that inhibit viral replication including endoribonucleases that degrade viral RNA, as well as other proteins which inhibit viral replication. Additionally, type I IFNs increase the cellular immune response to infection, promote synthesis of MHC I at the cell surface so viral peptides can be presented to CD8 T cells, and activate NK cells to kill virus-infected cells.

Two IFN-α drugs include **peginterferon alfa-2a (Pegasys®)** and **peginterferon alfa-2b (PegIntron®)**, both of which have been used in the treatment of Hepatitis C in combination with ribavirin. Depending on the HCV genotype, the patient sustained virologic response (SVR) rate is somewhere between 50 and 80%. Due to the development of newer Hepatitis C drugs such as sofosbuvir and ledipasvir which offer a much higher SVR rate of 96–98%, the use of the IFN drugs has declined. Both drugs have a 40 kDa polyethylene glycol chain added to increase their half-lives, making them long-acting. The dose of pegylated interferon alfa-2a is the same for all patients, regardless of weight or size, while the dosing of pegylated interferon alfa-2b is based on an individual's weight.

Common adverse effects of interferon drugs include flu-like symptoms, depression or other neurological-related symptoms, or irritability. Many Hepatitis C patients on a ribavirin/interferon combination complain of a side effect they call "Riba Rage." This depression, changes in mood or irritability is not a result of the ribavirin, but of the interferon.

Lastly, **IFN-beta (Avonex®)** is used mainly in Multiple Sclerosis to improve the integrity of the blood brain barrier. Like the interferon-α drugs, many patients also experience flu-like symptoms as an adverse effect of this drug.

From Bench to Bedside: Discovery of TNF Inhibitors

Initially, TNF inhibitors were developed for the treatment of Rheumatoid Arthritis (RA). Sir Marc Feldman, an Australian immunologist published his hypothesis in 1983 on the role of pro-inflammatory cytokines in the mechanism of autoimmune diseases. In 1984, a collaboration with Ravinder Maini at the Kennedy Institute of Rheumatology highlighted RA in particular, finding that impacted joints contained more pro-inflammatory cytokines than normal joints, in particular TNF-α. *In vitro* studies demonstrated that blocking TNF-α could indeed reduce its levels. Subsequent studies of TNF blockade would be done in patients who had failed current RA treatments. The first of these trials took place in 1992 at Charing Cross Hospital in London, using infliximab.

In 1993, RA patients began taking the fusion inhibitor etanercept as part of a Phase I study. In 1998, etanercept became the first TNF inhibitor to be approved by the FDA for moderate to severe RA. It subsequently received FDA approval for juvenile rheumatoid arthritis, psoriatic arthritis, plaque psoriasis and ankylosing spondylitis. Clinical trials using TNF inhibitors were able to show that inhibiting a single cytokine is enough to inhibit and gain control of the immune activation that leads to inflammatory symptoms in certain disease states. Subsequently, infliximab was approved by the FDA in 1998 for the treatment of Crohn's disease, particularly in patients where conventional therapies had failed, as well as RA. Several years later, adalimumab, the third TNF inhibitor, and first fully-human monoclonal antibody against TNF for RA was approved in 2002. It was branded Humira® (Human monoclonal antibody in RA). Two more TNF inhibitors were to follow. Certolizumab pegol was first approved in 2008 and is a recombinant humanized Fab fragment specific for TNF which was conjugated with a PEG molecule to enhance its half-life and bioavailability. One year later, golimumab (Simponi®) was approved for the treatment of severe RA, active psoriatic arthritis, and active ankylosing spondylitis. While golimumab may seem like another "me too" drug, it was prepared uniquely using transgenic mice with the human immunoglobulin locus. Among all of the TNF inhibitors, golimumab has the highest affinity for TNF, and lacks some of the immunogenicity of infliximab because, like adalimumab, it lacks mouse antibody fragments.

Certain biosimilars have also recently been gaining approval by the FDA. Etanercept-szzs (Erelzi®) was approved in 2016 and, like etanercept, is indicated for the treatment of RA, polyarticular juvenile idiopathic arthritis (JIA), psoriatic arthritis, and ankylosing spondylitis. Adalimumab-atto (Amjevita®) was also approved in 2016 for the treatment of seven inflammatory diseases, including plaque psoriasis, Crohn's, and moderate-to-severe RA. Infliximab-dyyb (Inflectra®) is yet another biosimilar approved in 2016 for Crohn's disease, RA, and several other inflammatory diseases. Due to patent litigation with the parent drugs and their manufacturers, only a couple of these biosimilars have launched onto the US market. Several more are already available on the European market.

For their work on TNF blockade and important contribution to the treatment of inflammatory disease, both Feldman and Maini received several awards including the Crafoord Prize, the Albert Lasker Award for Clinical Medical Research, and the Ernst Schering Prize, among others.

Summary

The primary purpose of the innate immune system is to mount an initial response to infection. Cells of the innate immune system are programmed to destroy invading pathogenic organisms, and thus, most routine infections are rapidly terminated by the innate immune response. In addition, innate immune cells also alert cells of the adaptive immune system to the presence of infection, initiating the development of adaptive immunity. During the initial response, and while the adaptive response is mounting, innate immune cells recognize nonspecific bacterial, viral, and fungal molecular patterns using Toll-like receptors (TLRs). When pattern recognition receptors such as the TLRs are bound to microbial products, they initiate downstream signaling pathways that activate transcription factors that result in production of pro-inflammatory cytokines and chemokines. These mediators recruit leukocytes to the sites of infection to phagocytose pathogens and kill pathogen-infected cells. Leukocyte recruitment is mediated by selectins and adhesion molecules expressed on both the leukocyte and the endothelial surface of blood vessels. This results in the slowing down of leukocytes and their exit from blood vessels into tissues.

Natalizumab and vedolizumab are integrin inhibitors which prevent the inappropriate recruitment of leukocytes into tissues in certain inflammatory diseases. The development of inflammation during immune-mediated diseases may be targeted by inhibiting specific cytokines that contribute to the pathology of the disease. There are several TNF inhibitors that are used in the treatment of several inflammatory diseases in which TNF-α plays a role in the disease pathophysiology. Most of these are monoclonal antibodies, with the exception of etanercept, which is a fusion protein, and certolizumab pegol, which is a pegylated humanized anti-TNF Fab fragment. These drugs must be injected either subcutaneously or intravenously due to their biological properties. Because TNF inhibitors are immunosuppressive, they are associated with an increased risk of infection. Monoclonal antibodies may also be used to inhibit the deleterious effects of IL-1, IL-6, and IL-12 either by binding directly to the cytokine, or acting as a competitive inhibitor by binding to the receptor. Lastly, while IFN-α therapies have been used in the treatment of hepatitis to promote antiviral immunity, they are being used less often with the advent of newer hepatitis antivirals with higher response rates. IFN-β is still used for relapsing multiple sclerosis and is discussed in Chap. 7.

Practice Questions

1. The increased metabolic rate of cells in an injured area can speed up healing if the _____ is increased.
   (a) heat
   (b) pain
   (c) vasodilation
   (d) swelling

2. Which of the following correctly describes the structure of infliximab?
   (a) It is a fully human antibody
   (b) It is a chimeric human/mouse antibody
   (c) It is a humanized antibody
   (d) It is a fusion protein

3. Which of the following conditions can be treated with etanercept?
   (a) Lupus
   (b) *C. diff* colitis
   (c) Rheumatoid arthritis
   (d) Crohn's disease

4. Which of these is a fully human anti-TNF-α monoclonal antibody?
   (a) Golimumab
   (b) Etanercept
   (c) Certolizumab
   (d) Infliximab

5. Patient MF is about to be put on infliximab for his psoriatic arthritis. Knowing the mechanism of action of this drug, what should be done prior to beginning this therapy?
   (a) MF should learn how to inject himself with this drug at home.
   (b) MF should be tested for latent TB infection.
   (c) MF should have a total WBC count done.
   (d) MF should be tested for Type I hypersensitivity for this drug.

6. Which of the following is true concerning ustekinumab?
   (a) It binds to the IL-6 receptor
   (b) It binds to both IL-12 and IL-23 receptors.
   (c) It is a biosimilar for adalimumab.
   (d) It is an IL-1 receptor antagonist.

7. Interferon-beta is used for which of the following conditions?

(a) Crohn's disease
(b) Chronic granulomatous disease
(c) Hepatitis C
(d) Multiple Sclerosis

8. Which of the following statements is true concerning Type I interferons?
   (a) They signal to CD4 T lymphocytes for perforin-mediated killing of the virally-infected cell
   (b) They signal through Toll-like receptors to activate downstream transcription of genes for cell death
   (c) They signal directly to the adaptive immune response for antigen presentation and clonal expansion
   (d) They signal through the JAK/STAT pathway to activate transcription of genes that inhibit viral replication

9. Which of these inhibits IL-6 by binding to its receptor?
   (a) Siltuximab
   (b) Ustekinumab
   (c) Rilonacept
   (d) Tocilizumab

10. Which of the following describes the mechanism of action of vedolizumab?
    (a) Anti-IL-12 monoclonal antibody
    (b) Inhibitor of $\alpha_4\beta_7$ integrin
    (c) Inhibitor of IL-6 receptor
    (d) IL-1 receptor antagonist

11. Which of the following cytokines are released by virally-infected host cells to activate NK cells to aid in killing virally-infected cells? (Select all that apply)
    (a) IFN-α
    (b) IFN-β
    (c) IL-8
    (d) IL-12

12. Which of the following TNF inhibitors does not contain an Fc region and also contains a pegol group?
    (a) Remicade®
    (b) Simponi®
    (c) Humira®
    (d) Cimzia®

Suggested Reading

Abreu MT. Anti-TNF failures in Crohn's disease. Gastroenterol Hepatol. 2011;7(1):37–9.

Bendtzen K. Immunogenicity of anti-TNF-α biotherapies: I. individualized medicine based on immunopharmacological evidence. Front Immunol. 2015;6:152.

Brennan FM, Chantry D, Jackson A, Maini RN, Feldmann M. Inhibitory effect of TNF-alpha antibodies on synovial cell interleukin-1 production in rheumatoid arthritis. Lancet. 1989;334:244–7.

Campa M, Mansouri B, Warren R, Menter A. A review of biologic therapies targeting IL-23 and IL-17 for use in moderate-to-severe plaque psoriasis. Dermatol Ther (Heidelb). 2016;6(1):1–12.

Cessak G, Kuzawinska O, Burda A, Lis K, Wojnar M, Mirowska-Guzel D, et al. TNF inhibitors—mechanisms of action, approved and off-label indications. Pharmacol Rep. 2014;66(5):836–44.

Chen R, Chen B. Siltuximab (CNTO 328): a promising option for human malignancies. Drug Des Devel Ther. 2015;9:3455–8.

Christmas P. Toll-like receptors: sensors that detect infection. Nat Educ. 2010;3(9):85.

De Paepe B, Creus KK, De Bleecker JL. The tumor necrosis factor superfamily of cytokines in the inflammatory myopathies: potential targets for therapy. Clin Dev Immunol. 2011;2012:369432.

Dinarello CA, van der Meer JWM. Treating inflammation by blocking interleukin-1 in humans. Semin Immunol. 2013;25(6):469–84.

Doss GP, Agoramoorthy G, Chakraborty C. TNF/TNFR: drug target for autoimmune diseases and immune-mediated inflammatory diseases. Front Biosci. 2014;19:1028–40.

Dubé PE, Punit S, Polk DB. Redeeming an old foe: protective as well as pathophysiological roles for tumor necrosis factor in inflammatory bowel disease. Am J Physiol Gastrointest Liver Physiol. 2015;308(3):G161–70.

Elliott MJ, Maini RN, Feldmann M, Kalden JR, Antoni C, Smolen JS, et al. Randomised double blind comparison of a chimaeric monoclonal antibody to tumour necrosis factor-alpha (cA2) versus placebo in rheumatoid arthritis. Lancet. 1994;344:1105–10.

Feldmann M, Maini RN. Anti-TNF-alpha therapy of rheumatoid arthritis: what have we learned? Ann Rev Immunol. 2001;19:163–96.

Feldmann M, Brennan FM, Maini RN. Role of cytokines in rheumatoid arthritis. Ann Rev Immunol. 1996;14:397–440.

Giancane G, Minoia F, Davì S, Bracciolini G, Consolaro A, Ravelli A. IL-1 inhibition in systemic juvenile idiopathic arthritis. Front Pharmacol. 2016;7:467.

Goldback-Mansky R. Blocking interleukin-1 in rheumatic diseases. Ann N Y Acad Sci. 2009;1182:111–23.

Gonzalez-Navajas JM, Lee J, David M, Raz E. Immunomodulatory functions of type I IFNs. Nat Rev Immunol. 2012;12:125–35.

Haanstra KG, Hofman SO, Lopes Estêvão DM, Blezer EL, Bauer J, Yang LL. Antagonizing the α4β1 integrin, but not α4β7, inhibits leukocytic infiltration of the central nervous system in rhesus monkey experimental autoimmune encephalomyelitis. J Immunol. 2013;190(5):1961–73.

Heinrich PC, Behrmann I, Muller-Newen G, Schaper F, Graeve L. Interleukin-6-type cytokine signaling through the gp130/JAK/STAT pathway. Biochem J. 1998;334:297–314.

Hennigan S, Kavanaugh A. Interleukin-6 inhibitors in the treatment of rheumatoid arthritis. Ther Clin Risk Manag. 2008;4(4):767–75.

Kalliolias GD, Ivashkiv LB. TNF biology, pathogenic mechanisms and emerging therapeutic strategies. Nat Rev Rheum. 2016;12:49–62.

Kim GW, Lee NR, Pi RH, Lim YS, Lee YM, Lee JM. IL-6 inhibitors for treatment of rheumatoid arthritis: past, present, and future. Arch Pharm Res. 2015;38(5):575–84.

Kishimoto J, Akira S, Taga T. IL-6 receptor mechanism of signal transduction. Int J Immunopharmacol. 1992;14:431–8.

Lukina GV, Sigidin Ya A. Certolizumab in therapy of rheumatoid arthritis. Sovrem Revmatol. 2012;2:44–9.

Mayadas TN, Culler X, Lowell CA. The multifaceted functions of neutrophils. Annu Rev Pathol. 2014;9:181–218.

Mclean LP, Shea-Donahue T, Cross RK. Vedolizumab for the treatment of ulcerative colitis and Crohn's disease. Immunotherapy. 2012;4(9):883–98.

Mihara M, Hashizume M, Yoshida H, Suzuki M, Shiina M. IL-6/IL-6 receptor system and its role in physiological and pathological conditions. Clin Sci. 2012;122(4):143–59.

Mosser DM, Edwards JP. Exploring the full spectrum of macrophage activation. Nat Rev Immunol. 2008;8(12):958–69.

Orrock JE, Ilowite NT. Canakinumab for the treatment of active systemic juvenile idiopathic arthritis. Expert Rev Clin Pharmacol. 2016;9(8):1015–24.

Perry AK. The host type I interferon response to viral and bacterial infections. Nat Cell Res. 2005;15(6):407–22.

Shealy D, Cai A, Staquet K, Baker A, Lacy ER, Johns L, et al. Characterization of golimumab, a human monoclonal antibody specific for human tumor necrosis factor α. MAbs. 2010;2:428–39.

Spooner CE, Markowitz NP, Saravolatz LD. The role of tumor necrosis factor in sepsis. Clin Immunol Immunopathol. 1992;62(1 Pt 2):S11–7.

Stone KD, Prussin C, Metcalfe DD. IgE, mast cells, basophils, and eosinophils. J Allergy Clin Immunol. 2010;125(2 Suppl 2):S73–80.

Taylor P. Developing anti-TNF and biology agents. The past, the present, and the future. Rheumatology. 2011;50(8):1351–3.

Trinchieri G. Interleukin-12: a proinflammatory cytokine with immunoregulatory functions that bridge innate resistance and antigen-specific adaptive immunity. Annu Rev Immunol. 1995;12:251–76.

Wajant H, et al. Tumor necrosis factor signaling. Cell Death Differ. 2003;10(1):45–65.

Zhang JM, An J. Cytokines, inflammation and pain. Int Anesthes Clin. 2007;45(2):27–37.

Modulation of the Adaptive Immune System

3

Doreen E. Szollosi, Clinton B. Mathias, and Jeremy P. McAleer

Learning Objectives

1. Briefly explain the process of lymphocyte development in the primary lymphoid organs.
2. Review the signals required for lymphocyte activation, differentiation, and effector function, including the role of innate immune cells.
3. Explain the benefits of secondary immune responses.
4. Define immunological memory and discuss the importance of recall responses during immune function.
5. Review the structure and function of antibodies.
6. Discuss the mechanisms of action of medications targeting the adaptive immune system.

D. E. Szollosi (✉)
Department of Pharmaceutical Sciences, School of Pharmacy and Physician Assistant Studies, University of Saint Joseph, Hartford, CT, USA
e-mail: dszollosi@usj.edu

C. B. Mathias
Department of Pharmaceutical and Administrative Sciences, College of Pharmacy and Health Sciences, Western New England University, Springfield, MA, USA
e-mail: clinton.mathias@wne.edu

J. P. McAleer
Pharmaceutical Science and Research, Marshall University School of Pharmacy, Huntington, WV, USA
e-mail: mcaleer@marshall.edu

Drugs discussed in this chapter

Drug	Classification
Abatacept (Orencia®)	Fusion protein, CTLA-4/IgG1 Fc
Aldesleukin (Proleukin®)	Recombinant IL-2
Anti-Rh IgG (RhoGAM®)	Anti-Rh monoclonal antibody
Atezolizumab (Tecentriq®)	Anti-PD-L1 monoclonal antibody
Basiliximab (Simulect®)	Anti-CD25 monoclonal antibody
Belatacept (Nulojix®)	Fusion protein, CTLA-4/IgG1 Fc
Belimumab (Benlysta®)	Anti-BAFF monoclonal antibody
Benralizumab (Fasenra®)	Anti-IL-5R monoclonal antibody
Brodalumab (Siliq™)	Anti-IL-17 monoclonal antibody
Cyclosporine (Neoral®, Sandimmune®)	Calcineurin inhibitor
Daclizumab (Zenapax®) [discontinued]	Anti-CD25 monoclonal antibody
Dupilumab (Dupixent®)	Anti-IL-4Rα monoclonal antibody
Glucocorticoids	Global immunosuppressive agents
Ixekizumab (Taltz®)	Anti-IL-17 monoclonal antibody
Mepolizumab (Nucala®)	Anti-IL-5 monoclonal antibody
Muromonab-CD3 (Orthoclone OKT3®)	Anti-CD3 monoclonal antibody
Nivolumab (Opdivo®)	Anti-PD-1 monoclonal antibody
Obinutuzumab (Gazyva®)	Anti-CD20 monoclonal antibody

© Springer Nature Switzerland AG 2020
C. B. Mathias et al., *Pharmacology of Immunotherapeutic Drugs*,
https://doi.org/10.1007/978-3-030-19922-7_3

Drug	Classification
Ocrelizumab (Ocrevus®)	Anti-CD20 monoclonal antibody
Ofatumumab (Arzerra®)	Anti-CD20 monoclonal antibody
Pembrolizumab (Keytruda®)	Anti-PD-1 monoclonal antibody
Rapamycin/Sirolimus (Rapamune®)	Anti-proliferative, mTOR inhibitor
Reslizumab (Cinqair®)	Anti-IL-5 monoclonal antibody
Rituximab (Rituxan®)	Anti-CD20 monoclonal antibody
Secukinumab (Cosentyx®)	Anti-IL-17 monoclonal antibody
Tacrolimus, FK506 (Prograf®, Protopic®)	Calcineurin inhibitor

Introduction

The adaptive arm of the immune system is critical for the development of life-long immunity in all vertebrates. In contrast to innate immune responses, adaptive immune responses are characterized by a specific, targeted response against specific pathogens that involves a memory of the antigenic characteristics of the organism, and the capacity to mount a faster, powerful response upon re-exposure to the antigen. This specificity is conferred by cell surface receptors known as **T-cell receptors (TCR)** or **B-cell receptors (BCRs)** on the surfaces of adaptive immune cells such as T and B lymphocytes. Gene rearrangement processes that occur during lymphocyte development provide the flexibility necessary for B cells and T cells to recognize foreign molecules that they have never encountered (Fig. 3.1). Thus, each newly formed lymphocyte is unique in terms of its antigen recognition capability. While T-lymphocytes are mainly involved in the development of cell-mediated responses, B-lymphocytes mediate the humoral or antibody response resulting in the secretion of various immunoglobulins. Secreted immunoglobulins, or antibodies, are able to travel throughout the bloodstream and other body fluids to bind to and inactivate pathogens and various microbial toxins. The binding of antibodies to a pathogen also marks the pathogen for removal by a phagocyte (opsonization). Lastly, the hallmark of adaptive immunity is its rapid and robust response to a second encounter with the same antigen. This is due to the activation of "memory" lymphocytes that were formed at the conclusion of the first encounter. These memory cells rapidly proliferate and differentiate into

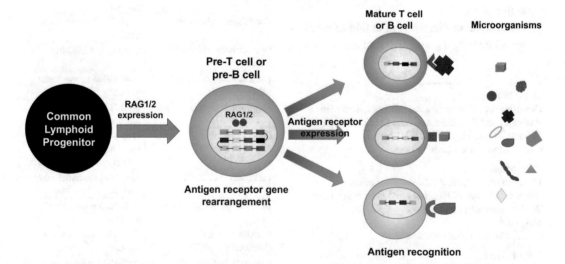

Fig. 3.1 Antigen receptor gene rearrangement provides lymphocytes with the flexibility to recognize microbial antigens they have never encountered. T cells and B cells derived from the common lymphoid progenitor express recombinase enzymes (RAG1, RAG2) that facilitate the random rearrangement of gene segments encoding the T cell receptor or B cell receptor, respectively. The vast variety of possible combinations leads to the expression of a surface antigen receptor unique for each lymphocyte. Some of these receptors are capable of recognizing antigens produced by microorganisms. Antigen recognition is the first step in lymphocyte activation and is required for adaptive immune responses

effector cells during secondary infections. Thus, adaptive immune responses are an adaptation to environmental antigens.

Development of the Adaptive Immune Response

Lymph and Lymphoid Organs

The generation and development of B and T lymphocytes occurs within the bone marrow and/or the thymus, which are referred to as primary lymphoid organs. From here, mature, **naïve lymphocytes** travel throughout the body's tissues via blood and lymphatic vessels, which are an interconnecting network of anastomosing vessels that are dedicated to the transport of lymph and connect the various lymphatic tissues and bone marrow. Lymph is a clear fluid which drains from the capillaries and interstitial fluid. Lymph fluid within the lymphatic vessels transports the various lymphocytes as well as other immune cells and helps facilitate immune responses by acting as a conduit between lymphoid organs and tissues. Lymphocytes derive their name by virtue of their presence within the lymph, of which they are the primary constituents. At various junctions throughout the body, lymphatic vessels give rise to lymph nodes, where mature, naïve lymphocytes survey the area for the presence of **antigen**. Lymph eventually drains into venous blood.

Lymphocytes begin their differentiation from common hematopoietic stem cells in the **bone marrow** as described in Chap. 1. B cells stay within the bone marrow and complete their maturation there. T-lymphocytes, however, migrate to the **thymus** and complete their maturation there.

On completion of their development in the primary lymphoid organs, lymphocytes travel to various secondary lymphoid organs (lymph nodes, spleen) where they mature, are activated to specific antigens, and differentiate into effector and memory cells. Depending on the site of infection or antigen entry into the body (systemic, connective, and mucosal), lymphocyte activation and differentiation can occur in the spleen, lymph nodes, tonsils, Peyer's patches of the gut, and **mucosa-associated lymphoid tissue (MALT)**. Activation of lymphocytes to blood-borne infections typically occurs in the spleen, while antigens within the connective and mucosal tissues will activate lymphocytes in lymph nodes draining those sites. For mucosal immunity, the MALT can be subcategorized based on the location of the tissue, which can exist in many locations in the body. Bronchus-associated lymphoid tissue (BALT) and gut-associated lymphoid tissue (GALT) are two subcategories of MALT. Other locations are found in the skin, larynx, and conjunctiva, among others. Lymph nodes are mainly found in the neck, abdomen, thorax, and pelvis, and contain both B- and T- lymphocytes. While the secondary lymphoid organs filter extracellular fluids including lymph, they also serve as locations where naive lymphocytes can encounter their antigen and become activated.

Development of T and B Lymphocytes

In contrast to the innate immune system, adaptive immune responses are not directly inherited in germline configuration from parents. Rather, the *potential* to mount a specific immune response against nearly any non-self target molecule is passed on from generation to generation. This flexibility occurs as a result of the somatic recombination of specific gene segments within developing lymphocytes, named **V**ariable, **D**iversity and **J**oining, which encode for the various surface antigen receptors for T and B cells (Fig. 3.2). As explained in Chap. 1, the adaptive immune system responds to specific **antigens** that are recognized as non-self by lymphocytes (B cells, T cells). Somatic recombination is a unique mechanism of gene rearrangement that only occurs in B and T lymphocytes. The term antigen originally derived from **anti**body-**gen**erating substance, but now includes targets that are recognized by T cell receptors as well as B cell receptors (Fig. 3.3). Many biologically relevant antigens are macromolecules (proteins, peptides, carbohydrates, lipids, nucleic acids) from microorganisms that interact with lymphocyte receptors. In addition, antigens can derive from the covalent attachment of small molecules to proteins. These are termed **haptens** and have a role in the pathogenesis of hypersensitivity responses or autoimmune

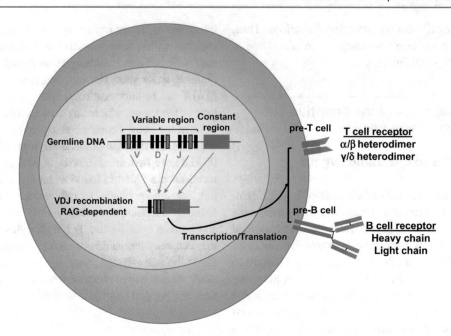

Fig. 3.2 Lymphocyte VDJ recombination generates a diverse antigen receptor repertoire. The expression of RAG enzymes in developing (pre-) T cells and B cells causes the random recombination of gene segments termed V, D and J in the genes encoding antigen receptors. During recombination, one of many V segments will randomly associate with a D and J segment, with the intervening DNA removed. The recombined VDJ region (green) in lymphocytes encodes for the antigen binding portion of the T cell receptor or B cell receptor, and is also referred to as the variable region. This is paired with a constant region that provides structural support for antigen receptors (blue), and also initiates intracellular signaling pathways upon receptor activation. T cell receptors are heterodimers composed of gene products from alpha, beta, gamma and delta loci. B cell receptors are composed of gene products from heavy and light chains, connected through disulfide bonds

disease. The **antigen receptor repertoire** determines the variety of different antigens that individuals are capable of generating an immune response towards. Although the repertoire is not fixed and depends on somatic gene rearrangements, healthy individuals typically have at least one lymphocyte capable of responding to nearly any non-self antigen. Lymphocytes are first activated by their antigen in lymph nodes and, as explained below, the requirements for activating B cells differ from T cells.

T-Cell Development

During **hematopoiesis**, some bone marrow-derived **common lymphoid progenitor cells (CLPs)** migrate to the **thymus** where they develop into **T cells** (Fig. 3.4). Stages of T cell development are identified by their expression of cell surface markers that define the T cell lineage as well as chromosomal rearrangements occurring at genetic loci encoding T cell antigen receptors (TCR α/β or γ/δ genes). These chromosomal gene rearrangements are catalyzed by enzymes that are encoded by genes named the **Recombination Activating Genes (RAG)-1** and **RAG-2**. T cell receptors are composed of **variable** and **constant** regions, referring to their antigen binding and surface membrane anchoring domains, respectively. The variable region is further subdivided into sections named **V**, **D** and **J**, which are abbreviations for variable, diversity and joining segments. Germline cells contain many distinct V, D, and J segments in TCR α and β genetic loci. When CLPs enter the thymus and express RAG enzymes, one D gene segment randomly joins with one J segment, with the intervening DNA removed. This is a somatic recombination event that occurs in thymocytes expressing RAG-1 and RAG-2 but not other cell types. Once the D-J recombination event is complete, one of many V segments is randomly selected to join the DJ region. VDJ recombination is not unique to T cell receptors and also occurs in genes encoding the B cell receptor variable region, as described below. Following VDJ recombination, **thymocytes**

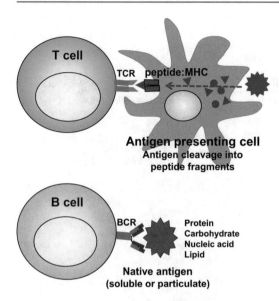

Fig. 3.3 Antigen recognition by T cells and B cells. T cell receptors (TCRs) recognize peptides presented on major histocompatibility complex (MHC) molecules by antigen presenting cells. The peptides are derived from proteins that are acquired (internalized) by antigen presenting cells and subsequently processed. B cell receptors (BCRs) recognize macromolecules (proteins, carbohydrates, nucleic acids, lipids) in their native conformation

expressing a functional T cell receptor survive and progress to the next stage of development. In contrast, thymocytes that fail to express a T cell receptor undergo programmed cell death. This is termed **positive selection** and requires thymocytes to interact with antigen presenting cells (APCs) expressing **Major Histocompatibility Class I (MHC I)** or **MHC II** on their surface (Fig. 3.5). At this stage of development, thymocytes are termed "**double-positive**," meaning they express both **CD4** and **CD8** co-receptors that identify specialized T cell subsets. Thymocytes expressing TCRs that recognize MHC I will downregulate CD4 and become CD8 single-positive cells. This is because the CD8 co-receptor recognizes a region on MHC I that strengthens its interactions with the TCR. Conversely, thymocytes expressing a TCR recognizing MHC class II will downregulate CD8 and become CD4 single-positive cells. Thus, CD8 and CD4 T cells are referred to as being MHC class I-restricted or MHC class II-restricted, respectively. This distinction becomes important for peripheral immune responses, as MHC class II is only expressed by certain cell types (mostly APCs)

and differs from MHC class I with respect to the antigens it presents to T cells in lymph nodes.

The next stage in thymocyte development is termed **negative selection** and eliminates self-reactive T cells from the repertoire, protecting people from autoimmune diseases. Since VDJ recombination is a random process and can generate T cells expressing receptors that recognize self-antigens, it is important for the immune system to have a mechanism that eliminates self-reactive thymocytes. A transcription factor named **Autoimmune Regulator (AIRE)** induces the expression of genes that are primarily restricted to peripheral tissues, such as the pancreas, adrenal glands, and thyroid, among others. Developing thymocytes that react strongly to these antigens will undergo **apoptosis** and become eliminated from the repertoire (Fig. 3.6). Loss-of-function mutations in AIRE predispose people to Autoimmune Polyendocrine Syndrome Type 1 (APS-1) a disease characterized by susceptibility to chronic mucocutaneous candidiasis, adrenal insufficiency and hypoparathyroidism. In addition, some APS-1 patients suffer from hypothyroidism or type 1 diabetes, illustrating the importance of T cell negative selection in protection from systemic autoimmune diseases. Thymocytes surviving the positive and negative selection processes in the thymus mature into single-positive CD4 or CD8 T cells that populate peripheral lymphoid tissues including lymph nodes and the spleen.

B-Lymphocyte Development

Two different B cell lineages have been identified: B-1 and B-2 (Fig. 3.7). While B-1 cells develop neonatally and have a restricted antigen receptor repertoire, B-2 cells are bone marrow-derived and have a more diverse repertoire. Similar to T cells, B-2 cells develop from the common lymphoid progenitor; however, their development is completed in the bone marrow where stromal cells provide stem-cell factor, stromal cell-derived factor 1 and other growth factors such as IL-7. B cell differentiation occurs under the control of the transcription factor Pax-5 and different stages of B cell development are identified by their surface expression of markers that define the B cell lineage such as CD19, CD20, CD45R and the IL-7

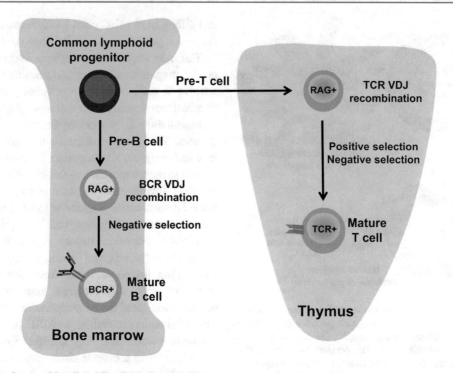

Fig. 3.4 Stages of B cell and T cell development. Bone marrow-derived common lymphoid progenitor cells have the potential to develop into B cells or T cells. These processes are dependent on the expression of RAG enzymes that facilitate VDJ recombination in the genes encoding antigen receptor variable regions. Pre-B cells are retained in bone marrow, where VDJ recombination takes place on genes encoding antibody heavy and light chains. On the other hand, Pre-T cells migrate to the thymus, where VDJ recombination occurs in the genes encoding the T cell receptor (TCR) alpha and beta chains. Once VDJ recombination has taken place, antigen receptors are expressed on the cell surface. Lymphocytes then undergo positive selection, in which only the cells expressing a functional antigen receptor (BCR, TCR) receive survival signals, followed by negative selection in which recognition of self antigens results in apoptosis. Pre-B cells and pre-T cells surviving the positive and negative selection process become mature lymphocytes that exit the bone marrow and thymus, respectively, and populate secondary lymphoid tissues

receptor. These stages include pro-B cells, pre-B cells, and immature B cells. The pro-B cell stage is characterized by V, D, J gene recombination events that generate the variable region of the immunoglobulin heavy chain. During this stage, the recombined V, D, J region attaches to the constant region encoding IgM. In pre-B cells, the heavy chain is tested for compatibility with a surrogate light chain comprising of the VpreB and λ5 segments resulting in the formation of the pre-B cell receptor. Cells which express an incompatible IgM heavy chain undergo apoptosis at this point, resulting in the halting of B cell development within these cells. The light chain genes are rearranged during the pre-B cell stages via V and J recombination. Successful recombination results in the generation of an IgM molecule comprising of both heavy and light chains with the ability to bind a variety of antigens. At this stage,

developing B cells are referred to as immature B cells. Once IgM has been acquired, developing B cells go through **negative selection**, where they are tested for their ability to bind various resident and migrating self-antigens that enter the bone marrow via circulation and lymph. Any immature B cells that recognize self-antigens are either rendered anergic or given the chance to further rearrange their light chain genes, which is termed as **receptor editing**. Immature B cells that are unsuccessful at generating a new receptor that is tolerant to self-antigens are eliminated by apoptosis. Following negative selection, the heavy chain genes in IgM-expressing immature B cells undergo alternative splicing to the IgD constant region, resulting in the co-expression of IgD on these cells. The IgM and IgD expressing B cells are now referred to as mature B cells, which enter the circulation. **Positive selection** of B cells

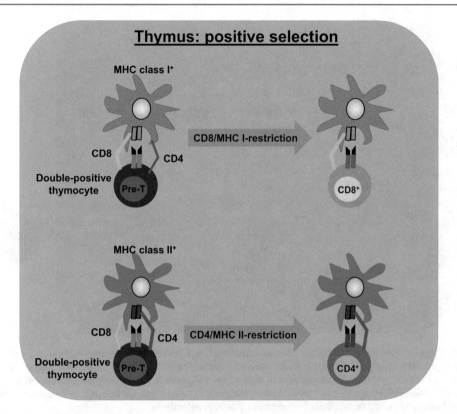

Fig. 3.5 T cell positive selection in the thymus establishes MHC-restriction. T cell development includes a double-positive stage in which pre-T cells express both CD8 and CD4 co-receptors. Following VDJ recombination, T cell receptors that preferentially interact with MHC class I molecules on antigen presenting cells will have the interaction strengthened by CD8 (top panel). This results in the downregulation of CD4 and development of a CD8 single-positive thymocyte. Alternatively, T cell receptors that preferentially interact with MHC class II will have the interaction strengthened by CD4 and downregulate CD8, resulting in CD4 single-positive thymocytes (bottom panel)

occurs within the secondary lymphoid organs. Here, they compete with other B cells for entry into the primary lymphoid follicles, where they interact with follicular dendritic cells and receive survival signals such as lymphotoxin (LT) and **B cell activating factor (BAFF)**. BAFF is particularly important for the growth and survival of B cells after their activation has occurred in secondary lymphoid organs. Here, they also further complete their maturation, resulting in the formation of germinal centers, and various activation-related events such as somatic hypermutation, affinity maturation, and isotype switching. For immune responses against T cell-dependent antigens, many of these processes are facilitated by interactions with follicular helper T cells which provide cytokines and costimulation. These interactions induce an enzyme named **activation-induced**

cytidine deaminase (AID) in B cells, which plays an important role in the induction of somatic hypermutation and class switching of the IgM heavy chain to other isotypes.

Primary and Secondary Immune Responses

Primary Response

The **clonal selection** theory explains how the adaptive immune system is capable of responding to antigens it has never encountered while still maintaining tolerance to self-antigens. This theory is based on four principles that relate to the lymphocyte receptor diversity necessary for recognizing antigens from foreign pathogens. The first principle

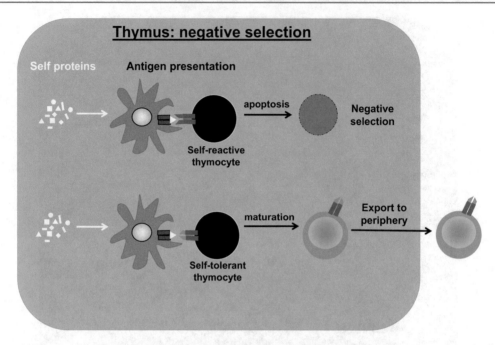

Fig. 3.6 Negative selection in the thymus eliminates autoreactive T cells from the repertoire. During T cell development, antigen presenting cells display peptides derived from self-protein on MHC molecules. Strong interactions between the TCR and peptide/MHC complexes in thymocytes will result in apoptosis. Weak interactions between the TCR and peptide/MHC complexes will provide survival signals to thymocytes, leading to T cell maturation. Negative selection helps to minimize the number of autoreactive T cells in individuals

dictates that under normal regulatory conditions, lymphocytes with BCRs or TCRs that recognize self-antigens are deleted during development, termed negative selection. The second principle states that a single type of BCR or TCR exists on individual B- or T-lymphocytes, each with a unique specificity created through VDJ recombination during development (Fig. 3.2). These lymphocytes are then activated upon the binding of an antigen to its receptor. This usually occurs through interactions with APCs. For instance, dendritic cells display peptides collected from sites of infection on MHC class II to T cells, some of which may express a specific receptor recognizing that antigen. The third principle supports the notion that effector cells derived from the proliferation of activated lymphocytes will also express BCRs or TCRs of the same specificity. This is termed **clonal expansion** and the activated antigen-specific cells proliferate into thousands of clones retaining the same receptor for antigen recognition (Fig. 3.8). Clonal expansion is accompanied by lymphocyte **effector differentiation** in which cells acquire specialized functions for fighting infections. For instance,

T cells differentiate into helper or cytotoxic subsets, while B cells differentiate into antibody-producing plasma cells. The antibodies will bind to pathogens or their toxins, resulting in their **opsonization** or neutralization, respectively. Following the expansion phase, most of the effector cells die by apoptosis; however, a small population of **memory cells** persists, capable of providing a rapid and vigorous response following a second exposure to the same antigen (Fig. 1.7). Due to the low precursor frequency of antigen-specific lymphocytes and the time required for clonal expansion and effector differentiation, adaptive immune responses take several days to develop.

Secondary Response

The hallmarks of adaptive immunity are antigen specificity and immunological memory. Antigen specificity refers to the immune response targeting microbes expressing the same antigen, while **memory** refers to long-lived cells that are prepared to react against any future exposure to the

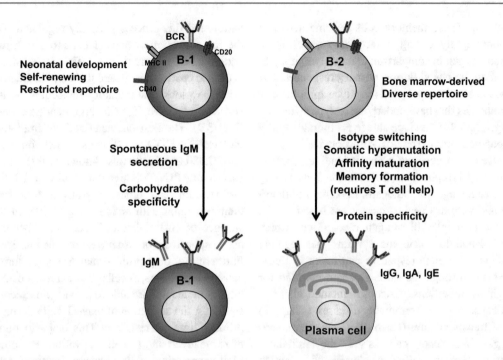

Fig. 3.7 Characteristics of the major B cell lineages. B-1 cells develop neonatally and produce natural IgM antibodies that bind to conserved carbohydrate structures on microorganisms. This population is thought to have self-renewing capability. B-2 cells are bone marrow-derived and have a greater diversity in antigen recognition capability. Following their activation, B-2 cells undergo isotype switching and somatic hypermutation to generate IgG, IgA and IgE isotypes with greater affinity for their antigen. Following their activation, B-2 cells are capable of terminal differentiation into memory cells or antibody-producing plasma cells

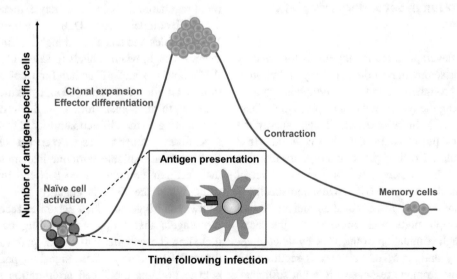

Fig. 3.8 **Phases** of primary lymphocyte responses following activation. Primary immune responses are initiated when naive T cells or B cells are activated with antigen. The inset shows a T cell interacting with a dendritic cell presenting an antigen recognized by the TCR. Dendritic cells provide other signals (costimulation, cytokines) that stimulate full T cell activation, leading to their clonal expansion and differentiation into specialized effector cell subsets. These processes are required for increasing the number of lymphocytes that are capable of attacking pathogens expressing their cognate antigen. Following clonal expansion, most of the effector cells undergo apoptosis during the contraction phase. A small population of antigen-specific memory cells persists in the individual, capable of responding robustly to a second encounter with the same antigen

antigen. These memory cells become activated more rapidly during a secondary exposure to their antigen in comparison to naive lymphocytes that are activated during primary responses. For instance, memory B cells produce high affinity antibodies that have undergone isotype switching (IgA, IgG, IgE) and are able to proliferate rapidly upon activation. The goal of prophylactic **vaccination** is to generate a pool of antigen-specific memory lymphocytes that provide long-lasting protection against pathogens. Personalized therapeutic vaccines against cancer are based on the same principles of antigen recognition (Chap. 10). Breakdowns in the systems that regulate adaptive immune responses can result in tissue damage through the same mechanisms used for fighting infections. Examples include allergies (Chaps. 4–6), autoimmune diseases (Chap. 7) and transplantation (Chap. 8). Thus, pharmacologic treatments can target the initiation, reactivation or effector phases of adaptive immune responses.

T Cell Activation and Function

Activation in Secondary Lymphoid Organs

T cell development in the thymus is followed by their dissemination to the periphery and circulation throughout secondary lymphoid organs including the lymph nodes and spleen (**see** Chap. 1, Fig. 1.8). In these organs, T cells survey the antigens presented by dendritic cells on MHC molecules. T cells expressing a receptor that recognizes the antigen:MHC complex will interact with the dendritic cell (DC), while non-specific T cells continue searching for their antigen or exit the lymph node and circulate to the next. Although stimulation of the TCR by its complementary antigen:MHC complex is required for initiating immune responses, it is not sufficient. The activation of a naïve T cell is a pivotal event since it is committed to a specific antigen for the duration of its life and may have the potential to cross-react with self-antigens. Thus, a significant amount of energy is expended towards T cell acti-

vation and this process is tightly regulated. For the full activation of naïve T cells to occur, two additional signals are required. The second signal is termed **costimulation** and involves the interaction of various costimulatory molecules on the surfaces of naïve T cells and dendritic cells (Fig. 3.9). The best characterized costimulatory molecule is CD28 on T cells, which interacts with CD80 and CD86 (also known as B7) on the surface of APCs. This signal is required for T cell proliferation and clonal expansion following their activation with antigen (Fig. 3.10). In the absence of costimulation, T cells may become non-responsive, or **anergic**, to the antigen. Furthermore, only professional APCs (dendritic cells, macrophages, B cells) that express costimulatory molecules are able to provide this second signal for the activation of naïve T cells during a primary immune response. This helps to minimize inadvertent T cell activation by other MHC-expressing cells. Several costimulatory molecules have been identified that stimulate (CD28, CD40L, ICOS, OX40, 4-1BB) or suppress (**CTLA-4**, 4-1BB) proliferation, and are pharmacologic targets for T cell-mediated diseases. CTLA-4 functions as an immune checkpoint regulator and is constitutively expressed on T cells. It competes with CD28 for the binding to B7 molecules and has a much higher affinity for them. As such, when it binds to CD80/CD86 on APCs it acts as an "off" switch for T cell activation. In addition to costimulation, cytokines provide a third signal for T cell activation, contributing to the differentiation of T cells into specialized subsets, as described below. **Cytokines** are soluble hormone-like molecules that facilitate communication between immune cells. When the TCR is engaged, a signaling pathway is triggered which generates secondary messengers that propagate signaling cascades including the **calcineurin-NF-AT** pathway and the **mTOR** pathway. These signaling pathways help to promote the T cell proliferation signal, resulting in the production of IL-2, a critical cytokine for T cell proliferation and clonal expansion.

Programmed cell death protein 1 (PD-1) is another member of the CD28/CTLA4 family and

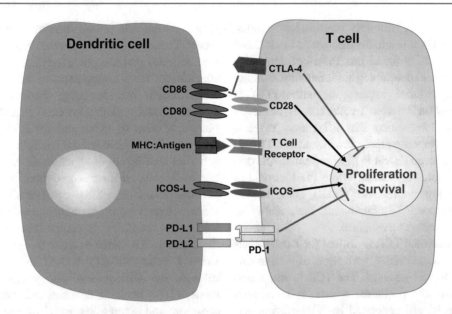

Fig. 3.9 Costimulatory molecules regulating T cell activation. Antigen recognition is not sufficient for stimulating T cell proliferation, clonal expansion and survival. Costimulatory molecules provide a second signal that promotes (CD28, ICOS) or suppresses (CTLA-4, PD-1) T cell activation and adaptive immune responses. Overall, the balance of signals received from the T cell receptor, costimulatory molecules and cytokines (not shown) determines the activation status and growth of a clonal T cell population

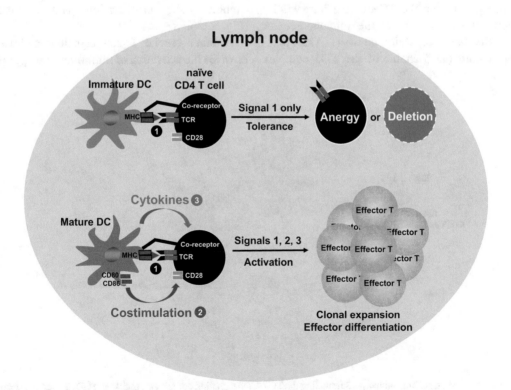

Fig. 3.10 Three signal model for the activation of naive T cells. The activation of naive T cells in lymph nodes requires antigen recognition by the T cell receptor (TCR; signal 1), costimulation (CD28 and others; signal 2) and cytokines (IL-2 and others; signal 3). The presence of signal 1 alone leads to T cell anergy or deletion, resulting in immunological tolerance to the antigen (top panel). The presence of all three signals induces their proliferation, clonal expansion, survival and effector differentiation (bottom panel)

functions as an inhibitory co-stimulatory molecule. PD-1 was originally discovered in 1992 and studies in 1999 found that PD-1-deficient mice were prone to developing autoimmunity, defining it as a negative immune regulator. PD-1 is expressed on activated T cells, B cells, and macrophages, suggesting that PD-1 may regulate immune responses more broadly than CTLA-4. PD-1 has been shown to have protective and deleterious roles in disease. While PD-1 can aid in suppressing autoreactive T cells, some tumors also express PD-1, facilitating their ability to escape immune surveillance.

A functional TCR is critical for T cell development, homeostasis, activation, as well as tolerance to self-antigens. The TCR is comprised of TCRα and β chains, which, as mentioned previously, are generated by VDJ recombination and are responsible for antigen recognition. In addition, the TCR associates with the CD3 complex, consisting of transmembrane proteins with cytoplasmic domains that transmit signals from the TCR to the intracellular compartment. Of these, the immunoreceptor tyrosine-based activation motifs (ITAMs) present within the ζ chains of the CD3 complex

play a pivotal role in transmission of the TCR signal. These sequences consist of various tyrosine residues that are phosphorylated by tyrosine kinases when engagement of the TCR and costimulation has occurred. Further downstream phosphorylation events include the binding of other signaling proteins that result in the generation of intracellular calcium. Calcium is a vital component of signaling in the activation of T cells and is released from the endoplasmic reticulum. This cytoplasmic Ca2+ influx activates a protein phosphatase known as calcineurin, resulting in dephosphorylation of the transcription factor **nuclear factor of activated T cells (NF-AT)**. NF-AT then translocates to the nucleus and, along with **AP-1**, binds to DNA response elements to induce transcription and expression of IL-2 and other genes responsible for T cell activation. Overall, the signaling pathways that are activated by signals 1 (TCR), 2 (costimulation) and 3 (IL-2 receptor) during T cell activation cooperate to support their proliferation and survival (Fig. 3.11).

Another crucial T cell signaling pathway involves the activation of **mammalian target of**

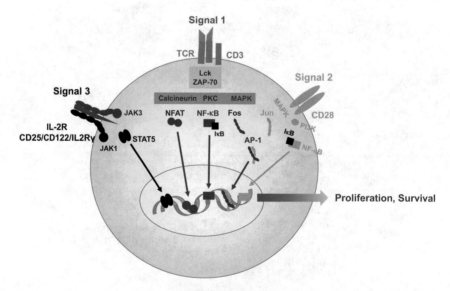

Fig. 3.11 T cell signaling pathways. Stimulating the TCR/CD3 signaling complex (signal 1) and CD28 (signal 2) leads to the activation and nuclear translocation of NFAT, NF-κB and AP-1 transcription factors. These transcription factors cooperatively induce many genes that support T cell proliferation and survival. Of these, IL-2 has an important role as an autocrine growth factor that activates its receptor complex (IL-2R; signal 3) to induce STAT5 nuclear translocation

rapamycin (mTOR). This kinase regulates T cell proliferation, growth, and metabolism through external stimuli, growth factors, and cytokines. When the TCR has bound to its antigen on the MHC complex, mTORC1 and mTORC2 are activated through the PI3K/Akt and Ras/ERK1/2 pathways. Studies using rapamycin, a compound originally described in 1975 and produced by bacteria isolated from the soil of Easter Island, demonstrated its inhibitory effects on the proliferation of eukaryotic cells. With regard to adaptive immunity, rapamycin was found to induce T cell anergy by inhibiting mTORC1, which is intrinsically more sensitive to rapamycin than mTORC2. In contrast, enhanced mTOR signaling prevents T cell anergy.

In summary, mature naïve T cells circulate throughout secondary lymphoid organs searching for their antigen. Once their TCR is engaged, costimulatory molecules, proliferation signals, and cytokines promote their full activation while the absence of these signals can lead to tolerance, or non-responsiveness, to the antigen.

Roles of T Cells in Host Defense

People suffering from T cell deficiencies are susceptible to opportunistic infections from fungi, bacteria, and viruses, demonstrating indispensable roles for T cells in protection against pathogenic microorganisms. To combat the variety of pathogens with differing portals of entry into the body and life cycles, the immune system is compartmentalized at the organ, tissue and cellular levels. As such, two major T cell subsets (CD4, CD8) are specialized for combating both extracellular and intracellular pathogens. These are termed helper T cells and cytotoxic T cells, respectively, and differ in the types of antigens they recognize as well as their mechanisms used to clear pathogenic microorganisms from the body. Below is a brief description of these subsets.

CD4 T Cell Subsets

CD4 T cells contribute to host defense against both extracellular and intracellular pathogens. They help to direct the removal of pathogens by other immune cells, including neutrophils, macrophages and antibody-producing B cells. CD4 is the co-receptor necessary for interacting with MHC II on the surfaces of DCs, B cells, and macrophages. Effector CD4 T cells are termed "helper" T cells because they facilitate pathogen clearance by activating other immune cells. Following their development and maturation in the thymus, naïve T cells migrate throughout the blood and lymphatic systems and primarily reside in secondary lymphoid organs such as the lymph nodes and spleen. Following antigen recognition in these organs, CD4 T cells differentiate into specialized helper T cell subsets, termed T_H1, T_H2, T_H17, and T_{FH} as well as regulatory T cells (T_{regs}) (Fig. 3.12). Other helper T cell subsets have also been proposed including the T_H9 and T_H22 subsets. The type of T cell subset they differentiate into depends on the cytokine signals they receive during their activation with antigens.

T_H1 Cells

T cell activation in the presence of IL-12 induces the expression of a transcription factor named **T-bet**, programming T_H1 differentiation. $\mathbf{T_H1}$ cells are important for immunity to intracellular bacteria, as demonstrated by people with loss-of-function mutations in the IFN-γ signaling pathway or experimental animal models. A primary function of **IFN-γ** is to activate macrophages, augmenting their microbicidal activity. In addition to IFN-γ (the primary signal), CD40 binding on the macrophage to **CD40 ligand (CD40L)** on the T_H1 cell is also required for macrophage activation. This binding results in a greater expression of CD40 as well as TNF receptors on the surface of the macrophage, which helps to activate it. This results in their production of nitric oxide and reactive oxygen species, enhancing the intracellular killing of ingested pathogens. Thus, T_H1 cells primarily function to help cell-mediated immune responses.

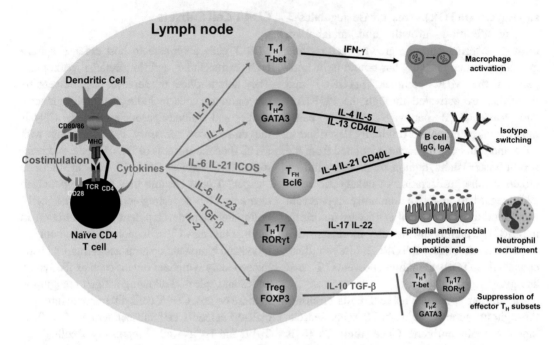

Fig. 3.12 Effector CD4 T cell differentiation into specialized subsets depends on cytokine signals received during their activation in lymph nodes. CD4 T cells that recognize antigens presented by DCs in lymph nodes will differentiate into effector T cell subsets in the presence of costimulation and cytokines. T cell activation in the presence of IL-12 induces differentiation into T_H1 cells that secrete IFN-γ. This subset activates macrophages among other cells and is important for host defense against bacterial pathogens. IL-4 induces T_H2 cell differentiation. T_{FH} cells have functions that are complementary to that of T_H2 cells in that they express CD40L and cytokines to induce antibody class switch recombination and affinity maturation. T_H2 cells also protect against parasitic organisms. T cell activation in the presence of IL-6, IL-23 and TGF-β induces T_H17 cell differentiation. This subset is important for host defense on mucosal surfaces due to their production of IL-17 and IL-22. These cytokines act on epithelial cells to induce the production of antimicrobial peptides, as well as chemokines that recruit neutrophils to the site of infection. The combination of TGF-β and IL-2 induces regulatory T cell (T_{reg}) differentiation, an anti-inflammatory subset that is required for resolving inflammation and protection against autoimmune diseases. Each CD4 T helper cell subset is associated with their expression of a transcription factor that promotes the expression of specialized genes associated with each subset

T_H2 Cells

Alternatively, T cell activation in the presence of IL-4 induces T_H2 cell differentiation through the induction of the **GATA3** transcription factor. This population is required for host defense against parasitic organisms. The activation of T_H2 cells results in the secretion of cytokines such as IL-3, IL-4, IL-5, IL-13, IL-9, and IL-10 which help coordinate the IgE-mediated response against parasitic organisms. **IL-4** both drives T_H2 differentiation and also serves to activate naïve B cells to the parasitic antigen. **IL-5** is important for the differentiation and activation of eosinophils. Both IL-4 and IL-13 induce isotype class switching from IgM to IgE. Furthermore, **IL-13**

also stimulates mucus secretion, smooth muscle hyperreactivity and epithelial cell turnover. Lastly, IL-3, IL-9, and IL-10 act as mast cell growth factors.

T_{FH} Cells

The differentiation of T_{FH} cells is promoted by IL-6 and engagement of the costimulatory molecule **inducible costimulator (ICOS)**, resulting in expression of a transcription factor named **Bcl-6**. T_{FH} cells produce IL-4 and IL-21, cytokines which facilitate naive B cell activation and antibody responses. These interactions between T_{FH} cells and B cells occur in lymph nodes where they recognize antigens derived from the same pathogen, with the resulting cross-talk involving both cytokines and surface-bound receptors. Initially, antigen binding to B cell receptors (BCRs) leads to its receptor-mediated endocytosis, where it is processed into peptide fragments and presented by MHC class II molecules on the surface of B cells. Lymph node-resident T_{FH} cells survey the peptides presented by B cells. Recognition of the cognate antigen will result in T_{FH} cells stimulating the CD40 costimulatory molecule on B cells with their own CD40L. The activation of CD40 on B cells induces their expression of activation-induced cytidine deaminase (AID), an enzyme required for antibody somatic hypermutation and isotype switching, as described below. In addition, T_{FH} cells release important cytokines such as IL-4, IL-5, IL-6 and IL-21, which aid in the proliferation and differentiation of B cells into antibody-producing plasma cells. In particular, IL-21 is important for T_{FH} cell differentiation and the formation of B cell germinal centers. Overall, T_{FH} cells contribute to humoral immunity by stimulating the production of high affinity, isotype-switched antibodies from B cells. Immune responses involving the activation of CD40 on B cells are said to be "T cell-dependent."

T_H17 Cells

T_H17 cells were described in the late 2000s as a third lineage of T helper cells that produce IL-17 and IL-21. An important function of T_H17 cells is to help strengthen the epithelial barrier on surfaces in the respiratory tract, GI tract, and skin. Thus, this subset has important roles in host defense against extracellular bacteria and fungi. IL-17 produced by T_H17 cells stimulates epithelial cells to secrete antimicrobial peptides and chemokines that can recruit neutrophils in response to infection or injury. Overactivity of T_H17 cells is associated with the development of several autoimmune diseases, as described in Chapters 5, 6, and 7. T_H17 differentiation occurs when CD4 T cells are activated in the presence of TGF-β and IL-6. Activation of the IL-6 receptor leads to STAT3 nuclear translocation and the production of IL-21, an autocrine cytokine that supports T_H17 differentiation. Additionally, the

IL-23 receptor is upregulated during T_H17 cell differentiation, and stimulation with IL-23 induces a positive feedback loop to promote their survival. The combined actions of IL-6 and TGF-β induce the expression of a transcription factor named RORγt, defining the T_H17 subset. This transcription factor is required for IL-17 secretion. Depending on the cytokine milieu in which T cells are activated, phenotypically diverse T_H17 subsets may be produced. For example, "regulatory"-type T_H17 cells may be formed in TGF-β-dominant environments, whereas pro-inflammatory environments with cytokines such as IL-1β, IL-22 and IFN-γ may induce more "pathogenic"-type T_H17 cells which contribute to chronic inflammatory diseases. A role for intestinal microbiota in regulating T_H17 cell functions has been identified, possibly implicating them as a contributing factor in autoimmune diseases.

Regulatory T Cells (T_{regs})

The primary function of T_{regs} is not to serve as an effector CD4 T cell, but to suppress pro-inflammatory immune responses mediated by effector T_H cell subsets and other cell types. T_{regs} have important roles in resolving inflammation following immune responses against microorganisms, maintaining self-tolerance and protecting against autoimmune diseases. The suppression of inflammation by T_{regs} prevents adverse effects that would otherwise occur with overactive immune responses. These important functions are dependent on their direct contact with antigen-specific helper T cells and production of TGF-β and/or IL-10, which suppress T cell proliferation and cytokine production (Fig. 3.13). In addition, T_{regs} express high levels of CTLA-4, a negative costimulatory molecule which can outcompete effector T cells for access to CD80/CD86 on APCs, dampening the CD28 costimulatory signal that is required for effector T cell activation. T_{regs} are identified by their expression of the transcription factor **FOXP3** and can arise in the thymus or peripheral tissues. Thymus-derived T_{regs} are referred to as natural T_{regs}, while those in the periphery are termed induced T_{regs} and require TGF-β for their differentiation. Expression of

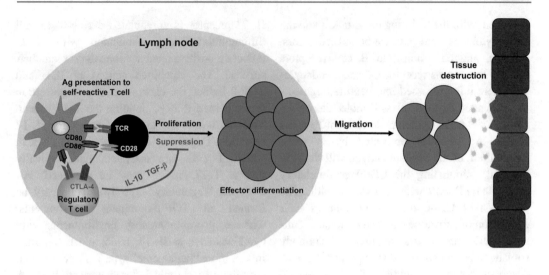

Fig. 3.13 Suppression of autoreactive T cells by T_{regs}. Regulatory T cells (T_{regs}) protect against tissue destruction caused by autoreactive T cells. This occurs through production of anti-inflammatory cytokines (IL-10, TGF-β) and by competing with effector T cells for the costimulatory ligands CD80/CD86

FOXP3 is required for the induction and maintenance of T_{regs}. Phenotypic characterization initially showed that cells expressing the IL-2 receptor α chain CD25 are enriched for T_{regs}, but newer research has identified CD25-expressing cells that lack suppressive activity. Furthermore, CD25 is transiently upregulated early during effector T cell differentiation. To identify T_{regs}, a combination of markers is recommended, including CTLA4, PD-1, and glucocorticoid induced TNF receptor (GITR). Essential roles for T_{regs} in maintaining self-tolerance are demonstrated in people born with FOXP3 deficiencies. These individuals rapidly develop a severe autoimmune disease termed immunodysregulation polyendocrinopathy enteropathy X-linked syndrome (IPEX).

CD8 T Cells

CD8 T cells recognize antigens presented on MHC class I molecules. Antigens produced inside cells are shuttled to the MHC I presentation pathway, which is present in all nucleated cells. Thus, CD8 T cells are particularly important for host defense against viruses and tumors. These subjects are discussed in greater detail in Chaps. 9

and 10, respectively. Following their activation by APCs in lymph nodes, CD8 T cells differentiate into cytotoxic effector cells and migrate out of secondary lymphoid organs to survey the peripheral environment including mucosal surfaces. Once they recognize their antigen presented by a target cell, CD8 T cells release cytotoxic granules containing perforin, granzymes, granulysin, and serglycin (Fig. 3.14). **Perforin** forms pores in target cell membranes, disrupting their osmotic balance. Membrane integrity is further disrupted by the detergent-like substances granulysin and serglycin. **Granzyme** molecules, which are serine proteases, now enter through the pores and activate caspase enzymes that induce programmed cell death, or apoptosis. CD8 T cells can also express **Fas ligand (FasL)**, which binds to the death receptor Fas expressed on many cell types. Fas-FasL interactions also result in the activation of caspases within the target cell, resulting in apoptosis. In this way, cytotoxic effector CD8 T cells provide immune surveillance against antigens produced in intracellular compartments. CD8 T cells also release cytokines including IFN-γ and TNF-α which contribute to macrophage activation and inflammation. Some viruses are able to escape immune recognition by mutating their antigens. Chronic infections that are not

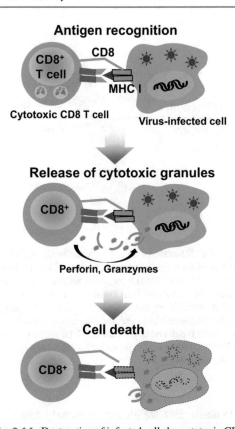

Antigen recognition

CD8⁺ T cell

CD8

MHC I

Cytotoxic CD8 T cell   Virus-infected cell

Release of cytotoxic granules

CD8⁺

Perforin, Granzymes

Cell death

CD8⁺

Fig. 3.14 Destruction of infected cells by cytotoxic CD8 T cells. Intracellular infections result in the presentation of antigens on surface MHC class I molecules. Effector CD8 T cells recognizing the antigen will release cytotoxic granules containing perforin and granzymes, resulting in apoptosis of the target cell. In this way, CD8 T cells prevent viral replication and dissemination

efficiently cleared by the immune system can lead to the exhaustion of antigen-specific CD8 T cells, resulting in the failure of T cells to kill antigen-expressing target cells.

B Cell Immunity

B cells are derived from the common lymphoid progenitor and are the only cell type that produces antibodies. The primary function of antibodies is to protect against viruses and extracellular pathogens, although patients with autoimmune diseases produce antibodies that recognize self-antigens and contribute to chronic inflammation. Thus, B cells are pharmacologic targets for vaccines and autoimmunity.

Activated B cells form germinal centers in lymph nodes, consisting of actively dividing cells in the interior and resting cells near the periphery. Antibodies are modified during germinal center reactions, so the antigen-binding variable region acquires mutations that increase binding affinity, termed **somatic hypermutation** and **affinity maturation**. In addition, **isotype switching** occurs in which the gene encoding the constant region of the antibody changes, resulting in B cells producing IgG, IgA, or IgE isotypes rather than IgM (Fig. 3.15). The functional specialization of antibodies is described below. Both

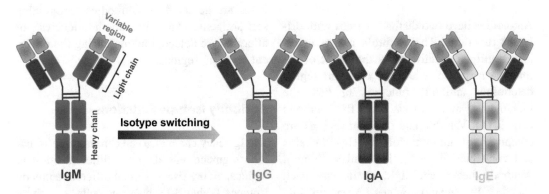

Fig. 3.15 Antibody isotypes. IgM is the initial isotype produced by newly developed B cells. Isotype switching is an irreversible T cell-dependent process that follows antigen recognition, and results in the constant region of IgM being replaced with the constant region of another isotype, i.e. IgG, IgA or IgE. Isotype switching is also accompanied by affinity maturation, in which the variable region acquires mutations that increase its binding affinity for antigens (not depicted)

somatic hypermutation and isotype class switching require the function of an enzyme named
Activation-Induced Cytidine Deaminase (AID).
The expression of AID in B cells is induced by
signals from CD4 T cells in secondary lymphoid
organs, notably CD40L. Thus, antibodies produced in a T cell-dependent manner tend to have
a high affinity for antigen and have undergone
isotype switching. Microbial products can also
activate B cells independently of T cells; however, T cell-independent antibodies are lower-
affinity IgM molecules (Fig. 3.7). These natural
IgM antibodies produced in the absence of
co-stimulation typically recognize conserved
carbohydrate residues on fungi or bacteria.
Signals provided by T_H2 or T_{FH} cells induce germinal center reactions, resulting in the terminal
differentiation of B cells into plasma cells which
are specialized for secreting high amounts of
antibodies. Memory B cells resulting from this
clonal expansion phase persist for years in people. Upon re-exposure to their antigen, memory
B cells rapidly differentiate into antibody-secreting plasma cells and help to clear re-infections
before the symptoms are noticed. The exquisite
specificity of antibodies for their target antigen
provided impetus for the engineering and development of therapeutic monoclonal antibodies, as
described below.

Antibody Structure and Specificity

Antibodies have two distinct regions with different functions. The **variable** region determines antigen specificity, or the target of the
immune response, while the **constant** region
determines antibody function, or how the
immune system reacts to the antigen
(Fig. 3.16). Variable and constant regions are
composed of immunoglobulin (Ig) domains
and connected by a flexible linker (hinge).
Antibody heavy and light chains are each
encoded by separate genes. A single IgG
molecule contains two identical heavy chains
and two identical light chains covalently
attached by disulfide bonds. With each Ig
domain having a molecular weight of 25 kDa,

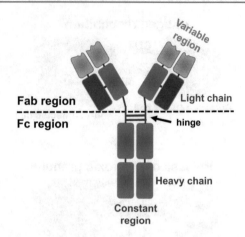

Fig. 3.16 Structure of an antibody molecule. Individual
antibodies are a dimer of dimers, with two identical heavy
chains and two identical light chains encoded by separate
genes. The heavy and light chain each have an antigen-
binding variable region (green) as well as a constant
region (purple or blue). The variable region is unique for
each naive B cell and is generated by VDJ recombination,
while the constant region is similar for all B cells expressing the same isotype

IgG antibodies weigh approximately 150 kDa.
This property helps to identify them by serum
protein electrophoresis. The binding properties of serum antibodies are also analyzed by
ELISA or Western blot for diagnostic purposes. For instance, the presence of antibodies
recognizing certain pathogens through their
variable regions can be indicative of previous
infections or vaccinations, autoimmune diseases are detected by antibodies recognizing
self-antigens,   and   immunodeficiencies   or
allergies are detected by measuring the different constant regions.

Antibody Isotype Functions

The Ig heavy chain locus on chromosome 14 has
nine segments encoding the different constant
regions, giving rise to several different antibody
isotypes (Table 3.1). Naïve B cells, e.g. those
cells that have not yet been activated by antigen
through their B cell receptor, express IgM and
IgD. IgM exists as a bulky pentamer and is
extremely effective at fixing complement and

Table 3.1 Functions of human antibody isotypes

Antibody functions	Human isotypes								
	IgA1	IgA2	IgD	IgE	IgG1	IgG2	IgG3	IgG4	IgM
Antibody-dependent cellular cytotoxicity					+++	+	+++		
Complement activation	+	+			+++	+	+++		+++
Mast cell sensitization				+++	+		+		
Neutralization	++	++			++	++	++	++	+
Opsonization					+++		++	+	

inducing opsonization following antigen binding; however, it does not get into tissues as easily as other isotypes. In contrast, monomeric IgG molecules are multifunctional antibodies that are effective at complement activation, opsonization, and neutralization (**see** Chap. 1, Fig. 1.9). As discussed in Chaps. 1 and 2, **complement** activation through the classical pathway occurs when IgM or IgG antibodies coat the surface of pathogens or infected cells, resulting in cellular destruction. IgG antibodies have comparatively greater binding affinity for cognate antigens than IgM. This is due to the somatic hypermutation and affinity maturation processes that occur in variable regions while B cells are undergoing isotype switching. There are four subtypes of IgG (Table 3.1), with IgG1 being the most common, and IgG4 being the least common. **Opsonization** refers to antibodies labeling pathogens for their uptake and destruction by phagocytic cells. In particular, macrophages express Fc receptors that bind to IgG constant regions. Thus, IgG-coated pathogens are easy targets for macrophages to recognize. **Neutralization** refers to preventing toxins, molecules or viruses from interacting with their receptor(s) or attaching to host cells. IgA is the most predominant isotype produced in mucosal lymphoid tissue and primarily functions through neutralization. Molecules of IgA can exist as a monomer or a dimer.

Once antibodies are secreted, they function independently of B cells and humoral immunity can even be transferred from one person to another. A common example of this occurs during pregnancy when the placenta expresses the FcRn or Brambell receptor, allowing IgG to cross the placenta and enter the fetal circulation. FcRn is a specialized receptor that prevents the endocytic degradation of IgG in tissues and increases its half-life in the circulation. The transplacental transfer of antibodies is a form of passive immunity in which antibodies protecting the mother from certain infections can also protect the fetus which has an undeveloped immune system. In a similar manner, immunocompromised patients who are unable to produce antibodies may receive prophylactic serum Ig injections to minimize their risk of infections. An important cell type for anti-tumor immunity, NK cells, expresses Fc receptors. As explained in Chapters 1 and 2, NK cells survey peripheral tissues for signs of unhealthy cells. They can recognize antibody-coated tumors or virus-infected cells, resulting in their degranulation and release of perforin and granzyme, leading to apoptosis of the unhealthy cell. This is termed **antibody-dependent cellular cytotoxicity (ADCC)** and is an important mechanism for how therapeutic monoclonal antibodies help to clear tumors or chronic virus infections. Mast cells express another type of Fc receptor that has high affinity for IgE. Serum levels of IgE are typically low since most of these antibodies are bound to the surface of tissue-resident mast cells, sensitizing them. Secondary exposures to the antigen recognized by IgE will then activate mast cells, resulting in their degranulation and release of vasoactive amines including histamine. In this way, IgE-dependent mast cell degranulation contributes to type 1 allergic reactions, also termed **immediate hypersensitivity** (further explained in Chap. 4). These mechanisms of opsonization, ADCC and type I hypersensitivity provide examples of how the adaptive and innate immune systems interact with each other to promote pathogen clearance.

Therapeutic Monoclonal Antibodies

The exquisite specificity of antibodies for their targets is exploited to produce clones recognizing therapeutic targets. Since individual B cells produce antibodies of a single specificity, monoclonal antibodies can be derived from mice or rabbits immunized with the antigen of interest. Following immunization, B cells are isolated from secondary lymphoid tissues such as the spleen or lymph nodes, and then cultured individually. Supernatants containing secreted antibodies are assayed for bioactivity against the target antigen. Therapeutic monoclonal antibodies are typically IgG and function through neutralization, complement activation, ADCC or opsonization (**see** Chap. 1, Fig. 1.9). Antibodies that recognize a cellular receptor can either activate their target as an agonist, or inactivate it as an antagonist. B cells with the most desirable activity against their target are fused with myeloma cells to generate a stable clone producing the antibody, termed **hybridoma**. These immortalized cells are used to produce massive amounts of the antibody. To minimize the risk of hypersensitivity or the immune-mediated rejection of antibodies derived from other species, the regions not involved in antigen binding can be engineered to replace the mouse sequence with that of human IgG.

The generation of antibodies for research and clinical use has come a long way in the past several decades. Antibody production through phage display was first described by George Smith and colleagues in 1985. The first publications describing phage display libraries were published in 1990. Production of antibodies through this method requires genetic engineering of bacteriophages and allows for antigen-guided selection *in vitro* of monoclonal antibodies for almost any desired target. To construct a phage library, RNA from a human cell source (usually peripheral blood mononuclear cells) is extracted and transcribed into cDNA. Polymerase chain reaction (PCR) of Variable Heavy and Variable Light (V_H and V_L) regions are amplified with primers specific for those sequences. The constructs that result reflect all of the antibody specificities from that individual. Next, the PCR product of the V_H and V_L chains, which represent the portion of the

antibody which contains the antigen binding site, are ligated into a phage display vector. The vector is fused into the capsid protein of a bacteriophage for *E. coli*. What results is a phage library displaying various monoclonal antibodies on their surfaces. Subsequent steps of the process involve selection of monoclonal antibodies of interest by several rounds of what is called panning. Panning involves pulling out antigen-binding clones via ELISA, washing away clones that don't bind, and then eluting the clones that are bound. After several rounds of washing and selection, the monoclonal antibodies of the phage clones undergo functional and genetic analysis. Libraries can be made specific for IgG, IgA, and IgE. Due to its relative ease of getting into tissues and to its targets, most therapeutic antibodies made are IgG.

The first monoclonal antibody used in therapy, muromonab (which targets CD3), was approved by the Food and Drug Administration (FDA) in 1985 and was 100% mouse in origin. Its name is a contraction of the phrase "*mur*ine *mon*oclonal *antib*ody targeting *CD3*" and was named before the development of the World Health Organization's (WHO's) nomenclature of monoclonal antibodies. Newer mouse antibodies end in the suffix -momab or -omab. Because its structure is fully mouse-derived, some individuals may develop hypersensitivity towards it. Thus, newer technologies were developed to replace some mouse sequences with human sequences. Chimeric antibodies are composed of human constant region fused to mouse variable region, resulting in an antibody that is approximately 65% human in composition and thus has reduced immunogenicity. Based on the nomenclature of monoclonal antibodies, chimeric antibodies usually end in the suffixes –imab or –ximab. Humanized antibodies are made by grafting sequences of mouse variable regions onto human antibodies, resulting in an antibody that is approximately 95% human. Humanized antibodies typically end with the suffix –zumab. Humanized and chimeric monoclonal antibodies have reduced antigenicity, leading to a longer half-life. Lastly, fully human antibodies can be produced using phage libraries or transgenic mice. These antibodies usually end in the suffix -umab of -mumab. As indicated, the names of monoclonal antibody therapies are based on their source (mouse, human, or a combination) as well as their target (Table 3.2). For example, bevacizumab is a humanized monoclonal antibody with a cardiovascular target.

B Cell Activation

T Cell-Derived Signals Promote B Cell Activation

The BCR on newly-developed B cells consists of surface-bound IgM and IgD immunoglobulins. Recognition of antigen by surface bound IgM on B cells results in the endocytosis of the antigen and

Table 3.2 Monoclonal antibody nomenclature

Target		Source		Suffix
-li	Immune system	-mo	Mouse	-mab
-tu	Tumor	-xi	Chimeric	
-ci	Cardiovascular	-zu	Humanized	
-ki	Interleukin	-mu	Human	
-vi	Virus			

Most antibody names contain the general biological target and source of the antibody (human, mouse, or a combination of the two), followed by the suffix "mab." For example, a monoclonal antibody targeting tumor cells that is humanized may contain the stem "-tuzumab." A fully human monoclonal antibody with a target in the immune system may be referred to as "-limumab"

processing and presentation on MHC class II molecules to CD4 T cells. If helper T cells recognize these antigens, their membrane-bound CD40 ligand (CD40L) molecules will activate CD40 on B cells (Fig. 3.17). The CD40L/CD40 interaction is essential for B cell isotype switching and affinity maturation in germinal centers and induces AID expression in B cells. This enzyme removes amine groups from cytidine residues, and the cell's machinery subsequently recognizes this as damaged DNA. The DNA repair process has a high error rate, resulting in the random incorporation of mutations into variable region genes encoding the antigen binding site. In addition to somatic hypermutation, AID facilitates isotype switching. This occurs when the IgM constant region is removed and replaced with that of IgG, IgA or IgE. The cytokines produced by T cells help to determine which isotype is expressed.

Memory B-Cells in the Secondary Immune Response

Upon a secondary exposure to an antigen, memory B cells are poised to respond quicker than naive B cells and proliferate to great numbers. Their antibody affinity is also much higher. A secondary antibody response usually results in some production of IgM, higher amounts of IgG. IgA as well as IgE may also be produced

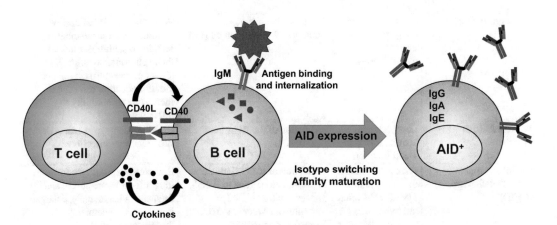

Fig. 3.17 Activation of B cells by helper T cells. Antigen recognition by the BCR (IgM) results in receptor-mediated endocytosis, followed by its proteolytic processing into peptides that are presented on MHC class II molecules. If effector CD4 T cells recognize the antigen, they will activate CD40 on the B cell surface and produce cytokines, resulting in AID expression, isotype switching and affinity maturation

depending on the antigen. Memory B cells that were primed during the first exposure also express higher levels of MHC class II, which enhances their antigen uptake and promotes improved antigen presentation. Thus, memory B cells can interact with T helper cells with less antigen present. Memory B cells also are able to recirculate throughout the secondary lymphoid compartment follicles of the spleen, lymph nodes, and Peyer's patches. It is important to note that secondary responses and any responses thereafter are conducted only by memory lymphocytes, not by naive ones. In fact, naive B cells are blocked from participation in a subsequent immune response. This typically happens when IgG antibodies produced by memory B cells binds inhibitory Fc receptors such as FcγRIIb on naïve B cells and prevents their activation by helper T cells.

Adaptive Immune Deficiencies

As is seen in the innate immune system, defects in one or more genes necessary for the response of the adaptive immune system can result in severe immunodeficiencies. Many of these are manifested by recurrent infections. Table 3.3 describes selected immunodeficiencies, but is by no means a comprehensive list. There are many different types and subtypes of immunodeficiencies, however, many of them are considered to be quite rare.

Table 3.3 Primary immunodeficiencies affecting the adaptive immune system

Disease	Immune deficiency	Mutation	Clinical manifestations
SCID (severe combined immunodeficiency)	Severe defect in T- and in some cases B-lymphocyte development	Most common form is X-linked (IL2RG) Other genes affected included JAK3, RAG1/RAG2, CD45, ARTEMIS, or CD3 delta or epsilon	Chronic diarrhea, failure to thrive, fever, recurrent respiratory infections, sepsis, recurrent ear infections, persistent thrush in the throat/mouth
Agammaglobulinemia	Low levels of IgM, IgA, IgG	BTK (X-linked)	Recurrent bacterial infections
Hyper IGM	Low IgG, IgA, IgE due to the inability to switch antibody isotypes	CD40 or CD40L	Opportunistic infections, liver damage, neutropenia
DiGeorge syndrome	T-cell deficiency, congenital heart disease, hypocalcemia	Deletion in chromosome number 22 at position 22q11.2	Wide phenotypic variability including: Cardiac anomalies, learning disabilities, unusual facial characteristics, small or absent thymus resulting in poor T-cell production resulting in increased susceptibility to infections
Wiskott-Aldrich syndrome	Low platelets, abnormal B- and T-cell function	Mutation of the WAS gene (X-linked)	Bleeding tendency, eczema of the skin, recurrent infections
Common variable immune deficiency (CVID)	Lack of functional IgG, IgA, and/or IgM. B cells often fail to become plasma cells	Mutation of ICOS (inducible costimulation) gene in B cells necessary for antibody production. Mutation of TACI, a receptor on B cells necessary for receiving a signal to undergo isotype switching, has also been implicated	Recurrent respiratory infections, lung infections are severe and frequent, splenomegaly, enlarged lymph nodes, anemia/thrombocytopenia

Drugs That Affect Adaptive Immunity

Pharmacologic T Cell Suppression

Chronic inflammatory diseases can result from a combination of factors that may include both deficiencies in immune cells as well as the impairment of regulatory or tolerance mechanisms due to hereditary defects or environmental triggers. In the latter case, the causative events may often be attributed to the failure of regulatory mechanisms governing antigen-specific T cell-mediated effects. As such, a number of drugs have been developed with the aim of specifically targeting T cells and their various subsets and mediators. T cell activation is a multi-step process involving antigen recognition, costimulation, tissue migration, and cytokine secretion. Each of these steps allows for pharmacologic intervention, with immunosuppressive agents used for treating autoimmune diseases, organ transplantation, and hypersensitivity (Fig. 3.18).

T Cell Signaling Inhibitors

Orthoclone OKT3 (Muromonab-CD3) was approved by the FDA in 1985 and was the first monoclonal antibody in history to be approved for human use. Muromonab is a murine IgG2a antibody which blocks TCR signaling by preventing signal transduction downstream of the CD3 receptor. Its target, CD3, is a 17–20 kDa molecule complex found on mature T cells as well as medullary thymocytes. The CD3 complex exists near the TCR and its interaction with the TCR is necessary for T cell activation. By binding to CD3, muromonab inhibits this interaction and thus, inhibits T cell activation. Muromonab is given as an IV infusion and is often used for treatment of acute rejection in patients who have received an organ transplant. T cells can become undetectable within minutes to hours after initial administration with muromonab, and can reappear within 48 h of discontinuation of the drug. Because muromonab binds to T cells, it may cause them to release cytokines such as TNF-α or IFN-γ. Skin reactions, fatigue, fever, headaches, and GI upset are common manifestations of this cytokine release syndrome (CRS). To reduce the risk of CRS, glucocorticoids or diphenhydramine may be given before the infusion. Because this is a murine antibody, it should not be used in patients with allergies to mouse proteins. It should also not be used in women who are pregnant or lactating.

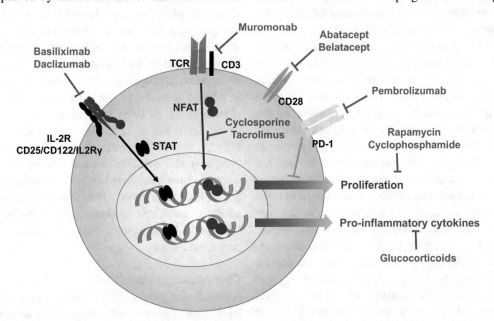

Fig. 3.18 Pharmacologic suppression of T cell activation. Several receptors and signaling pathways that regulate T cell proliferation and cytokine production are pharmacologic targets for inflammatory diseases (indicated in red)

Cyclosporine (Neoral®, Sandimmune®) and **tacrolimus (Prograf®, Protopic®)** suppress TCR signaling by inhibiting the phosphatase calcineurin. Cyclosporine is a cyclic peptide antibiotic consisting of 11 amino acids which is isolated from the fungus *Tolypocladium inflatum*. Tacrolimus is a macrolide antibiotic isolated from *Streptomyces tsukubaensis*. Cyclosporine and tacrolimus both inhibit calcineurin in T-cell signaling by binding to cyclophilin, which as mentioned earlier, is a phosphatase necessary for the activation of the transcription factor NFAT (Fig. 3.11).

This inhibits downstream transcription of T-cell cytokines including IL-2 through the transcription factor NF-AT, further preventing more activated T cells. This also results in decreased TNF-α, IL-4, IL-3, GM-CSF, and IFN-γ. While their primary action is on T_H cells, regulatory T cells and cytotoxic cells may also be affected. Cyclosporine can also increase levels of anti-inflammatory TGF-β. Both cyclosporine and tacrolimus can be used in autoimmunity as well as for the prevention of transplant rejection. Adverse effects tend to be more common in transplant patients versus patients taking these drugs for autoimmunity due to the higher doses used for prevention of transplant rejection. Long-term, nephrotoxicity can be a significant issue with both cyclosporine and tacrolimus. Acute nephrotoxicity may manifest as an increase in plasma creatinine which should be monitored while on one of these drugs. This can be reversed by decreasing the dose. Chronic renal disease is usually irreversible. It is for this reason that other drugs known to possibly be nephrotoxic should be avoided while using cyclosporine or tacrolimus. Hypertension due to renal vasoconstriction and sodium retention may also develop in the first few weeks on therapy. Gastrointestinal adverse effects can include nausea, vomiting, diarrhea, and abdominal discomfort, with patients on tacrolimus being more likely to encounter these GI effects. Other adverse effects can include increased risk of infection, increased risk of malignancy, neurotoxicity, altered mental state, or metabolic abnormalities.

Cyclosporine comes in oral, IV, and ophthalmic formulations while tacrolimus is available in oral, IV, and topical formulations. Because they are metabolized extensively by CyP450 CYP3A4, drugs that inhibit CYP3A4, as well as grapefruit and grapefruit juice should be avoided concomitantly. The risk of these drugs in pregnancy cannot be ruled out. If use of cyclosporine during pregnancy is absolutely necessary to the extent that the mother's health is threatened by her inflammatory disease, the smallest possible dose should be used, and the mother's renal function should be monitored closely. Tacrolimus has been safely used in pregnancy as an alternative to more cytotoxic drugs, but risk of fetal harm still cannot be 100% ruled out. Both drugs seem to be compatible with breastfeeding.

Sirolimus (Rapamune®), also known as **rapamycin** is a macrolide compound which suppresses signaling through the IL-2, IL-4 and IL-6 receptor by inhibiting **mammalian target of rapamycin (mTOR)**. Through this mechanism, sirolimus inhibits the activation of T- and B-lymphocytes. This compound is a macrolide antibiotic produced by the soil bacterium *Streptomyces hygroscopicus* and was first found in 1972 on Easter Island (also known natively as Rapa Nui, which lent a portion of its name to the newly-discovered compound named rapamycin). While rapamycin was first studied as an antifungal agent, research showed that it was a potent immunosuppressive/antiproliferative agent, resulting in it being approved by the FDA for renal transplant rejection in 1999. In contrast to the calcineurin inhibitors, sirolimus is less toxic to the kidneys. Some adverse effects include thrombocytopenia and impaired wound healing. Thus, after an organ transplant surgery, sirolimus may not be used right away. Other common adverse effects may include headache, abdominal pain, GI upset, hypertension, fever, anemia, and peripheral edema.

Costimulation Inhibitors

As mentioned previously, T cells need a costimulation signal from the interacting APC in addition to the MHC/peptide/TCR interaction in order to become active. The costimulation inhibitors

abatacept (Orencia®) and **belatacept (Nulojix®)** are CTLA-4/IgG1 fusion proteins that suppress T cell activation by binding to CD80 and CD86 on APCs, blocking their interaction with CD28 on T cells. Abatacept is a recombinant fusion protein consisting of the extracellular domain of CTLA4 fused to human IgG Fc region. Abatacept is given as an IV infusion and is a treatment option for rheumatoid arthritis. Common adverse effects include hypersensitivity, infusion-related reactions, and increased risk of malignancy. Belatacept is also a fusion protein which only differs from abatacept by two amino acids. Belatacept is used for prophylaxis of kidney transplant rejection and is also given intravenously. Common adverse effects include neutropenia, anemia, headache, and peripheral edema. Because both of these drugs increase the threshold for T cell activation, the treated T cells do not produce cytokines, do not undergo cell division, and often undergo apoptosis, thus resulting in T cell anergy.

IL-2 Inhibitors

T cell proliferation is suppressed with agents that regulate IL-2 production or function. Interleukin-2 is an autocrine cytokine produced by activated T cells that functions as a growth factor. The IL-2 receptor is a heterotrimeric protein containing α (CD25), β (CD122) and γ subunits (CD132, common gamma chain). The γ subunit is used by other cytokine receptors involved in lymphocyte development including IL-7 and IL-15. Activated T cells upregulate IL-2R α to form a high affinity receptor that contributes to proliferation and clonal expansion. T cell proliferation is blocked by **basiliximab (Simulect®)** and **daclizumab (Zinbryta®, Zenapax®**, both of which are which are no longer on the market), humanized monoclonal antibodies that recognize the alpha chain (CD25) and prevent its activation by IL-2.

IL-17 Inhibitors

Research has suggested that a disruption in the balance of T_{regs} and T_H17 cells is correlated with development of autoimmune diseases such as rheumatoid arthritis (RA), psoriatic arthritis, inflammatory bowel disease and Crohn's disease,

multiple sclerosis (MS), and systemic lupus erythematosus. In addition to stimulating epithelial cells to produce antimicrobial peptides and chemokines for the recruitment of innate immune cells, IL-17 exerts its effects on several other cell types. IL-17 stimulates macrophages and DCs to release TNF-α, IL-1, and IL-6, resulting in inflammation. In the endothelium, IL-17 promotes coagulation, IL-6 production and the release of matrix metalloproteinases (MMPs), resulting in vessel activation and thrombosis. IL-17 is thought to play a role in MS and Crohn's disease by stimulating fibroblasts to release IL-6, chemokines, growth factors, and MMPs. Its effects on osteoblasts and chondrocytes promote RANKL and MMPs, leading to bone erosion and cartilage destruction seen in RA. As such, several monoclonal antibodies are on the market that bind to and inhibit IL-17 produced by T_H17 cells that may contribute to inflammation and tissue damage. **Ixekizumab (Taltz®)** and **secukinumab (Cosentyx®)** both bind to IL-17A and are given as subcutaneous injections. While ixekizumab is approved for moderate to severe plaque psoriasis, secukinumab is also used for ankylosing spondylitis, and psoriatic arthritis. **Brodalumab (Siliq™)** was approved in February 2017 and is a monoclonal antibody against IL-17 receptor. Brodalumab is given subcutaneously and is approved for moderate to severe plaque psoriasis.

Glucocorticoids

Glucocorticoids, or corticosteroids, bind to the glucocorticoid receptor, regulating the expression of steroid-responsive genes including cytokines. The anti-inflammatory functions of glucocorticoids are conducted through binding of the glucocorticoid to the glucocorticoid receptor to form a complex which subsequently binds to glucocorticoid response elements (GRE) in gene promoter regions. Other transcription factors such as NF-κB or AP-1 may also be affected. This mechanism may inhibit proinflammatory molecules including cytokines, chemokines, or adhesion molecules. Additionally, anti-inflammatory cytokines may also be upregulated. Due to the immunosuppression caused by these agents, there is an increased risk for infection. Additionally, there are several other adverse effects that limit their use, particularly long-term. Some of these possible adverse effects may include (but are not limited to) osteoporosis, diabetes, weight gain, impaired wound healing, glaucoma, cataracts, avascular necrosis, and hypertension. Because of their widespread use in conditions and disorders that require varying levels of immunosuppression, the glucocorticoids will appear in several subsequent chapters of this textbook.

Pharmacologic T Cell Stimulation

IL-2 (Proleukin®) is human IL-2 produced using recombinant DNA technology in *E. coli*. It differs slightly from endogenous human IL-2, in that it is not glycosylated, nor does it have an N-terminal alanine. As mentioned earlier, IL-2 activates and promotes proliferation of T cells to promote clonal expansion. Similarly, aldesleukin (Proleukin®) binds to the IL-2 receptor leading to dimerization of IL-2R β and γ chain cytoplasmic regions. This activated receptor complex leads to recruitment of cytoplasmic signaling molecules, resulting in growth and differentiation of T cells. It may also enhance the cytotoxic activity of effector CD8 T cells. While IL-2 may be used in cancer treatment, it is associated with many adverse effects, and is thus often reserved unless needed. Adverse effects include fever, chills, dry skin, mouth sores, and severe nausea and vomiting. Because of the severity of side effects caused by high-dose IL-2, patients receiving this therapy are often monitored through hospitalization. Low-dose IL-2 may be used in some regimens and is thought to promote the survival of regulatory T cells; thus, some schools of thought suggest that it may be beneficial in treating autoimmunity.

PD-1/PD-L1 Checkpoint Inhibitors
As mentioned earlier, **programmed cell death protein 1 (PD-1)** is an inhibitory co-stimulatory molecule on the T cell surface and is a member of the CD28/CTLA4 family of T cell regulatory proteins. It can be expressed on activated T cells, B cells, and macrophages. This suggests that PD-1 regulates immune responses more broadly than CTLA-4. While PD-1 can suppress autoreactive T cell activity and autoimmunity, expression of PD-1 is upregulated on some tumors. The expression of immunosuppressive molecules is one mechanism that allows tumors to escape immune surveillance; thus, blocking PD-1/PD-L1 interactions with monoclonal antibodies such as atezolizumab, pembrolizumab, and nivolumab is a novel therapeutic target in cancer. These therapies are referred to as checkpoint inhibitors. **Pembrolizumab (Keytruda®)** is a humanized monoclonal antibody against PD-1 located on lymphocytes and is used for metastatic melanoma as well as non-small cell lung cancer. This mechanism essentially inhibits the inhibition of lymphocytes, allowing the immune system to kill abnormal cells. **Nivolumab (Opdivo®)** is a human IgG4 monoclonal antibody and is also a PD-1 inhibitor. It is often used with ipilimumab for metastatic melanomas that do not have a mutation in BRAF.

Atezolizumab (Tecentriq®) is a humanized monoclonal against PD-L1, which is the ligand for PD-1. Thus, the mechanism of action of atezolizumab is similar to the action of pembrolizumab and nivolumab because it still inhibits the inhibitory activity of the PD-1/PD-L1 binding, allowing lymphocytes to kill tumor cells.

In general, the checkpoint inhibitors may induce severe inflammation due to their mechanism of action. This inflammation may occur in the lungs, colon, liver, kidneys, intestines, and thyroid. More common adverse effects of these drugs include skin rash, pruritis, fatigue, cough, nausea, or loss of appetite.

CTLA4 Inhibition
Ipilimumab (Yervoy®) was approved by the FDA in 2011 and is a fully human monoclonal antibody against CTLA4. The normal role of CTLA4 is to act as an inhibitory molecule for T cells. Shutting off this inhibitory signal allows for cytotoxic T lymphocytes (CTLs) to maintain their cytotoxicity and kill cancer cells. Its adverse effects include stomach pain, bloating, fever, and breathing problems (for which the risk versus benefit must be weighed). Other severe side

effects may include inflammation of the intestines leading to intestinal tears, liver inflammation/damage, as well as inflammation of the skin or eyes. Ipilimumab is given intravenously and is approved for treatment of unresectable or metastatic melanoma, and renal cell carcinoma.

B Cell Pharmacologic Suppression

Cell Surface Molecules
CD20 is the molecular target of monoclonal antibodies **rituximab (Rituxan®)** and **ofatumumab (Arzerra®)** used to treat B cell lymphomas. Rituximab is a chimeric antibody and was the first biologic developed which binds to CD20 found on the surface of B cells, resulting in complement-dependent cytotoxicity. CD20 is necessary for B cell cycle initiation and may also function as a calcium channel. Removal of autoreactive B cells may help alleviate symptoms of certain autoimmune diseases in which autoantibodies are being produced against self-antigen, such as RA, and is also used in certain cancers. Rituximab is given as an IV infusion and can sometimes cause a serious infusion reaction which can be fatal. Other adverse effects seen with rituximab include cardiovascular events such as peripheral edema, cardiac arrhythmias, and hypertension. Because rituximab is a human-mouse chimeric antibody, the patient often develops anti-chimeric antibodies during the course of treatment. To get around this immunogenicity, humanized and fully human antibodies have been developed against CD20. These are considered to be second-generation anti-CD20 monoclonal antibodies. Ofatumumab is a fully human anti-CD20 antibody and binds to an epitope on CD20 different from that of rituximab and is said to promote better complement-dependent cytotoxicity than rituximab. Other humanized anti-CD20 antibodies include **ocrelizumab** and **obinutuzumab**. These have overlapping epitopes on CD20 with rituximab.

Inhibition of B Cell Growth Factors
Therapeutic monoclonal antibodies can target B cell development, maintenance and function. **Belimumab (Benlysta®)** is a fully human IgG antibody which neutralizes the function of B-cell activating factor (BAFF) also known as B lymphocyte stimulator (BLyS) and is used to induce B cell death in patients with active systemic lupus erythematosus (SLE). In 2011, it became the first drug approved for SLE in more than 50 years. BLyS is a part of the TNF superfamily and is expressed by many cell types including dendritic cells, monocytes, and macrophages. While it can be membrane-bound, the biologically active form is soluble. B-cells express three types of BLyS receptors (BR3, TACI, and B-cell maturation antigen). When BLyS binds to BR3 (also known as BAFF receptor), it promotes the survival of B-cells by preventing them from undergoing apoptosis. BLyS that is bound to belimumab is unable to bind to BR3, thus allowing for autoreactive B-cells to undergo negative selection and apoptosis.

Inhibition of Naive B Cells
RhoGAM,® also known as anti-D IgG, is used in pregnancy to prevent hemolytic disease of the newborn. This disorder can occur in second and subsequent pregnancies in fetuses that have Rh+ erythrocytes with mothers who are Rh−. Hemolytic disease of the newborn, also sometimes referred to as erythroblastosis fetalis, is caused by antibody-mediated destruction of fetal red blood cells and can result anemia, or in severe cases, fetal death due to heart failure. RhoGAM® (anti-D antibodies) consists of polyclonal antibodies purified from individuals who have been immunized with Rh factor (D polypeptide). Women who lack this antigen on erythrocytes and who are pregnant with an Rh+ baby should receive RhoGAM® at around the 27th week of pregnancy to prevent sensitization of her immune system against the RhD antigen. Following treatment, anti-D antibodies bind to Rh+ erythrocytes that cross the placenta from the fetal circulation into the mother's, inhibiting naive B cell activation against the D polypeptide. This treatment is effective at suppressing the production of higher affinity IgG antibodies against D polypeptide that may cross the placenta and damage fetal erythrocytes. In order to protect fetuses in subsequent pregnancies, RhoGAM® would need to be readministered during each pregnancy. While it is

thought that RhoGAM® is capable of crossing the placenta, the dose administered is not sufficient to cause fetal hemolysis.

Inhibitors of the Type 2 Immune Response

IL-4 and IL-13 Inhibitors

IL-4 and IL-13 are two cytokines critical for the development of type 2 immunity. Disease states in which the scales are tipped towards type 2 immunity, such as allergic asthma and eczema, represent disorders in which inhibition of IL-4 and IL-13 may be beneficial. **Pitrakinra** is a 15 kDA recombinant IL-4 protein consisting of two point mutations which allow it to act as an IL-4/IL-13 antagonist. It is under investigation as an inhaled therapy for asthma but can also be delivered subcutaneously. **Dupilumab (Dupixent®)** is a monoclonal antibody which binds to IL-4Rα subunit and is used for eczema and asthma. Because IL-4 and IL-13 share the IL-4Rα subunit, dupilumab blocks signaling of both of these cytokines. Dupilumab was approved in 2017 for adults with moderate to severe atopic dermatitis and received another indication in 2018 for ages 12 and older as an add-on therapy for asthma. Adverse effects reported are usually mild to moderate, and can include nasopharyngitis, infection of the upper respiratory tract, injection site reactions, skin infections, or conjunctivitis.

Tralokinumab is a human monoclonal antibody against IL-13 and thus prevents it from binding to both IL-13Rα1 and IL-13Rα2, resulting in the inhibition of IL-13 signaling which may be useful in decreasing airway inflammation, mucus production, as well as airway hyper-responsiveness and airway remodeling seen in asthma. Tralokinumab is currently in phase III clinical trials. Lebrikuzumab, another anti-IL-13 monoclonal antibody did not perform well in clinical trials for asthma, but is currently being studied for atopic dermatitis.

IL-5 Inhibitors

IL-5 is a cytokine which is necessary for the maturation, activation, survival, and prolifera-

tion of eosinophils. Thus, antibodies against IL-5 have been developed to combat eosinophilic inflammation, a common characteristic of both acute and chronic inflammation in asthma. Currently, three IL-5 monoclonal antibodies are available. **Mepolizumab (Nucala®)** binds the IL-5α chain and prevents its association with the IL-5 receptor while **reslizumab (Cinqair®)** binds to circulating IL-5, preventing it from binding to eosinophil receptors. Both have been shown to decrease exacerbations in asthma and improve symptoms. **Benralizumab (Fasenra®)** is a monoclonal antibody against the IL-5 receptor and has shown to decrease eosinophils in the airways, sputum, bone marrow, and peripheral blood. Common adverse effects seen with the IL-5 inhibitors include headache and nasopharyngitis.

Summary

The adaptive immune system defends the body against specific foreign invaders via TCRs and BCRs which recognize a wide range of possible antigens. After an initial adaptive response, memory T and B cells are generated which can become activated much more rapidly to fight a subsequent exposure to the same pathogen before symptoms develop. The mechanism of introducing an antigen to the body to create immunological memory is the basis for immunization. There are several pharmacological targets in the adaptive immune response which can be utilized to suppress the aberrant adaptive response in the case of autoimmunity or chronic inflammatory diseases. Many of these targets lie within T cell activation, including T cell signaling, inhibition of T cell cytokines such as IL-2, and inhibition of co-stimulation needed for T cell activation. B cell activity can be inhibited by binding to cell surface molecules such as CD20, or by inhibition of B cell growth factors. In certain types of cancer, it is beneficial to stimulate the adaptive immune response as an effort to remove abnormal cells.

Case Study: RhoGAM®

Carrie Jones is 24 weeks pregnant with her first child. During one of her OB-Gyn visits, laboratory findings revealed that Carrie's blood type is B−. Her doctor explained that if her baby is Rh+, then her body could produce an immune reaction against her baby's red blood cells. He suggests an injection of RhoGAM in her 28th week. At 39 weeks, Carrie delivered a healthy baby girl via Cesarean section. The baby was found to have the blood type AB+. Carrie's doctor suggested that Carrie receive another injection of RhoGAM 72 h post-delivery.

Questions

1. What kind of antibody is RhoGAM?
2. How does RhoGAM prevent the production of anti-Rh antibodies?
3. Which disease is RhoGAM intended to prevent?
4. Does RhoGAM cross the placenta?
5. If Carrie decides to have another baby, should she receive RhoGAM?
6. Is RhoGAM indicated for every expecting mother who is Rh−?

From Bench to Bedside: Development of Monoclonal Antibody Therapy

Commentary by Daniella D'Aquino

Monoclonal antibodies, or mabs, are antigen-recognizing glycoproteins that are made by identical immune cells, all of which are clones of a unique parent B cell. Due to their specificity, monoclonal antibodies embody the promise of precision medicine, which is to develop therapies that are tailored to a specific molecular target. These therapies encompass a number of indications such as autoimmune disorders, infectious diseases, and oncology. This concept has been around since the late nineteenth century when Paul Ehrlich coined the term "magic bullet". He envisioned personalized and tailored drugs that would seek out specific molecular defects in the body.

The first licensed monoclonal antibody was Orthoclone OKT3 (muromonab-CD3) which was approved in 1986 for use in preventing kidney transplant rejection. It is a monoclonal mouse IgG2a antibody whose cognate antigen is CD3. It works by binding to and blocking the effects of CD3 expressed on T lymphocytes. It was produced using murine hybridoma technology made famous by Nobel winning scientists Kohler and Milstein. This a multi-step process that involves injecting the mice with a particular antigen which stimulates the mouse's immune system to create antibodies against the antigen. However, these antibody-producing cells are short-lived. To ensure that there will be a mass production of therapeutic antibodies; the antibody-producing mouse cells were isolated and fused with immortalized myeloma tumor cells. This produces hybrid cells that can produce antibodies with the explicative properties of tumor cells. Since the human immune system is designed to attack anything that is foreign like muromonab, which is mouse in origin, many patients experienced limited efficacy and many serious adverse effects that led to limited use of muromonab and other fully murine antibodies.

The continued desire for monoclonal antibodies led scientists to minimize non-human sequences by creating other antibodies with limited animal exposure. These new categories are: chimeric, humanized, and fully human. Chimeric monoclonal antibodies contain antibodies from two different species, usually mouse and human. Chimeric antibodies contain the antigen-specific variable domain from a mouse, while the constant region is human in origin. Since the resulting chimeric antibody is approximately two-thirds human in origin, the risk of an immune reaction to foreign antibodies is reduced. These are usually produced using recombinant DNA technology.

Humanized monoclonal antibodies use the same technology as chimeric antibodies, in which the variable region complementarity-determining regions (CDRs), or segments of the variable region that are able to bind to the target antigen, are inserted into a human antibody. The addition of human parts in the antibody led to lower levels of adverse effects compared to the chimeric monoclonal antibodies, since the human immune system recognizes the human constant region. However since there was still the inclusion of the animal species in the variable region, adverse effects were still present. Another issue that arose was unintended consequences of monoclonal antibody specificity leading to a decreased ability of the antibody to interact with the antigen.

Fully human monoclonal antibodies were generated to minimize severe adverse effects and to ensure optimal antigen-antibody binding. These can be made in two ways. The first method is similar to the hybridoma process. Mice used to produce fully human monoclonal antibodies have been genetically altered to carry human antibody genes rather than mouse antibody genes to ensure that there will only be human-derived genes giving rise to the antibodies. The other way to generate fully human monoclonal antibodies is called phage display. Phage display was first described by George Smith at the University of Missouri in 1985. His work at Duke University the year prior with Robert Webster began the groundwork for the creation of the phage display method. This technique was further developed by scientists at Scripps Research Institute, the Laboratory of Molecular Biology in Cambridge, England, as well as the German Cancer Research Center. Both George Smith and Greg Winter from the Laboratory of Molecular Biology were awarded the Nobel Prize in Chemistry in 2018 for their contribution to the development of phage display. Phage display helps to identify optimal CDRs, a part of the variable region that is responsible for antigen binding. The first step involves inserting genetic libraries of CDRs into a virus that infects bacteria, known as bacteriophages. The phage then expresses CDRs which allows for easy screening of the CDRs exhibiting the strongest antigen binding. Once the best CDRs are displayed they are then fused onto a human antibody scaffold. Fully monoclonal antibodies have the lowest incidence of adverse effects but still have immune responses associated with the various human monoclonal antibodies.

Practice Questions

1. A patient with high levels of IgM and low levels of IgA, IgG, IgE may have a defect in:
   (a) T-cell co-stimulation
   (b) Isotype class switching
   (c) Negative selection
   (d) Calcineurin signaling

2. Which of the following drugs would stimulate T-cell activation?
   (a) Mepolizumab
   (b) Ixekizumab
   (c) Proleukin
   (d) Keytruda®

3. Which of the following cell types all express MHC II?
   (a) B-cells, NK cells, and T-cells
   (b) Macrophages, B-cells, and Dendritic cells
   (c) T-cells, Dendritic cells, and Basophils
   (d) Hepatocytes, Macrophages, and B-cells

4. Which statement best describes a biologic therapy ending in "kizumab"?
   (a) Fully human antibody with a cardiovascular target
   (b) Chimeric antibody with an immune target
   (c) Humanized antibody with a cytokine target
   (d) Humanized antibody with a tumor antigen target

5. Costimulation inhibitors bind to _____ on antigen presenting cells.
   (a) CD20
   (b) CD3
   (c) CD45
   (d) CD80/86

6. Which of the following is a PD-1 inhibitor?
   (a) secukinumab
   (b) pembrolizumab
   (c) brodalumab
   (d) basiliximab

7. Rituximab and ofatumumab bind to which cell surface molecule on B cells?
   (a) CD3
   (b) iCOS
   (c) CD20
   (d) CD80

8. Today, antibodies for clinical applications are **primarily** made via which method?
   (a) Antisera from rabbits
   (b) Hybridoma
   (c) Recombinant DNA technology

9. Dupilumab is a monoclonal antibody against which of the following cytokine targets?
   (a) IL-2
   (b) IL-5
   (c) IL-17
   (d) IL-4

10. RhoGAM directly inhibits which of the following cell types?
    (a) Eosinophils
    (b) Dendritic cells
    (c) Naive B cells
    (d) Memory B cells

11. Which of the following drugs inhibit both IL-4 and IL-13 signaling? (Select all that apply)
    (a) Mepolizumab
    (b) Daclizumab
    (c) Pitrakinra
    (d) Dupilumab
    (e) Tralokinumab

Suggested Reading

Bao K, Reinhardt RL. The differential expression of IL-4 and IL-13 and its impact on type-2 immunity. Cytokine. 2015;75(1):25–37.

Brinc D, Lazarus AH. Mechanisms of anti-D action in the prevention of hemolytic disease of the fetus and newborn. Hematology Am Soc Hematol Educ Program. 2009:185–91.

Dubey AK, Handu SS, Dubey S, Sharma P, Sharma KK, Ahmed QM. Belimumab: first targeted biological treatment for systemic lupus erythematosus. J Pharmacol Pharmacother. 2011;2(4):317–9.

Durandy A, Kracker S. Immunoglobulin class-switch recombination deficiencies. Arthritis Res Ther. 2012;14(4):218.

Fernandez-Ramos AA, Marchetti-Laurent C, Poindessous V, Antonio S, Laurent-Puig P, Bortoli S, Loriot MA, Pallet N. 6-mercaptopurine promotes energetic failure in proliferating T cells. Oncotarget. 2017;8:43048–60.

Gaud G, Lesourne R, Love PE. Regulatory mechanisms in T cell receptor signalling. Nat Rev Immunol. 2018;18:485–97.

Gooderham MJ, Hong HC, Eshtiaghi P, Papp KA. Dupilumab: a review of its use in the treatment of atopic dermatitis. J Am Acad Dermatol. 2018;78(3S1):S28–36.

Gorentla BK, Zhong X-P. T cell receptor signal transduction in T lymphocytes. J Clin Cell Immunol. 2012;2012(Suppl 12):005.

Hammers CM, Stanley JR. Antibody phage display: technique and applications. J Invest Dermatol. 2014 Feb;134(2):e17.

Huynh Du F, Mills EA, Mao-Draayer Y. Next-generation anti-CD20 monoclonal antibodies in autoimmune disease treatment. Auto Immun Highlights. 2017;8(1):12.

Kennedy BK, Lamming DW. The mechanistic target of rapamycin: the grand conducTOR of metabolism and aging. Cell Metab. 2016;23(6):990–1003.

Kopecky O, Lukesova S. Genetic defects in common variable immunodeficiency. Int J Immunogenet. 2007;34(4):225–9.

Norman DJ. Mechanisms of action and overview of OKT3. Ther Drug Monit. 1995;17(6):615–20.

Oakley RH, Cidlowski JA. The biology of the glucocorticoid receptor: new signaling mechanisms in health and disease. J Allergy Clin Immunol. 2013;132:1033–44.

Puig L. Brodalumab: the first anti-IL-17 receptor agent for psoriasis. Drugs Today (Barc). 2017;53(5):283–97.

Ramamoorthy S, Cidlowski JA. Corticosteroids-mechanisms of action in health and disease. Rheum Dis Clin North Am. 2016 Feb;42(1):15–31.

Smith-Garvin JE, Koretzky GA, Jordan MS. T cell activation. Annu Rev Immunol. 2009;27:591–619.

Tan LD, Bratt JM, Godor D, Louie S, Kenyon NJ. Benralizumab: a unique IL-5 inhibitor for severe asthma. J Asthma Allergy. 2016;9:71–81.

Zwick MB, Shen J, Scott JK. Phage-displayed peptide libraries. Curr Opin Biotechnol. 1998;9(4):427–36.

Respiratory Disorders of the Immune System and Their Pharmacological Treatment

4

Clinton B. Mathias

Learning Objectives

1. Describe the immune components of the respiratory tract and explain the mechanisms involved in immune defense.
2. Describe the types of hypersensitivity reactions and discuss the roles of immune cells and mediators.
3. Explain the differences between IgE-mediated and non-IgE-mediated allergic reactions.
4. Identify and discuss various genetic polymorphisms involved in the development of asthma.
5. Identify environmental triggers resulting in the development of asthma.
6. Discuss the immune mechanisms involved in the pathophysiology of asthma.
7. Explain the roles of immune cells and mediators responsible for the development of asthma.
8. Discuss the immune mechanisms involved in the pathophysiology of chronic obstructive pulmonary disease (COPD).
9. Identify and discuss the pharmacology of the various bronchodilators used in the treatment of asthma and COPD.
10. Identify and discuss the pharmacology of the various anti-inflammatory agents used in the treatment of asthma and COPD.

Drugs discussed in this chapter

Drugs	Classification
Albuterol (ProAir®, Proventil®, Ventolin®)	Short-acting β₂-agonist
Levalbuterol (Xopenex®)	Short-acting β₂-agonist
Metaproterenol (Alupent®)	Short-acting β₂-agonist
Salmeterol (Serevent Diskus®)	Long-acting β₂-agonist
Formoterol (Perforomist®)	Long-acting β₂-agonist
Indacaterol (Arcapta Neohaler®)	Long-acting β₂-agonist
Arformoterol (Brovana®)	Long-acting β₂-agonist
Olodaterol (Striverdi Respimat®)	Long-acting β₂-agonist
Ipratropium bromide (Atrovent®)	Short-acting muscarinic antagonist
Tiotropium (Spiriva Respimat®; Spiriva Handihaler®)	Long-acting muscarinic antagonist
Glycopyrronium (Seebri Neohaler®)	Long-acting muscarinic antagonist
Aclidinium (Tudorza Pressair®)	Long-acting muscarinic antagonist
Umeclidinium (Incruse Ellipta®)	Long-acting muscarinic antagonist
Beclomethasone (Qvar Redihaler®; Beconase AQ®)	Inhaled/intranasal corticosteroid
Budesonide (Pulmicort Flexhaler®; Rhinocort®)	Inhaled/intranasal corticosteroid
Ciclesonide (Alvesco®; Omnaris®)	Inhaled/intranasal corticosteroid
Fluticasone (Flovent®; Flonase®)	Inhaled/intranasal corticosteroid
Mometasone (Nasonex®; Asmanex Twisthaler®)	Inhaled/intranasal corticosteroid

C. B. Mathias (✉)
Department of Pharmaceutical and Administrative Sciences, College of Pharmacy and Health Sciences, Western New England University, Springfield, MA, USA
e-mail: clinton.mathias@wne.edu

© Springer Nature Switzerland AG 2020
C. B. Mathias et al., *Pharmacology of Immunotherapeutic Drugs*,
https://doi.org/10.1007/978-3-030-19922-7_4

Drugs	Classification
Triamcinolone (Nasacort®; Kenalog®)	Inhaled/intranasal corticosteroid
Methylprednisolone (Medrol®)	Oral/systemic corticosteroid
Prednisone (Deltasone®)	Oral/systemic corticosteroid
Hydrocortisone (Cortef®)	Oral/systemic corticosteroid
Budesonide and formoterol (Symbicort®)	Combination steroid inhaler and β_2-agonist
Fluticasone and salmeterol (Advair®)	Combination steroid inhaler and β_2-agonist
Mometasone and formoterol (Dulera®)	Combination steroid inhaler and β_2-agonist
Fluticasone and vilanterol (Breo-Ellipta®)	Combination steroid inhaler and β_2-agonist
Glycopyrrolate and formoterol (Bevespi Aerosphere®)	Combination steroid inhaler and muscarinic antagonist
Theophylline (Theo-24®; Elixophylline®; Theochron®)	Phosphodiesterase inhibitor
Aminophylline (Somophyllin®)	Phosphodiesterase inhibitor
Montelukast (Singulair®)	Leukotriene receptor antagonist
Zafirlukast (Accolate®)	Leukotriene receptor antagonist
Zileuton (Zyflo®)	5-lipoxygenase inhibitor
Omalizumab (Xolair®)	Anti-IgE
Mepolizumab (Nucala®)	Anti-IL-5
Reslizumab (Cinqair®)	Anti-IL-5
Benralizumab (Fasenra®)	Anti-IL-5 receptor
Dupilumab (Dupixent®)	Anti-IL-4 receptor α
Roflumilast (Daliresp®)	Phosphodiesterase 4 inhibitor
Cromolyn sodium (Gastrocrom®)	Mast cell stabilizer
Brompheniramine (Bromfed®; Dimetapp®)	H_1R (H_1 receptor) antagonist
Chlorpheniramine (Chlor-Trimeton®)	H_1R inverse agonist
Dexchlorpheniramine (Polaramine®)	H_1R antagonist
Carbinoxamine maleate (Arbinoxa®; Carbihist®)	H_1R antagonist
Clemastine fumarate (Tavist®; Dayhist®)	H_1R antagonist
Cyproheptadine (Periactin®)	H1R antagonist; serotonin antagonist
Diphenhydramine (Benadryl®)	H_1R antagonist
Promethazine (Phenergan®)	H_1R antagonist (acts as antiemetic)

Drugs	Classification
Azelastine, intranasal (Astelin®)	H_1R antagonist
Cetirizine (Zyrtec®)	H_1R antagonist (second-generation)
Desloratadine (Clarinex®)	H_1R inverse agonist (second generation)
Fexofenadine (Allegra®)	Peripheral H_1 blocker (second generation)
Levocetirizine (Xyzal®)	H_1R antagonist (second generation)
Loratadine (Claritin®)	H_1R antagonist (second generation)

Introduction

The primary function of the human respiratory system is the facilitation of gas exchange, including the oxygenation of blood and the elimination of carbon dioxide. The execution of this task, which is essential in order to maintain survival, necessitates that the respiratory tract be in continuous exposure to the outside environment, with the potential of being exposed to numerous environmental antigens of both plant and animal origin, as well as other non-living particulate matter, which can damage the respiratory mucosa and/or impair function and survival. As such, the respiratory tract must maintain a delicate balance that involves the surveillance of a wide variety of antigens resulting in either the tolerance of non-harmful, innocuous antigens such as plant matter or the rejection of potential pathogenic species such as invading bacteria or viruses. The default state of the mucosal immune system in the respiratory tract tends towards tolerance with a response dominated by alveolar macrophages producing immunosuppressive cytokines such as IL-10 and a helper T cell profile skewed towards anti-inflammatory responses. Breaching of these surveillance mechanisms due to impaired inflammatory responses to invading pathogens, unregulated antigenic responses to innocuous antigens or damage to immune system components caused by chemicals and some drugs, can lead to the development of chronic inflammation and immunological disorders of the respiratory system.

Disorders of the Respiratory System

Diseases of the respiratory system may be categorized into but are not limited to **obstructive lung diseases**, **restrictive lung diseases**, and abnormalities of the vasculature. Obstructive diseases include disorders of the airways such as **asthma** and **chronic obstructive pulmonary disease (COPD)**, as well as bronchiectasis and bronchiolitis. The primary pathologic characteristic of obstructive diseases is the difficulty associated with the expiration of inhaled air due to bronchoconstriction and chronic airway inflammation. In contrast, restrictive diseases which include parenchymal lung diseases, abnormalities of the chest wall and pleura, and neuromuscular disease, are associated with declines in both inspiration and expiration due to diminished lung capacities. Vasculature abnormalities can include pulmonary embolism and pulmonary hypertension. Anti-inflammatory processes resulting from the damage caused to the respiratory system by pathogens, environmental stimuli, and neoplasms can lead to the development of chronic inflammation and pathologic abnormalities which may fall in either or all of the above categories. In this chapter, we will focus on the pathophysiology and the drugs used to treat the two most common obstructive lung diseases, asthma and COPD, for which the immunological basis of the disease is well-established. A major characteristic of both these diseases is the presence of chronic inflammation in the airways, which drives the phenotype of the disease, including the manifestation of symptoms, as well as the response to treatment such as corticosteroid therapy. Asthma alone can be categorized into different sub-types depending on the types of immune cells prominent within that subtype. Furthermore, in patients with both asthma and COPD, overlapping symptoms attributed to common cellular culprits may often be found to be present. This necessitates a more thorough understanding of the different types of immune cells and their mediators present in each disease type as well as the many varied functions performed by them.

The Respiratory System and Its Immune Environment

The Human Respiratory Tract

In adult humans, the respiratory tract has an approximate combined surface area of 70 m² which consists of an epithelial cell layer that is covered with cilia and bathed in mucus and an underlying mucosa that houses **lymphoid follicles** and other **bronchial associated lymphoid tiss**ue (BALT). The lungs form a major component of the lower respiratory tract, and together with the upper respiratory tract which includes the nose, mouth and pharynx, they allow and regulate the passage of air through the body (Fig. 4.1). The primary function of the lungs is the exchange of gases needed for cellular respiration. However, they also participate in other activities such as the filtering of systemic blood and the production of vasoactive substances. The lungs contain approximately 12% of the body's total blood volume that is continuously passaged to the left atrium and this allows for the passage of numerous nutrients, cells and factors that can modulate the lung environment. In addition to the lungs, the lower respiratory tract contains the trachea, the bronchi, the bronchioles, and millions of **alveoli** that represent the gas-exchange surface (Fig. 4.1).

The various airways are lined with several different types of epithelial cells, while the bronchioles are typically lined with Clara, ciliated, and basal cells. The bronchiolar mucosal layer is surrounded by a basement membrane, the lamina propria, elastic tissue and smooth muscle, and an adventitial layer connecting the alveoli and interstitium. The epithelium contains two major types of glands, serous glands that secrete bactericidal substances, and mucus glands that produce mucin. The surface of the mucus glands is highly innervated, leading to the initiation of cough reflexes and mucus secretion when irritated by antigens and other stimuli.

Pulmonary Defense

The upper and lower airways combined represent the largest epithelial surface exposed to foreign substances including antigens of bacterial, viral,

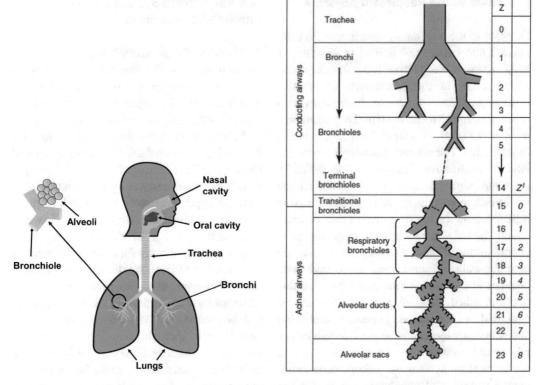

Fig. 4.1 Diagram of the Human Respiratory Tract. **Left**: The human respiratory system consists of the upper respiratory tract comprising the nose, mouth and pharynx, and the lower respiratory tract comprising the lungs, trachea, bronchi, bronchioles and alveoli. The lobar bronchi divide into segmental bronchi, which continue to bifurcate into non-respiratory bronchioles and respiratory bronchioles, until the terminal bronchiole opens into the alveolar ducts. The ducts have about 300 million alveoli where gas exchange occurs. **Right**: Diagram representing branching of the respiratory tree into conducting airways and terminal respiratory units over an average of 23 generations. The numbers at the bottom represent the approximate number of generations from trachea to alveoli. The first 14 generations are purely conducting. Transitional airways lead into acinar airways, which contain alveoli and thus participate in gas exchange (Right: Reprinted with permission from: The Structural and Physiologic Basis of Respiratory Disease, by Matthias Ochs MD and Hugh O'Brodovich MD, Kendig's Disorders of the Respiratory Tract in Children, 6, 63–100.e2)

and fungal origin. While the upper airways are continuously exposed to foreign matter, the lower airways are essentially sterile. This is achieved *via* an efficient defense network comprising of both innate and adaptive immune mechanisms that destroys harmful pathogens and induces the elimination of foreign particles.

Pulmonary defense is carried out by mechanisms either in the airways or in the alveoli (Fig. 4.2). Highly organized lymphoid tissue is distributed throughout the lower airways, comprising of several lymph nodes adjacent to the trachea as well as the major bronchi and a wide network of lymphatic vessels throughout the connective tissue. The expulsion of harmful foreign

substances is coordinated *via* both anatomical barriers and the muco-ciliary network. Airway mucus consists of a dense network of mucins which are heavily glycosylated glycoproteins that trap invading particles and also facilitate the transport of bactericidal substances and dimeric IgA. In particular, dimeric IgA attached to mucin molecules on the apical surface of epithelial cells *via* the secretory component of the poly Ig receptor plays a critical role in mucosal defense. The epithelial cells of the mucosa and sub-mucosa also play important roles during the development of inflammation. They can up-regulate adhesion molecules such as ICAM-1 and can recruit other cells by releasing chemokines. They also play a

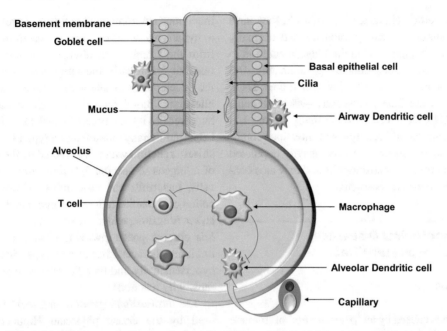

Fig. 4.2 Cells and molecules contributing to pulmonary host defense. Immune defense in the respiratory system is mediated by a number of cells and molecules. Mucins and mucus produced by goblet cells help trap invading pathogens. Epithelial cells sense the presence of infection and send signals to dendritic cells and other immune cells. T and B cells are activated in the mediastinal lymph nodes and reside within the lamina propria, bronchial associated lymphoid tissue and lymphoid follicles where they interact with pathogen components. Alveolar macrophages conduct phagocytosis and produce a number of anti-inflammatory substances including defensins, nitric oxide and superoxide radicals. Heterogeneous populations of macrophages and dendritic cells residing in the alveolus, interstitium, and the airways mediate both pro- and anti-inflammatory reactions (figure contributed by Dylan Krajewski)

key role in the initiation of immune responses by secreting alarmin molecules such as the cytokines **IL-33**, **IL-25** and **thymic stromal lymphopoietin (TSLP)**, which subsequently induce the activation of **type 2 innate lymphoid cells (ILC2s)** and pulmonary dendritic cells (DCs). A major component of the mucosa and sub-mucosa also includes a large network of DCs that lie above and below the basement membrane. These are in the immature state and act as sentinels for antigen capture. The distribution of the DC population is not constant and their profile changes during infections with the presence of increasing numbers of mature DCs. After the DCs capture antigen, they acquire migratory properties by upregulating CCR7 and home to the mediastinal lymph nodes where they encounter naïve T cells.

The immune response in the alveolar spaces consists of **alveolar macrophages (AMs)**, lymphocytes, neutrophils, eosinophils, mast cells and basophils. Resident AMs are the major compo-

nent of the alveoli, representing 85% of the **bronchoalveolar lavage (BAL) fluid** under normal conditions. Their function is to rapidly neutralize or phagocytose any invading substances, although they are normally immunosuppressive. During an inflammatory process however, the recruitment of monocytes and DCs makes them stimulatory and they contribute to a growing inflammatory cascade. This is largely accomplished by the release of numerous mediators such as IL-1 or TNF-α which promote the induction of adhesion molecules and the release of chemokines and growth factors that contribute to inflammation. They are also involved in lung modeling and repair, by producing or inhibiting factors such as matrix metalloproteinases (MMP)-1 and-2, and releasing fibroblast growth factors like TGF-β and platelet derived growth factor (PDGF). Pathogens are typically eliminated by the release of bactericidal substances like defensins, lysozyme, nitric oxide radicals or complement. Although AMs may acquire certain characteristics of DCs, they have poor antigen presenting capacity and normally suppress DC functions in the lung. In addition to AMs, the alveoli also contain approximately 10% of lymphocytes, about half of which are CD4 T cells, 30% are CD8 T cells and 5–9% are B cells. The CD4/CD8 T cell ratio is usually around 1.5. Depending on different types of infectious conditions, the alveoli may become heavily populated with neutrophils or eosinophils and may also contain mast cells and basophils.

Immunological Diseases of the Respiratory Tract

Asthma

Asthma is caused by an '*overreaction*' of immune cells in the respiratory system to harmless environmental antigens resulting in the development of inflammation, bronchoconstriction, and in severe cases, airway remodeling, which involves the restructuring of respiratory organs and tissues. Such overreactions of the immune system to innocuous environmental antigens are referred to as hypersensitivities or 'allergic' reactions derived from the Greek word **allergy** meaning 'altered reactivity'. Similarly, the antigens responsible for the development of allergic reactions are termed **allergens**. Based on Coomb's classification of hypersensitivity reactions (Table 4.1), asthma has been traditionally classified as a type I **hypersensitivity reaction** which is triggered by the binding of allergens to specific **IgE antibodies** on **mast cells, basophils** and **eosinophils**. However, the pathogenic manifestations of asthma include both an *early* IgE-dependent acute phase as well as a *late* chronic phase involving CD4 T cells, thus imbibing characteristics of both type I immediate hypersensitivity and type IV delayed type hypersensitivity reactions.

The term *asthma* (*panting* in Greek) was first used by the Greek physician Hippocrates to describe recurrent episodes of breathlessness and wheezing. Clinical and experimental observations have led to the association of several cardinal characteristics with the manifestation of the disease (Table 4.2): *bronchial inflammation* consisting predominantly of eosinophils, lymphocytes

Table 4.1 Hypersensitivity reactions

Hypersensitivity Type (*causative antigen*)	Immune mechanisms	Example
Type I immediate (*soluble antigens*)	• IgE-mediated • Mast cell and basophil activation	• Allergic asthma • Allergic rhinitis • Systemic Anaphylaxis to insect stings, venoms, food allergens, or drugs such as penicillin
Type II (*cell or matrix associated antigens or cell surface receptors*)	• IgG-mediated • Complement, phagocyte or NK cell activation	• Some drug allergies such as to penicillin • Chronic urticaria
Type III (*soluble antigens*)	• IgG-mediated • Immune complex activation • Complement and phagocyte activation	• Serum sickness caused by drugs or other foreign substances
Type IV (*soluble or cell-associated antigen*)	• T_H1, T_H2, or CTL mediated • Activation of macrophages, eosinophils • CD8 T cell-mediated cytotoxic reactions	• Contact dermatitis (T_H1 cells or CTL) • Tuberculin reaction (T_H1 cells) • Chronic asthma (T_H2 cells)

Hypersensitivity reactions are divided into four types depending on the inducing antigen and the immune mechanism involved. Immediate reactions are mediated by IgE antibodies and cells such as mast cells. Type II reactions are mediated by IgG antibodies in response to novel epitopes produced as a result of modifications of cell-associated or surface antigens. Type III reactions are mediated by IgG containing immune complexes resulting in complement activation and phagocytosis. Type IV reactions are mediated by helper T cells to soluble antigens such as pollen or tuberculin or cytotoxic T cells to novel cell-associated antigens produced as a result of covalent linking with chemical haptens

Table 4.2 Cardinal characteristics of asthma

Cardinal characteristics of asthma
• Reversible airway construction
• Bronchial smooth muscle hyperreactivity (BHR)
• Chronic airway inflammation (eosinophilia in IgE-mediated allergic syndromes)
• Mucus plugging
• Airway remodeling

According to the World Health Organization (WHO), IgE-mediated allergic asthma is characterized by the presence of the following defining criteria: airway obstruction that can be reversed spontaneously or by pharmacologic treatment; smooth muscle airway hyperreactivity resulting in bronchoconstriction; airway inflammation dominated by **eosinophilia**; **mucus hypersecretion** giving rise to the presence of mucus plugs; airway remodeling occurring due to structural changes resulting from fibrosis and epithelial cell turnover

and degranulated mast cells; *reversible airway obstruction* and *airway hyperresponsiveness (AHR)* also referred to as **bronchoconstriction** to non-specific stimuli; *mucus cell hyperplasia* along with sub-basement membrane thickening, resulting in loss of the structural integrity of the airways; elevated levels of *serum IgE*; and *airway remodeling* occurring as a result of chronic inflammatory and repair mechanisms. However, although these characteristics have been found to be associated with asthma, they are only surrogate markers of the expression of the disease and the intensity of expression of particular phenotypes has been found to vary between individuals depending on a number of criteria including but not limited to the type of allergic exposure, immune status of the patient, and host genetic background. Clinical observations have also led to the characterization of two different types of asthma: *extrinsic* or *atopic* **asthma**, which is allergic in nature and often begins in childhood; and *intrinsic* or *non-atopic* **asthma** which may develop in adulthood and is not always associated with elevated IgE levels.

Asthma Epidemiology

According to the WHO, about 235 million people worldwide suffer from asthma, resulting in frequent episodes of breathlessness and wheezing of varying severity and often accompanied by short to prolonged hospitalizations and even death in severe cases when left untreated and unmanaged. Annually, asthma results in over 330,000 deaths worldwide and management of the disease requires enormous constraints to the economy. In the United States alone, 25 million people were affected in 2009, out of which 1 in 10 were children under the age of 18. Asthma related health care costs were 56 billion in the United States in 2007.

Over the last few decades, the frequency of asthma (and other allergic diseases) seems to have increased significantly in westernized and developed nations. In the United States alone, the prevalence of asthma from 1980 to1994 increased by 75%. In comparison, the low baseline levels of asthma in developing countries has not changed too much. This rapid shift in asthma epidemiology in the last 40 years indicates that the prevalence of disease may not be attributable to heredity alone but may also include environmental components. One prominent explanation that has often been provided for the exponential increase in allergic diseases has been the **Hygiene Hypothesis**. Proponents of this theory argue that the development of allergic diseases in the western world may be directly attributed to several practices that have resulted in a deviation of the immune response from one which is geared towards fighting infections to one that mediates allergic reactions. Exposure to microbial antigens in early childhood and the induction of immunity is thought to counter-regulate a predisposition toward T_H2 responses that is already present in neonates. This is supported by a number of studies that demonstrate an inverse relationship between infections acquired during childhood and sensitivity to allergens. For example, infants in developing countries who have been exposed to multiple pathogens during childhood and whose intestinal tracts are colonized earlier than their counterparts from developed countries are less susceptible to developing allergic diseases later in life. Similarly, antibiotic overuse as well as exposure to tuberculosis or the *Bacille Calmette-Guerin* (BCG) vaccine has been linked to deviation of the immune response from a pro-allergic T_H2 response to a favorable T_H1-type cell-mediated response. Other studies suggest that the increased allergic response in

Western countries may be a consequence of decreased exposure to parasitic helminth worms in these nations, which are normally eliminated by an IgE-mediated response that is coordinated by T_H2 cells. Conversely, however, certain viral infections such as influenza virus infection or infection with respiratory syncytial virus appear to exacerbate the risks for developing allergic diseases such as asthma. Thus, both microbial exposure and an individual's previous immunological experience has the potential to increase or decrease the risk of developing allergic diseases such as asthma.

The Hygiene Hypothesis
Commentary by Kaitlin Armstrong

The hygiene hypothesis is the proposition that the increased incidence of hypersensitivity reactions and autoimmune disorders over the past few decades can be attributed to changes in sanitation, exposure to microbes, and antibiotic overuse in developed countries. Without the introduction of common infections and parasites during childhood—specifically helminths—the immune system does not exercise appropriate responses to foreign agents and instead becomes hyperreactive to harmless environmental antigens that do not pose a threat.

Some tenets of the hygiene hypothesis include:

1. *Improved sanitation*, which reduces childhood exposure to pathogens and parasites that the immune system evolved to fight.
2. *Improvements in public health*, have resulted in declining exposure to infections such as tuberculosis that typically provoke potent cell-mediated responses.
3. *Overuse of antibiotics*, which gives the immune system fewer opportunities to fight infections unaided from start to finish and additionally disrupts the gut microbiome.

The Genetic Basis of Asthma
The genetic predisposition or tendency to develop allergies to common innocuous environmental allergens is termed as **atopy**. Atopy is derived from the Greek word for '*peculiar*' or '*out of place*' and is associated with the ability to produce copious amounts of IgE antibodies to a wide variety of environmental allergens, including pollen, cockroach antigen, **house dust mite (HDM) antigen** and cat dander. Most allergens are typically low-molecular weight proteins or haptens that can elicit allergic responses (Table 4.3). The reason why these molecules induce an allergic response in some but not all individuals is not yet understood, but the discovery that some of these proteins (example, Der p2) are enzymes or have enzymatic activity that could provide a T_H2 bias, suggest that they may act by disrupting normal immune regulation.

Numerous population studies have verified the role for heredity in asthma acquisition. The single strongest risk factor for asthma development is atopy itself. Individuals with a first-degree relative with atopy are at high risk, but those with two atopic parents are at even higher risk. This has been confirmed in the studies of monozygotic and dizygotic twins. However

Table 4.3 Examples of common environmental triggers of asthma

Environmental triggers of asthma
• House dust mite
• Pollen
• Animal dander
• Cockroach antigen
• Fungal spores
• Viral infections (respiratory syncytial virus, influenza)
• (ozone, sulfur dioxide, tobacco smoke, cold air)
• Drugs (aspirin, NSAIDs)
• Occupational stimuli (hay mold, flour dust, papain)

A number of diverse environmental antigens and gases have the potential to trigger various endotypes of asthma. Low-molecular weight allergens such as pollen and house dust mite antigens are potent inducers of IgE-mediated allergic asthma. Other environmental factors such as ozone or tobacco smoke may contribute to non-IgE-mediated manifestations of asthma such as those observed in patients with chronic asthmatic symptoms atopy alone is not sufficient to induce asthma, because many atopic individuals do not have asthmatic symptoms. Also, since symptoms vary from individual to individual, determination of the genes involved must focus not only on 'symptoms' of the disease but also take into account the overall pattern of disease expression and various indices of atopy in different populations. Studies have linked the following loci to an atopic phenotype (Fig. 4.3): *IL-3, IL-4, IL-5, IL-13, IL-9* in the T_H2 cytokine gene cluster on chromosome 5, the **high-affinity IgE receptor (*FcεRI*)** on chromosome 11, and a large region on chromosome 12 spanning several candidate genes (*STAT-6, IFN-γ, stem cell factor and nitric oxide synthase*). Interestingly, while the T_H2 cytokine genes and the IgE receptor have been directly linked to asthma development, the IFN-γ gene has been inversely linked to the development of disease.

In addition to the above genes, other novel susceptible genes have also been identified. These include: *C5* (complement factor 5) and *TIM1* (T-cell immunoglobulin and mucin-domain containing molecules) which may be involved in T_H2 differentiation processes (through as yet undefined mechanisms); *ADAM33* (a disintegrin and metalloproteinase 33) which is primarily expressed on airway smooth muscle and fibroblasts and may contribute to the remodeling process in the asthmatic lung; and *DPP10* (dipeptidyl peptidase 10) which is thought to modulate the activity of many chemokines and cytokines that regulate the inflammatory process. Lastly, recent studies have elucidated the roles of novel mediators such as *IL-25* and *IL-33* in the activation of innate lymphoid cells and the development of airway inflammation. A cartoon depicting the probable targets of some of these genes is shown in Fig. 4.3. Inheritance of any of these loci

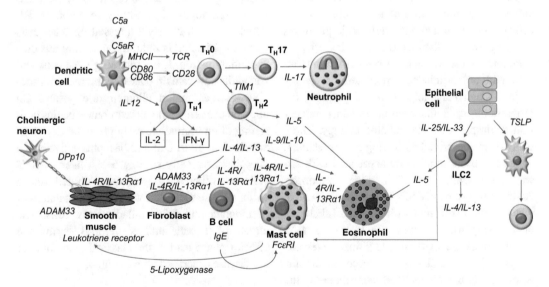

Fig. 4.3 Cartoon depicting the association of various genes with asthma pathogenesis. Development of asthma requires T cell activation which is induced by presentation of allergen *via* MHC class II on DCs to the T cell receptor and the engagement of co-stimulatory molecules on T cells (CD28 or CTLA-4) with CD80 or CD86 on DCs. T cells then acquire a T_H2 phenotype characterized by the production of IL-4, IL-5, and IL-13 as opposed to T_H1 cells which produce IFN-γ and IL-2 and are present in non-atopic individuals. IL-13 interacts with its receptor IL-4R and IL-13Rα1 on various cell types in the airway wall contributing to asthma pathogenesis. IL-4 and IL-5 act on T cells and eosinophils respectively inducing survival and proliferation. C5 and TIM1 may act in the Th2 differentiation pathway in as yet undefined ways. Additionally C5a can also induce the production of IL-12 from DCs. ADAM 33 is thought to contribute to lung remodeling and dipeptidyl peptidase (DPP)10 is thought to modulate the activity of many different chemokines and cytokines. Epithelial cells can produce IL-25 and IL-33 which activate ILC2s and mast cells and thymic stromal lymphopoietin (TSLP) which activates DCs (figure contributed by Dylan Krajewski)

may form a common genetic basis for different atopic diseases. Overall, the emerging consensus from genetic studies implies a strong T_H2 bias in the development of asthma.

Pathophysiology of Asthma

In the vast majority of asthma patients, the development of asthma is atopic in nature and dependent on the activation and recall responses of allergen-specific T_H2 cells. These patients typically develop chronic inflammation, which may extend from the trachea down towards the peripheral airways, and exhibit the cardinal characteristics of asthma defined earlier, including eosinophilic inflammation, bronchial smooth muscle hyperreactivity, narrowing of the airway lumen and mucus plugging, reversible airway obstruction, and airway remodeling. The development of asthmatic symptoms and airway inflammation is driven by a combination of factors, including chronic inflammation mediated by T_H2 cells secreting IL-4, IL-5 and IL-13, the activation and degranulation of mast cells, and the activation of neuronal and cholinergic pathways resulting from inflammation. The majority of symptoms in these patients is responsive to treatment with oral or inhaled corticosteroids.

In a small percentage (5%) of patients, the progression of inflammation remains uncontrolled, despite maximal inhaled therapy. These patients are described as having severe asthma, which has been found to be associated with airway neutrophils and T_H17-type responses. Additionally, some patients have intrinsic asthma, which is not associated with elevated IgE levels or T_H2 responses. Despite the lack of a T_H2-specific response in these individuals, elevated levels of IL-5 and IL-13 are present in the airways of these patients, and contribute to the development of airway eosinophilia and AHR. Recent evidence suggests that the asthmatic phenotype in these patients may be driven by a subset of innate lymphoid cells, ILC2 cells, that produce IL-33 in response to epithelial cell injury caused by protease allergens.

The effector functions of T_H2 cells in asthma are controlled by a complex interplay of interactions between innate and adaptive immune components, and major players from both arms of immunity play a role in the development of the disease (Fig. 4.4). In atopic individuals, sensitization to allergens first occurs when allergens are captured by immature DCs at sites of exposure and are presented to naïve T cells in secondary lymphoid organs, resulting in the generation of allergen-specific effector T_H2 cells and follicular Th cells or T_{FH} cells. T_{FH} cells are an important subset of helper T cells, whose primary function is to stimulate the activation and maturation of naïve B cells in the T-B cells areas of secondary lymphoid organs. The production of IL-4 by these cell types as well as the delivery of costimulatory signals such as CD40L-CD40 interactions is critical for the differentiation of naïve B cells into allergen-specific B cells that can produce elevated levels of allergen-specific IgE. Both IL-4 and IL-13 produced by T_H2 cells play a role in switching the immunoglobulin isotype from IgM to IgE. The release of high levels of circulating IgE by plasma cells is followed by the binding of IgE to its high affinity receptor, FcεRI, which is constitutively expressed on mast cells and basophils and is induced on eosinophils during inflammation. IgE-expressing mast cells and basophils now remain poised to interact with specific allergens upon allergen re-exposure. On allergen challenge, the effector phase begins consisting of an immediate early phase mostly characterized by mast cell and basophil activation, a late phase typically starting 6–9 h later when T cells and other leukocytes are recruited, and a chronic phase thereafter with the accumulation of eosinophils and other inflammatory cells. The effects of T cells and eosinophils during the effector phase lead to the classical symptoms of the disease described above (Fig. 4.5).

The Immediate Allergic Response: Acute Effects Mediated by IgE-Activated Mast Cells and Basophils

Historically, mast cell activation mediated by IgE antibodies is thought to play a critical role in the induction of allergic asthma. This is supported by linkage and pedigree analysis in humans which suggest an important role for IgE in atopy . Under normal conditions, IgE is the least abundant

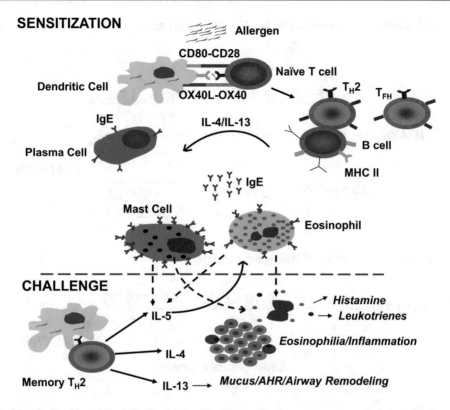

SENSITIZATION

Allergen

CD80-CD28

Naïve T cell

Dendritic Cell

OX40L-OX40

T_H2 T_{FH}

IgE

IL-4/IL-13

Plasma Cell

B cell

MHC II

IgE

Mast Cell

Eosinophil

CHALLENGE

IL-5

Histamine

Leukotrienes

IL-4

Eosinophilia/Inflammation

Memory T_H2

IL-13 ⟶ *Mucus/AHR/Airway Remodeling*

Fig. 4.4 Allergic Sensitization and Challenge. Sensitization to allergens occurs when atopic individuals encounter allergens for the first time and helper T cells are activated to the offending allergen. T_H2 cells produce cytokines resulting in the activation of B cells and the production of IgE antibodies. During re-exposure, mast cells bearing IgE are activated causing acute asthma attacks. Chronic airway inflammation and bronchoconstriction result from the activation of eosinophils and the action of cytokines such as IL-13 which induce airway hyperreactivity and mucus hypersecretion

antibody isotype in serum its levels can range from 0.6 to 10 ng/mL. In atopic individuals however, the levels rise from 100 to 1000 ng/mL. Similarly, patients with asthma also have elevated numbers of mast cells in their airways. Upon activation, either through IgE-dependent mechanisms or non-IgE dependent stimuli such as neuropeptides and complement components, mast cells can release a number of mediators (Fig. 4.6). These include preformed mediators such as **histamine**, proteoglycans, and serine proteases which can induce vasodilation, smooth muscle contraction, increased vascular permeability, mucus production, anticoagulant and anticomplement effects, and various enzymatic activities. In addition to pre-formed mediators, mast cells can also produce *de novo* synthesized mediators several hours after activation, which

contribute to the **late-phase response**. Prominent among these are the lipid mediators such as **cysteinyl leukotrienes** which induce a wheal and flare response, bronchoconstriction and constriction of smooth muscle, enhanced vascular permeability and mucus secretion, and **prostaglandin D2** which is a potent bronchoconstrictor; cytokines like TNF-α, IL-6, IL-1α, IL-3, GM-CSF, IL-4, IL-5, IL-13, all of which have potent effects on the on-going immune response by influencing recruitment and activation of Th2 cells; and chemokines like MCP-1, MIP-1β, MIP-1α, and RANTES which serve to attract eosinophils and other leukocytes.

IgE-induced mast cell activation occurs when polyvalent antigen crosslinks IgE molecules bound to FcεRI on the surface of tissue mast cells. This results in the immediate degranulation of

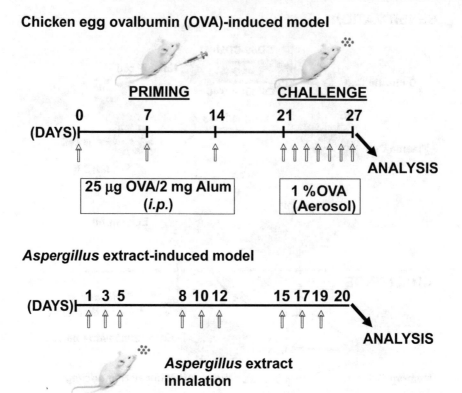

Fig. 4.5 Mouse models of acute allergic inflammation. Many of the key roles played by cells and molecules of the immune system in the pathophysiology of asthma were uncovered using animal models. While not perfectly resembling all the features of human asthma, various types of animal models have been developed to study both T$_H$2- and mast cell-dependent phases of asthma and the associated inflammation. The primary characteristic is typically to replicate the sensitization and challenge phases described above. This is usually done by either systemically priming mice (*i.p.* injections) with a low molecular weight antigen such as chicken egg ovalbumin followed by multiple intransal exposures or directly sensitizing them intransally with allergen extracts such as with intranasal house dust mite allergen, cockroach antigen or *Aspergillus* extract. Represented above are examples of OVA (Yiamouyiannis et al. 1999) and *Aspergillus*-induced (Mathias et al. 2009) models of allergic inflammation

mast cells and the release of vasoactive mediators and TNF-α, and an activation-induced signaling cascade that is dependent on FcεRI and other signaling molecules. The high affinity FcεRI receptor for IgE is present on a variety of cell types in humans including mast cells, basophils, and eosinophils and has also been shown to be expressed on DCs. A low affinity receptor for IgE, FcεRII or CD23, is also present on B cells and follicular DCs, and is found to be elevated in atopic individuals but decreased during remission.

The local effects of mast cell activation include vascular permeability leading to edema, and loss of intravascular fluid which causes erythema (Fig. 4.7). The cytokines IL-3, IL-4, IL-5 and IL-13 play pivotal roles during the development of asthma. IL-3 is an autocrine growth factor for mast cells and basophils; IL-4 causes upregulation of VLA-4 on epithelial surfaces promoting recruitment of T cells, monocytes and eosinophils; IL-5 is the key T$_H$2 cytokine involved in the differentiation, proliferation and migration of eosinophils; and IL-13 induces AHR, mucus hypersecretion, as well as fibrosis. Both IL-4 and IL-13 are also crucial for class switching of the IgM isotype to IgG and IgE on B cells.

Basophils, a population of bone marrow derived blood granulocytes that are distinct from mast cells, also play an important role during

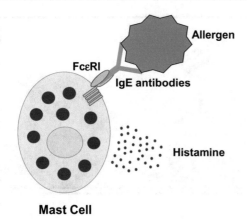

Mast Cell

Fig. 4.6 Mast cell activation. Mast cells are round or elongated granulocytes which mature in the periphery and are distributed throughout the connective tissue of the respiratory and gastrointestinal tracts and skin. They act as sentinel cells whose prototypical functions include sensing pathogens and alerting the immune system to presence of infection. Mast cells constitutively express the high affinity receptor for IgE, FcεRI. Upon sensitization, allergen-specific IgE is bound to FcεRI, ready to engage the allergen upon re-exposure. Allergen challenge results in cross-linking of bound IgE molecules and the induction of signaling cascades that result in mast cell degranulation and the release of pre-formed mediators within minutes after activation. Subsequently, activated mast cells also produce de novo synthesized mediators which include cytokines and cysteinyl leukotrienes (figure contributed by Jeffrey Rovatti)

allergic responses. Like mast cells, they also require IL-3 for their development, express FcεRI, and are activated upon IgE binding. Similarly, degranulation of basophils also results in the release of various vasoactive mediators, enzymes, and cytokines. More recently, basophils have been studied extensively for their role as initiators of the allergic response, since they are recruited to the lungs and nose soon after allergen challenge and can make copious amounts of IL-4 and IL-13. Additionally, they constitutively express both CD40L and CCR3 on their surface, indicating their potential for trafficking and activation. Their ability to produce extensive amounts of IL-4 has led some immunologists to hypothesize that they may be the key innate immune cell type that is involved in the sensitization of T_H2 cells. However, while a number of studies suggest their importance during allergic inflammation, this still remains to be established.

Did You Know: *Some People Ingest Worms to Cure Their Asthma?*

Many immunologists think the T_H2 arm of the immune system and its effector mechanisms, IgE-mediated mast cell and eosinophil responses, evolved to mediate host defenses against parasitic infections. In the absence of parasites, it is thought that T_H2 cells develop abnormally resulting in dysregulated responses to allergic substances. These insights have led to efforts by some patients and clinicians to reprogram their immune system by exposing it to parasites such as helminth worms. The goal of this type of therapy is to lessen the impact of allergic diseases by promoting anti-parasitic responses in allergic individuals.

Chronic Allergic Inflammation: The Role of CD4 T Cells

While mast cells play a critical role in the development of acute allergic episodes, treatments aimed at inhibiting mast cell function alone do not provide complete relief from symptoms. Patients with allergic asthma often exhibit AHR to non-specific stimuli even during asymptomatic phases. Over the years, it gradually became apparent to physicians and scientists studying allergic responses, that a more chronic inflammation was present in the airways of allergic patients, that appeared to be dominated by T_H2-specific lymphocytes, eosinophils, and other immune cells. Support for T cells as a principal mediator of asthma pathogenesis has come from a number of different studies (Fig. 4.8 and Table 4.4). Activated lymphocytes have been found to be present in the peripheral blood of asthmatics and T cells have been demonstrated in mucosal biopsies in patients with fatal asthma . In addition, asthmatic patients have been shown to have markedly increased numbers of CD4 T cells which are positive for CD25, VLA-1, and HLA-DR. A direct correlation between the numbers of activated T cells and activated eosinophils was also demonstrated. Furthermore, the

Fig. 4.7 Local effects of mast cell activation. When an allergen enters the epidermis or the dermis, mast cells are activated leading to a localized allergic response. At the injection site, heat, pain and swelling occur due to blood vessel dilation, an increase in vascular permeability and fluid extravasation (figure contributed by Jeffrey Rovatti)

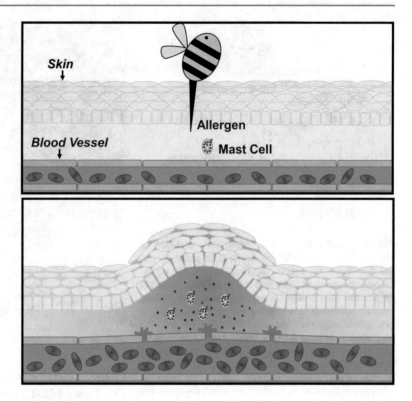

Asthma and the T$_H$2 hypothesis

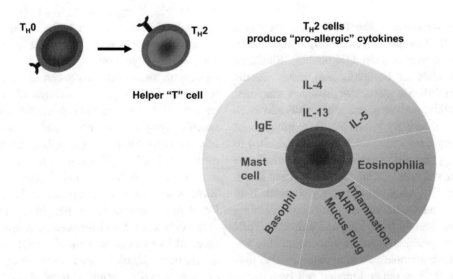

Fig. 4.8 T$_H$2 cells drive the allergic response. T$_H$2 cells produce a number of pro-allergic cytokines which drive the course of allergic inflammation. IL-4 induces the activation of B cells and serves as a positive regulator of T$_H$2 activation. Both IL-4 and IL-13 induce the class-switching of antibodies from IgM to IgE. IL-13 plays a central role in the development of AHR, mucus hypersecretion and fibrosis, also contributing to airway remodeling. IL-5 is critical for the differentiation, activation and survival of eosinophils. IL-9 and IL-10 promote mast cell proliferation and activation

Table 4.4 Key studies demonstrating a critical role for T_H2 cells in asthma

Study	Finding
Corrigan CJ, Hartnell A, Kay AB. *T lymphocyte activation in acute severe asthma*. Lancet **1988**; 1:1129–32.	Examination of T cell subsets in the peripheral blood of asthmatic patients demonstrated increased numbers of activated T cells
Azzawi M, Bradley B, Jeffery PK, Frew AJ, Wardlaw AJ, Knowles G, et al. *Identification of activated T lymphocytes and eosinophils in bronchial biopsies in stable atopic asthma*. Am Rev Respir Dis **1990**; 142:1407–13.	Examination of bronchial biopsies from asthmatic patients demonstrated the presence of activated T cells and increased numbers of eosinophils
Walker C, Kaegi MK, Braun P, Blaser K. *Activated T cells and eosinophilia in bronchoalveolar lavages from subjects with asthma correlated with disease severity*. J Allergy Clin Immunol **1991**; 88:935–42.	The broncholaveolar lavage of asthmatic patients contains increased numbers of activated T cells and eosinophils which can be correlated to disease severity.
Robinson DS, Hamid Q, Ying S, Tsicopoulos A, Barkans J, Bentley AM, et al. *Predominant TH2-like bronchoalveolar T-lymphocyte population in atopic asthma*. N Engl J Med **1992**; 326:298–304.	The bronchoalveolar lavage of asthmatic patients is characterized by expression of the cytokines IL-2, IL-4, IL-5, and GM-CSF, which is representative of a Th2 profile.
Gavett SH, Chen X, Finkelman F, Wills-Karp M. *Depletion of murine CD4+ T lymphocytes prevents antigen-induced airway hyperreactivity and pulmonary eosinophilia*. Am J Respir Cell Mol Biol **1994**; 10:587–93.	Depletion of CD4 T cells in mice results in attenuation of airway hyperreactivity and eosinophilia in a mouse model of asthma.
Brusselle GG, Kips JC, Tavernier JH, van der Heyden JG, Cuvelier CA, Pauwels RA, et al. *Attenuation of allergic airway inflammation in IL-4 deficient mice*. Clin Exp Allergy **1994**; 24:73–80.	The development of eosinophilia and airway inflammation was attenuated in mice deficient in IL-4 in a mouse model of asthma. This was further corroborated in mice deficient in MHC II, which lack mature CD4 T cells.
Foster PS, Hogan SP, Ramsay AJ, Matthaei KI, Young IG. *Interleukin 5 deficiency abolishes eosinophilia, airways hyperreactivity, and lung damage in a mouse asthma model*. J Exp Med **1996**; 183:195–201.	The development of eosinophilia, lung damage and airway hyperreactivity was abolished in IL-5 deficient mice in a mouse model of asthma. In contrast, reconstitution with IL-5 restored these features in allergic mice.
Hamelmann E, Oshiba A, Schwarze J, Bradley K, Loader J, Larsen GL, et al. *Allergen-specific IgE and IL-5 are essential for the development of airway hyperresponsiveness*. Am J Respir Cell Mol Biol **1997**; 16:674–82.	The transfer of allergen-specific IgE and IL-5 induces the development of airway hyperreactivity in a mouse model of allergic sensitization. AHR is only induced when allergen-specific IgE and not unrelated IgE is transferred.
Grunig G, Warnock M, Wakil AE, Venkayya R, Brombacher F, Rennick DM, et al. *Requirement for IL-13 independently of IL-4 in experimental asthma*. Science **1998**; 282:2261–3	Selective neutralization of IL-13 abolished the development of eosinophilia, AHR, and mucus production in a mouse model of asthma. Administration of IL-4 or IL-13 was able to induce an asthma-like phenotype in T cell-deficient mice.
Wills-Karp M, Luyimbazi J, Xu X, Schofield B, Neben TY, Karp CL, et al. *Interleukin-13: central mediator of allergic asthma*. Science **1998**; 282:2258–61.	IL-13 plays a critical role in the development of asthma by promoting AHR and mucus production. The development of asthma is completely inhibited in mice lacking IL-13.
Zhang DH, Yang L, Cohn L, Parkyn L, Homer R, Ray P, et al. *Inhibition of allergic inflammation in a murine model of asthma by expression of a dominant-negative mutant of GATA-3*. Immunity **1999**; 11:473–82.	Transgenic mice bearing a dominant-negative mutation in GATA-3 in a T cell specific fashion exhibit reduced levels of IL-4, IL-5, and IL-13 in a mouse model of asthma resulting in attenuation of eosinophilia, AHR, and mucus production.

Naïve CD4 T cells stimulated with antigen produce IL-2 and subsequently differentiate into various subsets including the T_H1 phenotype, characterized by the production of IL-2, TNF-β, IFN-γ, and dependent on the transcription factor T-bet, as well as the T_H2 phenotype characterized by the production of IL-4, IL-5, IL-9, IL-10 and IL-13 and dependent on the transcription factor GATA-3. Additional Th phenotypes include the T_H9, T_H17 and T_{FH} subsets, all of which have been implicated in the development of asthma. Evidence for the role of T_H2 cells in asthma has come from a number of studies done in both animals and humans. A brief synopsis of key studies demonstrating a role for T_H2 cells and its mediators is provided
Table contributed by Dylan Krajewski

T_H2 phenotype of these T cells was demonstrated by showing a positive correlation with expression of mRNA for IL-5 in the lung and for IL-3, IL-4, IL-5 and GM-CSF in the BAL. Animal models have also elucidated a role for CD4 T_H2 cells and the T_H2 cytokines IL-4, IL-5, IL-9, IL-10 and IL-13 in asthma development. Mice deficient in the Th1-inducing transcription factor, **T-bet**, develop exaggerated immune responses characteristic of a T_H2 phenotype suggesting that in these animals the naïve T cells are automatically programmed to become T_H2. In contrast, mice deficient in IL-4, IL-5, IL-13, **STAT-6** and **GATA-3**, which are T_H2-associated factors, do not develop asthma, further proving that T_H2 cells are essential for asthma development. Similarly, the dependence of eosinophilia, AHR, mucus hyperplasia and airway remodeling on the T_H2 cytokines IL-4, IL-5 and IL-13 is well-established. Recent evidence further demonstrates the importance of the T_H2 cytokines IL-3, IL-9 and IL-10 in driving mast cell expansion and activation during the allergic response. Taken together, the development of chronic allergic inflammation in asthmatic patients is critically dependent on the activation and function of allergen-specific T_H2 cells in the airways.

IL-5 and The Development of Eosinophilia

In addition to mast cell and basophil activation, the activation of IL-5-dependent eosinophils is a hallmark of allergic responses. Under normal conditions, the numbers of eosinophils in the bone marrow and tissues is very low. During parasitic infections and atopy, their numbers highly increase and they are present in tissues and blood where they can perform effector functions and release various mediators that can amplify the response. Eosinophils can be identified *in vivo* and *in vitro* by the presence of their many granules which have an affinity for acidic stains like eosin. They can also be identified by immunohistochemical staining for eosinophil-specific proteins such as **major basic protein** (MBP). Upon activation, eosinophils can release various toxic substances including MBP, eosinophil peroxidase, as well as lipid mediators such as leukotri-

enes and prostaglandins. MBP, particularly, is very toxic and has been observed in many patients with asthma and other allergic disorders. Administration of MBP has been shown to directly damage the cell membrane of target cells and induce AHR in animals. MBP can also activate platelets, mast cells, and basophils, and induce histamine release. Like mast cells, activated eosinophils also release a variety of cytokines and chemokines. These include IL-1β, IL-2, IL-3, IL-4, IL-5, IL-6, IL-8, IL-10, IL-12, IFN-γ, TNF-α, TGF-β, **RANTES** and MIP-1α which can have varying effects on the immune system and can act as growth factors for various cells. The recruitment of eosinophils to the airways and blood, and their extravasation to tissues depends on a number of factors in addition to IL-5, IL-3, and GM-CSF. This includes the expression of adhesion molecules such as ICAM-1 and VCAM-1 and the presence of many chemoattractants like RANTES, **eotaxin**, MIP-1α, MCP-3, and MCP-4. Once in the airways, activated eosinophils undergo degranulation and produce cytokines, promoting the release of various toxic factors, possibly affecting AHR and amplifying the allergic response.

T_H17 Responses and Severe Asthma

In contrast to chronic allergic inflammation, the airways of patients with severe asthma and those experiencing asthma exacerbations exhibit inflammation that is dominated by elevated numbers of neutrophils and T_H17 cells, suggesting that the development of disease in these individuals is T_H17-dependent. Both the sputum and the airways of these patients is characterized by marked elevation of activated neutrophils as well the T_H17 cytokines IL-17A and IL-17F. The exact mechanisms of neutrophilic inflammation in these patients is not well-understood and may be related to treatment with high doses of corticosteroids as well as co-existing bacterial or fungal infections.

Non-T_H2 Asthma

In contrast to the T_H2 and IgE-dependent mast cell-mediated allergic responses described above, many patients exhibit asthma symptoms, that is not associated with elevated production of IgE antibodies. These patients still exhibit many features of asthma such as eosinophilia, AHR, and mucus plugging. A wide variety of immune cell types have been thought to contribute to physiologic manifestations of asthma in these individuals including subsets of IL-4, IL-5 and IL-13 producing invariant NKT cells, NK cells and $\gamma\delta$ T cells.

More recently, accumulating evidence suggests a critical role for IL-33-dependent ILC2 cells in the mediation of AHR to protease allergens. By virtue of the ability to produce T_H2 cytokines such as IL-4, IL-5, IL-9 and IL-13, these cell types can promote asthmatic inflammation independently of T_H2 cells; however, they also contribute to the development of allergic inflammation in T_H2-sensitized atopic patients.

The mediation of non-atopic or intrinsic asthma by ILC2s can occur when they are exposed to protease allergens, such as *Derp1* derived from house dust mite (HDM), or the plant-derived cysteine protease papain. *Derp1* is known to induce eosinophilia and bronchoconstriction in asthmatic patients, while papain is a common causative agent of occupational asthma. Exposure to proteases such as papain, induces injury in epithelial cells, leading to the production of *danger* or *alarmin* cytokines including IL-33, IL-25, and TSLP. These cytokines subsequently induce the activation of multiple cell types including ILC2s, DCs, basophils and mast cells, which can promote various symptoms of the allergic response.

Co-conspirators: Th2 Cells, Mast Cells, and Eosinophils Drive Symptoms Associated with the Annually Occurring Allergic Disease, *Allergic Rhinitis*

Allergic Rhinitis is a commonly occurring allergic disease that is prevalent throughout the United States and observed in both adults and children. It is commonly referred to as hay fever, which is associated with allergic reactions to seasonal allergens such as pollen and ragweed. However, it comprises of two forms, which includes both the seasonal manifestation as well as persistent allergic rhinitis which is induced by non-seasonal allergens such as house dust mite, cat dander, and mold.

The hallmark of allergic rhinitis is the IgE-triggered activation of nasal mast cells on allergen exposure, leading to the generation of a thick, viscous nasal discharge consisting of mucus and eosinophils. The immune reaction is a classic example of the coordination exhibited by T_H2 cells, B cells, mast cells, and eosinophils in driving the allergic response observed in conditions such as asthma. Activated T_H2 cells produce cytokines such as IL-4 and IL-5, which respectively induce B cell activation and nasal eosinophilia. IgE produced by B cells triggers the activation of mast cells which secrete a number of substances including histamine, leukotrienes, and prostaglandins, which contribute to the observed symptoms. Common symptoms associated with allergic rhinitis include clear rhinorrhea, sneezing, nasal congestion, post-nasal drip, and itching in the eyes, ears, nose or palate. Histamine can contribute to all of these, as well as inducing vasodilation, vascular permeability and increased nasal secretions. Leukotrienes and prostaglandin D2 enhance mucus secretion and cause nasal obstruction.

Chronic Obstructive Pulmonary Disease

Chronic obstructive pulmonary disease or COPD is currently the third leading cause of death in the United States. The majority of COPD cases worldwide occur due to cigarette smoking and may be prevented by abstaining from using tobacco. In contrast to asthma, the major characteristic of COPD is the development of *progressive* airflow limitation that increases with age, resulting in wheezing, dyspnea, chest tightness, and difficulty breathing. Both chronic inflammation and alveolar damage contribute to the development of chronic bronchitis and/or emphysema, which results in mucus hypersecretion and various structural changes within the lung tissue, severely restricting the passage of air and making breathing difficult. Pharmacologic therapy can reverse the broncho-constriction developed due to inflammation and mucus hypersecretion; however, the structural damage of lung tissue is irreversible.

Pathophysiology of COPD

COPD has been characterized as an abnormal inflammatory response to noxious particles and gases resulting in pathologic effects that cause small airway disease and parenchymal damage. The latter involves significant destruction of lung tissue and loss of elasticity over time. As a result, unlike asthma, the damage caused by COPD is not fully reversible. Historically, COPD has been classified in terms of either **chronic bronchitis** or **emphysema**. Chronic bronchitis refers to chronic or excessive mucus production accompa-nied by cough for most days of at least 3 months in a year, for at least 2 consecutive years, when other causes of cough have been ruled out. Emphysema is defined in terms of anatomic pathology, characterized by the loss of elastic recoil due to permanent damage to alveolar sacs. This occurs due to inflammation in the small air-ways, which leads to destruction of alveolar walls, resulting in enlargement of the air sacs and loss of elasticity. Most patients exhibit symptoms of both bronchitis and emphysema, precluding the clinical differentiation of COPD into either of these specific subsets. Acute exacerbations of COPD tend to have an infectious basis. Viruses are the most important initiators of COPD exac-erbations, but bacteria can also contribute. As such, patients who present with exacerbations are often treated with antibiotics.

Cigarette smoking is the primary cause of COPD in 85–90% of patients and COPD can continue to progress in these patients even after they have stopped smoking. Exposure to second hand smoke can also contribute to the develop-ment of COPD in some patients. Other causative factors include exposure to occupational dusts and chemicals, air pollution, and host genetic fac-tors such as a rare defect in α1-antitrypsin (AAT).

The latter has significantly enhanced our under-standing of the pathophysiology of the disease since patients with a hereditary defect in AAT spontaneously go on to develop emphysema at an early age, resulting in rapid declines in lung func-tion. AAT is a 42 kDa protein produced by hepa-tocytes and its major function is to inhibit the effects of elastase, produced by activated neutro-phils during inflammation. In the absence of AAT, the destructive effects of elastase are ampli-fied, resulting in damage to alveolar tissue and the loss of lung function.

The pathophysiology of COPD is understood in terms of damage caused by the persistent induction of inflammatory and repair mecha-nisms that are triggered by exposure to noxious particles such as cigarette smoke. The develop-ment of inflammation induces the release of sev-eral oxidants and proteinases leading to increases in oxidative stress and damage to tissue. This is accompanied by the action of endogenously pro-duced anti-oxidants and anti-proteinases, further contributing to the inflammation. The resulting inflammation causes the development of small airway disease characterized by airway inflam-mation and airway remodeling as well as paren-chymal destruction involving loss of alveolar attachments and decrease of elastic recoil. The role of proteolytic defenses is further highlighted by the fact that although smokers are 12–13 times more likely to die from COPD, only 15–20% of smokers develop the disease, suggesting that individuals who have deficient anti-proteolytic defenses maybe more susceptible.

Human COPD has been found to be associated with four anatomic lesions: emphysema, airway remodeling including goblet cell metaplasia, chronic bronchitis, and pulmonary hypertension. Wright and Churg in 1990 demonstrated that chronic smoke exposure led to progressive emphysematous changes, reflected by mucus metaplasia, epithelial hypertrophy, and fibrotic remodeling of small airways. Chronic exposure to tobacco components such as nicotine provokes a powerful inflammatory response consisting pri-marily of neutrophils, but also macrophages and lymphocytes such as T_H17 cells and CD8 T cells. This is accompanied by the release of degradative enzymes such as elastase, serine proteases, phosphodiesterase 4, and matrix metalloproteinases, as well as numerous cytokines and chemokines, including TNF-α, IL-1β, IL-18, IFN-γ and CXCR2,3,5,6, which promote inflammation. Every puff of smoke consists of over 4000 chemicals and $>10^{15}$ free radicals. Free radicals (reactive oxygen and nitrogen species) and reactive chemicals such as aldehydes are believed to be culprits that activate resident lung cells causing the release of chemotactic mediators which recruit additional inflammatory cells into the lung. Chronic exposure to smoke perpetuates this response, leading to the increased production of cytokines and degradative enzymes as well as effects in homeostatic mechanisms (inactivation of anti-proteases, anti-oxidants and repair mechanisms). Lung function progressively deteriorates due to structural remodeling (narrowing of airways due to peribronchiolar fibrosis and luminal obstruction by inflammatory mucus exudates). The parenchyma is destroyed due to proteolytic damage reducing the elastic drive and gas-exchange surface area as well as loss of alveolar wall support structures. Small airway remodeling includes increased matrix components, inflammatory cells and goblet cell metaplasia in the airway wall with luminal narrowing, distortion, and obstruction by mucus. Animal models further demonstrate that cigarette smoke induces low-grade chronic inflammation. It has a transient acute phase dominated by neutrophils in the first week and a progressive chronic phase composed of neutrophils, macrophages and lymphocytes infiltrating the lungs 1 month after exposure. The inflammation is very slow to resolve and persists even in the absence of cigarette smoke (Table 4.5).

Immunopharmacology of the Drugs Used to Treat Respiratory Disorders

The drugs used to treat respiratory disorders such as asthma and COPD fall into two main categories (Table 4.6): (1) **Bronchodilators** which are used to relieve symptoms associated with bronchoconstriction and relax the smooth muscles and (2) **Anti-inflammatory agents** which sup-

Table 4.5 Immune Mechanisms contributing to the pathophysiology of COPD

Immune mechanisms contributing to inflammation in COPD
• Chronic inflammation consisting of neutrophils, macrophages, T_H17 cells, and CD8 T cells
• Neutrophils release elastases which degrade lung tissue
• Release of nitric oxide and super oxide radicals which further damage lung tissue
• Increased production of cytokines and degradative enzymes
• Destruction of lung parenchyma by proteolytic enzymes
• Narrowing of airways due to peribronchiolar fibrosis and mucus exudates
• Small airway remodeling due to increased matrix components, inflammatory cells and goblet cell metaplasia

Continuous exposure to inflammatory agents such as nicotine induce a powerful immune response that eventually results in the destruction of lung tissue, airway narrowing and airway remodeling. Activated neutrophils, macrophages, T_H17 cells, and CD8 T cells respond to cigarette smoke inducing damaging effects on respiratory components. Structural damage is further propagated by the release of numerous oxidants which results in the continuous induction of repair mechanisms and anti-oxidative pathways

Table 4.6 The two main arms of therapeutic treatment of asthma

Bronchodilators	Anti-inflammatory agents
• β2-agonists(short-acting and long-acting) • Methylxanthines (theophylline) • Anti-muscarinics/ cholinergics	• Inhaled and oral corticosteroids • Leukotriene receptor antagonists • Mast cell stabilizers (cromolyn sodium) • Anti-IgE (Omalizumab) • IL-5 antagonists

Bronchodilators relieve bronchoconstriction inducing smooth muscle relaxation and the opening of the airways. Anti-inflammatory agents induce the pathologic features associated with inflammation such as eosinophilia, mast cell activation, mucus secretion and bronchoconstriction

press the underlying inflammation associated with bronchoconstriction.

Over the last few years, bronchodilators have become the main stay of asthma therapy and **β2-agonists**, which trigger the **β2-adrenergic receptors** on smooth muscle cells and other immune cells have become the most commonly prescribed drugs for asthmatic patients. While short-acting β_2-agonists such as **albuterol** are frequently used as *rescue inhalers*, drugs prescribed for control of asthma typically involve the combination of both β_2-agonists and **inhaled corticosteroids (ICS)** which suppress the inflammatory component of the asthmatic lung. Other drugs used in the treatment of asthma include the **anti-muscarinic/cholinergic** drugs such as **ipratropium bromide** for relief of bronchoconstriction and various anti-inflammatories such as **leukotriene receptor antagonists (LTRA)**, **mast cell stabilizers**, and novel immune modulators such as **anti-IL-5**.

Bronchodilators also represent the main stay of pharmacologic therapy for patients with COPD. Short acting β_2-agonists may be used initially for patients with mild or intermittent symptoms. However, long acting bronchodilators, including **long-acting β_2-agonists** and **anti-muscarinics** are recommended for patients with chronic and progressive COPD. The use of **glucocorticoids** or inhaled corticosteroids is controversial, since they have variable to no effects.

In addition to their use for the treatment of allergic asthma, anti-inflammatory agents are also used for the treatment of allergic rhinitis. These include **anti-histamines** such as **histamine-receptor antagonists**, nasal steroids, mast cell stabilizers and LTRAs. In addition, topical and oral decongestants are also commonly used by patients with allergic rhinitis.

Lastly, specific immunotherapy involving desensitization to commonly occurring allergens is a major focus of therapeutic options for diseases such as asthma and allergic rhinitis.

In the section below, we describe the most commonly prescribed FDA-approved drugs for the treatment of asthma, COPD, and allergic rhinitis, with an emphasis on the immunopharmacology of the drugs involved and their therapeutic action.

Agents Targeting Bronchoconstriction

The development of bronchoconstriction, also referred to as AHR or bronchial hyperreactivity (BHR) is a cardinal characteristic of asthma as defined by the World Health Organization. All patients with asthma present with bronchoconstriction and the extent of airway constriction is a critical parameter used to classify patients according to clinically-defined phases such as mild, moderate, persistent, and severe. The severity of AHR can be assessed using established spirometric tests to determine the peak expiratory flow rate (PEFR) as well as the forced expiratory volume 1 (FEV1) prior to and after being challenged with increasing doses of a non-specific bronchoconstrictor such as methacholine. Most normal individuals exhibit some bronchoconstriction when exposed to high doses of methacholine. However, this is significantly enhanced in asthmatic individuals whose airways are already constricted due to severe inflammation, mucus plugs, and airway remodeling.

Although AHR is a significant feature of patients with allergic asthma, it can also be induced in individuals with non-atopic asthma and can be brought on by other causative agents such as sulfur dioxide, ozone, exercise, cold air, and cigarette smoking. Furthermore, both immune and non-immune factors contribute to its development. Immune factors include T_H2 cytokines such as IL-13 which can enhance the development of AHR while also inducing mucus hypersecretion, fibrosis, and airway remodeling. Similarly, eicosanoids such as leukotrienes produced during the late phase of mast cell activation also have a potent broncho-constrictive effect. However, treatment with anti-inflammatory drugs does not completely resolve AHR in allergic patients, but it can be significantly diminished when treated with drugs that act as airway smooth muscle relaxants or that target muscarinic receptors. As such, depending on the patient's specific circumstances, drugs with differing modes of action may prove to be less or more efficacious in resolving AHR. This includes drugs in numerous categories such as **sympathomimetic agents** (β-adrenergic agonists), inhibitors of mast cell degranulation (anti-IgE, **calcium channel blockers**, **cromolyn sodium**), inhibitors of preformed and *de novo* synthesized mast cell mediators (anti-histamines and leukotriene receptor antagonists) and inhibitors of neuro-muscular interactions (muscarinic antagonists). Finally, prolonged therapy with anti-inflammatory agents such as inhaled corticosteroids (ICS) can subdue the inflammation associated with AHR and prevent re-exposure to allergen.

Sympathomimetic Agents

Sympathomimetic agents, also referred to as "relievers" or "bronchodilators" are among the most commonly used drugs for the management and treatment of asthma. The use of these drugs can cause immediate reversal of airway obstruction in asthma by stimulating adrenoreceptors on airway smooth muscle cells and preventing the development of AHR. The major effects of sympathomimetics are triggered *via* mechanisms underlying the functioning of the autonomous nervous system. Circulating neurotransmitters such as noradrenaline and adrenaline produced by the sympathetic nervous system bind to sympathetic receptors present throughout the body including β_1 and α receptors present in the cardiovascular system, β_2 receptors present on airway smooth muscle cells, and β_3 receptors present on adipose tissue, ensuring that the body is in a constant state of readiness against potential attack. Sympathomimetic agents such as β-agonists (also called as adrenergic agents) mimic the sympathetic neurotransmitters, inducing excitement and tachycardia when they bind β_1 receptors, and airway smooth muscle relaxation when they bind β_2 receptors. Commonly used sympathomimetic agents include ephedrine, epinephrine, isoproterenol, and the β_2-agonists.

Ephedrine: Ephedrine was first isolated in 1887 from a Chinese herb used to relieve symptoms of asthma for thousands of years. It is a non-selective α-adrenoreceptor and β-adrenergic agonist that has low potency, a long duration of activity, but pronounced systemic effects due to its ability to bind multiple receptors. As a result, its use has fallen out of favor, particularly with the increasing use of drugs such as selective β_2-agonists.

Epinephrine: Epinephrine is a rapidly acting bronchodilator that has potent effects and can stimulate both α and β_1 receptors on cardiovascu-

lar cells and β_2 receptors on smooth muscle cells. It is extremely effective when administered both *via* subcutaneous as well as inhalational routes with maximal bronchodilation achieved within 15 min of inhalation. Because it has systemic effects, inducing smooth muscle relaxation and the raising of systolic blood pressure, it is the drug of choice for circumventing acute episodes of anaphylaxis and shock. However, adverse effects including tachycardia, arrhythmias and the worsening of angina pectoris have led to the cessation of its use in asthma in favor of the selective β_2-agonists.

Isoproteronol (Isoprenaline): Isoproteronol is a potent non-selective β_1 and β_2-agonist. It is rarely used in the treatment of respiratory disorders, since high doses can lead to fatal cardiac arrhythmias. However, when used as a last resort, it can lead to maximal bronchodilation within 5 min, lasting for 60–90 min.

β_2-Agonists and Their Mechanism of Action

β_2-agonists are currently the drug of choice for management of asthma symptoms and the most widely prescribed drugs for the treatment of asthma. Their effects are mediated by selectively binding to β_2 adrenoreceptors in the lung and inducing a sequence of intracellular signals leading to increases in cyclic adenosine monophosphate (cAMP) and changes in levels of intracellular calcium. The β-receptor selectivity of these drugs is conferred by modifying the terminal amine in the catechol ring of epinephrine.

β_2 adrenoreceptors are present throughout the respiratory tract including airway smooth muscle cells, epithelial cells, endothelial cells, and mast cells. They belong to the seven transmembrane receptor superfamily which classically signals through heterotrimeric **G-protein coupled receptors**. These receptors act as molecular switches that regulate downstream cellular processes by alternating from an inactive guanosine diphosphate (GDP) state to an active guanosine triphosphate (GTP) state. The activated G-protein then regulates the activation of other mediators such as adenylyl cyclase, phospholipase C, and **protein**

kinase A (PKA). The presumed effects of β_2-agonists are mediated through the activation of adenylyl cyclase coupled to a stimulatory G protein (Gs) resulting in an increase in intracellular cAMP and the activation of PKA (Fig. 4.9). The activation of PKA has a number of effects on the cell including decreasing intracellular calcium levels and the phosphorylation of various proteins that control airway smooth muscle tone and induce relaxation. In airway smooth muscle, PKA can also inactivate myosin light chain kinase, while activating myosin light chain phosphatase, thus directly inhibiting the contraction of smooth muscles and promoting their relaxation instead. PKA also facilitates the opening of large conductance calcium-activated potassium channels by inducing Ca^{++}/Na^{+} exchange (which results in a decrease of intracellular Ca^{++}) and stimulating the Na^{+}/K^{+} ATPase. This causes hyperpolarization of

the airway smooth muscle and reduction of acetylcholine levels. Activation of adenylyl cyclase can also cause the downstream activation of *Epac*, a Rap1 guanine nucleotide exchange factor, which induces relaxation in a PKA-independent manner through the downregulation of Rho. The combination of events mediated by adenylyl cyclase leads to bronchial smooth muscle relaxation and bronchodilation. In addition to the above mechanisms which act to directly relax airway smooth muscle, β_2-agonists can also indirectly lead to bronchodilation by inhibiting the release of mediators from mast cells, preventing vasodilation and edema induced by histamine and leukotrienes, and increasing mucociliary clearance.

Short-acting β_2 agonists (SABAs): Inhaled short-acting β_2 agonists are the most commonly used bronchodilators and are the drug of choice

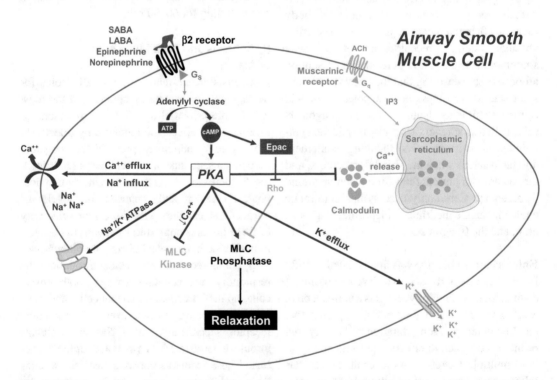

Fig. 4.9 The mechanism of action of β_2-agonists. Sympathomimetic agents such as β_2 agonists bind their receptors resulting in the activation of G-protein dependent adenylyl cyclase (AC). This results in the induction of protein kinase A (PKA), which inhibits the production of intracellular calcium, inhibits myosin light chain kinase and activates myosin light chain phosphatase, resulting in the relaxation of airway smooth muscle. PKA also enhances the activation of Ca^{++}-dependent K^{+} channels and increases K^{+} conductance resulting in the hyperpolarization of airway smooth muscle cells and decreased acetylcholine production. The grayed out areas represent activities that are inhibited through the actions of β_2-agonists (figure contributed by Jeremy P. McAleer)

121

for acute, severe asthma. They are also extremely effective when used to reduce bronchoconstriction caused by other factors such as cold air, exercise, and pollutants. They are typically used on an *as need* basis and not recommended for purposes of maintenance treatment. Drugs in this class include **albuterol (salbutamol)**, **terbutaline**, **metaproterenol**, and **pirbuterol**. Of these, albuterol is the most commonly used SABA in the United States. It is often used as a rescue inhaler, but may also be used as a nebulizing agent. Albuterol consists of a racemic mixture of active R and inactive S enantiomers. Based on some studies that suggested that the S isomer can promote AHR, a purified R isomer of the drug, **levalbuterol**, was developed. However, clinical studies have shown no increases in efficacy compared with albuterol, leading to the more infrequent use of the purified derivative. Of the above drugs, albuterol and terbutaline are available in oral form, and terbutaline may be given subcutaneously in cases of emergency when inhalation therapy is unavailable or is ineffective.

Long-acting β_2 agonists (LABAs): Catechol amines are normally degraded by the Catechol-O-methyltransferase and monoamine oxidase pathways. Modification of the amines to produce longer aliphatic chains results in resistance to degradation and a longer duration of action, leading to the development of the long-acting β_2-agonists. These drugs have a longer duration of action (12 h or more) as a result of high lipophilicity which allows these drugs to bind to the cell membrane at very high concentrations. Drugs in this class include **salmeterol** (which has a longer aliphatic chain) and **formoterol** (which has a bulky substitution in its aliphatic chain). Formoterol is a full agonist that has a rapid onset of action, while salmeterol has a slower onset of action and is partially agonistic. A stereoselective version of formoterol (**arformoterol**) has also been developed, but like levalbuterol has no clinical advantage over the racemic mixture. Due to the longer duration, these drugs only need to be taken twice a day compared to several doses of short acting agonists. However, since none of these drugs are anti-inflammatory, they must not be used as monotherapy. Long-term monotherapy using LABAs has been associated with adverse effects, including fatality in some patients. It is also thought that monotherapy results in the eventual downregulation of β_2 receptors on smooth muscle cells, leading to resistance and ineffectiveness of treatment. Instead, LABAs are often prescribed in conjunction with inhaled corticosteroids which selectively treat the underlying respiratory inflammation. Such combination inhalers are extremely effective, not only simplifying the ease of treatment, but also acting in a synergistic manner and enhancing the effects of both drugs in the asthmatic lung. Examples of combination inhalers that contain a LABA and an inhaled corticosteroid include **Advair® (fluticasone/salmeterol)** and **Symbicort® (budesonide/formoterol)**.

The use of inhaled drugs such as the β_2-agonists has significantly reduced side effects associated with systemic oral or intravenous therapy. However, adverse effects can occur especially when large doses are used. These include muscle tremors due to the stimulation of β_2 receptors in skeletal muscle, tachycardia and palpitations due to the stimulation of atrial β_2 receptors and/or β_1 receptors on cardiac cells, hypokalemia due to the entry of potassium into skeletal muscle leading to cardiac arrhythmias, and ventilation-perfusion mismatch.

Anti-muscarinic/Anti-cholinergic Agents

The primary rationale behind the use of anti-muscarinic agents is to target bronchoconstriction induced by parasympathetic mechanisms leading to the stimulation of acetylcholine muscarinic receptors on bronchial smooth muscle cells in the airways. Under normal scenarios, acetylcholine, a cholinergic neurotransmitter produced by post-ganglionic neurons of the vagal nerve stimulates muscarinic receptors leading to contraction of airway smooth muscle and increases in mucus secretion (see Fig. 4.10). Airway damage either *via* allergen exposure in allergic asthma or exposure to irritants such as ozone and sulfur dioxide in chronic asthma can enhance stimulation of the parasympathetic

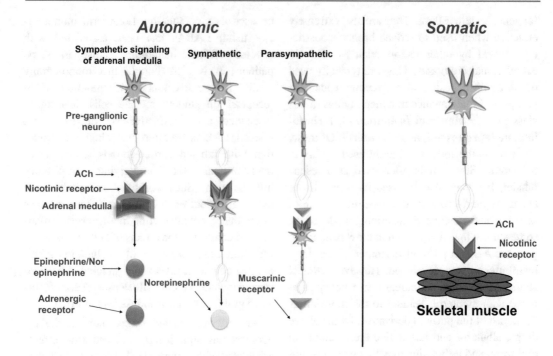

Fig. 4.10 The peripheral nervous system. The peripheral nervous system consists of the somatic and autonomic nervous system. The somatic nervous system is associated with the voluntary control of body movements via skeletal muscles and regulates sensory stimuli related to vision, smell, taste, temperature, and other senses. The effects of the somatic nervous system are mediated through neurotransmitters such as acetylcholine that act on effector cells. The autonomic nervous system on the other hand is associated with the involuntary control of bodily function that occurs below the level of conscious-ness. It consists of sympathetic nervous system which is typically associated with the *fight or flight* response and the parasympathetic system which is associated with the *rest, relaxation, and digestion.* The autonomic nervous system regu-lates body functions such as respiratory rate, heart rate, and digestion. Its effects are mediated via pre- and post-ganglionic neurons, which serve as a link between the central nervous system and effector cells. Pre-ganglionic neurons release acetyl-choline in the synaptic area, which then binds nicotinic cholinergic receptors at the postsynaptic membrane. In the sympa-thetic nervous system, post-ganglionic neurons release norepinephrine, which binds to α_1 receptors in the smooth muscles, β_1 receptors in the heart muscle, β_2 receptors in the smooth muscles, and α_2 adrenergic receptors. Similarly, stimulation of nicotinic receptors in the adrenal medulla results in the release of epinephrine, which binds adrenergic receptors in effector tissues. In contrast, the post-ganglionic neurons of the parasympathetic nervous system release acetylcholine, which binds muscarinic receptors in various tissues including the stomach, heart, and smooth muscles (figure contributed by Dylan Krajewski)

system leading to increased acetylcholine production and stimulation of muscarinic recep-tors. Induction of inflammation and production of proinflammatory cytokines such as TNF-α can further induce the secretion of acetylcholine by non-neuronic cells such as epithelial cells in the respiratory tract. Thus, a number of mechanisms, including both immunological and non-immunological can lead to vagal stimulation resulting in muscarinic receptor stimulation and contraction of airway smooth muscle. Anti-muscarinic agents used in asthma or COPD

selectively block the stimulation of muscarinic receptors in the respiratory tract, thus inhibiting smooth muscle contraction and increased mucus secretion.

Atropine, a purified plant alkaloid, has been widely used to curtail the effects of parasympa-thetic system resulting in reduced smooth muscle contraction. It acts by competitively inhibiting the binding of acetylcholine to its receptor, thus preventing muscarinic stimulation. However, atropine, is widely absorbed into circulation and readily enters the central nervous system by

Table 4.7 Bronchodilators used in the treatment of asthma and COPD

	Mechanism of action	Adverse effects	MDI	DPI	Nebulizing solution	Tablet	Syrup
Short Acting β_2-Agonists (SABA)							
Albuterol (ProAir®, Proventil®, Ventolin®)	Relaxes smooth muscle of bronchial passages by activating β_2 adrenergic receptors in the lungs.	• Tremors • Tachycardia and palpitations • Hypokalemia • Nervousness and restlessness • Metabolic effects	X		X	X	
Levalbuterol (Xopenex®)			X		X		
Metaproterenol (Alupent®)						X	X
Long Acting β_2-agonist (LABA)							
Salmeterol (Serevent Diskus®)	Relaxes smooth muscle of bronchial passages by activating β_2 adrenergic receptors in the lungs.	• Tremors • Tachycardia and palpitations • Hypokalemia • Nervousness and restlessness • Metabolic effects		X			
Formoterol (Perforomist®)					X		
Indacaterol (Arcapta Neohaler®)				X			
Arformoterol (Brovana®)					X		
Olodaterol (Striverdi Respimat®)			X				
Short acting muscarinic antagonist (SAMA)							
Ipratropium bromide (Atrovent®)	Relaxes smooth muscle of bronchial passages by inhibiting acetylcholine at type 3 muscarinic receptors (M_3) in the lungs.	• Dry mouth • Bronchitis • Myocardial infarction	X		X		
Long acting muscarinic antagonist (LAMA)							
Tiotropium (Spiriva Respimat®; Spiriva Handihaler®)	Relaxes smooth muscle of the bronchial passages by inhibiting acetylcholine at type 3 muscarinic receptors (M_3) in the lungs.	• Dry mouth • Constipation • Urinary retention	X	X			
Glycopyrronium (Seebri Neohaler®)				X	X		
Aclidinium (Tudorza Pressair®)				X			
Umeclidinium (Incruse Ellipta®)				X			

Table contributed by Kaitlin Armstrong; *MDI*: metered dose inhaler; *DPI*: dry powder inhaler

crossing the blood-brain barrier. In contrast, **ipratropium bromide** (Table 4.7).

(Atrovent®), a selective quaternary ammonium derivative of atropine is poorly absorbed from the respiratory and gastrointestinal tracts and does not cross the blood-brain barrier, in effect, serving as a much more potent inhibitor of muscarinic receptors for patients with asthma and COPD. It binds to the M_1-M_3 receptors which are expressed throughout the bronchial smooth musculature as well as nerve ganglion endings. For example, both the M_1 and M_2 receptors are expressed in parasympathetic ganglia, where the M_1 receptors facilitate neurotransmission, thus enhancing bronchoconstriction, and the M_2 receptors inhibit acetylcholine, thus contributing to feedback inhibition. M_2 receptors are also present in the heart. M_3 receptors are present on smooth muscle cells, where their stimulation causes bronchoconstriction and enhanced mucus secretion. Ipratropium bromide has varied effects on bronchodilation in patients with asthma with both modest to potent effects observed. In patients with acute severe asthma, it is effective when given in conjunction with inhaled albuterol. Ipratropium bromide only targets the parasympathetic system, and in terms of efficacy of bronchodilation, it is far less superior to β_2-agonists. This may be due to the fact that bronchoconstriction in asthma is a complex result of a number of factors including immunological stimuli such as leukotrienes and IL-13 produced by mast cells and Th2 cells, as well as, non-immunological stimuli resulting from fibrosis and airway remodeling. In contrast, ipratropium bromide is extremely effective as a bronchodilator in patients with COPD who have partially reversible bronchoconstriction.

Longer acting antimuscarinic agents such as **tiotropium** and **aclidinium** have now been approved as maintenance therapy for COPD patients. Tiotropium (Spiriva ®) is a potent selective anti-muscarinic agent, because although it binds all 3 muscarinic receptors, it rapidly dissociates from the M_2 receptor, thus not engaging the M_2-mediated negative feedback pathway, which normally results in increased acetylcholine production. As such, tiotropium is much more effective than ipratropium, and is becoming a bronchodilator of choice for COPD patients due to its potency and ease of use. Anti-muscarinic agents are usually well-tolerated although there has been some concern about increased dryness, especially in the mouth, due to decreased mucus secretion.

Methylxanthines

Methylxanthines, particularly **theophylline**, are some of the most widely prescribed drugs for the treatment of asthma worldwide, due to their ease of availability and low cost. Theophylline, a dimethylxanthine, is present in trace amounts in tea and cocoa beans and has been used in the treatment of asthma since 1922. However, despite the widespread use of methylxanthines globally, their use in developed countries as a mainstay of asthma treatment has fallen out of favor due to the high number of toxicities associated with increased concentrations of the drug, and with the advent of the use of more effective bronchodilators. Intravenous **aminophylline** in particular, a diethylene salt of theophylline, was previously widely used for the treatment of acute, severe, asthma, but is less commonly used now, due to the efficacy of inhaled β_2-agonists. Instead, theophylline and other methylxanthines are now used more commonly as add-on therapy in patients with uncontrolled asthma despite the use of inhaled corticosteroids, and in patients with COPD unresponsive to bronchodilator therapy. Oral rapid release theophylline tablets exist, but these result in wide fluctuations in plasma levels of the drug and are not recommended. Instead, slow-release preparations, which are very effective, are more commonly used, especially in the treatment of nocturnal asthma. In patients with chronic asthma, theophylline may often be added as adjunct therapy along with inhaled corticosteroids, providing better symptom control and lung function than increasing the dose of ICS by itself.

At low concentrations, theophylline has been shown to have several anti-inflammatory effects in both asthma and COPD. However, relatively higher concentrations are required for its efficacy as a bronchodilator, also increasing the risk of toxic side effects. Several mechanisms have been proposed for the effects of theophylline on the inhibition of inflammation and relaxation of airway smooth muscle, and it is likely that the anti-inflammatory pharmacologic effects are the cumulative result of a number of mechanisms rather than a single mode of action.

Mechanism of Action of Theophylline

Phosphodiesterase inhibition: At low concentrations, theophylline is a weak, non-selective inhibitor of **phosphodiesterase (PDE)** enzymes, which are required for the breakdown of cyclic nucleotides within the cell. As such, inhibition of

PDE results in enhanced levels of both intracellular cAMP and cGMP (in some tissues). Cyclic AMP in particular plays an important role in controlling airway smooth muscle tone *via* effector signaling molecules such as PKA and in decreasing activation of inflammatory genes by suppressing intracellular calcium. Inhibition of PDE3 has been shown to be important in relaxing airway smooth muscle, while PDE4 appears to be involved in regulating the release of immune cytokines and chemokines. Of note, inhibition of PDE has also been shown to result in increased concentrations of IL-10, which may account for some of the protective regulatory effects observed. While the anti-inflammatory effects mediated by PDE inhibition can be observed at low concentrations, much higher levels are required for maximum bronchodilator effect.

Adenosine Receptor Antagonism: Adenosine has been shown to have potent effects on airway mast cells resulting in the release of histamines and leukotrienes, thus contributing to increases in bronchoconstriction in asthmatic patients. Theophylline antagonizes the adenosine receptors A_1 and A_2 but is much less potent at blocking A_3 receptors. Furthermore, blockade of A_1 receptors can have serious side effects, including cardiac arrhythmias and seizures, which have been typically associated with high doses of theophylline.

Inhibition of immune gene activation and cell survival: At high concentrations, theophylline has also been shown to prevent the degradation of IκB, likely through PDE inhibition, thereby preventing the translocation of NF-κB into the nucleus and the subsequent activation of various T_H2 cytokine genes. It has also been shown to decrease levels of the anti-apoptotic protein BCl_2 and promote the apoptosis of T_H2 cells and neutrophils, thus decreasing cell survival. Similarly, low dose theophylline has been shown to inhibit the late asthmatic response and eosinophil influx after inhaled allergen exposure, as well as reduce the numbers of eosinophils in the BAL and bronchial biopsies. In patients with COPD, it can also reduce the number of neutrophils in induced sputum and decrease the concentrations of CXCL8, a chemokine required for neutrophil migration.

Histone Deacetylase Activation: A primary event during the activation of various immune genes is the acetylation of core histone proteins, that have been turned on by the activity of transcription factors such as NF-κB. The anti-inflammatory effects of corticosteroids are mediated by histone deacetylases such as HDAC2, which have been recruited to the gene complex through the activation of glucocorticoid receptors. HDAC2 deacetylates core histones turned on by histone acetyl transferases (HATs), resulting in the suppression of inflammatory genes. Theophylline, similarly, turns on HDAC2 at extremely low concentrations, by selectively inhibiting PI3K-δ, which is activated by oxidative stress and can inhibit HDAC2 activity by inducing increases in the concentrations of phosphorylative radicals.

Phosphodiesterase 4 (PDE4) Inhibitors

PDE4 inhibitors such as **roflumilast** have recently been approved for the treatment of COPD. Like theophylline, roflumilast inhibits PDE4, resulting in raised levels of cAMP within the cell and increased PKA activation, leading to smooth muscle relaxation. Roflumilast is effective in severe COPD associated with smoke-induced inflammation and emphysema. Although it reduces exacerbations, it is not effective at improving lung function in COPD patients. It is not an effective bronchodilator for the treatment of asthma.

Agents Targeting Inflammation

Corticosteroids

A key defining characteristic of asthma is that its pathophysiology is underscored by a complex interplay of many different immune mechanisms, including various cell types as well as both pro- and anti-inflammatory mediators that induce subtle variations in the manifestation of the disease and that contribute to both acute and chronic episodes of asthma. This sophisticated cross-talk between immune cells such as activated T_H2 cells, B cells, and mast cells and the action of diverse cytokines such as IL-4, IL-5, and IL-13 contribute both to the development and degree of the severity of eosinophilic inflammation, airway hyperreactivity, mucus plugging and airway remodeling in patients with asthma. The absence of a single anti-inflammatory agent that inhibits all the inflammatory symptoms associated with asthma further underscores this fact. Hence, the advent of the use of corticosteroids which significantly suppressed inflammation during various stages of asthma including acute and chronic, was a significant breakthrough in asthma pharmacotherapy and its management. Indeed, corticosteroids are the most effective treatment in the management of asthma and inhaled corticosteroids (ICS) are considered the first line treatment for children and adults with chronic asthma.

Mechanism of Action of Corticosteroids

Although the overall mechanism of action of corticosteroids is poorly understood, several recent studies suggest that corticosteroids have diverse effects on inflammatory pathways during asthma leading both to the activation and repression of genes involved in immune activation.

Since corticosteroids suppress the function of a number of immune cytokines as well as increase the activation of anti-inflammatory mediators during asthma, it was thought that they acted by directly targeting the genes for these molecules. Some of the effects of corticosteroid treatment include: decreased expression of adhesion molecules, resulting in decreased emigration of leukocytes; induction of endonucleases resulting in apoptosis of lymphocytes and eosinophils; decreased production of phospholipase A2 and cyclooxygenase type 2 resulting in decreased production of prostaglandins and leukotrienes; decreased production of nitric oxide synthase; decreased production of IL-1, TNF-α, IL-3, IL-4, IL-5 among other cytokines resulting in a net decrease in inflammation.

However, it is now clear that corticosteroids act by two different mechanisms (Fig. 4.11): one by directly inducing the binding of glucocorticoid

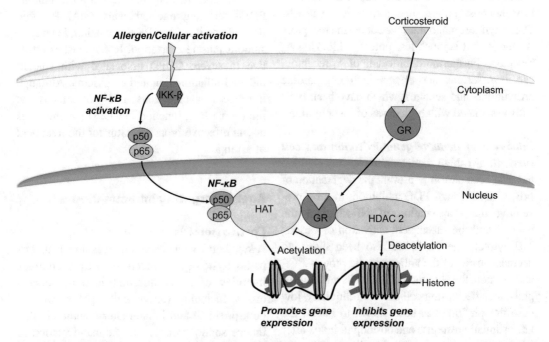

Fig. 4.11 Mechanism of action of corticosteroids. Corticosteroids diffuse through the plasma membrane into the cytoplasm where they bind glucocorticocoid receptors (GR). The steroid-receptor complex then moves into the nucleus where they bind DNA sequences in the promoter regions of various genes conferring steroid responsiveness. Additionally, the steroid-receptor complex also binds histone acetyl transferases (HATs) inhibiting their activity and instead promotes the recruitment of histone deacetylases resulting in suppression of gene expression (figure contributed by Dylan Krajewski)

response elements (GRE) in a gene that results in increased transcription of a gene, and two, by binding to transcriptional co-activators that result in suppression of transcription of a particular gene.

These processes are initiated by the diffusion of corticosteroids through the plasma membrane into the cytoplasm where they bind specific glucocorticoid receptors (GRs). These receptors are normally present bound to cytoplasmic molecular chaperone proteins. Binding to the glucocorticoid results in a conformational change in the receptor, leading to dissociation of the molecular chaperone, and exposure to nuclear localization signals, resulting in transport of the corticosteroid-receptor complex to the nucleus. Here they may bind directly to GREs which are specific DNA sequences present in the promoter regions of several genes that confer steroid responsiveness. The number of genes directly regulated by corticosteroids can range from 10 to 100, usually resulting in increased transcription and protein synthesis. Examples of genes that may be directly activated during asthma include antiproteases, IL-10, and IκB-α.

However, the primary mechanism by which suppression of inflammation is achieved by corticosteroids is the inhibition of histone acetylation which is required for the activation of genes that are turned on by proinflammatory transcription factors. In particular, the transcription factor nuclear factor-kappa B (NF-κB) plays a critical role in the activation of several genes that are turned on in T_H2 cells, mast cells, and eosinophils during allergic responses. NF-κB is normally present in the cytoplasm bound to the cytoplasmic protein IκB. When cells are activated *via* receptors such as toll-like receptors (TLRs), the T cell receptor, FcεRI, or other receptors such as the ST2 receptor for IL-33, complex signaling cascades are initiated that are punctuated by a series of phosphorylative events that typically terminate in the phosphorylation and degradation of IκB. The degradation of IκB results in the release and the migration of NF-κB to the nucleus where it turns on the genes for a number of cytokines, including IL-1, TNF-α, and the various T_H2-specific cytokines. When NF-κB is activated in the nucleus, it not only binds to specific DNA

sequences in the genes for immune cytokines, but also to coactivator molecules that have intrinsic histone acetyl transferase (HAT) activity and act as molecular switches of gene transcription. Increased acetylation increases the transcription of the activated genes and induces their production, which is reversed by corticosteroids by suppressing histone acetylation. Activated glucocorticoid receptors can also bind to coactivators directly and decrease their HAT activity, but additionally, they also recruit histone deacetylases such as HDAC2, which deacetylate the histones and repress gene transcription.

Thus a combination of both gene activation and gene repression is involved in the mechanism by which corticosteroids suppress inflammation during asthma. In addition to its anti-inflammatory effects, corticosteroids have also been found to increase β adrenergic responsiveness and enhance the effects of β agonists. In a similar manner, β agonists have also been found to enhance the activity of corticosteroids by enhancing the transport of glucocorticoid receptors to the nucleus. Thus, it is likely that when used in combination, both corticosteroids and β agonists synergistically lead to improvement of lung function in asthma. However, it must be noted, that the use of neither represents a cure and only provides temporary relief, since the cessation of administration results in renewal of symptoms. Moreover, as mentioned earlier, monotherapy with LABAs without treating the underlying inflammatory component is contraindicated in the treatment of asthma.

While glucocorticoids are extremely effective at controlling the inflammation present in asthma, they can have significant adverse effects when administered orally, systemically, or for long periods of time. In addition to inducing immunosuppression, corticosteroids can also disrupt pathways involved in other systems due to its effects in decreasing cortisol secretion from the pituitary gland. This can result in a number of serious long-term side-effects including among others: fluid retention, increased appetite, weight gain, osteoporosis, hypertension, and psychosis.

Commonly used systemic corticosteroids include **prednisone, prednisolone,** and **dexamethasone**. These were developed by modification of the structure of hydrocortisone (cortisol), the endogenous glucocorticoid secreted by the adrenal cortex. **Methylprednisolone** is used intravenously. Oral corticosteroids include prednisone and prednisolone. Inhaled corticosteroids (ICS) are most effective at avoiding the adverse effects associated with systemic or oral administration and directly target the lung. Commonly used ICS include: **beclomethasone dipropionate, triamcinolone, budesonide, fluticasone, fluticasone propionate, mometasone furoate,** and **ciclesonide**. In addition to systemic, oral, and inhaled steroids, a number of intranasal steroids are used in the treatment of allergic rhinitis (Table 4.8).

Mast Cell Stabilizers (Cromolyn Sodium)

Mast cell stabilizers have been an attractive therapeutic option due to their specific effects on IgE-mediated mast cell activation and low side effect profile. **Cromolyn sodium (sodium cromoglycate)**, a derivative of *khellin* (an Egyptian herbal remedy) was once widely used in children and adults for relief associated with asthma. Its putative mechanism of action includes a dose-dependent inhibition of inflammatory mediators by mast cells post IgE-activation and the blocking of early and late responses in mast cells. Although it does not reverse bronchoconstriction, it has been found to be useful for the treatment of allergen or exercise-induced asthma. However, due to its low solubility and absorption from the gastrointestinal tract, as well as the more potent

Table 4.8 Commonly used corticosteroids in the treatment of allergic diseases

Corticosteroids					
	Mechanism of action	**Adverse effects**	**Inhaled**	**Intranasal**	**Oral**
Beclomethasone (Qvar Redihaler®; Beconase AQ®)	Reduces inflammatory mediators by silencing the proinflammatory transcription factor NF-κB in airway structural cells and immune cells.	• Nose or throat irritation	X	X	
Budesonide (Pulmicort Flexhaler®; Rhinocort®)		• Cough • Oral thrush	X	X	
Ciclesonide (Alvesco®; Omnaris®)		• Adrenal suppression	X	X	
Fluticasone (Flovent®; Flonase®)		• Osteoporosis	X	X	
Mometasone (Nasonex®; Asmanex Twisthaler®)		• Hypertension • Cataracts or	X	X	
Triamcinolone (Nasacort®)		Glaucoma • Psychosis • Fragile skin or acne • Elevated blood glucose	X	X	
Methylprednisolone (Medrol®)		• Peptic ulceration			X
Prednisone (Deltasone®)		• Adrenal			X
Hydrocortisone (Cortef®)		suppression • Osteoporosis • Hypertension • Cataracts or Glaucoma • Psychosis • Cushingoid appearance • Fragile skin or acne • Elevated blood glucose			X

Table contributed by Kaitlin Armstrong

effects exerted by other anti-inflammatory inhibitors such as ICS and leukotriene inhibitors, it is no longer used clinically.

Leukotriene Antagonists

Cysteinyl leukotrienes (cys LTs) are potent inflammatory mediators produced by mast cells and eosinophils during the late phase allergic response. They are derived from the **5-lipoxygenase** mediated pathway of arachidonic acid metabolism in contrast to prostaglandins which are derived through the cyclooxygenase pathway. The leukotrienes are a hundred times more potent than histamine and have similar functions, including inducing vasodilation, smooth muscle contraction, increased bronchial reactivity and mucus hypersecretion. Leukotriene (LT) C4 and LTD4 are primarily produced during the late phase asthmatic response. In contrast, LTB4 is implicated during COPD and is a potent attractor of neutrophils. The effects of leukotrienes are mediated by binding specific receptors on the surface of proinflammatory cells including immune cells such as T cells and smooth muscle cells. Leukotriene receptor antagonists (LTRAs) block the binding of leukotrienes to their receptors, thus inhibiting the development of inflammation, edema and smooth muscle hyperreactivity.

Drug development has resulted in the approval of several antagonists that inhibit the actions of leukotrienes (Fig. 4.12). **Zileuton** is a direct inhibitor of 5-lipoxygenase, whereas **montelukast** and **zafirlukast** are inhibitors of the cysteinyl leukotriene receptor 1 or the **LTD4 receptor**. Both classes of drugs have been shown to improve asthma control and reduce asthma exacerbations. Although they are less effective than ICS in reducing inflammation overall, they are very effective at preventing exacerbations. Additionally, they are extremely effective in patients with aspirin-sensitive asthma, who may experience bronchoconstriction and histamine release on aspirin consumption.

Anti-IgE (Omalizumab)

The production of allergen-specific IgE antibodies is a hallmark of allergic asthma and IgE-mediated mast cell activation and degranulation is a critical feature of acute episodes of asthma. Omalizumab is a humanized monoclonal antibody that was developed in the 1990s and approved by the FDA in 2003 for the treatment of severe persistent asthma in patients greater than 12 years. It was also approved in 2014 for the treatment of chronic spontaneous urticaria. Omalizumab specifically binds the Fc portion of soluble IgE, thus preventing its binding to both the high affinity IgE receptor FcεRI on mast cells, basophils, eosinophils and dendritic cells, and the low affinity receptor FcεRII (CD23) on B cells (Fig. 4.13). This not only results in the inhibition of immune cell activation *via* IgE and allergen cross-linking, but also diminishes the total IgE repertoire by affecting the levels of expression of both FcεRI and CD23. Furthermore, it inhibits the activation of mast cells by IgE-mediated mechanisms during future episodes of allergen exposure. Omalizumab treatment does not prevent the activation of mast cells *via* pre-bound IgE or non-IgE mediated mechanisms. Omalizumab is reserved for patients with severe asthma who do not respond to high doses of ICS and β_2-agonist treatment. While it is effective at significantly reducing asthma exacerbations, it needs to be administered subcutaneously every 2–4 weeks and rarely anaphylactic responses have been observed.

Cytokine Inhibitors

Advances in basic science research over the last few decades have led to significant insights into the mechanisms of allergic inflammation, leading to the development of several novel therapeutic targets aimed at eliminating asthma symptoms. Some of these which have already received FDA approval or are in the process of being approved include specific cytokine modulators, which target the proallergic cytokines produced by T_H2 cells and other immune cells during allergic inflammation.

IL-5 Antagonists

IL-5 is critical for the development of eosinophilia, contributing to chronic bronchial inflammation observed in the airways of asthmatic patients. The

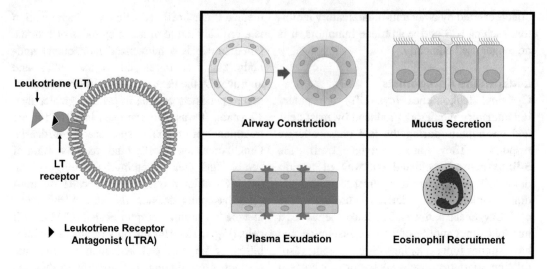

Fig. 4.12 Mechanism of action of leukotriene receptor antagonists (LTRA)s. Cysteinyl leukotrienes are produced as a by-product of the 5-lipoxygenase pathway of arachidonic acid metabolism. The leukotrienes LTD4 and LTE4 bind the LTD4 receptor inducing airway constriction, mucus secretion, plasma exudation and eosinophil recruitment. LTRAs such as montelukast and zafirlukast (black triangle) inhibit the binding of these leukotrienes, thereby preventing bronchoconstriction and reducing inflammation (figure contributed by Jeffrey Rovatti)

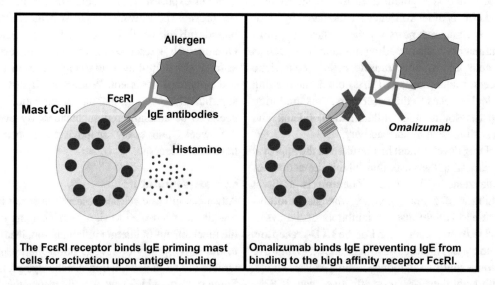

Fig. 4.13 Mechanism of action of Omalizumab. Omalizumab is a humanized IgG antibody specific for the Fc portion of IgE. Treatment with omalizumab prevents the binding of IgE to both FcεRI and FcεRII, thereby diminishing mast cell activation and suppressing the production of IgE antibodies (figure contributed by Jeffrey Rovatti)

development of airway eosinophilia is a key characteristic of allergic asthma and in many patients is linked to the development of other pathologic features including AHR and mucus production. However, the inhibition of eosinophilia, while providing relief from damage caused by eosinophils and decreasing airway inflammation, does not always result in the attenuation of bronchoconstriction. As such, anti-IL-5 treatment is focused on inhibition of eosinophilia in those patients who exhibit elevated levels of eosinophils and do not respond to standard corticosteroid therapy.

In these individuals, inhibition of IL-5 has been shown to have beneficial effects.

Cinqair (Reslizumab): Reslizumab is a humanized IL-5-targeting monoclonal antibody approved by the FDA in 2016. It prevents the induction of blood, airway, and sputum eosinophilia by specifically inhibiting the binding of IL-5 to its receptor on eosinophils. It is recommended as an add-on treatment for patients 18 years old and older with severe asthma and elevated eosinophil levels.

Nucala (Mepolizumab): Mepolizumab is also a humanized IL-5 antagonist that was approved in 2015 and prevents the binding of IL-5 to the IL-5Rα on eosinophils. Treatment with mepolizumab has been shown to reduce eosinophil levels in patients with blood eosinophils 150 cells/μL or greater. It is recommended as an add-on treatment for patients 12 years or older with elevated eosinophil levels and severe asthma.

Fasenra (Benralizumab): Lastly, benralizumab, a monoclonal antibody targeting the IL-5Rα on eosinophils was recently approved in 2018. It is an IgG antibody that targets IL-5Rα and binds FcγRIII (CD16) on NK cells, inducing killing of eosinophils by NK cells *via* antibody-dependent cellular cytotoxicity.

IL-4 and IL-13 Antagonists

In addition to the approved IL-5 antagonists, other biologics targeting IL-4 and IL-13 are currently being evaluated in clinical trials. Both these cytokines play critical roles in the development of allergic responses. IL-4 is important for the activation of Th2 cells and B cells and also promotes B cell class-switching to IgE. IL-13 is important for B cell class-switching, but also promotes BHR, mucus hypersecretion from goblet cells, and epithelial cell turnover resulting in fibrosis.

Dupilumab currently approved for the treatment of atopic dermatitis and moderate to severe asthma in adults and adolescents age 12 or older, is a fully human monoclonal antibody targeting the IL-4Rα subunit, a shared component of both IL-4 and IL-13 receptors. Treatment with dupilumab disrupts the IL-4/IL-13 signaling cascade, resulting in the attenuation of IL-4 and IL-13-mediated effects. In September of 2017, Regeneron and Sanofi announced positive results using dupilumab in patients with uncontrolled, persistent asthma. Dupilumab, when added to standard therapy, reduced severe asthma exacerbations and improved overall lung function. Similarly, pitrakinra (Aerovant), which is a mutated form of human IL-4 is being investigated in clinical trials for its ability to disrupt IL-4 and IL-13 signaling by binding to the IL-4Rα and preventing its assembly into either the IL-4 or IL-13 receptors.

In addition to drugs targeting both IL-4 and IL-13 signaling, a number of pharmaceutical companies are also investigating the efficacy of IL-13 antagonists in clinical trials. These include lebrikizumab (Genentech), tralokinumab (Astrazeneca), and anrukinzumab (Wyeth).

Anti-histamines

Histamine is a potent, biologically active amine that has complex physiologic effects on a number of tissues and cell types. In addition to the stored histamine found in mast cells and basophils, histamine may also be found in various tissues, including the brain, where it acts as an endogenous neurotransmitter controlling brain functions, such as cardiovascular regulation, sleep and arousal, and body weight regulation. Histamine is also stored and released by cells lining the stomach where it activates parietal cells in the mucosa to produce gastric acids. The biologic effects of histamine are mediated *via* binding to four distinct receptors belonging to the G-protein-coupled receptor family. These include the H_1 receptor which is expressed on smooth muscle, endothelium and the brain, the H_2 receptor which is expressed on gastric mucosa, mast cells, cardiac muscle and the brain, the H_3 receptor which is expressed on presynaptic neurons, and the H_4 receptor which is expressed on neutrophils, eosinophils and CD4 T cells. Activation of the H_1 receptors, especially during allergic reactions, induces vasodilation, vascular permeability and smooth muscle constriction, leading to symptoms such as sneezing, coughing, vomiting and itching. The H_2 receptors play an important role in gastric acid secretion. H_3 receptors play an important role in modulating the release of neurotransmitters and have been implicated in metabolic effects such as insulin resistance and energy expenditure. Lastly, H_4 receptors are expressed on a number of leukocytes and are thought to contribute to inflammation.

A number of competitive histamine-receptor antagonists have been developed to inhibit the actions of histamine and the consequent physiologic effects. Of these, the H_2-receptor antagonist, burimamide, was first developed to inhibit the gastric-acid inducing activity of histamine.

The H_1-receptor antagonists are the most commonly used drugs for the treatment of allergic conditions such as allergic rhinitis. A large number are marketed throughout the United States and are available both over the counter and *via* prescription. Two types of H_1-receptor antagonists are available. These include first generation agents which are non-selective and strongly sedative and second generation agents which are peripherally selective and less sedating due to decreased overall distribution in the central nervous system. While anti-histamines directly block the action of histamine by inhibiting its binding, the reversal of histamine-mediated effects occurs as a result of anti-cholinergic properties exhibited by these drugs. This includes drying effects such as reducing nasal and lachrymal secretions and inhibition of vascular permeability (Table 4.9).

Immunotherapy

Allergen-specific immunotherapy (SIT) is the only available curative treatment for allergic diseases such as allergic asthma and allergic rhinitis. Despite being in use since the early 1900s, it is the most underutilized treatment option for allergic diseases. The British physicians Leonard Noon and John Freeman first utilized the technique in 1911 as a means of inducing immunity to allergic 'toxins' by subcutaneously injecting them into patients with hay fever. The successful abolishment of allergic symptoms in these patients gained widespread attention and led to the adoption of the practice by many medical professionals. As immunologists began to gain a better understanding of the immune response and the basis of allergic reactions, the process began to be known as allergic *desensitization* or as it is sometimes called today hyposensitization. SIT involves exposing allergic patients to increasing doses of various allergens to which the patients have been sensitized. Historically, most of these

Table 4.9 Commonly used anti-histamines in the treatment of allergic rhinitis (the plus and minus denominators indicate the degree of potency); Rx = prescription; OTC: over the counter

Drug	Sedation	Anticholinergic	Availability
First generation—More lipophilic, non-selective, more sedating			
Brompheniramine	+	++	OTC
Chlorpheniramine (Chlor-Trimeton®)	+	++	OTC
Dexchlorpheniramine	+	++	Rx only
Carbinoxamine maleate	+++	+++	Rx only
Clemastine fumarate	++	+++	OTC
Cyproheptadine	+	++	Rx only
Diphenhydramine (Benadryl®)	+++	+++	OTC
Promethazine (antiemetic)	+++	+++	Rx only
Azelastine (intranasal)	−/+	−/+	Rx only
Second generation—peripherally-selective, non-sedating			
Cetirizine (Zyrtec®)	+/++	−/+	OTC
Desloratadine (Clarinex®)	−/+	−/+	Rx only
Fexofenadine (Allegra®)	−/+	−/+	OTC
Levocetirizine (Xyzal®)	+/++	−/+	OTC
Loratadine (Claritin®)	−/+	−/+	OTC

exposures occurred *via* the subcutaneous route although more recently the sublingual route has also been used. Over the course of therapy, which can sometimes last 3 years, the total levels of allergen-specific IgE are decreased, replaced by what is believed to be protective isotypes of IgG antibodies. In the last few years, several novel studies have shed further light regarding the mechanisms by which SIT modulates the allergic response. Particularly important are the roles of regulatory T cells secreting the cytokines IL-10 and TGF-β, while a shift of the T cell response from T_H2 to T_H1 has also been observed. The decrease in allergen-specific IgE antibodies accompanied by a concomitant increase in allergen-specific IgG4 antibodies results in diminished mast cell and basophil activation leading to resolution of the allergic response.

From Bench to Bedside: The Discovery of IgE Antibodies

The early association of IgE antibodies with the allergic response came from observations which demonstrated that hypersensitivity reactions could be passively transferred to individuals. The causative factor was initially termed as atopic reagin, and was later (1966) discovered to be IgE. Since then atopy has been come to be operationally associated with increases in serum IgE levels and skin reactivity to various allergens. Described below is a short synopsis of the journey from the discovery of reagin to the approval of the anti-IgE drug omalizumab.

In 1906, the scientist Clemens von Pirquet first expressed the belief that antigen-antibody reactions formed the basis of allergic disease. However, the hunt for the allergenic fraction of blood that gave rise to hypersensitivity reactions began several years later following the publication of a case report involving a patient with a mysterious asthma attack. In 1919, one of Dr. Maximilian Ramirez's patients suddenly developed an asthma attack while taking a horse ride in Central Park, New York. Subsequently, it was determined that the patient had recently received a blood transfusion from a donor who was allergic to horses, suggesting the presence of a horse-specific allergy-inducing substance that had been transferred from donor to recipient. In 1921, Carl Prausnitz confirmed the existence of such a substance by transferring serum from a colleague Heinz Kustner, who was allergic to fish, to himself and subsequently inducing allergic reactions to fish extract. This test of the capacity of serum components to transfer allergic reactions to unsensitized individuals was termed the Prausnitz-Kustner or P-K test and formed the basis of the study of hypersensitivity reactions for several decades to come. However, in the absence of sophisticated purification techniques such as chromatography, electrophoresis, centrifugation and filtration, the isolation of the reaginic substance in blood appeared to be elusive for many years.

Then in the early 1960s, the scientists Kimishige Ishizaka and Teruko Ishizaka first described experiments that attributed reaginic activity to a component in blood that they initially thought belonged to the recently discovered class of antibodies, IgA. However, subsequent experiments involving fractionation studies, enzymatic degradation, and assessment of immunization with reagin-containing serum in rabbits, revealed that the reagin-conferring substance was not IgA, but another molecule that they termed γE. At the same time, in Europe, the immunochemists Hans Bennich and Gunnar Johansson identified the presence of a mysterious immunoglobulin in a patient with multiple myeloma receiving regular blood transfusions. They named the immunoglobulin IgND after the initials of the patient. Subsequently, in collaboration with the scientists Denis Stanworth, Leif Wide and John Humphrey, they were able to demonstrate that the newly identified immunoglobulin was able to inhibit the PK test and develop an assay to quantify IgND. Further examination confirmed that IgND reacted with the Ishizakas' anti-γE and in 1967 both groups submitted reports to the World Health Organization allowing for the designation of a novel immunoglobulin class IgE.

In the 38 years since the classification of IgE, a number of breakthroughs in immunology have allowed us to understand the mechanisms by which it induces allergic reactions. This includes the discovery of the IgE receptors FcεRI and FcεRII and the ability of IgE to induce mast cell and basophil-mediated allergic reactions. The insight acquired from these studies led to the development of a novel anti-IgE monoclonal antibody that is able to inhibit IgE in vivo without causing anaphylactic reactions. This drug, omalizumab, binds the Fc portion of soluble IgE molecules, preventing their binding to IgE receptors on mast cells, B cells and other immune cells. Eventually, the production of both IgE and its receptors is diminished thus leading to a significant suppression of mast cell-mediated reactions. Omalizumab was FDA approved in 2003 for patients with severe persistent asthma and in 2014 for chronic spontaneous urticarial. It is currently being examined for treatment of severe food allergy.

Summary

The respiratory disorders allergic asthma and COPD represent a major fraction of the overall health care efforts expended in the United States. The rise in the incidence of these diseases over the last few years has gained significant attention in the medical community leading to several new advances in basic research examining the immunologic basis of these diseases and the development of new immunotherapeutic drugs for their management and treatment. It is now well-established that allergic asthma is a complex disease involving the contribution of many different cell types including T_H2 cells, mast cells, eosinophils, ILC2s, and their mediators. This cross-talk between immune cells and their mediators results in the pathophysiologic features of the disease including airway eosinophilia, bronchoconstriction, mucus hypersecretion and airway remodeling. Currently available drugs target both the bronchoconstriction and the inflammatory cells and mediators driving the disease. More recently, novel biologics targeting specific mediators have been developed. Similarly, recent advances in immunology research have refined our understanding of the inflammatory cause of COPD. While currently available drugs mostly target bronchoconstriction, providing temporary symptomatic relief, it is hoped that the elucidation of novel immunologic targets will lead to better therapeutic options.

Practice Questions

James Soros is a 30-year-old man who arrived in the emergency room with complaints of shortness of breath, difficulty breathing and slightly slurred speech. He claims that he has been waking up several times each night over the last few weeks, experiencing chest tightness and an inability to breathe. On these occasions, he has attempted to use his rescue inhaler, but without much success. His past medical history has involved seasonal bouts of allergic rhinitis and asthma and atopic dermatitis as a child. He complains that his asthma symptoms worsen during the Spring but improve if he goes away on vacation. His doctor has previously recommended treatment with Symbicort®, but he declined since he does not feel bad all the time.

1. Based on your understanding of the pathophysiology of asthma, which cells are responsible for the current symptoms James is experiencing? How are these cells activated? What mediators do they produce which may contribute to his observed symptoms?

2. You are the attending emergency room physician. You have been told that he is already on anti-allergic medication to treat symptoms caused by pre-formed mediators released by mast cells. But you are more interested in treating symptoms caused by *de novo* synthesized substances. Which of the following would you be most concerned about?:
   (a) Histamine
   (b) Heparin
   (c) Tryptase
   (d) Leukotriene D4
   (e) Mast cell proteases

3. James began to complain of increasing chest tightness and congestion making it very difficult for him to breathe. The emergency room physician is concerned that chronic inflammation in his airways is clogging his trachea, contributing to the wheezing and congestion. James mentioned that he had had a bronchoalveolar lavage (BAL) done in the past to assess the inflammation. When the doctor checked his electronic medical records, he learned that the majority of cells in the airway inflammatory infiltrate from James' BAL specimen were:
   (a) Mast cells
   (b) Macrophages
   (c) Neutrophils
   (d) Dendritic cells
   (e) Eosinophils

4. Which of the following statements regarding T cell involvement in asthma is correct? Select all that apply.
   (a) T_H2 cells mediate chronic allergic asthma through the release of cytokines
   (b) T_H17 cells and IL-17-mediated neutrophilia are observed in hyper acute episodes of asthma
   (c) T_H1 cells secrete IL-4 which activates B cells
   (d) Tregs normally suppress allergic responses in asthmatic patients

5. Which of the following statements regarding the mechanism of action of albuterol is correct?
   (a) Albuterol causes a decrease in myosin phosphatase activity

   (b) Albuterol produces an increase in intracellular Ca^{++} levels
   (c) Albuterol causes an increase in K^+ efflux *via* calcium-gated K^+ channels
   (d) Albuterol causes a decrease in PKA formation

6. All of the following are adverse effects associated with the use of a β_2-agonist except:
   (a) Tachycardia
   (b) Skeletal muscle tremor
   (c) Smooth muscle relaxation
   (d) Hyperkalemia

7. What role does IL-4 play in the development of asthmatic symptoms?
   (a) It induces eosinophilia
   (b) It activates mast cells
   (c) It is required for T_H2 activation and also activates B cells
   (d) It activates leukotrienes

8. Omalizumab is novel immunomodulatory drug for asthma that has been efficacious in patients with severe disease. The mechanism of action of omalizumab is represented by the blocking of which *target* below?
   (a) FcαRI
   (b) Soluble IgE antibodies
   (c) IL-5
   (d) IL-13

9. You are James' allergist, and you just became aware of the recent success of reslizumab. You recommend that James be put on a maintenance level of the drug with the hope of alleviating chronic asthma symptoms. What is the mechanism of action of reslizumab?
   (a) It blocks the binding of IgE to its receptor
   (b) It is an anti-IL-13 antibody
   (c) It blocks the development of eosinophilic inflammation by neutralizing IL-5
   (d) It blocks the activity of mast cells

10. Which of the following correctly describes the proposed mechanism of action of fluticasone?
    (a) It causes an increase in intracellular calcium
    (b) It inhibits signaling via leukotriene receptors

(c) It decreases gene transcription by activating histone deacetylases

(d) It inhibits phosphodiesterase 4

11. Which of the following correctly states the mechanism of action of theophylline in the treatment of asthma?

(a) Theophylline increases cell proliferation of immune cells

(b) Theophylline can increase cAMP production in smooth muscle cells

(c) Theophylline induces cortical arousal and alertness

(d) Theophylline activates phosphodiesterases

12. What are the effects of zafirlukast treatment? Select all that apply.

(a) It binds the receptor for LTD4

(b) It inhibits LTB4

(c) It reduces bronchoconstriction caused by leukotriene E4

(d) It reduces bronchoconstriction caused by prostaglandins

13. Which of the following cell types may be activated to produce leukotrienes during the allergic response? Select all that apply.

(a) Mast cells

(b) Eosinophils

(c) T cells

(d) Dendritic cells

14. Four abstracts were presented at a scientific conference on novel therapeutics being developed for the treatment of allergic asthma. Which of these in your opinion validates the T_H2 hypothesis of asthma? Select all that apply.

(a) Treatment with ixekizumab, an IL-17 inhibitor, prevented the accumulation of neutrophils during hyper acute episodes

(b) Treatment with adalimumab, a TNF-α inhibitor blocked 50% of FeNO release from macrophages

(c) Treatment with belimumab, a drug blocking B cell proliferation, prevented the production of IgE antibodies

(d) Treatment with dupilumab, a drug blocking IL-4Rα, prevented the accumulation of eosinophils after allergen challenges

15. One of the goals of allergen desensitization is to:

(a) Promote T_H1 responses to allergens instead of T_H2 responses

(b) Suppress the generation of mast cells from the bone marrow

(c) Shift the antibody response from IgE to IgG4

(d) Activate cytotoxic T cells that kill Th2 cells

16. Inflammation in COPD is caused due to:

(a) Increased CD8 T cell activation with recruitment of activated macrophages and neutrophils

(b) Increased CD4 T cell activation with recruitment of eosinophils

(c) Mast-cell mediated effects with increased production of histamine

(d) Chronic T_H2 activation with production of IL-4, IL-5 and IL-13

17. One suggested mechanism for the pathogenesis of COPD in susceptible individuals is:

(a) Induction of anti-nicotine antibodies which then mediate destruction of the lung parenchyma via complement-mediated lysis

(b) Interactions between noxious particles in nicotine and anti-proteinases

(c) Suppression of T_H2 responses and defective immunity against bacteria

(d) Rapid absorption of nicotine by lung parenchymal cells, causing blockage of small airways and inability to absorb oxygen

18. Acute viral respiratory tract infections are known to precipitate exacerbations of asthma and chronic obstructive pulmonary disease. Sam complained that about 2 months ago, he had suffered from infection with the H1N1 influenza virus. You are conducting research on how cigarette smoking enhances long-term effects of virus-induced chronic airway inflammation in asthma and COPD. You think Sam would be a perfect subject for research and ask for his consent. Which of the following parameters would you NOT necessarily test?

(a) Composition of airway inflammatory cells

(b) Expression levels of the anti-oxidant gene *Nrf2* in Sam's airway epithelial cells

(c) Effectiveness of treating with glucocorticoids

(d) Gene expression levels of lipid mediators in mast cells

19. Which properties below of ipratropium bromide make it a better therapeutic agent for COPD compared to atropine? Select all that apply.

(a) It binds M_2 receptors

(b) It is a quarternary ammonium derivative of atropine

(c) It is poorly absorbed into circulation

(d) It is a non-competitive inhibitor of acetyl choline

20. Which statement below correctly describes the mechanism of action of tiotropium bromide?

(a) Its effects last longer because it slowly dissociates from M_1, M_2 and M_3 receptors

(b) It is rapidly absorbed into circulation

(c) It binds M_1, M_2 and M_3 receptors, but rapidly dissociates from M_2 receptors

(d) It binds M_1 receptors

Suggested Reading

Akbari O, Stock P, DeKruyff RH, Umetsu DT. Role of regulatory T cells in allergy and asthma. Curr Opin Immunol. 2003;15:627–33.

Arthur G, Bradding P. New developments in mast cell biology: clinical implications. Chest. 2016;150:680–93.

Artis D, Spits H. The biology of innate lymphoid cells. Nature. 2015;517:293–301.

Azzawi M, Bradley B, Jeffery PK, Frew AJ, Wardlaw AJ, Knowles G, et al. Identification of activated T lymphocytes and eosinophils in bronchial biopsies in stable atopic asthma. Am Rev Respir Dis. 1990;142:1407–13.

Azzawi M, Johnston PW, Majumdar S, Kay AB, Jeffery PK. T lymphocytes and activated eosinophils in airway mucosa in fatal asthma and cystic fibrosis. Am Rev Respir Dis. 1992;145:1477–82.

Barnes PJ. Molecular mechanisms and cellular effects of glucocorticosteroids. Immunol Allergy Clin N Am. 2005;25:451–68.

Barnes PJ. Theophylline. Am J Respir Crit Care Med. 2013;188:901–6.

Barnes PJ. Inflammatory mechanisms in patients with chronic obstructive pulmonary disease. J Allergy Clin Immunol. 2016;138:16–27.

Barnes PJ. Cellular and molecular mechanisms of asthma and COPD. Clin Sci (Lond). 2017;131:1541–58.

Barnes PJ, Adcock IM. How do corticosteroids work in asthma? Ann Intern Med. 2003;139:359–70.

Barnes KC, Neely JD, Duffy DL, Freidhoff LR, Breazeale DR, Schou C, et al. Linkage of asthma and total serum IgE concentration to markers on chromosome 12q: evidence from Afro-Caribbean and Caucasian populations. Genomics. 1996;37:41–50.

Barnes PJ, Shapiro SD, Pauwels RA. Chronic obstructive pulmonary disease: molecular and cellular mechanisms. Eur Respir J. 2003;22:672–88.

Barnes PJ, Burney PG, Silverman EK, Celli BR, Vestbo J, Wedzicha JA, et al. Chronic obstructive pulmonary disease. Nat Rev Dis Primers. 2015;1:15076.

Begin P, Nadeau KC. Epigenetic regulation of asthma and allergic disease. Allergy Asthma Clin Immunol. 2014;10:27.

Brusselle GG, Kips JC, Tavernier JH, van der Heyden JG, Cuvelier CA, Pauwels RA, et al. Attenuation of allergic airway inflammation in IL-4 deficient mice. Clin Exp Allergy. 1994;24:73–80.

Burton OT, Oettgen HC. Beyond immediate hypersensitivity: evolving roles for IgE antibodies in immune homeostasis and allergic diseases. Immunol Rev. 2011;242:128–43.

Busse WW, Lemanske RF Jr. Asthma. N Engl J Med. 2001;344:350–62.

Busse WW, Lemanske RF Jr. Management of asthma exacerbations. Thorax. 2004;59:545–6.

Busse WW, Coffman RL, Gelfand EW, Kay AB, Rosenwasser LJ. Mechanisms of persistent airway inflammation in asthma. A role for T cells and T-cell products. Am J Respir Crit Care Med. 1995;152:388–93.

Busse WW, Lemanske RF Jr, Gern JE. Role of viral respiratory infections in asthma and asthma exacerbations. Lancet. 2010;376:826–34.

Cazzola M, Page CP, Rogliani P, Matera MG. beta2-agonist therapy in lung disease. Am J Respir Crit Care Med. 2013;187:690–6.

Chatila TA. Interleukin-4 receptor signaling pathways in asthma pathogenesis. Trends Mol Med. 2004;10:493–9.

Choby GW, Lee S. Pharmacotherapy for the treatment of asthma: current treatment options and future directions. Int Forum Allergy Rhinol. 2015;5(Suppl 1):S35–40.

Cohn L, Elias JA, Chupp GL. Asthma: mechanisms of disease persistence and progression. Annu Rev Immunol. 2004;22:789–815.

Corrigan CJ, Hartnell A, Kay AB. T lymphocyte activation in acute severe asthma. Lancet. 1988;1:1129–32.

Das J, Chen CH, Yang L, Cohn L, Ray P, Ray A. A critical role for NF-kappa B in GATA3 expression and TH2 differentiation in allergic airway inflammation. Nat Immunol. 2001;2:45–50.

Deckers J, De Bosscher K, Lambrecht BN, Hammad H. Interplay between barrier epithelial cells and dendritic cells in allergic sensitization through the lung and the skin. Immunol Rev. 2017;278:131–44.

Epstein MM. Do mouse models of allergic asthma mimic clinical disease? Int Arch Allergy Immunol. 2004;133:84–100.

Finkelman FD. Identification of IgE as the allergy-associated Ig isotype. J Immunol. 2017;198:3–4.

Foster PS, Hogan SP, Ramsay AJ, Matthaei KI, Young IG. Interleukin 5 deficiency abolishes eosinophilia, airways hyperreactivity, and lung damage in a mouse asthma model. J Exp Med. 1996;183:195–201.

Fulkerson PC, Rothenberg ME, Hogan SP. Building a better mouse model: experimental models of chronic asthma. Clin Exp Allergy. 2005;35:1251–3.

Galli SJ, Tsai M. Mast cells: versatile regulators of inflammation, tissue remodeling, host defense and homeostasis. J Dermatol Sci. 2008;49:7–19.

Galli SJ, Tsai M. IgE and mast cells in allergic disease. Nat Med. 2012;18:693–704.

Gavett SH, Chen X, Finkelman F, Wills-Karp M. Depletion of murine CD4+ T lymphocytes prevents antigen-induced airway hyperreactivity and pulmonary eosinophilia. Am J Respir Cell Mol Biol. 1994;10:587–93.

Gould HJ, Sutton BJ, Beavil AJ, Beavil RL, McCloskey N, Coker HA, et al. The biology of IGE and the basis of allergic disease. Annu Rev Immunol. 2003;21:579–628.

Gross NJ, Barnes PJ. New therapies for asthma and chronic obstructive pulmonary disease. Am J Respir Crit Care Med. 2017;195:159–66.

Grumelli S, Corry DB, Song LZ, Song L, Green L, Huh J, et al. An immune basis for lung parenchymal destruction in chronic obstructive pulmonary disease and emphysema. PLoS Med. 2004;1:e8.

Grunig G, Warnock M, Wakil AE, Venkayya R, Brombacher F, Rennick DM, et al. Requirement for IL-13 independently of IL-4 in experimental asthma. Science. 1998;282:2261–3.

Gurish MF, Austen KF. The diverse roles of mast cells. J Exp Med. 2001;194:F1–5.

Halim TY, Steer CA, Matha L, Gold MJ, Martinez-Gonzalez I, McNagny KM, et al. Group 2 innate lymphoid cells are critical for the initiation of adaptive T helper 2 cell-mediated allergic lung inflammation. Immunity. 2014;40:425–35.

Hamelmann E, Gelfand EW. IL-5-induced airway eosinophilia--the key to asthma? Immunol Rev. 2001;179:182–91.

Hamelmann E, Oshiba A, Schwarze J, Bradley K, Loader J, Larsen GL, et al. Allergen-specific IgE and IL-5 are essential for the development of airway hyperresponsiveness. Am J Respir Cell Mol Biol. 1997;16:674–82.

Hamid Q, Azzawi M, Ying S, Moqbel R, Wardlaw AJ, Corrigan CJ, et al. Expression of mRNA for interleukin-5 in mucosal bronchial biopsies from asthma. J Clin Invest. 1991;87:1541–6.

Hammad H, Lambrecht BN. Barrier epithelial cells and the control of type 2 immunity. Immunity. 2015;43:29–40.

He JQ, Hallstrand TS, Knight D, Chan-Yeung M, Sandford A, Tripp B, et al. A thymic stromal lymphopoietin gene variant is associated with asthma and airway hyperresponsiveness. J Allergy Clin Immunol. 2009;124:222–9.

Hekking PP, Wener RR, Amelink M, Zwinderman AH, Bouvy ML, Bel EH. The prevalence of severe refractory asthma. J Allergy Clin Immunol. 2015;135:896–902.

Hershey GK, Friedrich MF, Esswein LA, Thomas ML, Chatila TA. The association of atopy with a gain-of-function mutation in the alpha subunit of the interleukin-4 receptor. N Engl J Med. 1997;337:1720–5.

Hirota N, Martin JG. Mechanisms of airway remodeling. Chest. 2013;144:1026–32.

Holt PG, Strickland DH, Wikstrom ME, Jahnsen FL. Regulation of immunological homeostasis in the respiratory tract. Nat Rev Immunol. 2008;8:142–52.

Johansson SG. The history of IgE: from discovery to 2010. Curr Allergy Asthma Rep. 2011;11:173–7.

Kabesch M, Tzotcheva I, Carr D, Hofler C, Weiland SK, Fritzsch C, et al. A complete screening of the IL4 gene: novel polymorphisms and their association with asthma and IgE in childhood. J Allergy Clin Immunol. 2003;112:893–8.

Kabesch M, Schedel M, Carr D, Woitsch B, Fritzsch C, Weiland SK, et al. IL-4/IL-13 pathway genetics strongly influence serum IgE levels and childhood asthma. J Allergy Clin Immunol. 2006;117:269–74.

Kalesnikoff J, Galli SJ. New developments in mast cell biology. Nat Immunol. 2008;9:1215–23.

Kawakami T, Blank U. From IgE to omalizumab. J Immunol. 2016;197:4187–92.

Kay DSRAB. Mechanisms of allergic asthma: a Th2 disease. In: Yssel JBH, editor. Immunotherapy in asthma. First ed. New York: Marcel Dekker, Inc; 1999. p. 19–41.

Kay MLAB. CD4 T lymphocytes in allergic asthma. In: Lambrecht BN, Hoogsteden H, Diamant Z, editors. The immunological basis of asthma. 1st ed. New York: Marcel Dekker, Inc; 2003. p. 53–81.

Kim HY, DeKruyff RH, Umetsu DT. The many paths to asthma: phenotype shaped by innate and adaptive immunity. Nat Immunol. 2010;11:577–84.

Knutsen AP, Bush RK, Demain JG, Denning DW, Dixit A, Fairs A, et al. Fungi and allergic lower respiratory tract diseases. J Allergy Clin Immunol. 2012;129:280–91; quiz 92–3.

Kubo M. Innate and adaptive type 2 immunity in lung allergic inflammation. Immunol Rev. 2017;278:162–72.

Lambrecht BN, Hammad H. Taking our breath away: dendritic cells in the pathogenesis of asthma. Nat Rev Immunol. 2003;3:994–1003.

Lambrecht BN, Hammad H. Biology of lung dendritic cells at the origin of asthma. Immunity. 2009;31:412–24.

Lambrecht BN, Hammad H. Lung dendritic cells in respiratory viral infection and asthma: from protection to immunopathology. Annu Rev Immunol. 2012;30:243–70.

Lee NA, Gelfand EW, Lee JJ. Pulmonary T cells and eosinophils: coconspirators or independent triggers of allergic respiratory pathology? J Allergy Clin Immunol. 2001;107:945–57.

Lemanske RF Jr, Busse WW. Asthma: clinical expression and molecular mechanisms. J Allergy Clin Immunol. 2010;125:S95–102.

Liang HE, Reinhardt RL, Bando JK, Sullivan BM, Ho IC, Locksley RM. Divergent expression patterns of IL-4 and IL-13 define unique functions in allergic immunity. Nat Immunol. 2011;13:58–66.

Lloyd CM, Hessel EM. Functions of T cells in asthma: more than just T(H)2 cells. Nat Rev Immunol. 2010;10:838–48.

Lloyd CM, Gonzalo JA, Coyle AJ, Gutierrez-Ramos JC. Mouse models of allergic airway disease. Adv Immunol. 2001;77:263–95.

Lotvall J, Akdis CA, Bacharier LB, Bjermer L, Casale TB, Custovic A, et al. Asthma endotypes: a new approach to classification of disease entities within the asthma syndrome. J Allergy Clin Immunol. 2011;127:355–60.

Lukacs NW, Strieter RM, Chensue SW, Kunkel SL. Interleukin-4-dependent pulmonary eosinophil infiltration in a murine model of asthma. Am J Respir Cell Mol Biol. 1994;10:526–32.

MacKenzie JR, Mattes J, Dent LA, Foster PS. Eosinophils promote allergic disease of the lung by regulating CD4(+) Th2 lymphocyte function. J Immunol. 2001;167:3146–55.

Martinez FD. Early-life origins of chronic obstructive pulmonary disease. N Engl J Med. 2016;375:871–8.

Mathias CB. Natural killer cells in the development of asthma. Curr Allergy Asthma Rep. 2015;15:500.

Mathias CB, Freyschmidt EJ, Caplan B, Jones T, Poddighe D, Xing W, et al. IgE influences the number and function of mature mast cells, but not progenitor recruitment in allergic pulmonary inflammation. J Immunol. 2009;182:2416–24.

Mattes J, Yang M, Siqueira A, Clark K, MacKenzie J, McKenzie AN, et al. IL-13 induces airways hyperreactivity independently of the IL-4R alpha chain in the allergic lung. J Immunol. 2001;167:1683–92.

Medoff BD, Thomas SY, Luster AD. T cell trafficking in allergic asthma: the ins and outs. Annu Rev Immunol. 2008;26:205–32.

Moller GM, Overbeek SE, Van Helden-Meeuwsen CG, Van Haarst JM, Prens EP, Mulder PG, et al. Increased numbers of dendritic cells in the bronchial mucosa of atopic asthmatic patients: downregulation by inhaled corticosteroids. Clin Exp Allergy. 1996;26:517–24.

Ober C. Susceptibility genes in asthma and allergy. Curr Allergy Asthma Rep. 2001;1:174–9.

Ober C, Leavitt SA, Tsalenko A, Howard TD, Hoki DM, Daniel R, et al. Variation in the interleukin 4-receptor alpha gene confers susceptibility to asthma and atopy in ethnically diverse populations. Am J Hum Genet. 2000;66:517–26.

Oettgen HC, Geha RS. IgE regulation and roles in asthma pathogenesis. J Allergy Clin Immunol. 2001;107:429–40.

Pejler G, Ronnberg E, Waern I, Wernersson S. Mast cell proteases: multifaceted regulators of inflammatory disease. Blood. 2010;115:4981–90.

Platts-Mills TAE. The continuing effect of the discovery of IgE by Kimishige Ishizaka. J Allergy Clin Immunol. 2018;142:788–9.

Platts-Mills TA, Rakes G, Heymann PW. The relevance of allergen exposure to the development of asthma in childhood. J Allergy Clin Immunol. 2000;105:S503–8.

Platts-Mills TA, Heymann PW, Commins SP, Woodfolk JA. The discovery of IgE 50 years later. Ann Allergy Asthma Immunol. 2016;116:179–82.

Polukort SH, et al. IL-10 enhances IgE-mediated mast cell responses and is essential for the development of experimental food allergy in IL-10-deficient mice. J Immunol. 2016;196:4865–76.

Postma DS, Rabe KF. The asthma-COPD overlap syndrome. N Engl J Med. 2015;373:1241–9.

Postma DS, Bleecker ER, Amelung PJ, Holroyd KJ, Xu J, Panhuysen CI, et al. Genetic susceptibility to asthma--bronchial hyperresponsiveness coinherited with a major gene for atopy. N Engl J Med. 1995;333:894–900.

Pulendran B, Artis D. New paradigms in type 2 immunity. Science. 2012;337:431–5.

Reynolds LA, Finlay BB. Early life factors that affect allergy development. Nat Rev Immunol. 2017;17:518–28.

Robinson DS, Hamid Q, Ying S, Tsicopoulos A, Barkans J, Bentley AM, et al. Predominant TH2-like bronchoalveolar T-lymphocyte population in atopic asthma. N Engl J Med. 1992;326:298–304.

Saluzzo S, Gorki AD, Rana BMJ, Martins R, Scanlon S, Starkl P, et al. First-breath-induced type 2 pathways shape the lung immune environment. Cell Rep. 2017;18:1893–905.

Scanlon ST, McKenzie AN. The messenger between worlds: the regulation of innate and adaptive type-2 immunity by innate lymphoid cells. Clin Exp Allergy. 2015;45:9–20.

Shirakawa I, Deichmann KA, Izuhara I, Mao I, Adra CN, Hopkin JM. Atopy and asthma: genetic variants of IL-4 and IL-13 signalling. Immunol Today. 2000;21:60–4.

Stanworth DR. The discovery of IgE. Allergy. 1993;48:67–71.

Torgerson DG, Ampleford EJ, Chiu GY, Gauderman WJ, Gignoux CR, Graves PE, et al. Meta-analysis of genome-wide association studies of asthma in ethnically diverse north American populations. Nat Genet. 2011;43:887–92.

Trejo Bittar HE, Yousem SA, Wenzel SE. Pathobiology of severe asthma. Annu Rev Pathol. 2015;10:511–45.

Umetsu DT, McIntire JJ, Akbari O, Macaubas C, DeKruyff RH. Asthma: an epidemic of dysregulated immunity. Nat Immunol. 2002;3:715–20.

van Rijt L, von Richthofen H, van Ree R. Type 2 innate lymphoid cells: at the cross-roads in allergic asthma. Semin Immunopathol. 2016;38:483–96.

Virchow JC Jr, Walker C, Hafner D, Kortsik C, Werner P, Matthys H, et al. T cells and cytokines in bronchoalveolar lavage fluid after segmental allergen provocation in atopic asthma. Am J Respir Crit Care Med. 1995;151:960–8.

Walker C, Kaegi MK, Braun P, Blaser K. Activated T cells and eosinophilia in bronchoalveolar lavages from subjects with asthma correlated with disease severity. J Allergy Clin Immunol. 1991;88:935–42.

Wenzel SE. Emergence of biomolecular pathways to define novel asthma phenotypes. Type-2 immunity and beyond. Am J Respir Cell Mol Biol. 2016; 55:1–4.

Wenzel SE, Balzar S, Ampleford E, Hawkins GA, Busse WW, Calhoun WJ, et al. IL4R alpha mutations are associated with asthma exacerbations and mast cell/IgE expression. Am J Respir Crit Care Med. 2007;175:570–6.

Wills-Karp M. Immunologic basis of antigen-induced airway hyperresponsiveness. Annu Rev Immunol. 1999;17:255–81.

Wills-Karp M. Interleukin-13 in asthma pathogenesis. Immunol Rev. 2004;202:175–90.

Wills-Karp M, Ewart SL. Time to draw breath: asthma-susceptibility genes are identified. Nat Rev Genet. 2004;5:376–87.

Wills-Karp Marsha HGKK. Immunological mechanisms of allergic disorders. In: Paul WE, editor. Fundamental immunology. Philadelphia: Lippincott-Raven Publishers; 2003. p. 1439–79.

Wills-Karp M, Luyimbazi J, Xu X, Schofield B, Neben TY, Karp CL, et al. Interleukin-13: central mediator of allergic asthma. Science. 1998;282:2258–61.

Wills-Karp M, Santeliz J, Karp CL. The germless theory of allergic disease: revisiting the hygiene hypothesis. Nat Rev Immunol. 2001;1:69–75.

Wright JL, Churg A. Cigarette smoke causes physiologic and morphologic changes of emphysema in the Guinea pig. Am Rev Respir Dis. 1990;142:1422–8.

Yiamouyiannis CA, Schramm CM, Puddington L, Stengel P, Baradaran-Hosseini E, Wolyniec WW, et al. Shifts in lung lymphocyte profiles correlate with the sequential development of acute allergic and chronic tolerant stages in a murine asthma model. Am J Pathol. 1999;154:1911–21.

Zhang DH, Yang L, Cohn L, Parkyn L, Homer R, Ray P, et al. Inhibition of allergic inflammation in a murine model of asthma by expression of a dominant-negative mutant of GATA-3. Immunity. 1999;11:473–82.

Zhu J, Yamane H, Paul WE. Differentiation of effector CD4 T cell populations (*). Annu Rev Immunol. 2010;28:445–89.

Inflammation of the Skin and Its Therapeutic Targets

5

Clinton B. Mathias

Learning Objectives

1. Describe the immune components of skin and discuss their role in host defense.
2. Discuss the mechanisms by which keratinocytes initiate immune responses in the skin.
3. Identify and explain the roles of various innate lymphoid cells and T cells in host defense.
4. Discuss the immune mechanisms involved in the pathophysiology of atopic dermatitis.
5. Explain the contributions of T cell subsets and their mediators to the development of atopic dermatitis.
6. Discuss the immune mechanisms involved in the pathophysiology of atopic psoriasis.
7. Explain the contributions of T cell subsets and their mediators to the development of psoriasis.
8. Identify and discuss the pharmacology of the immunotherapeutic drugs used in the treatment of atopic dermatitis and psoriasis.
9. Explain the pharmacology of novel immunomodulating biologics in the treatment of atopic dermatitis and psoriasis.

Drugs discussed in this chapter

Drugs	Classification
Acitretin (Soriatane®)	Retinoid (Vitamin A derivative)

C. B. Mathias (✉)
Department of Pharmaceutical and Administrative Sciences, College of Pharmacy and Health Sciences, Western New England University, Springfield, MA, USA
e-mail: clinton.mathias@wne.edu

Drugs	Classification
Adalimumab (Humira®)	Anti-TNF-α monoclonal antibody
Anthralin (Dithranol®, Dithrocream®, Zithranol®)	Anti-inflammatory agent
Apremilast (Otezla®)	Phosphodiesterase (PDE) 4 inhibitor
Betamethasone dipropionate 0.05% (Diprosone®; Diprolene®)	Topical corticosteroid
Betamethasone valerate 0.1% (Valisone®); 0.12% foam (Luxiq®)	Topical corticosteroid
Brodalumab (Siliq™)	Anti-IL-17R monoclonal antibody
Calcipotriene 0.005% (Dovonex®; Sorilux foam®; Calcitrene ointment®)	Vitamin D3 analog
Calcipotriene 0.005% and Betamethasone dipropionate 0.064% (Enstilar foam®; Taclonex®)	Combination of Vitamin D analog and steroid
Clobetasol propionate 0.05% (Clobex®; Olux®; Temovate®)	Topical corticosteroid
Crisaborole 2% (Eucrisa®)	PDE 4 inhibitor
Cyclosporine (Gengraf®; Neoral®)	Calcineurin inhibitor
Desonide 0.05% (Verdeso®; Desonate®)	Topical corticosteroid
Desoximetasone 0.05% (Topicort LP®); 0.25% (Topicort®)	Topical corticosteroid
Diflorasone diacetate 0.05% (Apexicon E®)	Topical corticosteroid
Dupilumab (Dupixent®)	Anti-IL-4Rα monoclonal antibody

Drugs	Classification
Etanercept (Enbrel®)	TNF-α inhibitor (Fusion protein)
Fluocinolone acetonide 0.01% (Derma-Smoothe®)	Topical corticosteroid
Fluocinonide 0.01% (Halog®); 0.05% (Lidex-E-cream®); 0.1% (Vanos®)	Topical corticosteroid
Fluticasone propionate 0.05% (Cultivate®)	Topical corticosteroid
Guselkumab (Tremfya®)	Anti-IL-23 p19 monoclonal antibody
Halobetasol propionate 0.05% (Elocon®; Ultravate®)	Topical corticosteroid
Hydrocortisone 0.5, 1.0, 2.0, 2.5% (Cortaid®; Nutracort®; Synacort®; others)	Topical corticosteroid
Infliximab (Remicade®)	Anti-TNF-α monoclonal antibody
Ixekizumab (Taltz®)	Anti-IL-17A monoclonal antibody
Methotrexate (Trexall®; Rheumatrex®; others)	Immunosuppressive drug; anti-metabolite
Mometasone furoate 0.1% (Elocon®)	Topical corticosteroid
Pimecrolimus 1% (Elidel®)	Calcineurin inhibitor
Secukinumab (Cosentyx®)	Anti-IL-17A monoclonal antibody
Tacrolimus 0.03%, 0.1% (Protopic®; Prograf®)	Calcineurin inhibitor
Tazarotene (Tazorac®; Fabior®; others)	Retinoid
Tildrakizumab (Ilumya®)	Anti-IL-23 p19 monoclonal antibody
Triamcinolone acetonide 0.025% (Aristocort A®; Kenalog®)	Topical corticosteroid
Ustekinumab (Stelara®)	Anti-IL-12/IL-23 p40 monoclonal antibody

Introduction

The skin is a highly complex organ that performs diverse essential functions including barrier maintenance, physical sensing, temperature control, and defense against pathogens. It is composed of a number of highly specialized cells and structures that serve to aid the body in fighting pathogens and constitute a formidable and effective barrier against infection. When this barrier is breached, either due to an opening in the skin or as a consequence of a hereditary defect in barrier

function, the immune defenses of the skin are compromised, resulting in infection or disease. Nonetheless, the process of infection itself does not ensue unless the epidermal barrier is fully broken and the soft tissues of the dermis and subcutaneous fatty acid layer are exposed to pathogens. Similarly, the immune response to skin irritants is regulated by a number of diverse immune cell types including **keratinocytes**, **Langerhans cells**, and T cells that drive the development of skin disease and chronic cutaneous inflammation. In this chapter, we will focus on the pathophysiology of two widely prevalent skin diseases mediated by immune cells, namely atopic dermatitis and psoriasis, and discuss the immunopharmacology of the drugs used to treat them.

Immunological Functions of the Skin

Skin Structure and Its Immune Composition

The skin serves as a highly effective barrier against pathogens and foreign irritants. Simplistically, the skin consists of three distinct compartments, the epidermis, the dermis, and a subcutaneous fatty region, each of which contributes to host defense (Fig. 5.1). Along with a host of both resident and migratory immune cells, the epidermis and dermis consist of a number of other structures that confer immunity including sweat and sebaceous glands, blood vessels, and lymphatics. Additionally, the epidermis is colonized by the normal microflora of the skin, which discourages the growth of competing foreign bacteria and opportunistic pathogens. Collectively, all these different components contribute to the development of healthy skin and confer protection from foreign or infectious material.

The epidermis serves as the outermost layer of the skin, consisting of a highly cornified keratinized layer called the *stratum corneum*. This layer consists of terminally differentiated keratinocytes called corneocytes. Beneath this layer is the *stratum granulosum* which consists of living cells that form tight junctions, followed by the *stratum*

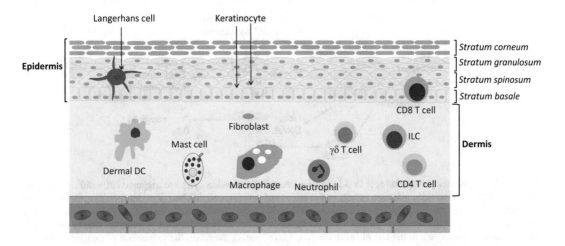

Fig. 5.1 The immunological functions of the skin. Human skin consists of an outer epidermal layer comprising of several layers of differentiated keratinocytes followed by a dermal layer comprising of mostly fibroblasts and resident as well as migrating immune cells. This is followed by a subcutaneous layer of fat which lies beneath the dermis. Immune function in the skin is mediated by a number of immune cells residing in both the epidermal and dermal layers. Langerhans cells in the epidermis capture antigens and migrate to secondary lymph nodes where they activate naïve T cells. Keratinocytes sense the presence of injury or infection and release various anti-pathogenic substances as well as cytokines and chemokines which serve to activate and recruit immune cells. Dermal dendritic cells initiate adaptive immune responses. A number of other immune cells such as mast cells, γδ T cells, and various subsets of innate lymphoid cells and T cells contribute to distinct facets of immune responses

spinosum, and finally a basal layer, attached to the basement membrane. The stratum corneum and stratum granulosum contribute to barrier protection, whereas the cornified layer of the epidermis serves as a scaffold for the microflora.

Keratinocytes Act as Early Sensors of Infection and Initiate Host Defense

Mounting evidence now suggests that keratinocytes play a vital role in the initiation of host defense including the detection of pathogens and the activation or recruitment of leukocytes (Fig. 5.2). Keratinocytes express a number of pathogen sensors including pattern recognition receptors such as the toll-like receptor (TLR) and nucleotide-binding oligomerization domain-like (NOD) receptors, as well as C-type lectins such as dectin. In response to infection, they produce a number of microbicidal agents including antimicrobial peptides such as defensins and bacterial cell-wall digesting enzymes such as lysozyme. They also produce a vast array of cytokines and

chemokines that serve to signal other immune cells such as T cells or macrophages and induce their recruitment and effector function. These include among many others CXCL9, CXCL11, CCL20, TNF-α, IL-1, IL-6, IL-33, and thymic stromal lymphopoietin (TSLP). TSLP and IL-33 are critical for the initiation of T_H2 responses by stimulating dendritic cells, and also potently stimulate type 2 innate lymphoid cells (ILC2 cells) in the skin. In addition to keratinocytes, the epidermis consists of a number of immune cells including αβ T cells, Langerhans cells (which are the dendritic cells of the epidermis), and γδ T cells.

Myeloid Cells of the Skin

In contrast to the epidermis, the dermis is not as densely packed with cells, consisting mostly of extracellular matrix components such as elastin and collagen fibers, as well as numerous fibroblasts. However, a number of resident and migratory immune cells reside in the dermis including

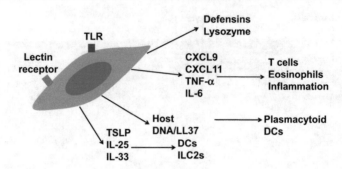

Fig. 5.2 Keratinocytes play a vital role in skin immune responses. Keratinocytes are triggered early during infection, trauma, or injury to the skin. Infection results in the release of several antimicrobial peptides including defensins and lysozyme. Cytokines like TSLP and IL-33 activate nearby cells such as dendritic cells and ILC2s. During inflammation, the production of proinflammatory cytokines and chemokines further alert the immune system and induce the recruitment of various leukocytes to the site of inflammation. Lastly, during psoriasis, the production of complexes of self-nucleic acids and **cathelicidins** by keratinocytes is critical for the activation of plasmacytoid dendritic cells

mast cells, macrophages, dendritic cells, innate lymphoid cells, and various subsets of T cells. These travel through the lymphatics in the dermis to various lymph nodes serving the skin throughout the body, where the activation and differentiation of naïve T and B cells can occur.

Together with keratinocytes and other innate cells such as mast cells and innate lymphoid cells, the dendritic cells of the skin play a vital role in the initiation of immunity. The Langerhans cells of the epidermis have long been known to be important in the capture and processing of antigenic material. They are able to extend their dendrites through the various layers of the epidermis, including the tight junctions of the stratum granulosum, enabling antigen capture and subsequent processing. However, their role in immune priming of the skin is not absolute, and a number of resident and migratory dendritic cell subsets play a role in the initiation of adaptive immunity in the skin. Migratory immature dendritic cells capture antigen in the skin and travel to secondary lymphoid organs such as lymph nodes, during which they undergo maturation and express high levels of T cell costimulatory molecules and MHC Class I or II. In addition to Langerhans cells and monocyte-derived dendritic cell subsets, plasmacytoid dendritic cells may also be recruited to the skin during infection or inflammation, serving as a vast source of type I interferon. This is especially important in

psoriasis, where they produce type I interferon in response to complexes of antimicrobial peptides such as **LL37** with self-nucleic acids that are released by keratinocytes.

The Role of Innate Lymphoid Cells in Skin Immunity

Innate lymphoid cells (ILCs) are newly discovered immune cell populations that play essential roles in innate immunity and the activation of adaptive immune cells (Fig. 5.3). Three classes of cells have been described. **ILC1**s express the transcription factor, T-bet, make IFN-γ, and respond to cytokines such as IL-12 and IL-18. They include cell types such as NK cells, but also other non-cytolytic populations. They are important in immunity to viruses. **ILC2** populations express the transcription factor GATA-3, produce T_H2 cytokines such as IL-5 and IL-13, and respond to the cytokines IL-25 and IL-33. They include cell types such as nuocytes and natural helper cells, which are among the first cell types to be activated during type 2 immune responses. ILC2s play critical roles in helminth responses and tissue repair, but also mediate allergic diseases such as asthma and atopic dermatitis. **ILC3** populations express the transcription factor **RORγt** and produce cytokines such as IL-22, IL-17A, and some IFN-γ in response to IL-1β

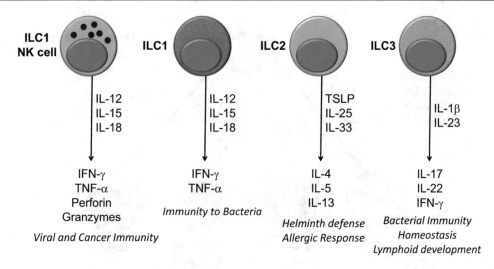

Fig. 5.3 Innate lymphoid cell populations and their roles in immune defense. Innate lymphoid cells have been classified into three distinct subsets based on the transcription factors they express, the cytokines they produce, and their
effector function. ILC2s play a pivotal role in allergic responses such as atopic dermatitis by producing the cytokines
IL-5 and IL-13, which induce allergic inflammation

and IL-23. They also participate in neutrophilic
responses to bacteria and the development of
lymphoid tissue.

ILC1 cell types such as NK cells have been
detected in healthy skin, but their functions are not
well understood. A small number have been
detected in the inflamed skin in psoriasis. ILC2s
have been better described in non-cutaneous
inflammation. They are characterized on the basis
of a number of lineage-negative markers and the
expression of molecules such as CD45, ICOS, and
the IL-33-receptor ST2. When stimulated by cytokines such as TSLP, IL-25 and IL-33, ILC2s make
prodigious amounts of IL-5 and IL-13, which
drive allergic inflammation, especially in atopic
dermatitis. These cytokines regulate the development of eosinophilia, mucus production, and fibrosis in skin tissue. Lastly, ILC3 cells are present in
the skin during inflammatory conditions, but their
functions have not been well studied.

The Skin Is Populated
with Heterogenous Subsets
of Resident T Cells

Mouse dendritic epidermal γδ T cells play an
important role in wound healing, immunity, and
tumor immunosurveillance. They express the

receptor NKG2D, which recognizes stress proteins such as Rae1 during viral infections or
tumorigenesis, express TLRs, and are required
for wound healing and keratinocyte proliferation.
Some γδ T cells may also serve as antigen presenting cells. In psoriasis, γδ T cells play an
important role in driving inflammation by producing IL-17A.

Lastly, both the epidermal and dermal layers
of the skin consist of a vast number of αβ T cells
including subsets of CD4 (Fig. 5.4), CD8, and
Foxp3-expressing regulatory T cells. Of these,
the vast majority of T cells are CD8-expressing
tissue-resident memory (TRM) T cells, mostly
present in the epidermis. These do not recirculate
between organs or enter circulation, but provide
effective effector and memory function capability
within skin tissue. Similar TRM populations are
also present within other organs. The CD4 T cell
population is more heterogeneous, consisting of
both circulating and resident populations.

Atopic Dermatitis

Atopic Dermatitis (AD) or **eczema** as it is
more commonly known is one of the most
widely prevalent allergic diseases in the West,
with incidences of up to 25% in children and 7%

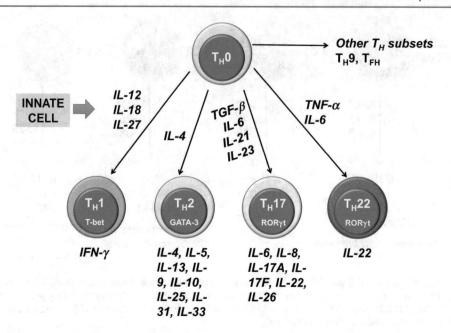

Fig. 5.4 Helper T cell subsets implicated in the pathogenesis of AD and psoriasis. Naïve T cells require three signals in order to be activated and perform effector function: Signal 1 is comprised of interactions between the T cell receptor and MHC plus peptide on an antigen presenting cell (APC). Signal 2 is mediated by costimulatory interactions between molecules on APCs and T cells including those involving B7 with CD28 and OX40L with OX40. Signal 3 is provided by immunomodulatory cytokines produced by innate cells, which drive the differentiation of T cell subsets. Four main helper T cell subsets have been implicated in the pathogenesis of atopic dermatitis and psoriasis. The differentiation of naïve CD4 T cells into T_H1 cells is driven by IL-12, which is produced by macrophages and dendritic cells at the onset of inflammation. IL-12 induces the activation of the transcription factor T-bet, leading to the generation of antigen-specific T_H1 cells, which produce the T_H1-associated cytokines IL-2, TNF-α, and IFN-γ. In contrast, the development of T_H2 cells is dependent on the transcription factor GATA-3 and differentiation in the presence of IL-4, which is produced by innate cells such as basophils or natural killer T cells. Activated T_H2 cells produce a number of proallergic cytokines including IL-4, IL-5, and IL-13. T_H17 cell differentiation occurs in the presence of IL-1, IL-6, and TGF-β produced by innate cells as well as through the autocrine production of IL-21 by T_H17 cells. T_H17 cells are characterized by the expression of the transcription factor retinoic acid receptor-related orphan receptor-(RORγt). Activated T_H17 cells produce high levels of the IL-17 family of cytokines (IL-17 A-F) as well as the IL-10 family of cytokines which includes IL-19, IL-20, IL-22, IL-24, and IL-26. In humans, a specific helper T cell subset producing IL-22 can be identified and is named as the T_H22 subset. This subset is driven by the production of IL-6 and TNF-α by innate cells. Both IL-17 and IL-22 have diverse effects on epithelial cells and keratinocytes. IL-17 is a proinflammatory cytokine that coordinates immune responses to infection by inducing the release of antimicrobial peptides, enhancing granulopoiesis, and inducing neutrophil accumulation in peripheral tissues. In contrast, IL-22 is predominantly an anti-inflammatory cytokine, maintaining the homeostatic integrity of organs and tissues. The maintenance and establishment of RORγt-positive T_H17 cells is driven by IL-23, a cytokine produced by dendritic cells. IL-23 also aids in the production of IL-22 by T_H17 cells. In addition to these subsets, T helper cells also differentiate into follicular helper T cells (T_{FH}) and T_H9 cells, which also modulate immune responses

in adults. Eczema symptoms characteristically start in children within the first 5 years of life and may last for several decades after manifestation, although a significant majority of patients outgrow the disease into adolescence and beyond. The disease is often associated with a family history of allergy and many patients with AD go on to develop other allergic diseases including allergic rhinitis, asthma, and food allergy, referred to as the *atopic march*. In addition, AD along with psoriasis, is also commonly categorized within the cluster of diseases comprising the *inflammatory skin march*. Diseases belonging to this category are frequently associated with a number of comorbidities such as cardiovascular disease.

Fig. 5.5 Pathologic manifestation of atopic dermatitis. This photograph depicts the skin about the anterior aspect of a patient's left knee, which displayed an erythematous, crusty appearance due to an immune-mediated inflammatory skin disorder, referred to as eczema, or more correctly termed atopic dermatitis. Credit: CDC, Public Health Image Library

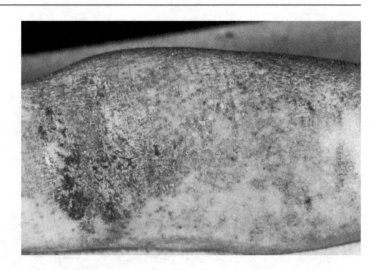

The hallmark of AD pathogenesis is skin barrier dysfunction and the most common symptom is pruritus or itching. Atopic lesions are characterized by itchy, inflamed skin, which can induce intense pruritus in patients, leading to severe pain, irritability, and loss of quality of life (Fig. 5.5). Pruritus also leads to the development of erythematous areas involving crusting, scaling, and lichenification of skin. Pruritic lesions in infants are especially disconcerting to both patients and their parents, resulting in painful itching often throughout the night and severe distress for the entire family. Furthermore, constant itching leads to further disruption of the epidermal barrier and the potential exposure to opportunistic pathogens resulting in the induction of secondary infections and superinfections. Susceptibility to *Staphylococcus aureus* infections in particular are extremely prevalent and a significant cause of concern. Lastly, although disease flare-ups are extremely painful, the progression of AD is often intermittent, involving periods of exacerbation followed by remission. This may be a consequence of regulation by a number of diverse helper T cell subsets, including T_H2, T_H1, T_H17, and **T_H22** cells.

Both skin barrier dysfunction and CD4 T cell-mediated chronic inflammation are major characteristics of the development of disease (Fig. 5.6). Evidence from a number of animal and human studies implicate genes that are typically involved in epidermal barrier integrity and T cell-mediated function. These include the genes for the epidermal barrier protein **filaggrin** as well as T cell cytokines such as IL-4, IL-5, IL-13, IFN-γ, IL-10, TNF-α, IL-17 and **IL-22**. Filaggrin especially is extremely important in at least 30% of patients, in whom deficiency of this gene is associated with disease persistence. However, not all patients with AD exhibit filaggrin deficiency, suggesting the possibility of involvement of other epidermal genes such as *loricrin* or *SPINK5*. Furthermore, the phenotypic development of the disease may differ depending on *filaggrin (FLG)* mutations, IgE levels, race, and age. For example, African American patients with AD rarely exhibit filaggrin mutations and many patients with these mutations outgrow the disease. Similarly, different disease phenotypes may be present depending on whether the development of AD is extrinsic (IgE-associated) or intrinsic (non-atopic). Patients with extrinsic disease have high total levels of IgE and the disease is characterized by severe infiltration with eosinophils. They also have a personal family history of allergy. In patients with intrinsic disease, normal levels of IgE are observed, and along with high T_H2 activity, increased T_H17 and T_H22 activity are also observed. Likewise, increased T_H17 activity is also observed in Asian patients with AD compared with European Americans. Lastly, distinct T cell profiles are observed in pediatric versus adult AD with differing T cell subsets predominating at various stages.

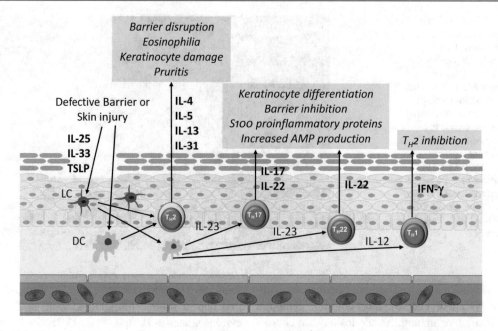

Fig. 5.6 The pathophysiology of atopic dermatitis. The development of atopic dermatitis is mediated via a complex interplay of various factors including mutations in epidermal barrier proteins such as filaggrin, environmental insults such as infection or wounds which induce mechanical injury and introduce antigens into the skin, as well as immune mediators released by activated immune cells. Keratinocytes sense the presence of injury and release cytokines such as IL-25, IL-33, and TSLP, which stimulate ILC2s and induce dendritic cell maturation. APCs such as Langerhans cells and dendritic cells capture antigen and activate naïve T cells in secondary lymphoid organs. T_H2 cells play a predominant role in acute AD and are associated with the production of high levels of IgE antibodies. They induce eosinophilia, dermatitis, and itching. Other T helper cell subsets are present during chronic stages of AD and may predominate in patients with intrinsic AD, which is not associated with elevated IgE. Distinct T cell subsets may also predominate in pediatric vs. adult patients. Abnormal levels of the cytokines IL-17 and IL-22 by T_H17 and T_H22 cells further contribute to inflammatory lesions by disrupting the normal processes of keratinocyte differentiation, antimicrobial peptide generation, and cytokine production

Pathophysiology of AD

The primary function of the skin is to serve as an effective barrier against pathogens and other foreign chemicals and irritants such as allergens. The skin also plays a vital role in regulating the loss of water. The barrier function of the skin is performed by keratinocytes in the epidermis, which regulate the entry of foreign substances into the skin. A primary molecule involved in this function is the filaggrin protein, which is derived from profilaggrin encoded for by the *FLG* gene. Filaggrins are critical for epidermal differentiation and mediate terminal differentiation of the skin and formation of the stratum corneum. Filaggrin breakdown products are also natural moisturizers, which serve to retain water in the

epidermis and hydrate the skin. Mutations in the *FLG* gene result in a loss of function resulting in deficiencies in skin permeability and defective barrier function. When the barrier function of skin is compromised, high molecular weight allergens such as pollen and food particles are able to traverse the skin much more easily, inducing the activation of immune cells. This is further enhanced by intense scratching of the skin, which can induce the development of mechanical injury and further damage the epidermal barrier, resulting in enhanced cutaneous penetration of allergens, and consequently immune sensitization and inflammation. Mechanical injury also increases transepidermal water loss, resulting in dry, itchy skin. However, skin barrier dysfunction alone is not responsible for the predisposition to develop AD. Atopic patients often also have other skin-associated immune defects such as the decreased production of **antimicrobial peptides (AMPs)** and consequently increased susceptibility to skin infections.

Injury to the skin instantly activates epidermal keratinocytes, which begin to secrete a number of protective cytokines. Predominant among these are the cytokines TSLP, IL-1, IL-6, and **TGF-β**. Recent evidence further indicates that they also produce prodigious amounts of IL-25 and IL-33. TSLP, in particular, has a profound effect on the Langerhans and dendritic cells of the skin, conferring on them the ability to skew CD4 T cells towards a T_H2 phenotype. Increased TSLP levels are found in the skin lesions of patients with AD. Allergen-laden dendritic cells mature and subsequently migrate to draining lymph nodes, where they encounter naïve CD4 T cells, and induce them to pivot towards a predominantly T_H2 phenotype in the presence of the cytokine IL-4.

T_H2 cells are the predominant T cell type in AD lesions and have long been known to be the culprit in all known endotypes of AD. The T_H2 cytokines IL-4, IL-5, and IL-13 in particular play a central role in the pathogenesis of AD, inducing allergen sensitization, driving inflammatory cascades, and impairing skin barrier function. IL-4 is critical for the skewing of naïve T cells towards a T_H2 phenotype and plays an important role in activating B cells and the subsequent class switching of IgM to IgE and IgG. Similarly, IL-13 induces mucus hypersecretion, enhances fibrosis by inducing epithelial cell turn over, and aids in antibody class switching. IL-5 is critical for the differentiation and proliferation of eosinophils. Additionally, the T_H2 cytokines IL-9 and IL-10 enhance mast cell function, and **IL-31** induces pruritus.

Evidence for the role of T_H2 cells comes from many laboratory studies and the successful therapeutic outcome of T cell targeting drugs (Table 5.1). Increased numbers of CD4 T cells including those producing high levels of IL-4 and IL-13 have been found in the circulation of AD patients and in AD lesions. Increased levels of these cytokines have also been found in atopic lesions where they cause keratinocytes and

Table 5.1 Evidence for the role of T_H2 cells in atopic dermatitis

- Increased numbers of CD4 T cells producing IL-4 and IL-13 are present in the blood and skin lesions of AD patients
- IL-4 and IL-13 stimulate the production of chemokines such as eotaxin by keratinocytes and fibroblasts
- Transgenic mice overexpressing epidermal IL-4 or IL-13 develop AD-like lesions, epidermal thickening, pruritis, and high IgE levels
- Transgenic mice overexpressing STAT6 (a transcription factor required for IL-4 and IL-13 signaling) develop an AD-like disease
- IL-4 and IL-13 inhibit epidermal barrier proteins such as filaggrin
- IL-4 and IL-13 inhibit the production of antimicrobial peptides enhancing susceptibility to cutaneous infections
- Inhibition of IL-5 reduces epidermal thickening and eosinophilia in AD lesions
- T_H2 cells induce keratinocyte damage and enhance cell death

T_H2 cells play a critical role in the development of AD. Cytokines produced by T_H2 cells drive the pathogenic manifestations of the disease including eosinophilia, thickened lesions, and pruritis

fibroblasts to release numerous chemokines for T cells and eosinophils, especially eotaxin. The importance of IL-4 and IL-13 has been demonstrated in a number of studies. Transgenic mice overexpressing epidermal IL-4 spontaneously develop signs and symptoms of AD including AD lesions and high IgE levels. Similarly, transgenic IL-13 mice also develop AD lesions, pruritus, epidermal thickening, and high IgE levels. Signaling by IL-4 and IL-13 results in the activation of the STAT6/JAK pathway. In transgenic mice modified to constitutively activate STAT6, an AD-like disease develops, which is reversed by inhibition of either IL-4 or IL-13. IL-4 and IL-13 also inhibit several of the epidermal barrier proteins including filaggrin, involucrin, and loricrin, and destabilize the tight junctions in the stratum. Furthermore, they inhibit the production of AMPs such as β-defensins and cathelicidins, increasing susceptibility to cutaneous infections with *S. aureus* and herpes simplex virus. IL-5 is also an important T_H2 cytokine driving the activation and proliferation of eosinophils. Inhibition of IL-5 in animal studies results in reduced epidermal thickening and decreased skin eosinophilia. However, clinical trials with mepolizumab, an anti-IL-5 monoclonal antibody approved in asthma, have not been very promising, with reduction of circulating eosinophils, but no attenuation of overall AD severity in patients. In the skin, activated T_H2 cells also directly impair epidermal function, where T_H2 cells express Fas L and TNF-α, which subsequently induce damage to keratinocytes and enhance cell death.

Despite the predominance of T_H2 cells in AD lesions and in the development of AD, emerging evidence suggests a more complex picture with a role for other Th cell types including T_H1, T_H17, and T_H22 cells. For example, T_H17-associated molecules such as IL-17 and CCL20 are consistently elevated in both acute and chronic AD lesions. Here they serve to upregulate the production of AMPs such as β-defensins and downregulate the expression of *FLG* and tight junction genes. Interestingly, however, when IL-4 and IL-13 are present, the antimicrobial activity of T_H17 cells is inhibited. T_H17 cells also contribute to increases in IL-22 and S100A proteins, which have antimicrobial and proinflammatory properties. IL-22 signals by binding its receptor which is a heterodimer consisting of IL-10β and IL-22R. While IL-10β is widely expressed, expression of IL-22R in humans is limited to epithelial cells. Here, it modifies the expression of several genes involved in tissue differentiation, repair, and survival. It also increases the production of antimicrobial peptides and peptides of the S100 family by keratinocytes. Through activation of the STAT3 pathway, it also has profound effects on the differentiation and turnover of keratinocytes, decreasing expression of epidermal barrier genes such as profilaggrin and hence inhibiting keratinocyte differentiation but promoting their proliferation. IL-17A can also have similar effects on keratinocytes. Finally, IL-22 activates anti-apoptotic pathways and promotes wound healing.

Recent evidence indicates that along with T_H2 cells, T_H22 cells also predominate in acute and chronic AD lesions. Conversely, in chronic lesions, the activity of T_H17 cells decreases and instead mixed lesions consisting of T_H2, T_H22,

and T_H1 are present. It is thought that IgE cross-linking causes dendritic cells to produce large amounts of IL-12, promoting IFN-γ-producing T_H1 activity.

What Are T_H22 Cells?

IL-22 is an important homeostatic cytokine, which is necessary for maintaining the integrity of tissues and organs such as the skin. It is a glycoprotein belonging to the IL-10 family and produced by both innate and adaptive cells including subsets of CD4 and CD8 T cells, $\gamma\delta$ T cells, and type 3 ILCs. While IL-22 is co-released along with IL-17 by mouse T_H17 cells, in humans this is limited. Instead, a specific Th subset T_H22 is responsible for releasing IL-22 along with TNF-α, but not IL-17, IFN-γ, or IL-4. T_H22 differentiation is driven by TNF-α and IL-6. However, IL-23, IL-12 and IL-18 are all required for the release of IL-22 by T_H17 cells.

Treatment of Atopic Dermatitis

The therapeutic approach in AD is focused on measures that include preventative, non-pharmacological, and pharmacological therapy. Control of symptoms such as itching during acute exacerbations is paramount. However, successful management of the disease requires not only clearance of skin lesions, but also the elimination of triggers, and monitoring of the patient throughout treatment.

Non-pharmacologic measures include the prevention of allergen exposure and appropriate skin care. These include the frequent application of moisturizers and emollients which soften skin tissue, the use of lukewarm baths, the use of unscented soaps for bathing and cleaning, the use of non-abrasive clothing such as cotton, and the use of appropriate over-the-counter therapy such as sedative anti-histamines to allow the child to sleep at night. Moisturizers are an important standard of care in AD and improve skin hydration by reducing transepidermal water loss. The use of occlusives which create an oily layer on the surface of the skin as well as emollients are recommended.

Pharmacologic Therapy

Corticosteroids

Topical corticosteroids remain the drug of choice for AD treatment. The immunopharmacology and mechanism of action of corticosteroids is described in detail in Chap. 4. Briefly, these drugs induce potent immunosuppression by inhibiting the activation and migration of immune cells and their mediators, thereby inhibiting inflammatory activity in the target area of application. Depending on the severity of the disease and the area of the body to be treated, different drugs and strengths may be used. For example, low potency **hydrocortisone 1%** may be used on the face, while medium-potency **betamethasone valerate 0.1%** may be used for the body. For short-term

treatments, mid-strength, high potency drugs are suitable, such as **betamethasone dipropionate 0.05%** or **clobetasone propionate 0.05%**. Adverse effects maybe both local and systemic, including but not limited to skin atrophy, acne, purpura, infections, hyperglycemia and growth retardation. However, adverse effects are dependent on the potency, duration of treatment, the site of application, and the percentage of body surface area covered.

Topical Calcineurin Inhibitors

Calcineurin inhibitors such as **tacrolimus ointment (Protopic®)** and **pimecrolimus cream (Elidel®)** are used as a second line treatment in AD and have been shown to reduce the extent, severity, and symptoms of AD in adults and children. Calcineurin inhibitors such as tacrolimus and **cyclosporine** directly block T cell function by binding to calcineurin and inhibiting the activation of the transcription factor NFAT (Fig. 5.7). Antigen-induced signaling *via* the T cell receptor initiates a signaling cascade that induces the

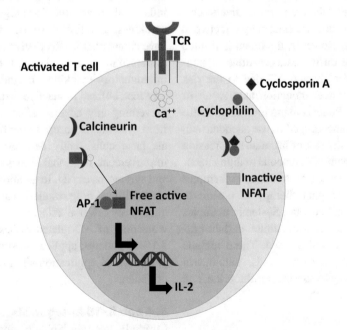

Fig. 5.7 Mechanism of action of calcineurin inhibitors. Calcineurin inhibitors are potent antagonists of T cell signaling. Signaling via the TCR results in various tyrosine-dependent phosphorylative events culminating in the rise of intracellular calcium levels. Calcium binds calcineurin, a phosphatase, which subsequently activates the transcription factor NFAT and induces the expression and activation of the gene for IL-2. Calcineurin inhibitors bind the calcineurin-binding proteins cyclophilins and FK506-binding protein 12, which prevent the activation of calcineurin by calcium, thus inhibiting the activation of NFAT and the production of IL-2

activation of the transcription factor NFAT and induction of the gene for IL-2. This signaling cascade involves a complex sequence of events including the upregulation of intracellular calcium and the activation of calcineurin, a calcium binding protein. Briefly, signaling *via* the T cell receptor induces the activation of the transcription factor AP-1 resulting in an increase in intracellular calcium levels. Increased calcium levels then activate calcineurin, a phosphatase that subsequently activates NFAT. Activated NFAT migrates to the nucleus where it binds with AP-1 to form an active transcription factor. Here, it promotes the activation of the IL-2 gene resulting in T cell activation and proliferation. The calcineurin inhibitors cyclosporine and tacrolimus exert their effects by binding cyclophilins and FK-binding proteins in the cytosol. These complexes subsequently bind calcineurin preventing the activation of NFAT and suppressing T cell activation.

The use of creams containing calcineurin inhibitors has been found to be efficacious in both adults and children. They are usually recommended in patients who are unresponsive to corticosteroid therapy and are extremely effective at relieving pruritus. However, treatment is limited to short-term use during exacerbations or noncontinuous use for chronic AD due to the risk associated with cancer induction as a result of T cell deficiency. Patients using topical calcineurin inhibitors are encouraged to use adequate sun protection due to the risk of immune suppression and the development of cutaneous malignancies.

Other pharmacologic treatment therapies include the use of phototherapy (exposure to ultraviolet light) and coal tar. Systemic therapies may also sometimes be used, although their efficacy has not been well studied. These include oral therapy with corticosteroids, calcineurin inhibitors such as cyclosporine, azathioprine, and methotrexate among others.

Immunotherapy

Oral Anti-histamines

Anti-histamines are widely used for the treatment of AD. However, they have mixed efficacy in patients. The mechanism of action of anti-histamines is described in Chap. 4.

Phosphodiesterase Inhibitors

Crisaborole ointment, 2% (**Eucrisa®; Pfizer**) is a topical, non-steroidal, small molecule drug that was approved by the Food and Drug Administration (FDA) in December 2016 for the treatment of mild to moderate AD in patients 2 years of age and older. Its beneficial effects are dependent on the inhibition of phosphodiesterase-4 (PDE4), an enzyme that is critical in the cellular regulation of NF-κB and NFAT transcription, resulting in modulation of cytokine secretion by immune cells. PDE4 is upregulated in the immune cells of patients with AD and its role in the control of cellular signaling is described in Chap. 4. Briefly, upregulation of PDE4 results in the enhanced degradation of adenosine cyclic monophosphate, resulting in the upregulation of NF-κB and NFAT activation and the production of proinflammatory cytokines. Treatment with crisaborole inhibits the PDE4-dependent degradation of cAMP resulting in the suppression of inflammation and the downregulation of T cell cytokines. Preclinical studies with crisaborole have shown that it effectively penetrates the skin at sites of treatment and inhibits the production of inflammatory cytokines. Furthermore, it is rapidly metabolized to inactive metabolites, thereby preventing any adverse effects that may result from systemic exposure to the drug. Clinical trials have consistently demonstrated an overall improvement in global disease severity scores and symptoms of AD. In addition, 48-week treatment with the drug resulted in an overall low frequency of adverse effects. These included the worsening of AD-related rashes or erythema in 3.1% of patients, application-site pain in 2.3% of patients, and application-site infections in 1.2% of patients.

IL-4 and IL-13 Antagonists

Currently, the only biologic approved for moderate-to-severe AD is **dupilumab (Dupixent®; Regeneron and Sanofi)**, which was approved by the FDA in 2017. It is approved for the treatment of adults with moderate-to-severe AD whose disease is not adequately controlled with topical

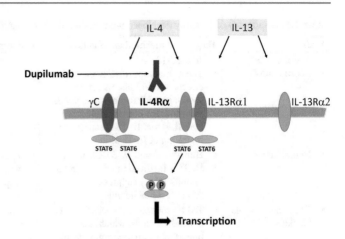

Fig. 5.8 Mechanism of action of Dupilumab. Dupilumab is a monoclonal antibody targeting IL-4Rα (blue oval), a shared component of both the IL-4 and IL-13 receptors. Inhibition of IL-4 and IL-13 signaling attenuates the progression of T_H2-mediated allergic responses, a major culprit in the development of AD

prescription therapies or when those therapies are not advisable. Dupilumab is a fully human monoclonal antibody that targets the IL-4Rα, which is shared by the receptors for both IL-4 and IL-13, thus blocking two key T_H2 cytokines that drive the development of AD (Fig. 5.8). IL-13 binds to a heterodimer that includes the IL-4Rα and IL-13Rα1 receptors, while IL-4 binds a receptor containing the IL-4Rα and γ chains. Treatment with dupilumab not only decreases T_H2 responses and T_H2-associated molecules such as CCL17, CCL18, and CCL26, but also suppresses molecules associated with T_H17 and T_H22 responses, such as S100A proteins and IL-23p19. Beck et al. showed that weekly treatment with dupilumab monotherapy (300 mg) for 12 weeks reduced skin disease severity, as measured by the Eczema Area Severity Index (EASI), by 74.0% compared with 23.3% with placebo. Also, a 60% reduction in the body surface area affected was observed and 40% of patients achieved disease clearance (Investigator's Global Assessment score of 0 or 1) at day 85. Patients treated with dupilumab also had fewer skin infections (0.05 infections per patient) overall.

Other Biologics Currently Under Investigation

In addition to dupilumab, a number of other drugs are currently undergoing investigation in clinical trials. These include drugs against the cytokines IL-4, IL-13, IL-31, IL-17, IL-12/IL-23p40 and IL-22 as well as inhibitors of TSLP, OX40L, CRTH2, PDE4, JAK kinases and H_4R.

A brief description of these is provided in Table 5.2 below. Of particular interest are the PDE4 and JAK kinase inhibitors which have been approved for the treatment of psoriasis. The **JAK–signal transducer and activator of transcription (JAK-STAT)** signaling pathway is critical for the development of cytokine-mediated responses and plays important roles in the generation of both innate and adaptive immune responses. Binding of cytokines such as IL-4 or IL-13 to its receptors results in the activation of JAK kinases including Jak1, Jak2, Jak3 and tyrosine kinase 2, which are a family of cytoplasmic protein tyrosine kinases. These then go on to activate the signal transducer and activator of transcription (STAT) proteins, which subsequently induce gene-specific activation and expression. The JAK-STAT pathway has been shown to have multiple effects in AD-associated allergic inflammation. This includes the induction of T_H2 polarization and skin barrier disruption, activation of eosinophils, induction of B cell maturation, upregulation of epidermal chemokines, and downregulation of AMPs.

Psoriasis

Psoriasis is a chronic inflammatory disease of the skin that affects approximately 2.5% of the population of North America and Europe. The disease is characterized by the presence of erythematous, thickened epidermal lesions that vary in intensity and in affected body surface area

Table 5.2   A summary of currently developed biologics for atopic dermatitis being evaluated in clinical trials

Drug	Target and mechanism of action	Outcome
• Tralokinumab • Lebrikizumab	• Anti-IL-13 • These drugs specifically block the effects of IL-13 and therefore should provide useful information regarding the effects of blocking both IL-4 and IL-13 compared to inhibition of IL-13 alone	• Completed phase II trials
• Nemolizumab	• Humanized anti-IL-31RA antibody • IL-31 is involved in pruritis and its inhibition may suppress AD-associated itching	• Phase I trials resulted in successful outcomes with decreased itching observed and improvement in nighttime sleep conditions
• TSLP and OX40L blockers	• TSLP production induces OX40L in dendritic cells, which is an important costimulatory molecule for T_H2 cells and is necessary for the maintenance of allergic inflammation.	• Phase I trials
• Fevipiprant	• CRTH2 (prostaglandin D2 receptor 2) inhibitor • CRTH2 is expressed by cutaneous T_H2 cells and are important for allergic skin inflammation. Polymorphisms in CRTH2 have been associated with allergic sensitization.	• Phase III trials • Favorable safety profile and promising outcomes with respect to pruritis
• Ustekinumab	• Anti-IL-12/IL-23p40 • The p40 subunit of IL-12 and IL-23 are important for the generation of T_H1 and T_H17/T_H22 responses	• Treatment with ustekinumab using the recommended dosing for psoriasis in AD patients in a clinical trial resulted in severe reductions in T_H2 responses along with expected decreases in T_H1, T_H17, and T_H22 responses. However, some of the outcomes compared to placebo were obscured likely due to background topical glucocorticoid usage by patients.
• ILV-094	• Anti-IL-22 • Inhibition of T_H22 and T_H17 responses	• In clinical trials
• Secukinumab	• Anti-IL-17A • Inhibition of T_H17 responses	• In clinical trials
• Apremilast • Crisaborole (topical)	• PDE-4 inhibitor • Increases cAMP levels resulting in decreased expression of IFN-γ, TNF-α, IL-12, IL-17, and IL-23, which play prominent roles in chronic AD pathophysiology	• Crisaborole has demonstrated a favorable safety profile and resulted in an improvement in clinical disease severity in phase III studies, both in children and adults with AD
• Tofacitinib (topical) • Baricitinib (oral) • Upadacitinib (oral)	• JAK kinase inhibitors	• Phase II trials • Promising results with improvement in pruritis and sleep outcomes
• ZPL389 (oral)	• Small molecule H_4R inhibitor • H_4R is involved in keratinocyte proliferation in AD patients	• 50% reduction in eczema lesions in a proof of concept study

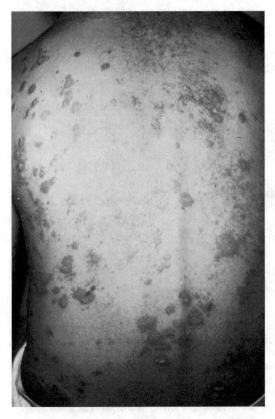

Fig. 5.9 Erythematous patches in Psoriasis. The back of this patient displayed numerous erythematous patches dispersed over the entirety of his back that was diagnosed as a case of psoriasis. Credit: CDC, Public Health Image Library

(Fig. 5.9). The lesions present as well-demarcated plaques with silvery white scales and are associated with variable levels of pruritis. This is often accompanied by changes in the fingernails (50% of patients) and toenails (35% of patients). The disease is extremely visible and in addition to pain and itching, often causes severe emotional distress in patients.

Plaque psoriasis, also known as **psoriasis vulgaris**, is the most common type of psoriasis in the US and has been observed in about 90% of patients. About 30% of patients also develop **psoriasis arthritis** (PsA). The disease is classified as mild, moderate or severe based on the assessment of various parameters such as symptom measures, affected body surface area, severity index, and quality of life measures using standardized evaluative tools.

The development of the disease is a consequence of a complex interaction of immune cells involving keratinocytes, multiple T cell subsets, and their corresponding cytokines (Fig. 5.10). Both genetic factors and environmental influences modulate the outcome of the disease, as prevalence of the disease is uncommon before age 9. Population studies as well as studies of monozygotic twins have identified psoriasis susceptibility genes and their variants such as the psoriasis susceptibility locus 1 (*PSORS1*) on chromosome 6p, which accounts for about 50% of disease heritability. Additionally, other genes such as those for TNF-α and IL-23 have also been reported to be involved.

The impact of environmental influences is not very well understood with variable causes triggering the development of the disease from patient to patient. Common triggers include injury or infection of the skin, streptococcal infections, drugs, smoking, alcohol consumption, obesity, and stress. The lesion often occurs on areas of the skin susceptible to friction or minor trauma, resulting in the induction of inflammation (also called as Koebner's phenomenon). The excessive production of proinflammatory cytokines in the lesional skin also has systemic effects by virtue of their release into circulation, leading to what is termed as the psoriasis march and the development of various comorbidities. In particular, comorbidities such as cardiovascular disease, endothelial dysfunction and insulin resistance (leading to type 2 diabetes and obesity) appear to be strongly associated with psoriasis. About 30% of patients also develop PsA approximately 10 years after the onset of lesional psoriasis, which is characterized by the progressive destruction of joint tissue, leading to severe disability if not treated.

Pathophysiology of Psoriasis

Historically, psoriasis was thought to occur as a result of dysregulated keratinocyte function leading to neutrophil accumulation, complement activation, and the hyperproliferation of epidermal cells. More recently, a more complex picture has

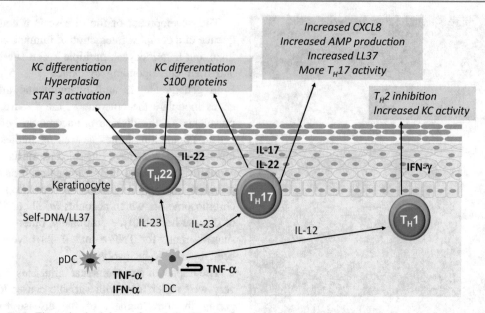

Fig. 5.10 The pathophysiology of psoriasis. The development of psoriasis is mediated *via* a complex interplay of diverse immune cells and their mediators which drive the development of the disease. Injury to keratinocytes results in the release of host DNA-cathelicidin complexes which serves to activate cells such as plasmacytoid dendritic cells. These cells then produce cytokines such as type I interferons and TNF-α, which can further activate myeloid dendritic cells and induce the activation of T helper cell subsets. The T_H cells that play a primary role in psoriasis include the T_H17, T_H22, and T_H1 subsets. T_H17 cells increase keratinocyte differentiation and induce the production of S100 proteins, AMPs, and CXCL8 which is a chemoattractant for neutrophils. IL-22 produced by T_H22 cells induces keratinocyte differentiation and hyperplasia. Lastly, T_H1 cells also increase keratinocyte activity and inhibit T_H2 functions

emerged, involving various subsets of helper T cells that drive key features of the pathophysiology of the disease (Fig. 5.10). Inflammation is thought to be initiated by the activation of **plasmacytoid dendritic cells (pDCs)** by keratinocytes producing complexes of host DNA and cathelicidins (LL-37). The pDCs subsequently produce type I interferons such as IFN-α and IFN-β, as well as TNF-α, which further induce the production of TNF-α, IL-12, and IL-23 by both pDCs and infiltrating myeloid dendritic cells. This combination of cytokines is also able to activate diverse T helper cell subsets including T_H1 and T_H17 cells, which participate in the progression and severity of the disease. Although the role of keratinocytes and neutrophils continues to be recognized to be of critical clinical importance, the identification of T_H1 and T_H17 subsets as major drivers of the inflammation has shifted the goal of therapeutic outcomes as well as the direction of basic and clinical research. Early studies with grafted human skin in mouse

models as well as the role of streptococcal superantigens in guttate psoriasis demonstrated the importance of T cells in mediating the development of disease. Since then, the role of T cells has become well-established through several studies in both mice and humans, and has also been borne out clinically through the efficacy of calcineurin inhibitors in treating the disease. More recent studies suggest that both T_H1 and T_H17 cells participate, with T_H17 cells playing a prominent role in driving the development of the disease. The T_H17 cytokine IL-22 in particular, which belongs to the IL-10 family of cytokines and the IL-20 subfamily, is critical for the proliferation of keratinocytes. Furthermore, IL-22, with the aid of IL-17, induces STAT3 activation, the production of CXCL8 (a chemoattractant for neutrophils), the production of the proinflammatory S100 proteins, and the formation of AMPs. IL-17 also binds to its receptor, IL-17 receptor, on keratinocytes and stimulates them to produce other cytokines such as GM-CSF, VEGF, and

TNF-α. In a similar manner, IL-17 also acts together with the T_H1 cytokine, IFN-γ, to stimulate keratinocyte activity. Conversely, the maintenance of T_H1 and T_H17 lineages in the skin is driven by IL-12 and IL-23 produced by myeloid dendritic cells activated by TNF-α as described above. Furthermore, IL-17 causes keratinocytes to further produce cathelicidins, resulting in increased TNF-α production and a vicious positive feedback loop, resulting in the production of more T_H17 cells.

Treatment Options and the Pharmacology of Immunotherapeutic Drugs

The management of psoriasis is based on the inclusion of both non-pharmacologic and pharmacologic therapies. Non-pharmacologic therapies aimed at reducing stress and improving skin hydration and healing as well as alleviating pruritis are often beneficial in psoriasis management and should always be considered as part of the treatment regimen and initiated whenever appropriate. In addition, preventive measures that decrease psoriasis exacerbation, such as the use of sunscreen protection or avoidance of harsh soaps and detergents, should always be recommended. Management of psoriasis-associated comorbidities should also be part of the treatment plan.

Pharmacologic therapy includes the use of topical and systemic agents, phototherapy, photochemotherapy, and various biologics (Table 5.3).

In most cases of mild to moderate psoriasis, the use of topical agents combined with phototherapy if necessary, is sufficient to control disease symptoms. Systemic agents are usually reserved for patients with moderate to severe psoriasis with or without topical treatment. The use of biologics is typically initiated in patients with moderate-to-severe disease who do not respond to systemic agents such as cyclosporine treatment, and/or those who present with comorbidities such as PsA.

Table 5.3 Classes of drugs used for treatment of psoriasis and psoriatic arthritis

Psoriasis type	Pharmacologic therapy	Drugs
Mild-to-moderate	Topical	• Topical corticosteroids • Vitamin D3 analogs (Calcipotriol) • Retinoids • Anthralin • Topical calcineurin inhibitors
Moderate-to-severe plaque psoriasis	• Systemic • Adjunctive topical therapy	• Acitretin • Cyclosporine • Methotrexate • Apremilast • Topical treatments
Moderate-to-severe plaque psoriasis who do not respond to systemic therapy	• Systemic • Adjunctive topical therapy	• TNF inhibitors • IL-17 inhibitors • IL-12/IL-23 inhibitors • Topical treatments
Psoriatic arthritis	• Systemic agents • Disease-modifying anti-rheumatic drugs	• Cyclosporine • Methotrexate • Apremilast • TNF inhibitors • IL-17 inhibitors • IL-12/IL-23 inhibitors • Sulfasalazine (Azulfidine)

Depending on the severity of psoriasis, both topical and systemic agents may be used for treatment. For treatment of mild-to-moderate psoriasis, topical therapy is usually sufficient. In contrast, the treatment of moderate-to-severe psoriasis may necessitate treatment with oral systemic agents as well as subcutaneously injected biologics. Systemic agents are also used for the treatment of psoriatic arthritis. In addition, disease-modifying anti-rheumatic agents such as the anti-inflammatory drug sulfasalazine may also be used

Topical Therapies

Approximately 80% of patients have mild-to-moderate psoriasis and can be treated with topical treatment alone. Additionally, topical treatments may be used as adjunctive therapy in patients also receiving systemic treatment. Topical agents include corticosteroids, vitamin D3 analogs, retinoids, anthralin, coal tar, and calcineurin inhibitors.

Corticosteroids

Topical corticosteroids remain the mainstay of therapy in the majority of patients with mild-to-moderate disease. Corticosteroids act by binding to corticosteroid receptors in immune cells as well as modulating gene expression resulting in the suppression of immune cell function and proliferation (see mechanism of action of corticosteroids in Chap. 4). A number of different topical corticosteroids with varying potencies may be used in the treatment of psoriasis. A list of some commonly used topical corticosteroids is provided in Table 5.4. These are usually well-tolerated in most patients, although adverse effects can occur such as the development of acne, contact dermatitis, skin atrophy, folliculitis, and purpura. Systemic adverse effects can occur with continued and widespread use.

Vitamin D3 Analogs

Absorption of vitamin D by skin cells results in the synthesis of its active metabolite, $1\alpha,25$-dihydroxyvitamin D_3 ($1,25(OH)_2D_3$ or calcitriol, which binds to the intracellular vitamin D receptor (VDR). VDR also acts as a nuclear transcription factor that changes conformation and together with another protein binds to genes called vitamin D response elements, resulting in the promotion or inhibition of gene transcription. Topical vitamin D3 analogs act by binding to the VDR in keratinocytes and other cutaneous cells, inhibiting their differentiation and proliferation in psoriatic lesions. They may also promote and stabilize keratinocyte turnover.

Topical vitamin D3 analogs include **calcipotriol (calcipotriene)**, **calcitriol** (the active metabolite of vitamin D), and **tacalcitol**, of which only calcipotriol is available in the U.S. They are usually well-tolerated and have a good safety profile, although mild adverse effects may occur.

Retinoids

Retinoids are derivatives of vitamin A that are prescribed by dermatologists for a number of skin diseases. **Tazarotene** is a topical retinoid that is used in the treatment of mild-to-moderate psoriasis. It acts by binding to nuclear retinoic acid receptors and inducing normal keratinocyte differentiation and proliferation while decreasing the extent of keratinocyte hyperproliferation. Adverse effects of tazarotene can include the development of intense irritation in the lesional site resulting in burning and pruritis. This effect is dose-dependent. Tazarotene is considered to be teratogenic and should not be used in pregnancy.

Anthralin

Anthralin or **dithranol** is a hydroxyanthone, anthracene derivative that is sometimes used to treat mild-to-moderate psoriasis. Although its exact mechanism of action in psoriasis is unknown, it inhibits keratinocyte proliferation and normalizes their differentiation. It is thought to act by accumulating in the mitochondria and disrupting cellular replication and division by interfering with the energy supply. Anthralin causes severe irritation and burning and is not to be used on the face. It is typically used as part of a short-acting regimen, where it is applied for about 10–30 min and then wiped off.

Coal Tar and Salicylic Acid

Both coal tar and salicyclic have keratolytic properties and inhibit the proliferation of keratinocytes. They may be used as part of ointments, creams, oils, and shampoos.

Table 5.4 Some commonly used topical corticosteroids classified according to their strengths

Brand	Generic	Potency
Clobex lotion/spray/shampoo, 0.05%®	Clobetasol propionate	Superpotent
Diprolene ointment, 0.05%®	Betamethasone dipropionate	Superpotent
Olux E foam, 0.05%®	Clobetasol propionate	Superpotent
Psorcon ointment, 0.05%®	Diflorasone diacetate	Superpotent
Topicort topical spray, 0.25%®	Desoximetasone	Superpotent
Ultravate cream/ointment/lotion, 0.05%®	Halobetasol propionate	Superpotent
Vanos cream, 0.1%®	Fluocinonide	Superpotent
Diprolene cream AF, 0.05%®	Betamethasone dipropionate	Potent
Florone ointment, 0.05%®	Diflorasone diacetate	Potent
Halog ointment/cream, 0.1%®	Halcinonide	Potent
Lidex cream/gel/ointment, 0.05%®	Fluocinonide	Potent
Psorcon cream, 0.05%®	Diflorasone diacetate	Potent
Topicort cream/ointment, 0.25%®	Desoximetasone	Potent
Cutivate ointment, 0.005%®	Fluticasone propionate	Upper mid-strength
Lidex-E cream, 0.05%®	Fluocinonide	Upper mid-strength
Luxiq foam, 0.12%®	Betamethasone valerate	Upper mid-strength
Cordran ointment, 0.05%®	Flurandrenolide	Mid-strength
Elocon cream, 0.1%®	Mometasone furoate	Mid-strength
Kenalog cream/spray, 0.1%®	Triamcinolone acetonide	Mid-strength
Synalar ointment, 0.03%®	Fluocinolone acetonide	Mid-strength
Topicort LP cream, 0.05%®	Desoximetasone	Mid-strength
Westcort ointment, 0.2%®	Hydrocortisone valerate	Mid-strength
Cordran cream/lotion/tape, 0.05%®	Flurandrenolide	Lower mid-strength
Cutivate cream/lotion, 0.05%®	Fluticasone propionate	Lower mid-strength
DesOwen lotion, 0.05%®	Desonide	Lower mid-strength
Pandel cream, 0.1%®	Hydrocortisone	Lower mid-strength
Synalar cream, 0.03%/0.01%®	Fluocinolone acetonide	Lower mid-strength
Aclovate cream/ointment, 0.05%®	Alclometasone dipropionate	Mild
Desonate gel, 0.05%®	Desonide	Mild
Synalar cream/solution, 0.01%®	Fluocinolone acetonide	Mild
Cortaid cream/spray/ointment®	Hydrocortisone	Least potent
Micort-HC cream, 2%/2.5%®	Hydrocortisone	Least potent
Nutracort lotion, 1%/2.5%®	Hydrocortisone	Least potent

Topical Calcineurin Inhibitors

Topical calcineurin inhibitors such as pimecrolimus 1% cream (Elidel®) are effective in the treatment of AD. Studies show that it may also be effective for plaque psoriasis and moderate-to-severe inverse psoriasis, and thus may be used as a safe and useful alternative for these conditions.

Systemic Agents

Systemic therapies are commonly used to treat moderate-to-severe plaque psoriasis with or without adjunctive topical therapy. They include the use of acitretin, cyclosporine, methotrexate, mycophenolate mofetil (MMF), hydroxyurea, and the biologics apremilast, etanercept, infliximab, adalimumab, ustekinumab, secukinumab, ixekizumab, brodalumab, guselkumab, and tildrakizumab.

Acitretin

Acitretin is an oral retinoid or vitamin A derivative that is used for the treatment of psoriasis. It is the active metabolite of etritenate. It is commonly used in combination with topical calcipotriol and may be efficacious in some cases of severe psoriasis. Common adverse effects of acitretin include mucocutaneous effects such as dryness of the eyes, nasal and oral mucosa, chapped lips, brittle nails, and burning or sticky skin.

Cyclosporine

Cyclosporine is a systemic calcineurin inhibitor that is effective in inducing psoriasis remission and is also used as part of maintenance therapy. The mechanism of action of cyclosporine is described above. A short course therapy of cyclosporine for 12 weeks or less is usually preferred to avoid adverse effects associated with nephrotoxicity.

Methotrexate

Methotrexate remains a mainstay of therapy for moderate-to-severe plaque psoriasis. It is slightly less efficacious than cyclosporine but is considered an overall safer alternative unless preexisting contradictions such as liver disease are present. Tolerance to methotrexate and its effectiveness is considered as a gold standard prior to switching to treatment with biologics.

Methotrexate is a potent folic acid analog that inhibits the activity of dihydrofolate reductase. Dihydrofolate reductase is a rate-limiting enzyme involved in the production of tetrahydrofolate, which is important for the synthesis of purines and pyrimidines, crucial components of the DNA molecule. Tetrahydrofolate also plays an important role in the methionine-homocysteine cycle, which is necessary for the addition of methyl groups during reactions such as DNA methylation. As such, the major application of methotrexate has been in the suppression of T cell turnover, which is a critical feature of inflammatory

diseases such as rheumatoid arthritis and leukocytic cancers. One consequence of the binding of methotrexate to the dihydrofolate reductase receptor results in the induction of enhanced extracellular adenosine levels, which have a profound effect on inflammatory responses. Depending on the interaction of adenosine with its various receptors, both pro- and anti-inflammatory effects may be observed, including the inhibition of chemokines and cytokines such as CXCL8, IL-6, IL-1 and TNF-α. Methotrexate has also been found to inhibit the recruitment of various inflammatory cells and induce their apoptosis. In addition, decreased levels of immune mediators have been observed in patients treated with methotrexate including prostaglandins and leukotrienes. Due to its potent anti-proliferative activity, a major adverse effect associated with methotrexate treatment is suppression of cellular turnover, often resulting in bone marrow suppression and stomatitis. Administration of folic acid has been found to reduce some of these side effects without compromising the anti-inflammatory effects.

Apremilast

Apremilast (Otezla®) is a small molecule inhibitor of phosphodiesterase 4 (PDE4) approved by the FDA in 2014 for the treatment of active psoriatic arthritis and moderate-to-severe plaque psoriasis. PDE4 is the dominant enzyme in inflammatory cells responsible for the breakdown of cAMP. Inhibition of PDE4 results in the enhancement of intracellular cAMP levels and increases in protein kinase A (PKA) resulting in the modulation of several immune mediators including TNF-α and IL-10. In general, treatment results in the preferential upregulation of cytokines such as IL-10 and downregulation of IL-17, IL-23, and TNF-α. Oral therapy with apremilast is associated with some adverse effects including diarrhea in 25% of patients as well as incidences of depression, suicidal thoughts, and mood disorders. The concurrent use of strong CYP3A4 inducers such as rifampin, phenytoin and St. John's Wort is contraindicated and may reduce the effectiveness of apremilast.

Biologics

With the discovery of novel immune cells and molecules involved in psoriasis, biologics have become important treatment options for moderate-to-severe plaque psoriasis. In the last two decades alone, several biologics have been approved by the FDA for the treatment of moderate-to-severe plaque psoriasis. In addition, many other drugs are in the pipeline or are undergoing clinical trials and emerging as therapeutic options. Classically, TNF-α was thought to be the main proinflammatory cytokine involved in psoriasis resulting in the approval of several anti-TNF inhibitors in the last 15 years. These include: *etanercept* (Enbrel®; Amgen, Thousand Oaks, Calif), *infliximab* (Remicade®; Janssen Biotech, Horsham, Pa), and *adalimumab* (Humira®; Abbvie, Lake Bluff, Ill), which received FDA approval for psoriasis in 2004, 2006, and 2008, respectively. More recently, with the emergence of the importance of the IL-17/IL-23 axis, approval has been granted to the IL-12/IL-23 inhibitor *ustekinumab* (Stelara®; Janssen Biotech) in 2009 and the IL-23 inhibitors *guselkumab* (Tremfya®; Janssen Biotech) in 2017 and **tildrakizumab** (Ilumya®; Sun Pharmaceuticals) in 2018, the IL-17A inhibitors *secukinumab* (Cosentyx®; Novartis Pharmaceuticals Corp, Basel, Switzerland) in 2015 and *ixekizumab* (Taltz®; Eli Lilly and Co, Indianapolis, Ind) in 2016, and the IL-17 receptor inhibitor **brodalumab** (Siliq™) in 2017. Additional biologics targeting the IL-17/IL-23 axis are currently in the pipeline.

Biologics are often used when systemic therapy with other agents has failed or is contraindicated, although treatment may sometimes be initiated in some patients as first line therapy. First line therapy may also be appropriate in certain patients with existing comorbidities. For example, treatment with the anti-TNFα inhibitors adalimumab or infliximab are beneficial for both psoriasis and PsA. Cost is a major factor when considering biologics for psoriasis treatment. The FDA has officially also approved biosimilars for the three anti-TNFα inhibitors, which should represent a potential costs savings.

Because of the nature of the immune cells and molecules being targeted by biologics, in general there is an increased risk for developing adverse effects related to immune suppression. This includes an increased risk of infection, including serious infections such as sepsis, new-onset or reactivation of tuberculosis (TB), and opportunistic infections such as histoplasmosis, cryptococcosis, aspergillosis, candidiasis, and pneumocystis. The use of live or live-attenuated vaccines during therapy is also generally contraindicated.

Tumor Necrosis Factor-α Inhibitors

TNF-α is a prominent proinflammatory cytokine that has pleiotropic effects during immune responses. During inflammation, it has potent effects on vasodilation and vascular permeability and mediates the upregulation of adhesion molecules on endothelial cells. It is involved in the activation of numerous immune cells and is a major player in the development of endotoxin-mediated septic shock. In psoriasis, TNF-α plays a major role in the induction of dendritic cells that produce IL-12 and IL-23 during inflammation. It can also induce T_H22 differentiation and can directly act on keratinocytes inducing the production of cathelicidins. Similarly, TNF-α is prominent cytokine that is involved in the pathogenesis of psoriasis arthritis. Elevated levels of TNF-α are present in the skin and serum of psoriasis patients, which is significantly correlated to the psoriasis severity index.

Etanercept (Enbrel®) was the earliest biologic approved for the treatment of psoriasis and PsA in 2002, and moderate-to-severe plaque psoriasis in 2004. It is also approved for the treatment of rheumatoid arthritis, juvenile rheumatoid arthritis, and ankylosing spondylitis. Etanercept is a soluble, recombinant, fully human fusion protein comprising of the extracellular domain of the TNF receptor 2 and the Fc portion of IgG1. It binds soluble and membrane-bound TNF, thereby inhibiting TNF-α activity. It is highly active and has been used in the treatment of rheumatological diseases for several years. Etanercept is given continuously, starting with a 50 mg subcutaneous dose twice weekly for the first 12 weeks, which is followed by 25 mg twice weekly or 50 mg once weekly. Clinical trials have showed significant improvement in approximately 50% of patients by week 12 and greater than 50% of participants by week 24; with continuing therapy, weaker responders continued to improve for up to 1 year. Etanercept has also been shown to be efficacious in children and adolescents (aged 4–17 years) with plaque psoriasis dosed at 0.8 mg/kg (maximum 50 mg) once weekly.

Infliximab (Remicade®) is a mouse-human chimeric monoclonal antibody consisting of mouse TNF-α specific variable regions and the constant region of human IgG1. It is specific for soluble and membrane-bound TNF and induces complement activation, resulting in opsonization and/or clearance. In addition to psoriasis and PsA, it is used for the treatment of ulcerative colitis, Crohn's disease, rheumatoid arthritis, and ankylosing spondylitis. Infliximab may be more efficacious than etanercept as suggested by a 2011 study which showed that psoriatic patients with an inadequate response to etanercept had rapid and sustained improvement when switched to infliximab. Infliximab is given as three *i.v.* infusions of 5 mg/kg over a 6-week induction period, followed by regular infusions every 8 weeks. Due to the chimeric nature of the antibody, the possibility of clearance by antibody induction exists. Thus, regular therapy is important. Clinical trials show an improvement in 80% of patients by week 10 of therapy, which dropped to about 50% by week 50.

Adalimumab (Humira®) is a fully human anti-TNF antibody that is specific for soluble and membrane-bound TNF-α and has been shown to be extremely effective and provide rapid control of psoriasis. Data from a number of clinical studies suggest dramatic results with significant improvements such as clearance of plaque psoriasis observed as early as 1 week after therapy and continuation of benefits over 1–3 years of maintenance therapy. It is given as 80 mg subcutaneously in the first week, followed by 40 mg during the second week, and 40 mg thereafter every other week.

A number of safety concerns need to be taken into account when treating with TNF inhibitors. Increased risk of infections is a major concern, most commonly including upper respiratory tract infections, and less commonly including serious infections such as sepsis, new-onset or reactivation TB, and opportunistic infections such as histoplasmosis, cryptococcosis, aspergillosis, candidiasis, and pneumocystis. Fatal reactions have occurred when these infections have not been properly recognized and appropriately treated. In addition to infections, there is the potential for the development or exacerbation of autoimmune diseases, specifically those of the central nervous system such as multiple sclerosis. An increased risk for the development of malignancies is also an important concern. These include lymphoma, melanoma, and other types of skin cancer. Adverse effects affecting the skin have also been observed such as vasculitis, granulomatous reactions, cutaneous infections, and psoriasiform eruptions. Lastly, TNF inhibitors are contraindicated in patients with preexisting moderate-to-severe chronic heart failure.

IL-12 and IL-23 Antagonists

Ustekinumab (Stelara®) is a fully human monoclonal antibody that targets the shared p40 subunit of the cytokines IL-12 and IL-23 (Fig. 5.11).

The cytokines IL-12 and IL-23 play critical roles in the generation of T_H1 and T_H17 responses in psoriatic lesions. IL-12 is a well-studied proinflammatory cytokine that is essential for the differentiation of CD4 T cells into the T_H1 subset, and also activates other cells such as CD8 T cells. It is made up of two subunits, p35 and p40, which together form the active heterodimer p70. The p40 subunit is also shared with the cytokine IL-23, which is essential for the establishment of IL-17-producing T_H17 cells. The biological activity of both cytokines as well as receptor binding is conferred by the shared p40 subunit. Similarly, the receptors for both cytokines consist of a common IL-12R1 chain which binds the IL-23R subunit to form the IL-23 receptor or the IL-12R2 subunit to form the IL-12 receptor. However, both cytokines have distinct and often opposing functions to each other.

Several studies in both humans and mice highlight the importance of the shared subunit p40 for the generation of T_H1 and T_H17

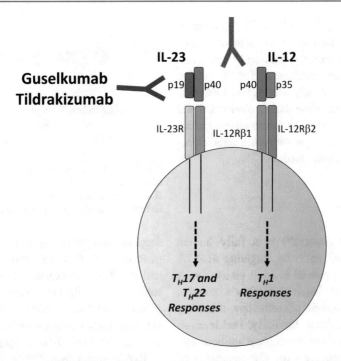

Fig. 5.11 Inhibition of IL-12 and IL-23-mediated signaling in psoriasis. Ustekinumab is a monoclonal antibody designed to bind the shared p40 subunit of IL-12 and IL-23 inhibiting the assembly of these cytokines and consequently their activity. In contrast, guselkumab and tildrakizumab bind the p19 subunit of IL-23, blocking its activity. The inhibition of IL-12 and IL-23 signaling has a profound impact on the development of T_H1 and T_H17 responses

responses. Studies of psoriatic lesions from patients show the presence of increased levels of the shared p40 subunit and the cytokines IL-12 and IL-23, which directly contribute to keratinocyte differentiation and proliferation. In addition, IFN-γ, IL-17A, IL-17F and IL-22 are also overexpressed in psoriasis plaques. Similarly, increased frequencies of IL-17- and IL-22- producing CD4 T cells have also been found in patients with PsA. Conversely, patients deficient in p40 succumb to overwhelming infections with mycobacteria, salmonella, staphylococci, and pneumococci, indicating the importance of T_H1 cells in controlling infection. The role of IL-23 has not yet been examined in these patients, since its functions are only now becoming known. However, animal studies demonstrate that mice deficient in p40 are protected from the development of autoimmune diseases such as arthritis and inflammatory bowel disease. Further examination showed that this protection occurred due to the loss of function of T_H17 cells and not T_H1, indicating the proinflammatory effects of T_H17 and IL-17 in driving

autoimmunity. Thus, blockade of the p40 subunit has the potential to ameliorate both T_H1 and T_H17 responses.

Ustekinumab is licensed for the treatment of both moderate-to-severe plaque psoriasis and PsA. It is also approved for the treatment of PsA in patients in whom anti-TNF inhibitors are contraindicated. It is given as a subcutaneous injection of 45 or 90 mg at weeks 0 and 4 and every 12 weeks afterwards. Some common adverse effects include upper respiratory infections, headache, fatigue, pruritus, back pain, injection site reactions, and arthralgia. Other serious adverse effects include those that are present for other biologics, including the risk of reactivation of TB and malignancies.

In 2017 and 2018, the FDA approved the use of **Guselkumab (Tremfya®)** and **Tildrakizumab (Ilumya®)** for the treatment of adults with moderate-to-severe plaque psoriasis who are candidates for systemic therapy or phototherapy (Fig. 5.11). Both these drugs target the p19 subunit of IL-23 (Fig. 5.11), preventing its signaling via the IL-23 receptor, and resulting in the inhibition of T_H17 and T_H22 responses. Guselkumab is administered subcutaneously as a 100 mg dose once during week 0 and week 4, followed by weekly treatments for 8 weeks. Tildrakizumab is similarly administered subcutaneously as a 100 mg dose during weeks 0, 4 and every 12 weeks thereafter. Some adverse reactions include upper respiratory infections, injection site reactions, and diarrhea.

IL-17 Inhibitors

Secukinumab (Cosentyx®) is a fully human IgG1k monoclonal antibody targeting IL-17A (Fig. 5.12). It is approved in adult patients with moderate-to-severe plaque psoriasis who are also candidates for systemic phototherapy, receiving FDA approval in 2015. Similarly, **Ixekizumab (Taltz®)** is a humanized monoclonal antibody targeting IL-17A approved for the treatment of moderate-to-severe plaque psoriasis. Blockade of IL-17A results in the inhibition of the effects of IL-17 on keratinocytes, preventing the production of various chemokines and antimicrobial peptides as well as the induction of neutrophils. This eventually leads to suppression of inflammation and normalization of keratinocyte differentiation. Head-to-head clinical studies of the anti-IL-17 inhibitors with both anti-TNF as well as ustekinumab show that both anti-IL-17 inhibitors are more efficacious. This resulted in

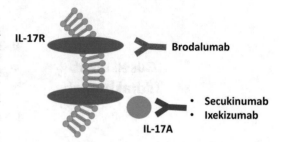

Fig. 5.12 The mechanism of action of IL-17 signaling inhibitors. IL-17 inhibitors directly target the cytokine IL-17A or its receptor, thereby inhibiting IL-17 activity and its associated inflammatory effects during psoriasis

secukinumab receiving FDA approval for the treatment of PsA in 2016. Treatment with anti-IL-17 inhibitors has been shown to result in some adverse effects including the development of mild candidiasis (which is normally controlled via T_H17-mediated neutrophil induction) as well as more uncommonly neutropenia.

Brodalumab (Siliq™) is a newly approved biologic (2017), which is a fully human monoclonal antibody targeting the IL-17A receptor (Fig. 5.12). It is approved for the treatment of moderate-to-severe plaque psoriasis in adult patients who are candidates for phototherapy and systemic therapy, and who have failed to respond to other systemic therapies. In clinical trials, it elicits a rapid response resulting in clearance of plaque psoriasis. However, it comes with a black box warning because of observed risks of suicidal ideation and behavior.

From Bench to Bedside: Discovery and Development of Dupilumab

Commentary by Kaitlin Armstrong

Dupilumab is a monoclonal antibody that was initially developed for the treatment of atopic dermatitis and is also being currently evaluated for the treatment of moderate-to-severe allergic asthma. Dupilumab targets the IL-4Rα receptor, an integral component of the receptors for the cytokines IL-4 and IL-13, which are critical for the mediation of the T_H2 inflammatory response that is characteristic of IgE-mediated diseases.

The development of dupilumab has been the culmination of a long process involving the work of countless scientists studying the pathophysiology of allergic asthma and its underlying immunological basis. The cytokine, IL-4, was first discovered in 1982 by two different laboratories, which simultaneously published papers describing the molecule. Howard et al. discovered a novel proliferating agent for B cells that was distinct from IL-2, which they initially named as BCGF or B cell growth factor and later changed to BSF-1 (B cell stimulating factor-1). In the same year, Isakson et al. also published the discovery of a molecule called BCDF-γ (B cell differentiating factor-gamma), which was shown to induce immunoglobulin class switching in B cells. The realization that the two laboratories were studying the same molecule did not happen until much later. Then, in 1985, through a collaboration emerging from both laboratories, it was shown that the two molecules were one and the same, an exciting discovery for many immunologists, who had until then believed that B cell proliferation and differentiation occurred *via* distinct cellular pathways. In 1986, after the successful cloning of the cytokine by various laboratories (Noma et al. and Lee et al.), it was first called IL-4.

Shortly thereafter, during the same year (1986), Mosmann et al. demonstrated the existence of two subsets of helper T cells, T_H1 and T_H2 cells, that could produce distinct sets of immune mediators. One of these was a factor called P600 that was shown to be produced by T_H2 cells by Cherwinski et al. Further characterization of this molecule would not come until 1992 when Morgan et al. demonstrated that P600 had similar activity as the recently discovered IL-4. It was therefore thought (Zurawski et al.) that the two molecules might share a common receptor component, leading to the successful cloning of P600 by McKenzie et al. and Minty et al. in subsequent studies. The new name given to the T_H2 derived factor was IL-13.

In the 1990s, a significant amount of progress was being made toward further dissecting the immunologic mechanisms underlying the pathophysiology of allergic asthma. In particular, T_H2 cells and its mediators came to increasingly be seen as major culprits in the pathogenesis of asthma. In 1992, Robinson et al. and Walker et al. demonstrated that IL-4 was a critical factor in the blood and bronchoalveolar-lavage fluid of patients with asthma. Several subsequent studies thereafter demonstrated the critical importance of IL-4 for the development of asthma. Much later, in 1998, the essential role of IL-13 in asthma was also elucidated through a series of elegant papers that examined its functions in mouse models of experimental asthma. Wills-Karp et al. demonstrated that the inhibition of IL-4 alone during allergen challenge did not prevent the development of AHR, a cardinal characteristic of allergic asthma, in allergic mice. In contrast, the inhibition of IL-13 dramatically reversed the development of AHR. They also demonstrated that the AHR mediated by IL-13 was independent of the levels of IgE and eosinophils, but that the secretion of mucus and subepithelial fibrosis in the airways was dependent on IL-13. Simultaneously, Grunig et al. also demonstrated using IL-4Rα deficient mice, that the IL-4Rα receptor pathway was essential for the development of AHR in allergic mice. These discoveries thus paved the way for the introduction of therapies targeting some of the specific molecules and receptors identified, including the IL-4Rα receptor.

Dupilumab is a fully human monoclonal antibody targeting the IL-4Rα on various immune cells. The first mouse monoclonal antibodies were developed in the 1970s using the hybridoma technique but weren't very successful clinically, due to their foreign origin. Mouse-derived monoclonal antibodies tended to activate immune responses in patients who developed human anti-mouse antibodies, which attached to the monoclonal antibody drugs, recognizing them as foreign entities in the body. To address this problem, chimeric monoclonal antibodies were then developed which were comprised of the variable regions of antigen-specific mouse antibodies and the constant regions of human antibodies. This was followed by the development of humanized monoclonal antibodies which were generated by merging the complementarity determining regions of mouse-derived antigen-specific antibodies with a human immunoglobulin scaffold. Eventually, the use of genetically modified mice and cells that were programmed to express human immunoglobulin genes, allowed the development of fully human monoclonal antibodies that do not contain any foreign components. The first fully human monoclonal antibody, adalimumab, was approved by the FDA in 2002 for the treatment of rheumatoid arthritis, paving the way for the development and approval of several others in the next decade.

Dupilumab, sold under the brand name Dupixent®, was developed through a collaboration between Regeneron Pharmaceuticals and Sanofi Genzyme. It entered clinical trials in 2012, and by 2014 was designated an investigational therapy for moderate-to-severe atopic dermatitis based on successful phase I and II trials. In March 2017, the drug was finally approved by the FDA for the treatment of moderate-to-severe AD. The drug has been hailed as a miracle drug by many anecdotal accounts from patients, many of whom have reported relief after using the drug. Its success in the treatment of eczema has also led to further evaluation of its efficacy in patients with persistent asthma. In March 2018, the FDA accepted the supplemental Biologics License Application (sBLA) for dupilumab to review its data supporting its use in moderate-to-severe asthma. This is supported by data from several clinical studies that demonstrate its safety and efficacy in patients with uncontrolled moderate-to-severe asthma, suggesting that it may be of benefit to patients with asthma.

Summary

Advances in the study of immunologic pathways over the last few decades have significantly enhanced our understanding of the pathophysiologic mechanisms involved in the development of immune-mediated dermatologic disorders. These studies paint a complex picture of the pathophysiology of AD and psoriasis, with the involvement of multiple subsets of T cells and various mediators produced by these subsets as well as other cell types such as keratinocytes. These novel breakthroughs in our understanding of the pathophysiology of these diseases have led to the development of several new immunotherapeutic drugs that have been tailored to inhibit specific aspects of disease progression. Included among these are several novel biologics that target cytokine signaling pathways resulting from the activation of T_H2, T_H17, T_H22 and other cell types. It is anticipated that further insight into the mechanisms regulating disease development will result in the approval of even more drugs for the treatment of AD and psoriasis. Many are already in the process of being evaluated in clinical trials and several more are undergoing investigation in preclinical studies.

Case Studies and Practice Questions

Case Study 1: Atopic Dermatitis

Janet Anderson is a 8-year-old Caucasian being seen in the Emergency room for her worsening eczema. In the last few weeks she has had several atopic dermatitis flare-ups that included the development of open skin lesions, erythema, and increased pruritis. She stated that her skin has been very itchy the last few weeks and she has been scratching it continuously. Physical examination revealed that her skin had become extremely red and that there were several infected lesions present on her hands and trunk. Some of these had been oozing a clear fluid forming crusts around the lesions. The presence of thickened plaques of skin were also noted in some areas suggesting the development of lichenification.

Janet's mother indicated that she had first been diagnosed with eczema when she was 3 months old and in the years since she has also been diagnosed with allergic rhinitis, asthma, and food allergy to eggs and shellfish. She stated that she also suffers from asthma and food allergy but the rest of the family does not seem to have any allergic disorders.

The doctor performed some skin cultures which turned out to be positive for *Staphylococcus aureus*. He also ordered some laboratory tests to assess the numbers of white blood cells (especially eosinophils) and her serum IgE levels. Janet was prescribed some oral antibiotics along with anti-histamines, a topical steroid, and a topical calcineurin inhibitor. Based on her previous history, the doctor suggested that Janet would be a good candidate for treatment with some new drugs called Eucrisa® and Dupixent® and should talk to her allergist about these.

1. Based on what you know about the pathophysiology of atopic dermatitis, why are topical steroids effective in reducing the eczema associated with the disease? Explain your answer in the context of specific cells and molecules involved in the development of the disease.
2. What is the atopic march? Why did the doctor ask Janet's mother about her previous medical history?
3. Why do patients with atopic dermatitis have elevated eosinophil counts? Explain your answer in the context of T cell-specific responses.
4. Briefly explain how mechanical injury contributes to the development of a T_H2 response during atopic dermatitis with specific mention of the cells and molecules involved.
5. Skin Langerhans cells play a pivotal role in initiating inflammation during the development of atopic dermatitis. Which of the following molecules produced by epithelial cells has been shown to skew Langerhans cell function in favor of eczema-associated T cell responses?
   (a) TNF-α
   (b) IL-6
   (c) TSLP
   (d) TGF-β
6. Defects in the following gene have been linked to failure of skin barrier function during atopic dermatitis:
   (a) *MHC II*
   (b) *IL-4*
   (c) *Filaggrin*
   (d) *IL-13*
7. What is the evidence for the role of T_H2 cells in the development of atopic dermatitis?
8. Why did the doctor check Janet for the presence of infection with *S. aureus*? How does bacterial infection exacerbate the development of eczema?
9. Why did the doctor suggest that Janet be treated with Dupixent®? What is its mechanism of action and how can it improve Janet's condition?
10. Crisaborole (Eucrisa®) is a recently developed drug for the treatment of atopic dermatitis. Its effects are exerted via the inhibition of:
   (a) IL-4
   (b) Phosphodiesterase 4
   (c) Eosinophils
   (d) IL-5

Case Study 2: Plaque Psoriasis

Sarah Harding, a 28-year-old woman, has had a several year history of mild plaque psoriasis. In the past, this was mostly controlled with coal tar treatments and the use of topical corticosteroids such as hydrocortisone and beclomethasone. More recently, however, she has been experiencing several more rashes that have been difficult to control. Her symptoms get worse during cold weather and have now begun to appear on several parts of her body, including her trunks, limbs, and vulva. She finds that they are significantly exacerbated when she is working out in the gym or participating in other athletic activities. In addition, she has noticed recently that her knee joints also hurt and look like they may be swelling up. She is extremely worried because she was just married a few months ago and she and her husband are planning on having a baby soon. Cutaneous examination of her symptoms revealed several well-demarcated erythematous plaques covering greater than 40% of her body surface area. These were also overlaid with silvery scales. Joint swelling and tenderness were also observed and the involvement of axial joint swelling was confirmed. The physician suggested that Sarah start with a quick short course therapy of oral cyclosporine for about 12 weeks starting at a dose of 5 mg/kg. He also wants her to get treated with a TNF inhibitor and is recommending weekly treatment with adalimumab. During this time, he wants her to continue taking oral contraceptives and not get pregnant. If there is any indication that she might be pregnant, he wants her to let him know immediately. He also wants her to be monitored every couple weeks for changes in blood pressure and renal function. If she has any symptoms indicating an infection, he wants her to report to him right away. He asks Sarah if she has recently traveled to another country. Sarah told the physician that she and her husband had spent several weeks in Bali, Indonesia for their honeymoon. The doctor wants her to get a PPD test before he starts the anti-TNF medication. He assures that her after a few months of treatment, she should feel a lot better and can start getting pregnant. Sarah got her PPD test which turned out to be negative and started therapy with cyclosporine and adalimumab. Five months later, both her psoriasis and joint swelling had significantly resolved. The doctor said that she could stop her medication and have the baby. During pregnancy, she had a few minor flare-ups which were controlled by topical corticosteroids. She began to re-experience some joint pain during the third trimester along with a few minor skin flare-ups. After the baby was born, she asked the doctor about Cosentyx®. She had seen several ads on television for it when she was pregnant. Her plaque psoriasis had also returned and seemed to be getting worse and her knee joints were hurting again too. The physician felt Sarah was a good candidate for treatment with Cosentyx® and started her on it with subcutaneous injections once a week for the first few weeks. After 2 months, he wants her to receive monthly treatment once a month. It has been 2 years since Sarah started on Cosentyx®. Her symptoms have mostly resolved and she has been feeling a lot better.

11. How would you classify Sarah's psoriasis symptoms?
12. Why did the physician initiate systemic therapy with both cyclosporine and adalimumab?
13. What are some contraindications with using adalimumab?
14. Why does the physician want Sarah to not get pregnant during therapy with adalimumab?
15. Explain the mechanism of action of cyclosporine.
16. Explain the mechanism of action of secukinumab.

17. Select all that apply. Which of the following is true regarding Etanercept?
    (a) It is pegylated
    (b) It consists of a TNF-II receptor
    (c) It inhibits soluble TNF-α
    (d) It is a humanized antibody against TNF-α
18. The development of psoriasis occurs as a result of chronic inflammation initiated in the skin. Ustekinumab is a novel biologic that was developed taking advantage of the fact that the functions of different immune cells can be targeted by inhibiting components that are shared across different molecules. The mechanism of action of ustekinumab is to:
    (a) block p40, a subunit common to IL-12 and IL-23, resulting in the inhibition of NK, T_H1 and T_H17 cells
    (b) block JAK kinases, important for IL-12 and IL-23 signaling, and thereby prevent the activation of NK, T_H1 and T_H17 cells
    (c) block the IL-12/IL-23 receptor, resulting in the inhibition of NK, T_H1 and T_H17 activation
    (d) block IL-17 production, resulting in the suppression of inflammation by NK, T_H1 and T_H17 cells

Suggested Reading

AbuHilal M, Walsh S, Shear N. The role of IL-17 in the pathogenesis of psoriasis and update on IL-17 inhibitors for the treatment of plaque psoriasis. J Cutan Med Surg. 2016;20:509–16.

Acosta-Rodriguez EV, Napolitani G, Lanzavecchia A, Sallusto F. Interleukins 1beta and 6 but not transforming growth factor-beta are essential for the differentiation of interleukin 17-producing human T helper cells. Nat Immunol. 2007;8:942–9.

Akdis CA, Akdis M. Immunological differences between intrinsic and extrinsic types of atopic dermatitis. Clin Exp Allergy. 2003;33:1618–21.

Akdis CA, et al. Diagnosis and treatment of atopic dermatitis in children and adults: European Academy of Allergology and Clinical Immunology/ American Academy of Allergy, Asthma and Immunology/PRACTALL consensus report. Allergy. 2006;61:969–87.

Amano W, et al. The Janus kinase inhibitor JTE-052 improves skin barrier function through suppressing signal transducer and activator of transcription 3 signaling. J Allergy Clin Immunol. 2015;136:667–77. e667.

Armstrong AW, et al. Effect of ixekizumab treatment on work productivity for patients with moderate-to-severe plaque psoriasis: analysis of results from 3 randomized phase 3 clinical trials. JAMA Dermatol. 2016;152:661–9.

Bao L, Zhang H, Chan LS. The involvement of the JAK-STAT signaling pathway in chronic inflammatory skin disease atopic dermatitis. JAKSTAT. 2013;2:e24137.

Beck LA, et al. Dupilumab treatment in adults with moderate-to-severe atopic dermatitis. N Engl J Med. 2014;371:130–9.

Bissonnette R, et al. Topical tofacitinib for atopic dermatitis: a phase IIa randomized trial. Br J Dermatol. 2016;175:902–11.

Blauvelt A, Chiricozzi A. The immunologic role of IL-17 in psoriasis and psoriatic arthritis pathogenesis. Clin Rev Allergy Immunol. 2018;55:379–90.

Blauvelt A, et al. Secukinumab is superior to ustekinumab in clearing skin of subjects with moderate-to-severe plaque psoriasis up to 1 year: results from the CLEAR study. J Am Acad Dermatol. 2017;76:60–9.e69.

Bonefeld CM, Geisler C. The role of innate lymphoid cells in healthy and inflamed skin. Immunol Lett. 2016;179:25–8.

Bruggen MC, et al. In situ mapping of innate lymphoid cells in human skin: evidence for remarkable differences between Normal and inflamed skin. J Invest Dermatol. 2016;136:2396–405.

Brunner PM, et al. A mild topical steroid leads to progressive anti-inflammatory effects in the skin of patients with moderate-to-severe atopic dermatitis. J Allergy Clin Immunol. 2016;138:169–78.

Brunner PM, Guttman-Yassky E, Leung DY. The immunology of atopic dermatitis and its reversibility with broad-spectrum and targeted therapies. J Allergy Clin Immunol. 2017a;139:S65–76.

Brunner PM, et al. Increasing comorbidities suggest that atopic dermatitis is a systemic disorder. J Invest Dermatol. 2017b;137:18–25.

Brunner PM, et al. Early-onset pediatric atopic dermatitis is characterized by TH2/TH17/TH22-centered inflammation and lipid alterations. J Allergy Clin Immunol. 2018;141:2094–106.

Castro M, et al. Dupilumab efficacy and safety in moderate-to-severe uncontrolled asthma. N Engl J Med. 2018;378:2486–96.

Chalmers JR, et al. Report from the fifth international consensus meeting to harmonize core outcome measures for atopic eczema/dermatitis clinical trials (HOME initiative). Br J Dermatol. 2018;178:e332–41.

Cherwinski HM, Schumacher JH, Brown KD, Mosmann TR. Two types of mouse helper T cell clone. III. Further differences in lymphokine synthesis between Th1 and Th2 clones revealed by RNA hybridization, functionally monospecific bioassays, and monoclonal antibodies. J Exp Med. 1987;166:1229–44.

Coffman RL. Converging discoveries: the first reports of IL-4. J Immunol. 2013;190:847–8.

Cole C, et al. Filaggrin-stratified transcriptomic analysis of pediatric skin identifies mechanistic pathways in patients with atopic dermatitis. J Allergy Clin Immunol. 2014;134:82–91.

Czarnowicki T, Krueger JG, Guttman-Yassky E. Skin barrier and immune dysregulation in atopic dermatitis: an evolving story with important clinical implications. J Allergy Clin Immunol Pract. 2014;2:371–9;. quiz 380-371.

Czarnowicki T, Krueger JG, Guttman-Yassky E. Novel concepts of prevention and treatment of atopic dermatitis through barrier and immune manipulations with implications for the atopic march. J Allergy Clin Immunol. 2017;139:1723–34.

Davis DM, Borok J, Udkoff J, Lio P, Spergel J. Atopic dermatitis: phototherapy and systemic therapy. Semin Cutan Med Surg. 2017;36:118–23.

Dong J, Goldenberg G. New biologics in psoriasis: an update on IL-23 and IL-17 inhibitors. Cutis. 2017;99:123–7.

Duhen T, Geiger R, Jarrossay D, Lanzavecchia A, Sallusto F. Production of interleukin 22 but not interleukin 17 by a subset of human skin-homing memory T cells. Nat Immunol. 2009;10:857–63.

Egawa G, Kabashima K. Multifactorial skin barrier deficiency and atopic dermatitis: essential topics to prevent the atopic march. J Allergy Clin Immunol. 2016;138:350–8.e351.

Egeberg A. Phase 3 trials of Ixekizumab in moderate-to-severe plaque psoriasis. N Engl J Med. 2016;375:2101–2.

Eichenfield LF, Stein Gold LF. Systemic therapy of atopic dermatitis: welcome to the revolution. Semin Cutan Med Surg. 2017;36:S103–5.

Eichenfield LF, et al. Long-term safety of crisaborole ointment 2% in children and adults with mild to moderate atopic dermatitis. J Am Acad Dermatol. 2017;77:641–9.e645.

Esaki H, et al. Early-onset pediatric atopic dermatitis is TH2 but also TH17 polarized in skin. J Allergy Clin Immunol. 2016;138:1639–51.

Eyerich K, et al. IL-17 in atopic eczema: linking allergen-specific adaptive and microbial-triggered innate immune response. J Allergy Clin Immunol. 2009a;123:59–66.e54.

Eyerich S, et al. Th22 cells represent a distinct human T cell subset involved in epidermal immunity and remodeling. J Clin Invest. 2009b;119:3573–85.

Eyerich S, et al. Mutual antagonism of T cells causing psoriasis and atopic eczema. N Engl J Med. 2011;365:231–8.

Eyerich K, Dimartino V, Cavani A. IL-17 and IL-22 in immunity: driving protection and pathology. Eur J Immunol. 2017;47:607–14.

Furue M, Kadono T. "Inflammatory skin march" in atopic dermatitis and psoriasis. Inflamm Res. 2017;66:833–42.

Ganguly D, et al. Self-RNA-antimicrobial peptide complexes activate human dendritic cells through TLR7 and TLR8. J Exp Med. 2009;206:1983–94.

Gisondi P, Girolomoni G. Apremilast in the therapy of moderate-to-severe chronic plaque psoriasis. Drug Des Devel Ther. 2016;10:1763–70.

Gittler JK, et al. Progressive activation of T(H)2/T(H)22 cytokines and selective epidermal proteins characterizes acute and chronic atopic dermatitis. J Allergy Clin Immunol. 2012;130:1344–54.

Glatzer F, et al. Histamine induces proliferation in keratinocytes from patients with atopic dermatitis through the histamine 4 receptor. J Allergy Clin Immunol. 2013;132:1358–67.

Gordon KB, Colombel JF, Hardin DS. Phase 3 trials of ixekizumab in moderate-to-severe plaque psoriasis. N Engl J Med. 2016a;375:2102.

Gordon KB, et al. Phase 3 trials of ixekizumab in moderate-to-severe plaque psoriasis. N Engl J Med. 2016b;375:345–56.

Gottlieb AB, et al. Efficacy, tolerability, and pharmacodynamics of apremilast in recalcitrant plaque psoriasis: a phase II open-label study. J Drugs Dermatol. 2013;12:888–97.

Griffin GK, et al. IL-17 and TNF-alpha sustain neutrophil recruitment during inflammation through synergistic effects on endothelial activation. J Immunol. 2012;188:6287–99.

Grunig G, et al. Requirement for IL-13 independently of IL-4 in experimental asthma. Science. 1998;282:2261–3.

Gutowska-Owsiak D, et al. IL-17 downregulates filaggrin and affects keratinocyte expression of genes associated with cellular adhesion. Exp Dermatol. 2012;21:104–10.

Guttman-Yassky E, Krueger JG, Lebwohl MG. Systemic immune mechanisms in atopic dermatitis and psoriasis with implications for treatment. Exp Dermatol. 2018;27:409–17.

Halim TY, et al. Group 2 innate lymphoid cells are critical for the initiation of adaptive T helper 2 cell-mediated allergic lung inflammation. Immunity. 2014;40:425–35.

Hamid Q, Boguniewicz M, Leung DY. Differential in situ cytokine gene expression in acute versus chronic atopic dermatitis. J Clin Invest. 1994;94:870–6.

Hamilton JD, et al. Dupilumab improves the molecular signature in skin of patients with moderate-to-severe atopic dermatitis. J Allergy Clin Immunol. 2014;134:1293–300.

Hanifin JM, Reed ML, Eczema P, Impact Working G. A population-based survey of eczema prevalence in the United States. Dermatitis. 2007;18:82–91.

He JQ, et al. Genetic variants of the IL13 and IL4 genes and atopic diseases in at-risk children. Genes Immun. 2003;4:385–9.

Hijnen DJ, ten Berge O, Timmer-de Mik L, Bruijnzeel-Koomen CA, de Bruin-Weller MS. Efficacy and safety of long-term treatment with cyclosporin A for atopic dermatitis. J Eur Acad Dermatol Venereol. 2007;21:85–9.

Howard M, et al. Identification of a T cell-derived b cell growth factor distinct from interleukin 2. J Exp Med. 1982;155:914–23.

Howell MD, et al. Cytokine modulation of atopic dermatitis filaggrin skin expression. J Allergy Clin Immunol. 2009;124:R7–R12.

Howell MD, Parker ML, Mustelin T, Ranade K. Past, present, and future for biologic intervention in atopic dermatitis. Allergy. 2015;70:887–96.

Irvine AD, McLean WH, Leung DY. Filaggrin mutations associated with skin and allergic diseases. N Engl J Med. 2011;365:1315–27.

Isakson PC, Pure E, Vitetta ES, Krammer PH. T cell-derived B cell differentiation factor(s). Effect on the isotype switch of murine B cells. J Exp Med. 1982;155:734–48.

Iwakura Y, Ishigame H, Saijo S, Nakae S. Functional specialization of interleukin-17 family members. Immunity. 2011;34:149–62.

Iwasaki M, et al. Association of a new-type prostaglandin D2 receptor CRTH2 with circulating T helper 2 cells in patients with atopic dermatitis. J Invest Dermatol. 2002;119:609–16.

Jones PT, Dear PH, Foote J, Neuberger MS, Winter G. Replacing the complementarity-determining regions in a human antibody with those from a mouse. Nature. 1986;321:522–5.

Kagami S, Rizzo HL, Lee JJ, Koguchi Y, Blauvelt A. Circulating Th17, Th22, and Th1 cells are increased in psoriasis. J Invest Dermatol. 2010;130:1373–83.

Khattri S, et al. Cyclosporine in patients with atopic dermatitis modulates activated inflammatory pathways and reverses epidermal pathology. J Allergy Clin Immunol. 2014;133:1626–34.

Khattri S, et al. Efficacy and safety of ustekinumab treatment in adults with moderate-to-severe atopic dermatitis. Exp Dermatol. 2017;26:28–35.

Kim BS, et al. TSLP elicits IL-33-independent innate lymphoid cell responses to promote skin inflammation. Sci Transl Med. 2013;5:170ra116.

Kim J, et al. Epidermal thymic stromal lymphopoietin predicts the development of atopic dermatitis during infancy. J Allergy Clin Immunol. 2016;137:1282–5. e1284.

Kopp T, et al. Clinical improvement in psoriasis with specific targeting of interleukin-23. Nature. 2015;521:222–6.

Kupetsky EA, Mathers AR, Ferris LK. Anti-cytokine therapy in the treatment of psoriasis. Cytokine. 2013;61:704–12.

Lande R, et al. Plasmacytoid dendritic cells sense self-DNA coupled with antimicrobial peptide. Nature. 2007;449:564–9.

Lande R, et al. The antimicrobial peptide LL37 is a T-cell autoantigen in psoriasis. Nat Commun. 2014;5:5621.

Langley RG, et al. Secukinumab in plaque psoriasis—results of two phase 3 trials. N Engl J Med. 2014;371:326–38.

Lebwohl M, et al. Phase 3 studies comparing brodalumab with ustekinumab in psoriasis. N Engl J Med. 2015;373:1318–28.

Lee F, et al. Isolation and characterization of a mouse interleukin cDNA clone that expresses B-cell stimulatory factor 1 activities and T-cell- and mast-cell-stimulating activities. Proc Natl Acad Sci U S A. 1986;83:2061–5.

Leung DY, Guttman-Yassky E. Deciphering the complexities of atopic dermatitis: shifting paradigms in treatment approaches. J Allergy Clin Immunol. 2014;134:769–79.

Levy LL, Urban J, King BA. Treatment of recalcitrant atopic dermatitis with the oral Janus kinase inhibitor tofacitinib citrate. J Am Acad Dermatol. 2015;73:395–9.

Lopez-Ferrer A, Vilarrasa E, Gich IJ, Puig L. Adalimumab for the treatment of psoriasis in real life: a retrospective cohort of 119 patients at a single Spanish centre. Br J Dermatol. 2013;169:1141–7.

Lopez-Ferrer A, Vilarrasa E, Puig L. Secukinumab (AIN457) for the treatment of psoriasis. Expert Rev Clin Immunol. 2015;11:1177–88.

Margolis DJ, et al. The persistence of atopic dermatitis and filaggrin (FLG) mutations in a US longitudinal cohort. J Allergy Clin Immunol. 2012;130:912–7.

McAleer MA, Irvine AD. The multifunctional role of filaggrin in allergic skin disease. J Allergy Clin Immunol. 2013;131:280–91.

McKenzie AN, et al. Interleukin 13, a T-cell-derived cytokine that regulates human monocyte and B-cell function. Proc Natl Acad Sci U S A. 1993;90: 3735–9.

Mease PJ, et al. Secukinumab inhibition of interleukin-17A in patients with psoriatic arthritis. N Engl J Med. 2015;373:1329–39.

Mease PJ, et al. Ixekizumab, an interleukin-17A specific monoclonal antibody, for the treatment of biologic-naive patients with active psoriatic arthritis: results from the 24-week randomised, double-blind, placebo-controlled and active (adalimumab)-controlled period of the phase III trial SPIRIT-P1. Ann Rheum Dis. 2017;76:79–87.

Mennini M, Dahdah L, Fiocchi A. Two phase 3 trials of dupilumab versus placebo in atopic dermatitis. N Engl J Med. 2017;376:1090.

Menter A, et al. Efficacy of ixekizumab compared to etanercept and placebo in patients with moderate-to-severe plaque psoriasis and non-pustular palmoplantar involvement: results from three phase 3 trials (UNCOVER-1, UNCOVER-2 and UNCOVER-3). J Eur Acad Dermatol Venereol. 2017;31:1686–92.

Minty A, et al. Interleukin-13 is a new human lymphokine regulating inflammatory and immune responses. Nature. 1993;362:248–50.

Montaldo E, Juelke K, Romagnani C. Group 3 innate lymphoid cells (ILC3s): origin, differentiation, and plasticity in humans and mice. Eur J Immunol. 2015;45:2171–82.

Moreno AS, McPhee R, Arruda LK, Howell MD. Targeting the T helper 2 inflammatory axis in atopic dermatitis. Int Arch Allergy Immunol. 2016;171:71–80.

Morgan JG, Dolganov GM, Robbins SE, Hinton LM, Lovett M. The selective isolation of novel cDNAs encoded by the regions surrounding the human interleukin 4 and 5 genes. Nucleic Acids Res. 1992;20:5173–9.

Morrison SL, Johnson MJ, Herzenberg LA, Oi VT. Chimeric human antibody molecules: mouse antigen-binding domains with human constant region domains. Proc Natl Acad Sci U S A. 1984;81:6851–5.

Mosmann TR, Cherwinski H, Bond MW, Giedlin MA, Coffman RL. Two types of murine helper T cell clone. I. Definition according to profiles of lymphokine activities and secreted proteins. J Immunol. 1986;136:2348–57.

Nakajima S, et al. Langerhans cells are critical in epicutaneous sensitization with protein antigen via thymic stromal lymphopoietin receptor signaling. J Allergy Clin Immunol. 2012;129:1048–1055 e1046.

Nast A, Jacobs A, Rosumeck S, Werner RN. Efficacy and safety of systemic long-term treatments for moderate-to-severe psoriasis: a systematic review and meta-analysis. J Invest Dermatol. 2015;135:2641–8.

Nemoto O, et al. The first trial of CIM331, a humanized antihuman interleukin-31 receptor A antibody, in healthy volunteers and patients with atopic dermatitis to evaluate safety, tolerability and pharmacokinetics of a single dose in a randomized, double-blind, placebo-controlled study. Br J Dermatol. 2016;174:296–304.

Nestle FO, Kaplan DH, Barker J. Psoriasis. N Engl J Med. 2009;361:496–509.

Niebuhr M, Scharonow H, Gathmann M, Mamerow D, Werfel T. Staphylococcal exotoxins are strong inducers of IL-22: a potential role in atopic dermatitis. J Allergy Clin Immunol. 2010;126:1176–83.e1174.

Noda S, Krueger JG, Guttman-Yassky E. The translational revolution and use of biologics in patients with inflammatory skin diseases. J Allergy Clin Immunol. 2015a;135:324–36.

Noda S, et al. The Asian atopic dermatitis phenotype combines features of atopic dermatitis and psoriasis with increased TH17 polarization. J Allergy Clin Immunol. 2015b;136:1254–64.

Nograles KE, et al. Th17 cytokines interleukin (IL)-17 and IL-22 modulate distinct inflammatory and keratinocyte-response pathways. Br J Dermatol. 2008;159:1092–102.

Nograles KE, et al. IL-22-producing "T22" T cells account for upregulated IL-22 in atopic dermatitis despite reduced IL-17-producing TH17 T cells. J Allergy Clin Immunol. 2009;123:1244–52.e1242.

Noma Y, et al. Cloning of cDNA encoding the murine IgG1 induction factor by a novel strategy using SP6 promoter. Nature. 1986;319:640–6.

Nomura I, et al. Cytokine milieu of atopic dermatitis, as compared to psoriasis, skin prevents induction of innate immune response genes. J Immunol. 2003;171:3262–9.

Oldhoff JM, et al. Anti-IL-5 recombinant humanized monoclonal antibody (mepolizumab) for the treatment of atopic dermatitis. Allergy. 2005;60:693–6.

Oliva M, Renert-Yuval Y, Guttman-Yassky E. The 'omics' revolution: redefining the understanding and treatment of allergic skin diseases. Curr Opin Allergy Clin Immunol. 2016;16:469–76.

Ong PY, et al. Endogenous antimicrobial peptides and skin infections in atopic dermatitis. N Engl J Med. 2002;347:1151–60.

Oppmann B, et al. Novel p19 protein engages IL-12p40 to form a cytokine, IL-23, with biological activities similar as well as distinct from IL-12. Immunity. 2000;13:715–25.

Paller AS, et al. Efficacy and safety of crisaborole ointment, a novel, nonsteroidal phosphodiesterase 4 (PDE4) inhibitor for the topical treatment of atopic dermatitis (AD) in children and adults. J Am Acad Dermatol. 2016;75:494–503.e496.

Papp KA, et al. A prospective phase III, randomized, double-blind, placebo-controlled study of brodalumab in patients with moderate-to-severe plaque psoriasis. Br J Dermatol. 2016;175:273–86.

Parham C, et al. A receptor for the heterodimeric cytokine IL-23 is composed of IL-12Rbeta1 and a novel cytokine receptor subunit, IL-23R. J Immunol. 2002;168:5699–708.

Perez-Aso M, et al. Apremilast, a novel phosphodiesterase 4 (PDE4) inhibitor, regulates inflammation through multiple cAMP downstream effectors. Arthritis Res Ther. 2015;17:249.

Pincelli C, Schafer PH, French LE, Augustin M, Krueger JG. Mechanisms underlying the clinical effects of apremilast for psoriasis. J Drugs Dermatol. 2018;17:835–40.

Puig L, Lopez A, Vilarrasa E, Garcia I. Efficacy of biologics in the treatment of moderate-to-severe plaque psoriasis: a systematic review and meta-analysis of randomized controlled trials with different time points. J Eur Acad Dermatol Venereol. 2014;28:1633–53.

Rabenhorst A, Hartmann K. Interleukin-31: a novel diagnostic marker of allergic diseases. Curr Allergy Asthma Rep. 2014;14:423.

Robinson DS, et al. Predominant TH2-like bronchoalveolar T-lymphocyte population in atopic asthma. N Engl J Med. 1992;326:298–304.

Samrao A, Berry TM, Goreshi R, Simpson EL. A pilot study of an oral phosphodiesterase inhibitor (apremilast) for atopic dermatitis in adults. Arch Dermatol. 2012;148:890–7.

Schafer P. Apremilast mechanism of action and application to psoriasis and psoriatic arthritis. Biochem Pharmacol. 2012;83:1583–90.

Schafer PH, et al. Apremilast is a selective PDE4 inhibitor with regulatory effects on innate immunity. Cell Signal. 2014;26:2016–29.

Schafer PH, Chen P, Fang L, Wang A, Chopra R. The pharmacodynamic impact of apremilast, an oral phosphodiesterase 4 inhibitor, on circulating levels of inflammatory biomarkers in patients with psoriatic arthritis: substudy results from a phase III, randomized, placebo-controlled trial (PALACE 1). J Immunol Res. 2015;2015:906349.

Schafer PH, et al. Phosphodiesterase 4 in inflammatory diseases: effects of apremilast in psoriatic blood and in dermal myofibroblasts through the PDE4/CD271 complex. Cell Signal. 2016;28:753–63.

Schurich A, Raine C, Morris V, Ciurtin C. The role of IL-12/23 in T cell-related chronic inflammation: implications of immunodeficiency and therapeutic blockade. Rheumatology (Oxford). 2018;57:246–54.

Sehra S, et al. IL-4 regulates skin homeostasis and the predisposition toward allergic skin inflammation. J Immunol. 2010;184:3186–90.

Silverberg JI. Persistence of childhood eczema into adulthood. JAMA Dermatol. 2014;150:591–2.

Silverberg JI. Association between adult atopic dermatitis, cardiovascular disease, and increased heart attacks in three population-based studies. Allergy. 2015;70:1300–8.

Silverberg JI, Simpson EL. Associations of childhood eczema severity: a US population-based study. Dermatitis. 2014;25:107–14.

Simon D. Systemic therapy of atopic dermatitis in children and adults. Curr Probl Dermatol. 2011;41:156–64.

Simon D, Bieber T. Systemic therapy for atopic dermatitis. Allergy. 2014;69:46–55.

Simpson EL, et al. Two phase 3 trials of dupilumab versus placebo in atopic dermatitis. N Engl J Med. 2016;375:2335–48.

Simpson EL, Akinlade B, Ardeleanu M. Two phase 3 trials of dupilumab versus placebo in atopic dermatitis. N Engl J Med. 2017a;376:1090–1.

Simpson EL, et al. When does atopic dermatitis warrant systemic therapy? Recommendations from an expert panel of the International Eczema Council. J Am Acad Dermatol. 2017b;77:623–33.

Slater NA, Morrell DS. Systemic therapy of childhood atopic dermatitis. Clin Dermatol. 2015;33:289–99.

Sofen H, et al. Guselkumab (an IL-23-specific mAb) demonstrates clinical and molecular response in patients with moderate-to-severe psoriasis. J Allergy Clin Immunol. 2014;133:1032–40.

Sonnenberg GF, Fouser LA, Artis D. Border patrol: regulation of immunity, inflammation and tissue homeostasis at barrier surfaces by IL-22. Nat Immunol. 2011;12:383–90.

Spertino J, Lopez-Ferrer A, Vilarrasa E, Puig L. Long-term study of infliximab for psoriasis in daily practice: drug survival depends on combined treatment, obesity and infusion reactions. J Eur Acad Dermatol Venereol. 2014;28:1514–21.

Suarez-Farinas M, et al. Intrinsic atopic dermatitis shows similar TH2 and higher TH17 immune activation compared with extrinsic atopic dermatitis. J Allergy Clin Immunol. 2013;132:361–70.

Thaci D, et al. Efficacy and safety of dupilumab in adults with moderate-to-severe atopic dermatitis inadequately controlled by topical treatments: a randomised, placebo-controlled, dose-ranging phase 2b trial. Lancet. 2016;387:40–52.

Torres T, Romanelli M, Chiricozzi A. A revolutionary therapeutic approach for psoriasis: bispecific biological agents. Expert Opin Investig Drugs. 2016;25:751–4.

Ulven T, Kostenis E. Novel CRTH2 antagonists: a review of patents from 2006 to 2009. Expert Opin Ther Pat. 2010;20:1505–30.

van de Kerkhof PC, et al. Secukinumab long-term safety experience: a pooled analysis of 10 phase II and III clinical studies in patients with moderate to severe plaque psoriasis. J Am Acad Dermatol. 2016;75:83–98.e84.

Veilleux MS, Shear NH. Biologics in patients with skin diseases. J Allergy Clin Immunol. 2017;139:1423–30.

Vena GA, Vestita M, Cassano N. Psoriasis and cardiovascular disease. Dermatol Ther. 2010;23:144–51.

Vilarrasa E, et al. ORBIT (outcome and retention rate of biologic treatments for psoriasis): a retrospective observational study on biologic drug survival in daily practice. J Am Acad Dermatol. 2016;74:1066–72.

Volf EM, Au SC, Dumont N, Scheinman P, Gottlieb AB. A phase 2, open-label, investigator-initiated study to evaluate the safety and efficacy of apremilast in subjects with recalcitrant allergic contact or atopic dermatitis. J Drugs Dermatol. 2012;11:341–6.

Walker C, et al. Allergic and nonallergic asthmatics have distinct patterns of T-cell activation and cytokine production in peripheral blood and bronchoalveolar lavage. Am Rev Respir Dis. 1992;146:109–15.

Wang YH, Liu YJ. Thymic stromal lymphopoietin, OX40-ligand, and interleukin-25 in allergic responses. Clin Exp Allergy. 2009;39:798–806.

Welsch K, Holstein J, Laurence A, Ghoreschi K. Targeting JAK/STAT signalling in inflammatory skin diseases with small molecule inhibitors. Eur J Immunol. 2017;47:1096–107.

Werfel T, Biedermann T. Current novel approaches in systemic therapy of atopic dermatitis: specific inhibition of cutaneous Th2 polarized inflammation and itch. Curr Opin Allergy Clin Immunol. 2015;15:446–52.

Werfel T, et al. Cellular and molecular immunologic mechanisms in patients with atopic dermatitis. J Allergy Clin Immunol. 2016;138:336–49.

Wills-Karp M, et al. Interleukin-13: central mediator of allergic asthma. Science. 1998;282:2258–61.

Wolk K, et al. IL-22 regulates the expression of genes responsible for antimicrobial defense, cellular differentiation, and mobility in keratinocytes: a potential role in psoriasis. Eur J Immunol. 2006;36:1309–23.

Wollenberg A, et al. Treatment of atopic dermatitis with tralokinumab, an anti-IL-13 mAb. J Allergy Clin Immunol. 2019;143:135–41.

Yiu ZZ, Warren RB. Novel Oral therapies for psoriasis and psoriatic arthritis. Am J Clin Dermatol. 2016;17:191–200.

Zheng T, et al. Transgenic expression of interleukin-13 in the skin induces a pruritic dermatitis and skin remodeling. J Invest Dermatol. 2009;129:742–51.

Ziegler SF, Liu YJ. Thymic stromal lymphopoietin in normal and pathogenic T cell development and function. Nat Immunol. 2006;7:709–14.

Zurawski SM, Vega F Jr, Huyghe B, Zurawski G. Receptors for interleukin-13 and interleukin-4 are complex and share a novel component that functions in signal transduction. EMBO J. 1993;12:2663–70.

Inflammatory Diseases of the Gastrointestinal Tract and Pharmacological Treatments

6

Clinton B. Mathias, Jeremy P. McAleer, and Doreen E. Szollosi

Learning Objectives

1. Describe the components of the gut-associated lymphoid tissue and explain the various effector mechanisms involved in mucosal immune responses
2. Explain the factors involved in the balance between tolerance and immunity in the mucosal immune system in the gastrointestinal tract
3. Explain mechanisms by which commensal bacteria modulate the outcome of mucosal immune responses
4. Describe and explain the effector immune mechanisms involved in anti-parasitic responses in the gastrointestinal tract
5. Describe and explain the differences between ulcerative colitis and Crohn's Disease
6. Explain the various effector mechanisms involved in the pathogenesis of inflammatory bowel disease (IBD)
7. Explain the mechanism of action of the drugs used for the treatment of IBD
8. Describe and explain the effector mechanisms involved in the pathogenesis of celiac disease
9. Describe and explain the effector mechanisms involved in the development of food allergy
10. Review the available and developing therapeutic options for the treatment of celiac disease and food allergy

Drugs discussed in this chapter

Drugs	Classification
6-mercaptopurine (6-MP, Purinethol®)	Anti-proliferative, purine analog
Adalimumab (Humira®)	Anti-TNF monoclonal antibody
Azathioprine (Imuran®)	Anti-proliferative, purine analog
Balsalazide (Colazal®)	5-aminosalicylate
Budesonide (Entocort®)	Glucocorticoid
Certolizumab pegol (Cimzia®)	Anti-TNF, antibody fragment
Glucocorticoids	Global immunosuppressive agents
Infliximab (Remicade®)	Anti-TNF monoclonal antibody
Mesalamine (Asacol®, Canasa®, Lialda®, Pentasa®, Rowasa®)	5-aminosalicylate
Methotrexate (Rheumatrex®)	Anti-proliferative, DNA replication inhibitor
Natalizumab (Tysabri®)	Anti-α_4 integrin monoclonal antibody

C. B. Mathias (✉)
Department of Pharmaceutical and Administrative Sciences, College of Pharmacy and Health Sciences, Western New England University, Springfield, MA, USA
e-mail: clinton.mathias@wne.edu

J. P. McAleer
Pharmaceutical Science and Research, Marshall University School of Pharmacy, Huntington, WV, USA
e-mail: mcaleer@marshall.edu

D. E. Szollosi
Department of Pharmaceutical Sciences, School of Pharmacy and Physician Assistant Studies, University of Saint Joseph, Hartford, CT, USA
e-mail: dszollosi@usj.edu

© Springer Nature Switzerland AG 2020
C. B. Mathias et al., *Pharmacology of Immunotherapeutic Drugs*,
https://doi.org/10.1007/978-3-030-19922-7_6

Drugs	Classification
Olsalazine (Dipentum®)	5-aminosalicylate
Sulfasalazine (Azulfidine®)	5-aminosalicylate
Thalidomide (Thalomid®)	Anti-inflammatory
Ustekinumab (Stelara®)	Anti-IL-12/23p40 monoclonal antibody
Vedolizumab (Entyvio®)	Anti-$\alpha_4\beta_7$ integrin monoclonal antibody
Metronidazole	Antibiotic
Ciprofloxacin	Antibiotic

Introduction

Our gastrointestinal (GI) tract, including the oral cavity, stomach, small intestine (duodenum, jejunum, ileum), cecum, large intestine (colon) and rectum, constitutes one of the largest surface areas in our body. In an adult human being, the GI tract is approximately 9 m in length, equivalent to the size of roughly two tennis courts. The primary function of the GI tract is the processing of ingested food into nutrients that are absorbed by the body and waste that is eliminated from the body. The absorption of dietary nutrients into the body is facilitated through a physical epithelial barrier consisting of numerous finger-like projections called villi. This same epithelial barrier also prevents bacterial invasion, a remarkable accomplishment, considering that trillions of bacteria normally live within the lumen of the gut, reaching densities of up to 10^{12} organisms per gram in the colon. These normal intestinal flora are termed microbiota, the composition of which varies from individual to individual, and play a pivotal role in the regulation of mucosal immune responses within the GI tract. The coordinated efforts of multiple cell types help to limit opportunistic infections caused by commensal bacteria and protect the body's GI surfaces from colonization by pathogens. Perturbations of normal immune homeostasis within the GI tract, either due to infection or injury, defects in barrier function, induction of autoimmune reactions, and disruption of commensal bacterial composition may lead to chronic inflammatory diseases such as inflammatory bowel disease, celiac disease, food allergy and other conditions. In this chapter, we will examine the inflammatory processes and immunotherapeutic drug targets involved in the development of these conditions.

Immune Responses in the Gastrointestinal Tract

Role of Mucus in Preventing Microbial Attachment to the GI Epithelial Layer

The organs of the GI tract, along with parallel organs in the respiratory and urogenital tracts, are collectively referred to as **mucosal** organ systems. A primary characteristic of these organ systems is the continuous bathing of surfaces by a thick, viscous fluid called mucus. This fluid is secreted by specialized mucosal epithelial cells throughout the GI tract. The viscosity of mucus is caused by numerous gigantic glycoproteins called mucins, which are a major constituent of the mucosal fluid.

The production and secretion of mucus plays an important role in the protection of our surfaces from infection and injury. In addition to mucin, the mucus consists of numerous proteoglycans, antimicrobial peptides (e.g. defensins), and other enzymes that protect the epithelial cells from damage and limit the development of infection. Bacteria within the mucus are quickly trapped by mucins, lysed through the activity of antibacterial peptides such as defensins, and neutralized with antibodies such as dimeric or secretory IgA. The activity of dimeric IgA in the lumen of the GI tract is facilitated by mucins. By attaching to IgA, mucins poise the antibodies to perform the neutralization or opsonization of pathogens and their products. The secretion of mucus is a dynamic process and consists of several polypeptides that are encoded by different genes. Hence, the viscoelastic properties of mucosal tissues may vary depending on the particular organ, the state of the organ with respect to health or disease, and specific functions associated with the particular organ. The replenishment of mucus occurs continuously throughout the body; as epithelial cells turnover every few days, old mucus containing microorganisms is expelled from the body.

Roles for Commensal Bacteria in the Digestion of Food and Protection Against GI Pathogens

The absorption of nutrients from food is a dynamic process that depends in part on numerous enzymes and commensal bacteria. Species residing in the oral cavity such as the mouth aid in the degradation of food particles by producing digestive enzymes. Food is then shuttled to the stomach followed by various compartments of the small and large intestines, where further interactions with commensal bacteria occurs. The major site for nutrient absorption is within the small intestine, whereas the large intestine is primarily for the storage, compaction, and elimination of waste. As food travels throughout the intestines, it comes into contact with increasing numbers of commensal bacteria, from approximately 10^8/mL in the small intestine to 10^{12}/mL in the large intestine. These bacteria aid in the digestion of food, produce metabolites such as vitamin K, inactivate toxins and other harmful enzymes, and limit the growth of opportunistic pathogens. The growth of the intestinal flora itself is a dynamic process, depending on interspecies competition for nutrients and resources as well as the production of antimicrobial peptides from epithelial cells. Disruption of the microbial composition as a result of antibiotic treatment or other processes can increase susceptibility to infections or mucosal inflammation. The population of commensal microorganisms is stabilized by expelling vast numbers of organisms in the feces every day.

Gut-Associated Lymphoid Tissue Mediates Host Defense in the GI Tract

Host defense in the GI tract depends on immune cells and the secondary lymphoid tissues present throughout the various organ systems. These are collectively referred to as the **gut-associated lymphoid tissue (GALT)**. These tissues include secondary lymphoid structures such as the Peyer's patches, specialized epithelial cells including M cells, and leukocytes that are present within the **lamina propria**, or loose connective tissue underlying the mucosal epithelium (Fig. 6.1). Furthermore, antigens from pathogens

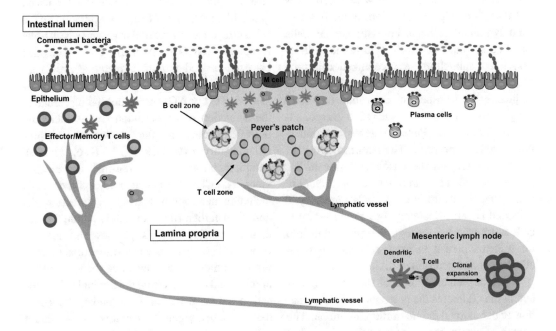

Fig. 6.1 Mucosal immune responses in the GI tract. Compartmentalization of the GI tract helps to facilitate immune responses while maintaining a physical barrier from microbial entry. Intestinal epithelial cells form a boundary between luminal contents and the underlying gut associated lymphoid tissue and lamina propria. Peyer's patches associated with the basolateral membrane of the epithelium are sites where immune responses are initiated. M cells interspersed between ciliated cells collect luminal antigens via phagocytosis. Dendritic cells and B cells residing in Peyer's patches then present antigens to T cells. Mesenteric lymph nodes are also sites where immune responses are initiated against intestinal antigens. Activated T cells undergo clonal expansion and migrate to the lamina propria where they provide effector functions. Antibody-producing plasma cells also reside in lamina propria, with IgA being the most predominant isotype produced in the GI tract

that invade the intestine are processed by antigen presenting cells and presented to naïve T cells within mesenteric lymph nodes, a large chain of lymph nodes within the mesentery, or connective tissue holding the gut in place.

Lymphoid tissues present in the mouth, tonsils and adenoids guard the entrance to the GI tract. They produce dimeric IgA that recognizes numerous oral microorganisms that individuals are exposed to, especially during the first few years of life. The presence of lymphoid tissue is most concentrated in the small intestine, which is also the major site of nutrient absorption. In the small intestine, finger-like projections called villi increase the surface area available for absorption. Numerous patches of discrete lymphoid tissue, named **Peyer's patches** after the scientist who discovered them, are present throughout the small intestine. These lymphoid organs vary in size, forming a dome-like structure containing numerous B cell follicles with germinal centers, interspersed with T cell areas and dendritic cells. In addition, numerous isolated lymphoid follicles consisting of B cells also line the intestinal wall. Within the follicle-associated epithelium, a specialized cell type called the microfold cell or **M cell** resides, which facilitates the transport of microbial and food antigens from the lumen of the gut to the secondary lymphoid tissue (Peyer's patches) and underlying lamina propria. The **lamina propria** directly underneath the basolateral side of the epithelium contains immune cells including macrophages, dendritic cells (DCs), memory T cells and B cells. Secretory IgA produced by B cells is transported through the epithelium into the lumen where it helps to prevent microbial attachment and neutralizes toxins.

A primary characteristic of the immune system in the GI tract is the prevention of inflammation under normal homeostatic conditions. The growth of commensal microorganisms is held in check by dimeric IgA and numerous effector cells within the lamina propria, which remain poised to defend against microbial invasion and quickly terminate pathogens. At the same time, tolerogenic mechanisms ensure that inflammation is primarily directed against pathogens rather than symbiotic microbes and does not contribute to unnecessary damage to the GI tract. For instance, unactivated DCs induce oral tolerance to food antigens and FoxP3-positive T_{reg} cells prevent and resolve inflammation. The mechanisms through which T_{regs} function include competing with naive T cells for costimulation, and producing anti-inflammatory cytokines (TGF-β, IL-10) which suppress the activation of effector T_H1, T_H2 and T_H17 cells.

Role of Individual Cell Types in Gastrointestinal Host Defense

The induction of immune responses in the gut is coordinated by a number of cell types. While their functions help to prevent and terminate colonization with pathogens, their activity must be tightly regulated in order to limit tissue damage caused by inflammation. Intestinal epithelial cells play a vital role by facilitating the uptake of nutrients and potential antigens from the lumen and sensing various microbial products with pattern recognition receptors. As described in Chap. 2, toll-like receptors (TLRs) are expressed on the cell surface and intracellularly, while NOD-like receptors (NOD1, NOD2) that recognize bacterial-derived muramyl dipeptide are localized to the cytoplasm. Signaling cascades initiated *via* TLR or NOD receptor binding results in the activation of transcription factors including NF-κB, leading to the production of pro-inflammatory cytokines (IL-1, IL-6, TNF-α), antimicrobial enzymes (defensins), and chemokines (CXCL8/IL-8) that attract other cells including neutrophils to sites of infection. As described earlier, M cells residing within the epithelium overlay Peyer's patches and isolated lymphoid follicles. They have numerous folds or ruffles on their surface, enabling the transcytosis of microbial antigens from the luminal side of the cell to the basal region. In secondary lymphoid tissues, these antigens are captured by DCs and B cells, and surveyed by T cells, leading to the initiation of adaptive immune responses.

Other important cell types in the GI tract include intestinal macrophages and dendritic cells. While macrophages are efficient in the capture and phagocytosis of microorganisms, they typically do so in a manner that elicits few proinflammatory cytokines and do not promote inflammation under steady-state conditions. The activation status of intestinal macrophages is regulated by cytokines such as TGF-β. Intestinal DCs play an important role in the activation of T cell-mediated immune responses. Under normal conditions, DCs induce tolerance by promoting T_{reg} differentiation. Infections lead to DC activation, including the upregulation of costimulatory molecules and production of cytokines. Thus, intestinal T cells recognizing pathogen-derived antigens presented by activated DCs will undergo differentiation into pro-inflammatory Th subsets.

T follicular helper cells (T_{FH}) are one of these subsets (Fig. 3.12). Their primary function is to promote isotype switching and somatic hypermutation in B cells recognizing antigens from the same pathogen. In the GI tract, this interaction usually leads to the production of dimeric IgA. Lymphocytes that are activated in mucosal lymphoid tissues preferentially reside within these tissues. This is due to their expression of certain adhesion molecules and chemokine receptors that are preferentially expressed in mucosal tissues. Thus, T and B cells activated in mesenteric lymph nodes or Peyer's patches will migrate to the epithelial and lamina propria compartments following their differentiation into effector cells. Specifically, activated lymphocytes lose the expression of CCR7 and gain the expression of CCR9. Ligands for these chemokine receptors are expressed in systemic secondary lymphoid organs and blood vessels supplying the GI tract, respectively. This process, termed **imprinting**, results in lymphocytes trafficking to the mucosal surfaces where the antigen was originally encountered. Cells in the lamina propria produce CCL25, serving as a chemoattractant for T and B cells expressing CCR9. DCs contribute to the imprinting of T cells and induce their expression of integrin $\alpha_4\beta_7$ in the GI tract. By interacting with **mucosal vascular addressin cellular adhesion molecule (MAdCAM-1)** expressed on intestinal endothelial cells, $\alpha_4\beta_7$ promotes the diapedesis of T cells and B cells into the intestinal parenchyma.

A variety of other immune cells also participate in GI host defense, including mast cells, γδ T cells, CD8 T cells, and a distinctive type of CD8 T cell, referred to as the **intraepithelial lymphocyte (IEL)**. Effector IELs integrate into the epithelial layer of the small intestine and help to confer immunity against a limited range of antigens. Unlike other T cell subsets, IELs possess both innate and adaptive immune characteristics and are thought to have been pre-activated against antigens. Upon their encounter with antigens, they immediately release various cytokines and induce the killing of target cells.

Anti-parasitic Immune Responses

A good illustration of how different cell types cooperate to provide host defense occurs during infections with parasites (Fig. 6.2). Helminth worms such as nematodes, trematodes, and cestodes are a major cause of debilitating diseases throughout the developing world. These infections are controlled by T_H2 responses, resulting in anti-parasitic IgE antibodies from B cells and the destruction of helminths coated with these antibodies by mast cells, basophils, and neutrophils. Infections with helminths results in production of cytokines such as IL-33 and TSLP by epithelial cells, leading to DC activation and the differentiation of naive T cells into T_H2 and T_{FH} subsets in draining lymph nodes. B cells that recognize helminth-derived antigens then undergo isotype switching to IgE under the direction of T cell-derived signals. When helminths are coated by IgE antibodies, innate immune cells are recruited to destroy the infectious organisms. Specifically, mast cells, basophils and eosinophils express a high affinity receptor for the constant region of IgE, named FcεRI. The activation of FcεRI on mast cells, basophils and eosinophils leads to their expulsion of granular contents such as histamine and various degradative enzymes including major basic protein. Degranulation also results in smooth muscle contraction, intestinal spasms, and diarrhea. This powerful response ensures the killing of helminth worms and their expulsion in the mucus and the feces. Overall, cytokines produced by T_H2 cells drive this process. IL-3, IL-9 and IL-10 drive mast cell expansion and function, IL-5 promotes eosinophil activation and survival, IL-4 promotes B cell activation and propagates the T_H2 response,

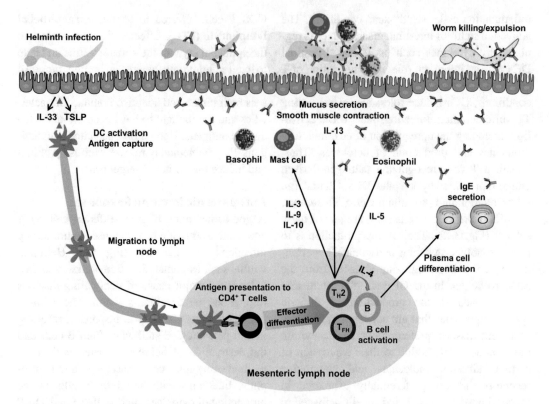

Fig. 6.2 T cell immune responses against parasites. Infections with helminth parasites stimulate epithelial cells to produce IL-33 and TSLP, resulting in DC activation and migration to lymph nodes. Antigen presentation to CD4 T cells results in their differentiation into T$_H$2 and T$_{FH}$ cells. Cytokines produced by T$_H$2 cells promote the activation of B cells, granulocytes and mast cells. T$_{FH}$ cells also help to induce the secretion of parasite-specific antibodies from B cells, namely IgE. This results in antibody coating the surface of parasites, marking them for attack by granulocytes and mast cells. Mucus produced in response to IL-13 also helps to prevent parasite attachment to epithelium

and IL-13 induces mucus hypersecretion, smooth muscle reactivity, and epithelial cell turnover. Collectively, these actions ensure the pathogen is driven out of the body by the combined activity of IgE-triggered mast cells and eosinophils.

In summary, the GI tract is a dynamic environment due to constant changes in food and nutrient availability, bacterial species growth, and activation of the immune system. Homeostasis refers to the remarkable ability of the GI tract to promote nutrient absorption while limiting pathogen colonization, repair injuries caused by inflammation, and maintain the epithelial lining. The role of the immune system in maintaining intestinal homeostasis has been demonstrated in studies showing that deficiencies in anti-inflammatory genes, notably IL-10, leads to spontaneous inflammatory

bowel diseases. On the other hand, pro-inflammatory cytokines including IL-6, IL-23 and TNF-α are therapeutic targets for IBD. Thus, maintaining intestinal homeostasis is a complex process that depends on a multitude of environmental (diet, microorganisms, allergens) and genetic factors. Injuries or disruptions to the epithelial barrier integrity can lead to acute or chronic inflammation, which is treated by various biologics that target the immune system, as described below.

Inflammatory Bowel Diseases

Inflammatory bowel disease (IBD) is an idiopathic disease thought to be caused by abnormal immune responses to host intestinal microbiota.

Two types of IBD have been described. They include **Ulcerative Colitis (UC)** which is typically confined to the colonic mucosal surface, and **Crohns's Disease (CD)** which may involve transmural inflammation along the length of the GI tract from the mouth through the anus (Table 6.1). Both diseases involve chronic inflammation that is relapsing-remitting in nature and can cause various complications including stenoses, abscesses, fistulas, extraintestinal manifestations, colitis-associated neoplasias, and cancer. The presence of blood in the stool, along with other symptoms, is a defining characteristic of IBD, aiding in distinguishing it from similar symptoms associated with irritable bowel syndrome. It is estimated that approximately 2.5 million people in the Western world suffer from IBD including UC and CD, with developing countries seeing more and more cases.

Ulcerative Colitis

In UC, the immune response and tissue damage is confined to the colon. The rectum is predominantly affected in 95% of patients, with variable degrees of proximal extension. Inflammation can be acute or chronic and is limited to the mucosa. Several immune cell types are involved, and the disease is characterized by ulceration, edema, hemorrhage along the length of the colon, crypt abscesses and goblet cell depletion (Fig. 6.3). Patients with UC typically present with bloody diarrhea accompanied by intense lower abdominal cramps, the severity of which increases during bowel movements. The disease can involve various parts of the colon resulting in fulminant colitis, leading to the development of peritonitis. The risk of colon cancer development in patients

Table 6.1 Differences observed between ulcerative colitis and Crohn's disease

Characteristic	Ulcerative colitis (UC)	Crohn's disease (CD)
Location of inflammation	Colonic mucosa, with the rectum affected in 95% of patients	Transmural inflammation can occur throughout the GI tract, from mouth to anus
Presence of skip areas	No	Yes
Symptoms	Bloody diarrhea; intense lower abdominal cramps	Determined by location, extent, and severity of inflammation *Ileocecal:* Abdominal pain *Small intestine:* Non-bloody, intermittent diarrhea, abdominal pain, weight loss *Colonic:* Bloody diarrhea, similar to UC *Gastroduodenal:* Nausea, vomiting, anorexia *Perianal:* Perirectal pain and rectal fistulas
Extra-intestinal manifestations observed	Yes	Yes

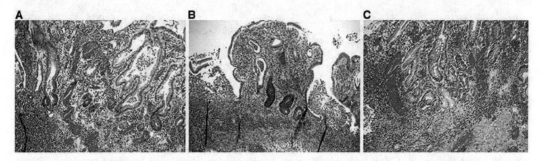

Fig. 6.3 Histologic evaluation of ulcerative colitis. Microscopic features of ulcerative colitis. (**a** and **b**): architectural distortion, including shortening of crypts, variation in the sizes and shapes of crypts, and basal lymphoplasmacytosis (**a** and **b**): H&E stain; ×100). (**c**) Paneth cell metaplasia and pyloric gland metaplasia in the left colon (H&E stain; ×100). Credit: Tom C. DeRoche, Shu-Yuan Xiao, and Xiuli Liu. *Histological evaluation in ulcerative colitis.* Gastroenterol Rep (Oxf). 2014 Aug; 2(3): 178–192. Reprinted under Creative Commons License Agreement (Attribution)

with UC increases from 2% in the first 10 years after diagnosis to 18% for those who have had UC for 30 years.

Crohn's Disease

In contrast to UC, CD can involve any part of the GI tract, and is characterized by the frequent separation of diseased segments of the GI tract from normal bowel areas, referred to as "skip" areas. The inflammation in CD is transmural and extends to the serosa, resulting in the formation of abscesses and fistulas. The disease often begins with inflammation and abscesses in the crypts, which then progresses to the formation of aphthoid ulcers (superficial ulcers over a Peyer's patch) and transverse, chronic inflammation extending into the submucosa, sometimes accompanied by non-caseating granulomas. The most common region for CD development is the ileocecal region, followed by the terminal ileum alone, diffuse small bowel, and isolated colonic regions. Transmural inflammation results in the development of lymphedema and thickening of the bowel wall and mesentery. The mesenteric lymph nodes are often enlarged, and the development of abscesses, fistulas, and strictures

often leads to obstruction of the bowel. Non-caseating granulomas, which may be observed in up to 50% of patients, can occur in the lymph nodes, peritoneum, and throughout the intestinal walls. In contrast to UC, the diagnosis of CD is subtle and often delayed since GI symptoms depend on the location, extent, and severity of the inflammation. In patients with ileocecal CD, the development of abdominal pain is usually post-prandial (occurring after consumption of a meal), and in children, may extend to the peri-umbilical area. CD of the small intestine often presents with non-bloody, intermittent diarrhea, abdominal pain, weight loss, and anorexia. In contrast, colonic CD presents with bloody diarrhea, making it indistinguishable from UC. Gastroduodenal CD presents with nausea, vomiting, and anorexia, and perianal CD can present with severe peri-rectal pain and discharge from rectal fistulas. Similar to UC, CD is associated with an increased risk of development of colon cancer, increasing from 3% at 10 years following diagnosis to 8% at 30 years. In Fig. 6.4 below, a biopsy specimen depicting pathologic changes consistent with Crohn's colitis is shown. Severe crypt atrophy and destruction can be observed, along with the accumulation of lymphoid cells and granulomas.

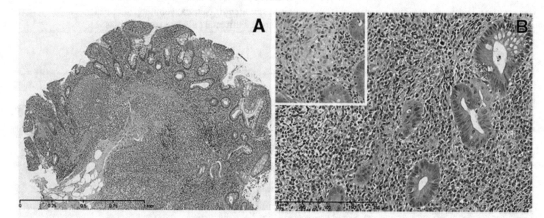

Fig. 6.4 Crohn colitis in a 10-year old child. Endoscopic biopsy specimen from right colon showing changes compatible with Crohn disease. (**a**) Colon mucosa with crypt atrophy and irregularity, and lymphoid hyperplasia (H&E, bar = 1 mm). (**b**) Higher magnification revealing crypt destruction and in the lamina propria severe accumulation of lymphocytes and plasma cells as well as a single small epithelioid cell granuloma (inset) (H&E, bar = 200 μm). Credit: Erling Peter Larsen, Allan Bayat and Mogens Vyberg. *Small duct autoimmune sclerosing cholangitis and Crohn colitis in a 10-year-old child. A case report and review of the literature.* Diagnostic Pathology 2012, 7:100. Reprinted under Creative Commons License Agreement (Attribution)

Extra-Intestinal Manifestations (EIM)

Both diseases are associated with various EIMs. Growth abnormalities and delayed sexual maturation are the most common in CD. Other systems affected include the skin (red scaly patches), joints (arthritis, ankylosing spondylitis), eyes (uveitis), and mouth (aphthous ulcers). The release of cytokines from immune cells, including TNF-α and IL-6, contributes to maintenance of the pro-inflammatory state and symptoms.

Pathogenesis of IBD

While the exact etiology of IBD is undetermined, several factors are thought to play a role in the development of the disease. This involves a complex interplay of distinct mechanisms including genetic, environmental, microbial, and immunologic influences (Fig. 6.5).

Genetics

Genome-wide association studies have identified more than 160 single nucleotide polymorphisms that may be associated with the development of IBD. Of these, the gene for *NOD2* (also called

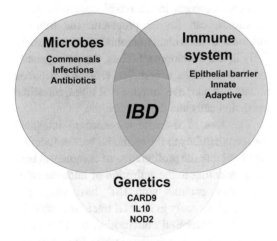

Fig. 6.5 Several factors contribute to the development of Inflammatory Bowel Diseases (IBDs) in susceptible individuals. IBDs are complex diseases that depend on interactions between the immune system, microorganisms and genetic susceptibility, giving rise to the manifestation of either ulcerative colitis or Crohn's Disease

CARD15) was the one first identified and holds one of the strongest associations. **Nucleotide binding oligomerization domain containing 2 (NOD2)** is a pattern recognition receptor (PRR) in the cytosol which helps the immune system recognize intracellular bacteria. It is expressed in Paneth cells of the intestinal epithelium, lamina propria immune cells, and other cell types. By detecting muramyl dipeptides in the peptidoglycan of bacterial cell walls, NOD2 stimulates innate immune functions including antigen presentation, antimicrobial peptides, bactericidal activity, and cytokines. Its role as a PRR helps to modulate the composition of normal gut flora. The immunological effects of NOD2 in the GI tract are complex, and a regulatory function has been identified due to its suppression of T_H17 responses that are driven by IL-23. T_H17 cells have roles in the development of both UC and CD, and IL-23 contributes to T_H17 cell differentiation and proliferation. Polymorphisms in the gene encoding for a subunit of the IL-23 receptor, *IL-23R*, have been implicated in IBD. Additional genes include *ATG16L1* and *IRGM* which are involved in autophagy, a cellular process that facilitates the lysosomal degradation and recycling of cellular components including organelles. In addition, autophagy can promote the lysosomal degradation of intracellular bacteria, limiting colonization with pathogens. Epithelial cells and dendritic cells with polymorphisms in these genes display defective antimicrobial responses, possibly leading to intestinal dysbiosis and susceptibility to IBD.

Environment

Several environmental factors are linked to the development of IBD, including cigarette smoking, the use of non-steroidal anti-inflammatory drugs (NSAIDs), antibiotics, frequent infections, and diet. Of these, smoking has been the most studied, and found to be inversely correlated with the development of UC, but positively correlated with CD. The use of NSAIDs such as aspirin at high doses or for prolonged or frequent use contributes to IBD symptoms. Antibiotics contribute to IBD by disrupting the composition of the normal microbial flora. While having a diverse microbiota is beneficial for GI homeostasis, antibiotics may kill protective species of bacteria and increase the space available for colonization with pathogens, promoting inflammation. Likewise, a lack of anti-inflammatory components in the diet as well as vitamin D deficiency have been implicated in development of the disease.

Microbial Factors

The human gut microbiome is established within the first 2 weeks of life, remaining relatively stable after that. While the intestines of healthy individuals are colonized by diverse species of bacteria, the intestines of patients with IBD exhibit remarkably reduced microbial biodiversity, with over-representation of enterobacteria in CD and increased numbers of *Escherichia coli* in UC. Residential intestinal bacteria are referred to as commensal microbiota and provide a number of important functions. Commensals aid in food digestion including dietary fiber, regulation of glucose homeostasis, and protection against infection from pathogens. Towards this, commensal bacteria compete with pathogens for nutrients or space in the gut, induce the secretion of antimicrobial peptides from intestinal Paneth cells, and stimulate adaptive immune responses including IgA production from B cells. Thus, interactions between commensal microbiota and our immune system help to maintain intestinal homeostasis in healthy individuals. Beneficial metabolites produced by the *Bacteroidetes* and *Firmicutes* phyla include short chain fatty acids, which have anti-inflammatory effects on immune cells. Several factors determine the composition of gut microbial species, including maternal transfer during birth, diet, antibiotic use, and potential drug/alcohol use. Further, the immune system shapes the composition of microbial species by producing antimicrobial peptides, IgA, and mucus which limits bacterial adhesion to the epithelial lining. The detection of microbes by pattern recognition receptors expressed on innate immune cells (see Chap. 2) may precipitate the inflammatory cascade in patients with a genetic susceptibility to IBD. As described earlier, genetic variants of NOD2 increase susceptibility to CD. By activating NF-κB and MAP kinases in monocytes, NOD2 induces the production of inflammatory cytokines. CARD9 contributes to innate immunity against fungi and intracellular pathogens by activating proinflammatory MAP kinases. These findings suggest that detection of commensal microbiota by the immune system is essential for maintaining intestinal homeostasis.

Immunologic Mechanisms

The immune system plays a critical role in the pathogenesis of IBD, and a number of factors have been proposed. These include chronic inflammatory responses against self-antigens or the intestinal commensal bacteria. A widely-held hypothesis is that environmental triggers including infections can lead to the loss of intestinal epithelial barrier integrity and oral tolerance to intestinal and microbial antigens. This results in the activation of DCs, which subsequently migrate to the mesenteric lymph nodes and induce the activation and differentiation of T_H1, T_H2, and T_H17 effector subsets which may recognize self or microbial antigens (Fig. 6.6). Potential target antigens in IBD may be derived from mucin, goblet cells or colonocytes. In addition, anti-neutrophil cytoplasmic antibodies (ANCA) and antibodies targeting neutrophil myeloperoxidase are associated with both CD and UC development. Changes in microbial composition, or dysbiosis, can further propagate the immune response to individual microbial species, particularly in UC development. Thus, the pathogenesis of IBD involves a complex crosstalk between innate and adaptive immune cell types, intestinal epithelial cells and the microbiome.

The loss of immune tolerance to intestinal antigens can impair the epithelial barrier function and facilitate the proliferation of commensal bacteria, resulting in the activation of immune cells. Moreover, patients with IBD have decreased microbial diversity in their GI tract, or **dysbiosis**, including decreased colonization by *Firmicutes* species, which can further impact food metabolism, vitamin synthesis, and nutrient absorption, and favor the development of microbial-specific immune responses. Several microbial species are thought to induce immune responses during IBD including viruses, protozoans, and specific bacte-

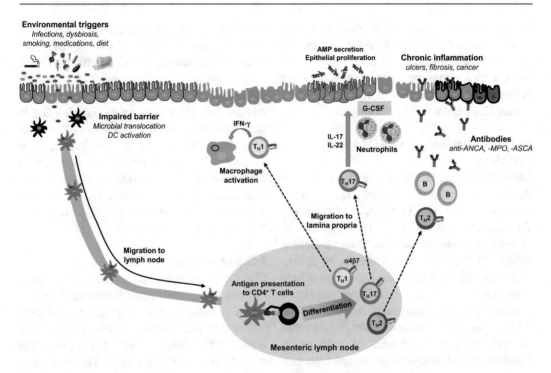

Fig. 6.6 Effector mechanisms of immune cells in IBD. In susceptible individuals, certain environmental triggers impair the intestinal barrier function, leading to microbial translocation across the epithelial layer and DC activation. This is followed by DC migration to lymph nodes, where they present antigens to T cells to induce differentiation into T_H1, T_H2 and T_H17 subsets. Effector differentiation is accompanied by their upregulation of the intestinal-specific integrin $\alpha_4\beta_7$, resulting in the migration of effector T cells to intestinal lamina propria. T_H1 cells mediate inflammation by secreting IFN-γ, resulting in macrophage activation and villus atrophy. Cytokines produced by T_H17 cells induce epithelial proliferation, antimicrobial peptide secretion and neutrophil recruitment. T_H2 cells induce B cell activation and antibody production against antigens commonly found in the GI tract. Chronic inflammation mediated by T cells results in cycles of epithelial cell injury followed by repair, impairing the epithelial barrier function, and leading to intestinal ulcers, fibrosis and cancer

rial species such as *Mycobacterium paratuberculosis*, *Mycobacterium avium*, *Listeria monocytogenes*, *Chlamydia trachomatis*, and *E. coli*. Antibodies to several commensal organisms have been detected in the sera of patients with IBD. In addition, circulating antibodies against *Saccharomyces cerevisiae* have also been found to be present. Due to the compromised mucosal barrier, increased numbers of bacteria adhere to the intestinal wall, increasing intestinal permeability and inflammation. This pro-inflammatory microenvironment can perpetuate IBD and lead to the development of intestinal ulcers, fibrosis, and increased susceptibility to the development of colon cancer. While the role for microbiota in the development of IBD in experimental rodent models is well-established, its significance in

human IBD development is variable. However, a subgroup of patients respond to fecal microbiota transplantation or antibiotic use, suggesting that the microbiota can regulate the severity of disease but may not be sufficient to cause IBD in otherwise healthy people. Lastly, studies in animal models demonstrate that the immune responses during IBD are associated with increased production of the pro-inflammatory cytokine TNF-α and decreased production of the anti-inflammatory cytokine IL-10. Interestingly, the development of colitis does not occur in germ-free animals, whereas IL-10-deficient mice can spontaneously develop colitis when housed in environments colonized by certain types of bacteria. Furthermore, the production of IL-10 by CD4 T_{reg} cells is particularly important in preventing the development of inflammation, suggesting that the induction of inflammatory and protective mechanisms is regulated *via* a delicate balance of immune processes that control the activation of inflammatory T_H1, T_H2, and T_H17 subsets and regulatory T_{reg} cell subsets.

Role of Macrophages and DCs in IBD Initiation

Macrophages and DCs in the lamina propria of the GI tract recognize microbes through pattern recognition receptors (TLRs, NLRs, C-type lectin receptors, and RIG-I-like receptors). These receptors activate transcription factors including NF-κB, MAP kinases, and interferon regulatory factors (IRFs), resulting in the production of pro-inflammatory cytokines, chemokines and type I interferons (IFNs). Macrophage activation in the GI tract can lead to the direct killing of microbes as well as the recruitment of neutrophils. Furthermore, the production of pro-inflammatory cytokines may activate intestinal DCs, promoting their antigen presenting function to T cells. Thus, the balance of pro-inflammatory (IL-6, IL-12, IL-23, TNF-α) and anti-inflammatory (IL-10) cytokines produced by lamina propria macrophages has potential to impact the inflammatory milieu. IL-10 is required to prevent spontaneous intestinal inflammation in response to microbiota and promotes regulatory T cell (T_{reg}) maintenance in the gut. In addition, IL-10 suppresses the production of IL-12/23 p40 from intestinal macrophages, leading to diminished T_H1 and T_H17 responses. In healthy individuals, pro-inflammatory responses to intestinal bacteria are transient and resolve over time. Intestinal macrophages appear to be able to distinguish between commensal microbiota and pathogens such that disease-causing bacteria are most likely to trigger inflammation. However, dysregulation of these pathways can enhance susceptibility to infections or produce the chronic inflammation characteristic of IBD. Several single nucleotide polymorphisms (SNPs) associated with IBD susceptibility are expressed in macrophages, including the genes encoding NOD2, NF-κB, IRF5, CARD9, IL-10, IL-12 and the IFN-γ receptor. The activation status of DCs can also modulate GI inflammation by inducing effector CD4 T cell differentiation. Various subsets of DCs can induce the differentiation of pro-inflammatory T cells (such as T_H1, T_H2, and T_H17) or anti-inflammatory cells (e.g. T_{reg}). DCs also positively regulate IgA production in the gut, helping to limit bacteria growth and adhesion to the epithelium. Secretory IgA (sIgA) facilitates antigen delivery to DCs and is significantly decreased in IBD, especially UC, although the serum levels of monomeric IgA may be elevated. Thus, both macrophages and DCs can contribute to inflammatory responses during IBD.

T Cell Immunity and IBD

CD4 T cells are central for driving gut inflammation and IBD pathogenesis. Following their activation by antigen presenting cells, CD4 T cells differentiate into specialized subsets in response to the cytokine milieu (Chap. 3). The production of IL-12 by innate cells induces T_H1 differentiation while the combination of IL-1β, IL-6, IL-23 and TGF-β promotes T_H17 differentiation. The differentiation of T_H2 subsets is driven by IL-4. Once activated within the mesenteric lymph nodes, effector T cells express the intestinal homing integrin $\alpha_4\beta_7$ and migrate to the gut where they secrete inflammatory cytokines. While these subsets are required for adaptive immunity, they contribute to pathogenic inflammation when directed against innocuous- or self-antigens. IFN-γ produced by T_H1 cells activates macrophages to augment their microbicidal properties, thus further amplifying the macrophage response. Similarly, IL-17 and IL-22 produced by T_H17 cells will stimulate the intestinal epithelium to proliferate, secrete various antimicrobial peptides and neutrophil-recruiting chemokines. Increased numbers of IFN-γ-producing T_H1 cells as well as IL-17-producing T_H17 cells have been selectively identified in patients with CD, suggesting a pathogenic role for these T_H subsets. In contrast, IL-5 and IL-13-producing T_H2 cells, as well as IL-13-producing NKT cells, are thought to be predominant in UC patients. However, the role of IL-13 in disease is complex, as it has been shown to have both pro- and anti-inflammatory effects in UC patients. The IL-23R and its signaling pathway appears to impact susceptibility to both CD and UC. Lastly, regulatory T cells (T_{regs}) contribute to tolerance in part by producing IL-10. Their protective role in CD is corroborated by studies demonstrating the efficacy of autologous T_{reg} transfer.

IBD Treatment

Given the many possible genetic, immune, environmental, and microbial interactions leading to the development of IBD, therapeutic approaches are aimed at either resolution of the inflammatory response or an attempt to suppress immune cell activation. As described below, the most commonly used drugs for inducing a state of remission are corticosteroids, methotrexate, sulfasalazine, azathioprine, cyclosporine, or TNF inhibitors. Initially, antibiotics such as **metronidazole** (Flagyl) or **ciprofloxacin** (Cipro) may be given, as many CD patients have increased levels of colonization with *E. coli, Serratia marcescens,* and/or *Candida tropicalis* in the GI tract. These may form a biofilm on the intestinal walls, precipitating inflammation.

Aminosalicylates (ASAs) exert their therapeutic efficacy in the colon after being chemically reduced from their prodrug form by coliform bacteria. **Sulfasalazine** and other 5-aminosalicylate drugs are effective at reducing inflammation and achieving remission in UC, but sulfasalazine's effects are more controversial in CD. This may be due to the sulfapyridine component of the drug, which is responsible for many of its adverse effects. While this component contributes to its therapeutic effects in rheumatoid arthritis, only the 5-ASA component is necessary for treating IBD. Thus, the use of the 5-ASA only drugs (Asacol, Colazal, and Delzicol, among others) are preferred over sulfasalazine.

Corticosteroids such as methylprednisolone, prednisone, hydrocortisone, or budesonide may be used to help relieve symptoms and flareups, as well as inducing remission. While these medications tend to work quickly, they are not used long-term due to adrenal suppression, and the patient should be gradually tapered off the drug.

While corticosteroids are often taken orally, methylprednisolone and hydrocortisone can be given locally in a rectal formulation for severe forms of the disease in the lower colon or rectum. Budesonide is given orally and targets inflammation in the distal small intestine and beginning of the large intestine.

Patients who are refractory to steroid therapy, 5-ASAs, or antibiotics may require therapy with calcineurin inhibitors, anti-metabolites, or biologics. For instance, TNF inhibitors (adalimumab, infliximab, certolizumab) may be used in combination with purine antimetabolites (thiopurines; azathioprine, 6-mercaptopurine). The class of antimetabolites function by inhibiting purine synthesis, which is required for cellular replication. Thus, dividing cells are most susceptible to antimetabolites and undergo apoptosis in their presence. In addition, it is thought that azathioprine may target Rac1, a small GTPase involved in CD4 T cell activation. When azathioprine is metabolized to 6-mercaptopurine and subsequently converted to 6-thioguanine, one of its metabolites (6-thio-GTP) binds to Rac1, acting as a competitive inhibitor of endogenous GTP, promoting apoptosis of the T cell.

Integrin-neutralizing monoclonal antibodies are used to suppress lymphocyte migration to the GI tract. By targeting α4 integrins, natalizumab blocks the function of $\alpha_4\beta_1$ and $\alpha_4\beta_7$ heterodimers. While $\alpha_4\beta_7$ is required for T cell migration to the gut, $\alpha_4\beta_1$ is involved in trafficking to the brain. By inducing immunosuppression in the brain, natalizumab comes with a risk of progressive multifocal leukoencephalopathy (PML), and patients must be monitored and tested for JC virus. Since vedolizumab specifically blocks the interaction of $\alpha_4\beta_7$ heterodimers with MAdCAM-1 on intestinal vascular endothelium, the risk of PML is thought to be much lower. Both drugs have demonstrated efficacy as Crohn's therapies by inhibiting/slowing leukocyte trafficking to the gut, thus suppressing inflammation and tissue damage.

Paying close attention to the diet and maintaining good nutrition may help decrease symptoms in CD patients and allow for the healing of tissues. Spicy or fibrous foods may lead to flareups, diarrhea, and impaired nutrient absorption.

Approximately 50–75% of patients with complications (fistulas, abscesses) whose condition is not well-controlled with medication require surgical resection of affected tissues within 10 years of their diagnosis. Even with surgery, up to 30% of patients may experience a recurrence within 3 years, with 60% experiencing a recurrence within 10 years.

Mechanism of Action of IBD Drugs

5-Aminosalicylates

Drug formulations containing 5-aminosalicylic acid (5-ASA) are often used as first line therapy for treating IBD and to maintain remission. Produced as inactive prodrugs, they must undergo chemical reactions in the gut to become active. This is essential because unformulated 5-ASA is mostly absorbed in the small intestine prior to reaching inflamed regions of the GI tract. The azo (sulfasalazine, olsalazine, balsalazide) and mesalamine formulations allow for high concentrations of the active drug to reach the terminal ileum and colon. **Olsalazine (Dipentum®)** contains two 5-ASA moieties bound through an azo bond, reducing its absorption from the small intestine. In the terminal ileum and colon, bacteria cleave the azo bond, releasing two active 5-ASA molecules. In **sulfasalazine (Azulfidine®)**, 5-ASA is bound to the inert compound sulfapyridine, which is metabolized by intestinal bacteria to yield free 5-ASA. In **balsalazide (Colazal®)**, 5-ASA is bound to 4-aminobenzoyl-beta-alanine. **Mesalamine formulations** deliver 5-ASA to different sections of the small or large bowel. **Pentasa®** contains microgranules that target 5-ASA release to the small intestine. **Asacol®** and **Lialda®** are coated in resins that dissolve at pH 7, releasing 5-ASA into the distal ileum and proximal colon. For treating inflammation confined to the distal colon or rectum, enema formulations (**Rowasa®**) and suppositories (**Canasa®**) are preferred for delivering high concentrations of 5-ASA to these regions. The mechanism through which 5-ASA provides anti-inflammatory action is not well understood, although it has structural similarity to the cyclooxygenase (COX) inhibitor acetylsalicylic acid (aspirin). Likewise, 5-ASA suppresses arachidonic acid metabolism into prostaglandins and leukotrienes, implicating a possible inhibitory effect on COX and lipoxygenase enzymes. Further, 5-ASA is a free radical scavenger and decreases oxidative stress. An animal model of colitis showed that 5-ASA inhibits NF-κB activation, an important transcription factor for pro-inflammatory cytokine production.

Glucocorticoids

Therapeutic glucocorticoids (GCs) are structurally similar to the endogenous hormone cortisol, which is involved in the stress response and has anti-insulin effects, increasing blood glucose levels. Their mechanism of action is described in detail in Chaps. 1 and 4 and is briefly alluded to below. The potent immunosuppressive properties of GCs render them very useful for treating inflammation, including moderate to severe relapses of UC and CD. GCs are lipophilic and largely bound to serum albumin or steroid binding globulin, while the free hormone passively diffuses through cell membranes. Cortisol is an essential hormone and nearly every cell in the body expresses the GC receptor. The initial interaction between GCs and the GC receptor occurs in the cytoplasm, resulting in the nuclear translocation of this complex and binding to genetic sequences called glucocorticoid response elements (GREs) (Fig. 6.7). In addition to directly regulating gene expression, the GC receptor interacts with other transcription factors including NF-κB and AP-1, antagonizing their activity. It is estimated that 10–20% of the human genome is positively or negatively regulated by GCs. The mechanism through which GCs suppress pro-inflammatory cytokines, prostaglandins, chemokines, and tissue damage involves the inhibition of NF-κB, COX-2, phospholipase A2, and nitric oxide synthase. The adverse systemic effects of GCs include adrenal suppression, acne, edema, glucose intolerance, osteoporosis and susceptibility to infection. While endogenous cortisol can bind to and activate the mineralocorticoid receptor, therapeutic GCs can be selected for their anti-inflammatory

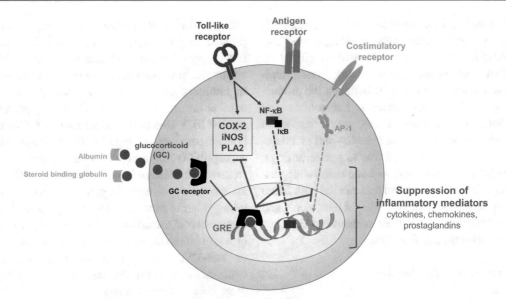

Fig. 6.7 Mechanism of action for therapeutic glucocorticoids. Immune cell activation is mediated by several types of receptors including those involved in antigen recognition, costimulation or pathogen detection (Toll-like receptor). Signaling through these receptors results in the activation of transcription factors that induce cell proliferation and the secretion of inflammatory cytokines and prostaglandins. Glucocorticoids are potent immunosuppressive agents that diffuse across cell membranes and activate cytoplasmic glucocorticoid receptors. This results in its nuclear translocation and binding to promoter regions in genes containing glucocorticoid response elements (GRE). Thus, glucocorticoids suppress immune cell functions by regulating gene expression

potency with minimal mineralocorticoid effects. Common IBD treatments are prednisone, prednisolone and budesonide. For active IBD in the rectum and distal colon, topical formulations of hydrocortisone or budesonide are used (enemas, foam, suppositories) since they produce fewer systemic side effects than oral or intravenous forms due to their poor absorption. **Budesonide (Entocort®)** binds to the GC receptor with 200-fold greater affinity than cortisol and 15-fold greater affinity than prednisolone. The bioavailability of budesonide is low due to its extensive first pass hepatic metabolism by CYP3A4, resulting in a low probability of systemic side effects. Entocort capsules are filled with enteric coated granules that dissolve when the pH is above 5.5, resulting in budesonide release into the distal ileum and colon.

Anti-proliferative Drugs

Purine Analogs
Azathioprine (Imuran®) and **6-mercaptopurine (6-MP, Purinethol®)** are purine anti-proliferative agents used for the induction and maintenance of remission in IBDs. Their inhibitory effect on DNA and RNA synthesis results in the apoptosis of proliferating cells, including T cells. Following administration, azathioprine is non-enzymatically converted to 6-MP, which is subsequently converted into several metabolites through the action of hypoxanthine-guanine phosphoribosyltransferase (HGPRT). The active metabolites, 6-thioguanine nucleotides and 6-methylmercaptopurine, inhibit the enzyme amidophosphoribosyltransferase (ATase), required for purine synthesis. Proliferating T cells treated with 6-MP have rapid reductions in intracellular ATP concentrations, leading to decreased catabolism of glucose and glutamine. Purine analogs can cause bone marrow depression, leading to leukopenia and increased susceptibility to infections. Adverse effects of purine analogs can be exacerbated by allopurinol through the inhibition of xanthine oxide, a major enzyme in the catabolism of 6-MP metabolites.

Methotrexate (Rheumatrex®) is a competitive inhibitor of dihydrofolic acid reductase, suppressing purine and pyrimidine biosynthesis.

This inhibits DNA replication in T cells and other actively proliferating cells including tumors and intestinal mucosa. In addition to its effects on DNA synthesis, methotrexate has anti-inflammatory properties by inducing the production of IL-10, IL-1 receptor antagonists, and adenosine secretion. These properties make methotrexate effective at inducing and maintaining remission in CD. Similar to purine analogs, methotrexate can result in bone marrow depression and leukopenia. Supplementation with folate may be able to reduce the risk of leukopenia and susceptibility to infections without impairing its anti-inflammatory functions.

Monoclonal Antibodies

Cytokine Targets

TNF produced by immune cells is a pharmacologic target in IBD. Initially synthesized as a plasma membrane-bound protein, **TNF-α converting enzyme (TACE)** cleaves the extracellular domain to release soluble TNF. The effects of soluble and membrane-bound TNF are mediated through TNF receptor I and II, respectively. Many cell types express TNF receptors, the activation of which results in the nuclear translocation of NF-κB, pro-inflammatory cytokine (IL-1, IL-6) production, leukocyte activation, fibroblast collagen production, endothelial adhesion molecule expression, and liver acute phase response proteins. These effects of TNF can promote intestinal tissue damage during IBD. Cellular responses to TNF are complex, as signaling pathways downstream of its receptors can promote either survival or apoptosis. Three monoclonal antibodies are used therapeutically to neutralize soluble and membrane-bound TNF, preventing it from interacting with its receptors. These treatments are typically used for patients that have inadequate responses to conventional anti-proliferative agents. In addition to neutralization, the full-length antibodies **infliximab** and **adalimumab** can lyse cells containing membrane-bound TNF in the presence of complement, destroying cellular sources of this cytokine. **Certolizumab pegol (Cimzia®)** is an antibody fragment with the variable region conjugated to polyethylene glycol and does not induce complement-mediated lysis. Anti-TNF antibodies have been shown to induce apoptosis in lamina propria-resident T cells, providing another mechanism through which they protect against IBD. Due to important roles for TNF in host defense, anti-TNF antibodies may increase susceptibility to infections and allow for the reactivation of latent infections. Adverse effects are most likely to occur in patients concurrently taking other immunosuppressive agents such as corticosteroids, anakinra, abatacept, rituximab or natalizumab. A large percentage of patients on anti-TNF therapy become non-responsive over time, resulting in treatments targeting other inflammatory pathways.

Interleukin-12 is a heterodimeric cytokine consisting of p35 and p40 subunits encoded by different genes. The p40 subunit is also used to form IL-23 when it dimerizes with the p19 subunit. Both IL-12 and IL-23 have been implicated in pre-clinical models of IBD. These cytokines are produced by antigen presenting cells including DCs and macrophages. Receptors for IL-12 and IL-23 are expressed on CD4+ T cells, CD8+ T cells, γδ+ T cells, NK cells and innate lymphoid cells. Stimulating CD4+ T cells with IL-12 or IL-23 results in their differentiation into inflammatory T_H1 and T_H17 subsets, respectively. Inflamed sections of the GI tract in IBD patients have elevated numbers of CD4+ T cells. In addition, IL-23 may promote intestinal inflammation by stimulating innate lymphoid cells. **Ustekinumab** is a human IgG1k monoclonal antibody against IL-12/23p40, preventing its binding to IL-12Rβ1 (Fig. 5.11). Thus, ustekinumab neutralizes the function of IL-12 and IL-23, both of which signal through IL-12Rβ1. This treatment is used for moderate to severe CD, including patients that have become non-responsive to anti-TNF therapy. Patients receiving ustekinumab should not receive live vaccines.

Integrin Targets

Integrins are adhesion molecules on the surface of leukocytes that interact with their ligands expressed on vascular endothelium, allowing circulating leukocytes to adhere to the vascular endothelium and migrate into the underlying tissue. Integrins are heterodimers consisting of α and β subunits. A subset of memory T cells express $\alpha_4\beta_7$, resulting in their migration to the GI tract. The ligand for $\alpha_4\beta_7$ is MAdCAM-1, which is expressed on intestinal endothelial cells. The $\alpha_4\beta_7$/MAdCAM-1 interaction facilitates T cell transmigration into the intestinal lamina propria, contributing to the pathogenesis of CD. **Natalizumab (Tysabri®)** recognizes α_4 subunits of integrins, inhibiting the interaction of $\alpha_4\beta_7$ with MAdCAM-1 on GI vascular endothelial cells (Fig. 6.8). In addition, natalizumab inhibits $\alpha_4\beta_1$ from interacting with vascular cell adhesion molecule-1 (VCAM-1) on activated vascular endothelium. By preventing the transmigration of leukocytes from endothelial to parenchymal tissue compartments, natalizumab reduces intestinal inflammation in IBD patients. **Vedolizumab (Entyvio®)** is specific for $\alpha_4\beta_7$ with no effect on $\alpha_4\beta_1$ integrins, and is used to decrease T cell accumulation into the intestine. Due to their inhibitory effects on leukocyte migration, these antibody therapies may increase susceptibility to infections.

Thalidomide (Thalomid®) suppresses proinflammatory cytokine production from immune cells and may be used in patients that fail to respond to anti-TNF therapy. Thalidomide is well known for causing embryo-fetal toxicity resulting in congenital limb abnormalities and should never be taken during pregnancy. Nonetheless, its anti-inflammatory properties are unrelated to embryo-fetal toxic effects, and thalidomide has been shown to induce a clinical response and remission in 70% and 55% of IBD patients, respectively. The most common side effects associated with thalidomide use in IBD patients include peripheral neuropathy and sedation.

Celiac Disease

Celiac Disease is a widely occurring autoimmune disorder of the small intestine that is prevalent in up to 1% of the world's population. In recent years, the incidence of the disease has been steadily increasing, and it is not just confined to industrialized countries in Western Europe or the United States, but has been found in populations throughout the world including North Africa, the Middle East, and India. The defining characteristic of celiac disease is a chronic inflammatory reaction in susceptible individuals to derivatives of the dietary component gluten, which are found in grains including wheat, barley, and rye. This reaction results in severe impairment and enteropathy of the small intestine, leading to villous atrophy, and the malabsorption of nutrients. Patients with celiac disease often present with either classic symptoms such as weight loss, chronic diarrhea, malabsorption, or failure to thrive (which is rare), or non-classical symptoms

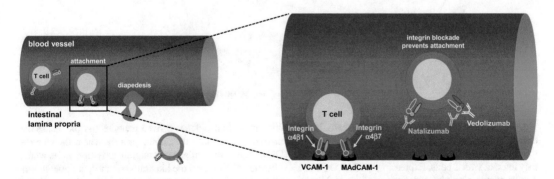

Fig. 6.8 Mechanism of action for anti-integrin antibodies. α_4 integrins are important for the migration of circulating T cells to the GI tract by facilitating attachment to VCAM-1 ($\alpha_4\beta_1$) and MAdCAM-1 ($\alpha_4\beta_7$) on intestinal blood vessels. The monoclonal antibodies natalizumab and vedolizumab neutralize α_4 integrins, preventing T cell attachment and entry into the GI tract

such as bloating, constipation, abdominal pain, iron deficiency, chronic fatigue, and osteoporosis. Both intestinal and extra-intestinal manifestations of celiac disease have been reported. Although celiac disease was first described in 1888, its relation to gluten components was only established in 1953, and the immunological basis of the disease is only now beginning to be appreciated.

Immune Mechanisms in the Pathogenesis of Celiac Disease

The primary immune triggers in the development of celiac disease are peptides generated from gluten components that induce CD4 T cell reactions to autoantigens in susceptible individuals. Gluten is a major component of the cereals wheat, rye, and barley, and is widely used in bread-making due to its elastic properties. The main components of gluten include glutenins, prolamins and gliadins in wheat, secalines in rye, and hordeins in barley. The presence of various glutamine and proline residues in gluten results in its incomplete digestion by intestinal gastric, pancreatic, and brush-border enzymes, giving rise to the formation of large, undigested peptides up to 33 amino acids in length. In susceptible individuals, gliadins interact with intestinal epithelial cells and disassemble the tight junctions between enterocytes (Fig. 6.9). This results in leakiness and impairment of the epithelial cell barrier, leading to transcytosis (probably via secretory IgA) of gluten components including gliadin peptides from the intestinal lumen to the lamina propria. Here, the gliadin peptides are deamidated by enzymes such as tissue transglutaminase. Deamidation increases the immunogenicity of these peptides in susceptible individuals, favoring their binding to the HLA molecules DQ2 and DQ8 on antigen presenting cells. The subsequent

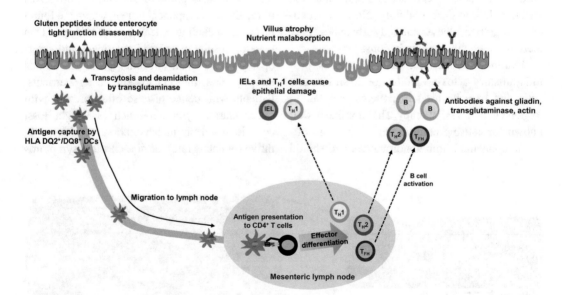

Fig. 6.9 Role of immune cells in celiac disease. In susceptible individuals, gluten-derived peptides (purple) cause the disassembly of enterocyte tight junctions, resulting in their translocation into the lamina propria where the enzyme transglutaminase deamidates the peptides. Dendritic cells (DCs) acquire this antigen and migrate to lymph nodes where they interact with T cells. Expression of HLA DQ2 or DQ8 by the DC increases the likelihood of antigen presentation. T cells recognizing gluten-derived peptides and receiving other signals required for activation will undergo effector differentiation into T_H1, T_H2 and T_{FH} subsets. B cell activation is associated with their production of antibodies recognizing gliadin, transglutaminase or actin. T cells migrating to the intestinal lamina propria promote inflammation in the presence of gluten, as shown. In this way, chronic exposure to gluten over time will result in villus atrophy and nutrient malabsorption in the GI tract in susceptible individuals

activation of naïve CD4 T cells against these peptides results in immune sensitization and the production of antibodies against gliadin peptides and the autoantigens tissue transglutaminase and actin. T_H1 cells producing IFN-γ, T_H2 cells and T_{FH} cells have been found to be implicated in the pathogenesis of celiac disease.

In addition to the adaptive immune response in the lamina propria, innate immune responses mediated by IELs also appear to be important for the formation of celiac lesions. These cells are able to acquire receptors characteristic of NK cells, including NKG2D, in an IL-15-dependent manner and directly contribute to epithelial cell damage. In fact, an increased density of IELs in celiac lesions is a hallmark of celiac disease.

While genome-wide association studies have identified non-HLA loci that may predispose to the development of celiac disease, the most important genetic risk factors are the genes encoding the α and β chains of HLA DQ2 and DQ8 molecules, respectively. Nearly all patients with celiac disease harbor specific variants of these genes, named *HLADQA1* and *HLADQB1*. Greater than 90% of celiac patients are DQ2-positive, with most of the others being DQ8-positive. The presence of these loci is not sufficient for the development of disease, however, as only 1–3% of individuals expressing these loci develop disease. This suggests a role for additional environmental factors in the development of disease, such as the early introduction of large doses of gluten to children, birth by cesarean section, various infections including rotavirus in children, *campylobacter* in adults, respiratory infections, antibiotic and proton pump inhibitor use, and microbial dysbiosis. With respect to the latter, increased concentrations of *Bifidobacterium bifidum* were found to be present in the feces of adults with celiac disease compared with healthy controls. Similarly, children with celiac disease were reported to have a greater proportion of duodenal gram-negative bacteria compared to healthy controls. Thus, genetic and environmental factors both contribute to celiac disease.

The presentation of celiac disease may be extremely heterogeneous. While patients with classic symptoms are easily diagnosed, those with atypical symptoms such as EIMs, silent or latent forms of the disease may be harder to diagnose. The latter typically exhibit serum IgA antibodies against tissue transglutaminase and harbor genetic risk factors without developing symptoms. Patients with refractory celiac disease, who exhibit persistent symptoms despite a gluten-free diet for a period greater than 1 year, are particularly challenging to treat. Patients with classical symptoms usually present in childhood, while those with atypical symptoms usually present as adults. Examples of EIMs associated with celiac disease include dermatitis herpetiformis (an inflammatory cutaneous disease resulting in diffuse, polymorphic lesions consisting of erythema, urticarial plaques, herpetiform vesiculae and blisters), type 1 diabetes, autoimmune thyroid disorders, autoimmune hepatitis, liver conditions, and other neurological conditions. The link between celiac disease and autoimmunity is further supported by the role of HLADQ2 and HLADQ8 genetic risk factors in thyroid disorders and antibodies to autoantigens such as actin in dermatitis herpetiformis. Other manifestations such as hepatic damage could occur due to increased entry of toxins and other factors into portal veins due to the defective intestinal barrier. Secondary manifestations caused by nutrient malabsorption can occur in celiac patients. Examples of these include osteoporosis due to insufficient calcium absorption or malignancies resulting from intestinal damage.

Celiac Disease Treatment

The most widely prescribed and effective treatment for celiac disease is the adoption of a gluten-free diet. Typically, clinical improvement is observed within weeks, and physiological improvement of intestinal tissues occurs within 1–2 years (Fig. 6.10). Early diagnosis and treatment in pediatric celiac disease is especially

A.   **B.**

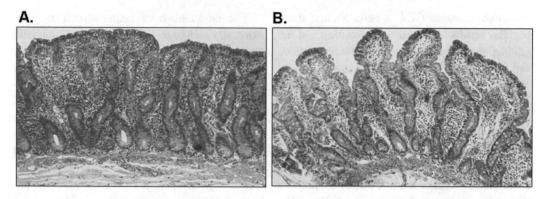

Fig. 6.10 Normalization of biopsy-proven changes in celiac disease after implementation of a gluten-free diet. (**a**) Biopsy-proven changes of untreated celiac disease. The villi are "flattened" and rudimentary, while the crypts are expanded and hyperplastic with increased numbers of epithelial cells and an increased mitotic index. The cellularity of the lamina propria is enhanced, and there is an increased number of plasma cells and lymphocytes. (**b**) Following implementation of a gluten-free diet, the villi are elongated, crypts are shortened, and the cellularity of the lamina propria is much reduced. Credit: Adapted from Hugh J. Freeman. *Adult Celiac Disease and Its Malignant Complications.* Gut and Liver, Vol. 3, No. 4, December 2009, pp. 237–246. CCLI attribution

beneficial, preventing the induction of many secondary conditions. Pharmacologic treatment options, especially in patients with refractory celiac disease, are limited and include immunosuppressants such as corticosteroids, azathioprine, and cyclosporine. Since the benefits derived from these are transient, a number of other pharmacologic agents are currently being evaluated. These investigational treatments include gluten degrading enzymes and the zonulin inhibitory octapeptide larazotide. Zonulin is a protein involved in the degradation of epithelial tight junctions. Inhibiting its function with larazotide has been found to be particularly promising, decreasing symptom scores and autoantibody levels during clinical trials. Other immunotherapeutic options being evaluated include the use of anti-IL-15 antibodies to induce apoptosis of IELs and tolerogenic vaccines containing gluten peptides.

Food Allergies

Food allergies are adverse health effects arising from an immune response that occurs reproducibly on exposure to a given food. The incidence of food allergy has been dramatically increasing throughout the developed world and constitutes a substantial public health burden in affected nations. It is estimated that approximately 3–6% of the population in the United States has a food allergy. The induction of food allergy occurs due to a breakdown of oral tolerance, resulting in immune sensitization to offending allergens and the activation of mast cells, T_H2 cells, and eosinophils. The most common allergen-containing foods include milk, egg, peanuts, wheat, soy and fish. In sensitized individuals, exposure to these foods can manifest in a range of clinical symptoms that involve the gastrointestinal tract, skin, lungs, and in severe cases, anaphylactic shock. Skin reactions include urticaria and angioedema manifesting as itching and hives, while gastrointestinal symptoms include intestinal spasms, vomiting, and diarrhea. Systemic anaphylaxis, resulting from allergen absorption into the bloodstream and systemic mast cell and basophil activation, affects several organ systems including the skin, GI, lung, and cardiovascular systems. This leads to a severe drop in blood pressure and is accompanied by tightening of the throat and difficulty breathing and swallowing, requiring immediate treatment with injected adrenaline or epinephrine.

Currently, food allergies can only be managed through allergen avoidance or treating the symptoms. While most allergies are identified during childhood, 15% are first diagnosed in adults. Many patients with food allergy naturally outgrow them over time; however, this depends on the causative allergen. For example, patients frequently outgrow hen and cow milk allergies, while peanut and tree nut allergies typically persist for life.

The development of food allergy has been linked to genetic susceptibilities as well as extrinsic factors that have the potential to modulate the immune response. Genetic susceptibility includes polymorphisms in a number of immune-related genes including IgE, the TCR, FoxP3, IL-4, IL-10, and IL-13. Extrinsic factors tend to be multifactorial, including early exposure to allergens and infections, microbial diversity within the GI tract, predisposing conditions including eczema due to cutaneous sensitization to food allergens, the type of diet, and vitamin D deficiency. A number of hypotheses have been postulated to explain how environmental factors regulate susceptibility to food allergies, including the dual-allergen hypothesis, the hygiene hypothesis, and the vitamin D hypothesis.

Mechanisms of Food Allergy

Although the term 'food allergy' is widely used among the public to refer to adverse reactions to food, the development of food allergy is a consequence of the breakdown of immunological tolerance to specific ingested antigens. A failure in oral tolerance is defined as the state of active systemic unresponsiveness to ingested food antigens. Adverse reactions not due to immune responses are referred to as food intolerances. The breakdown of tolerance can result in the development of IgE-mediated reactions to the ingested food, as well as non-IgE-mediated reactions such as eosinophilic esophagitis, allergic proctocolitis, and food-protein induced enterocolitis. Mixed reactions involving both IgE-dependent and IgE-independent mechanisms may be present during some types of food allergies.

Acute episodes of food allergy manifest as immediate hypersensitivity reactions that are triggered by the IgE-mediated activation of mast cells and basophils in target tissues (Fig. 6.11).

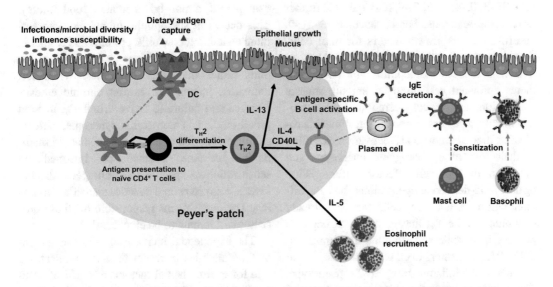

Fig. 6.11 Immune cell activation during food allergies. Susceptibility to food allergies is influenced by microorganisms in the GI tract. DCs that acquire dietary antigens and become activated can induce the differentiation of allergen-specific CD4 T cells into T_H2 cells that produce cytokines in the presence of the allergen. B cells activated under these conditions produce antigen-specific IgE antibodies that sensitize mast cells and basophils. Re-exposure to the allergen will result in their degranulation and subsequent tissue damage. IL-13 produced by T_H2 cells induces intestinal epithelial cell growth and mucus production, while IL-5 recruits eosinophils to the GI tract. Thus, T_H2 cells have a pathogenic role in the context of food allergies

Exposure to food allergens in sensitized patients results in the crosslinking of specific IgE molecules on mast cells and basophils, leading to their degranulation and release of preformed mediators including histamine, tryptase, and chymase, triggering vasodilation and smooth muscle contractions in the GI tract. Subsequently, mast cells and basophils produce substances (leukotrienes, prostaglandins, platelet activating factor (PAF)) that potentiate vasodilation, vascular permeability, smooth muscle contraction, mucus production and the activation of nociceptive nerves involved in pruritis. Cytokines secreted by these cells (IL-4, IL-5, IL-13) further propagate the inflammatory reaction, promoting the proliferation and survival of T_H2 cells and eosinophils. Specific roles for T_H2 cells, mast cells, basophils, and eosinophils in allergic responses are described in Chap. 4. The ensuing myriad of physiological reactions includes angioedema, oral pruritis, intestinal spasms, vomiting and diarrhea. These reactions are mediated by mast cell and eosinophil activation upon the recognition of allergens by IgE antibodies on sensitized cells. The cytokines produced by activated T_H2 cells (IL-3, IL-4, IL-5, IL-9, IL-10, IL-13) further drive these reactions. For instance, IL-3, IL-9, and IL-10 act as growth factors for mast cells, IL-4 promotes T cell survival and B cell activation, IL-5 induces eosinophilia, and IL-13 promotes epithelial cell turnover, smooth muscle contraction, and mucus secretion. Lastly, proinflammatory factors from the intestinal microbiota or diet can induce DC activation, resulting in their loss of a tolerogenic phenotype and induction of T_H2 cell effector differentiation against food-derived antigens rather than T_{reg} differentiation. In addition, cells that are already committed to the T_{reg} lineage cells can begin to produce IL-4 while still retaining the expression of FoxP3. Altogether, T cell responses are shifted towards an inflammatory T_H2 phenotype. Through these mechanisms, interactions between environmental, cellular and physiological processes drive acute inflammatory responses to ingested food antigens.

In contrast to acute episodes of food allergy, chronic allergic processes are responsible for the pathology of proctocolitis, food-protein induced enterocolitis, and eosinophilic esophagitis. While allergen-specific IgE is produced during these conditions, the pathological responses are primarily mediated by T cells. Eosinophilic esophagitis in response to food allergens is a chronic inflammatory condition characterized by epithelial cell hyperplasia. Patients typically present with gradual onset of gastro-esophageal reflux, dysphagia (difficulty swallowing), eosinophilic infiltrates in the esophagus, and esophageal strictures (narrowing of the esophagus). Patients have difficulty eating and express an aversion to various types of foods. The disease is driven by T_H2 cells producing IL-4, IL-5, IL-13, and chemokines promoting the inflammatory reaction. In particular, IL-5 promotes the proliferation and survival of eosinophils, which are responsible for the tissue damage and fibrosis associated with the disease. Epithelial cell-derived cytokines such as TSLP and IL-33 also play a role, promoting sensitization to various food allergens and T_H2 responses. In addition to eosinophils and T cells, mast cells have been observed in the esophagus of these patients. Allergic proctocolitis is another example of a non-IgE-mediated food allergy. This occurs in susceptible infants fed with formula containing cow milk proteins and results in rectal bleeding that is driven by mucosal eosinophils rather than IgE antibodies. When left untreated, infants can exhibit chronic emesis, diarrhea and failure to thrive. Similarly, in food protein-induced enterocolitis syndrome, patients exhibit eosinophil and T_H2 cell-mediated inflammation in the absence of IgE-mediated sensitization to specific food allergens, driving severe gastrointestinal reactions such as vomiting. The mechanisms responsible for these processes still remain to be elucidated.

The exponential increase in the development of food allergies in recent decades implicates a role for environmental factors in sensitization to food allergens. Such factors include commensal microbes and their metabolites, adjuvants in foods including peanuts, and other dietary components. The role of microbial factors has been extensively studied. While germ-free mice are prone to developing food allergies, certain species including

Clostridium confer protection against allergen sensitization. In susceptible individuals, the intestinal microbiota present at birth has been linked to food allergies. Factors that may regulate the diversity of microbial species include the route of birth delivery (vaginal or caesarian section), infections, diet, and antibiotics. Short chain fatty acids produced by intestinal microorganisms activate certain G-protein coupled receptors (GPCRs) on epithelial cells, mast cells and T cells, inducing their differentiation into T_{regs}. The mas-related G-protein-coupled receptor member X2 is a recently described GPCR on mast cells and binds to peptides and quinolone compounds. Activation of this receptor induces mast cell degranulation in the absence of IgE, implicating its potential role in food allergies.

Three hypotheses have been proposed to account for the factors contributing to food allergies, termed the dual-allergen hypothesis, vitamin D hypothesis, and hygiene hypothesis. Variables contributing to these hypotheses are summarized as the '5Ds'- dry skin, diet, dogs, dribble, and vitamin D.

The dual-allergen hypothesis (dry skin, diet) postulates that allergic sensitization to food allergens occurs in early life *via* disrupted skin barrier function, resulting in increased skin permeability to food antigens. In this way, transdermal sensitization leads to food allergies in the absence of oral consumption. This hypothesis is supported by multiple lines of evidence in both animal and human studies, including patients with eczema (atopic dermatitis). Mutations in skin barrier proteins such as filaggrin have been linked to both atopic dermatitis and food allergy. Mouse studies have shown that epicutaneous sensitization with allergens stimulates epithelial cells to secrete TSLP and IL-33, leading to the activation of T cells and eosinophils which drive the allergic reaction (described in Chap. 5). Additionally, the Learning Early About Peanut Allergy (LEAP) study was designed to induce oral tolerance in infants in order to prevent the development of peanut allergies. Data from this randomized controlled trial suggested that early introduction of peanuts lowers the risk of developing an allergy to this food later in life. This was in contrast to

guidelines issued in 2000 by the American Academy of Pediatrics and other organizations world-wide, which recommended to delay the introduction of solid allergenic foods to children. Several other trials, including the Enquiring About Tolerance (EAT) study, have since examined the effects of early introduction of other allergens including hen egg protein. Although these trials have yielded mixed results, most data supports early exposure to allergenic foods. Currently, North American guidelines recommend early peanut consumption in infants with atopic dermatitis in order to lower the risk of developing peanut allergies.

The Hygiene Hypothesis (dogs, dribble) postulates that allergies can result from a lack of exposure to infections or other microorganisms during early childhood. The tenets of the Hygiene Hypothesis are described in detail in Chap. 4. It is believed that the absence of infectious or other microorganisms during early childhood results in individuals having T cells that are biased towards differentiating into T_H2 cells following their activation during allergic sensitization. On the other hand, exposure to helminth worms can help to confer protection against IgE-mediated allergies involving mast cells and eosinophils. As described above, recent evidence suggests the microbiome can help to shape immune responses during allergies. Other factors associated with increased microbial exposure, such as living on a farm, attending daycare, having pets, vaginal delivery during birth, and the presence of older siblings, have been found to be protective.

Lastly, a number of studies suggest a role for vitamin D deficiency in the development of allergic responses, with some of these showing higher rates of food allergies in individuals living further from the equator compared to those living closer. Similarly, higher rates of food allergies are observed in individuals born during the Fall or Winter in contrast to those born during the Spring or Summer. These studies suggest that a lack of vitamin D by lieu of equatorial distance and/or seasonal birth may predispose to the development of food allergy. More direct evidence comes from the Australian HealthNuts study, which demonstrated a correlation between low levels of vitamin D in infants and the risk of developing food allergies. A number of mechanisms have been postulated to account for the role of vitamin D in preventing food allergies. Vitamin D is known to support intestinal T_{reg} responses and may also be important for the differentiation of effector T cell subsets. Further studies are needed to more fully understand its beneficial effects.

Did You Know: *A Recently Discovered Allergy Makes Some People Allergic to Steak?*

Commentary by Kaitlin Armstrong

Mammalian-meat allergy is an allergic reaction to meat characterized by hives and anaphylaxis hours after consuming the allergen. Unlike common food allergies (e.g. peanuts), mammalian-meat allergy is triggered by a lone star tick bite and can break an established tolerance—causing people to develop this allergy after eating meat their entire lives without mishap. This phenomenon was first observed in the 1990s but it wasn't until 2009 that the tick bite was identified as the sensitizing agent, shedding some light on the immunological mechanism of this novel allergy. The lone star tick bite functions similarly to a vaccine containing an antigen and an adjuvant. While the disaccharide galactose-alpha-1,3-galactose (alpha-gal) serves as the antigen, an enzyme in the mouth of the tick (dipeptidyl-peptidase) is the adjuvant, increasing the magnitude of immune responses against alpha-gal. The alpha-gal antigen is not present in the human body but is in the cell membranes of non-primate mammals, resulting in our immune system identifying it as a foreign antigen upon meat consumption. The reason why humans lost the enzyme required for producing this sugar is uncertain; however, it may be linked to protection against malaria infections. The malaria virus is coated in alpha-gal residues, resulting in a survival advantage for humans recognizing alpha-gal as a non-self antigen.

One of the most intriguing questions related to the rise in mammalian-meat allergy is why people have started developing this allergic response in the past 30 years even though ticks have been around for centuries. This phenomenon has been observed in the United States, Australia, Europe and elsewhere. One of the proposed reasons for this reaction is the idea that changes in the diet and antibiotic use have altered the human gut microbiome in such a way that increases susceptibility to developing allergic reactions against alpha-gal. Humans normally have circulating antibodies that recognize alpha-gal due to its production by intestinal microbiota. These naturally occurring antibodies are IgG or IgM, which do not produce allergic responses. Tick-derived compounds along with changes in the human microbiome may help to increase the likelihood of IgE class switching. Overall, the surge in cases of mammalian-meat allergy is an example of how environmental factors help to shape susceptibility to allergies.

Food Allergy Treatment

Strict avoidance of allergenic foods is currently the only realistic option for patients with food allergy. Patients at risk of developing severe reactions such as anaphylaxis must carry epinephrine auto-injectors for immediate self-treatment. Elimination diets, which consist of avoiding specific foods based on the patient's clinical history, are often utilized to identify the offending allergen. While mild allergic reactions can be controlled by over-the-counter drugs such as anti-histamines, anaphylactic shock requires the administration of epinephrine. The effects of epinephrine are rapid, reversing mast cell-mediated responses in various target tissues by binding β1 and β2- adrenergic receptors. This results in the restoration of bronchodilation, repair of tight junctions between epithelial cells, increases in systolic blood pressure, and the enhancement of myocardial function. Inhaled salbutamol and corticosteroids may be used as add-on medications during adrenaline therapy.

Although allergen avoidance is currently the only option available for preventing food allergies, a number of immunotherapeutic options are currently being examined. This includes oral allergen immunotherapy where patients are exposed to increasing concentrations of the allergen until a state of tolerance is achieved. Sublingual therapy and epicutaneous therapy, where patients are epicutaneously treated with allergens such as peanuts for several weeks, are also under investigation. Finally, the effects of biologics such as omalizumab, cytokine blockers or cytokine receptor blockers are also being examined.

From Bench to Bedside: Interferon-α and Hepatitis C

In 1957, two British scientists, Alick Isaacs and Jean Lindenmann, published a seminal paper in the Proceedings of the Royal Society (Biological Sciences). They had been focused for several years on understanding how inactivated influenza virus can interfere with the growth of live influenza viruses in the chorioallantoic membranes of chick embryos. Years of research by several investigators had established that the interference activity could not be attributed to the dose of the virus used, type of influenza strain, method of viral inactivation, time interval between inoculations, or the blockage of known cell surface receptors. To investigate this more fully, the British scientists suspended chick embryo membranes in buffered salt solution, allowing them to observe and manipulate the cells and fluid separately outside of the intact chick embryo. The scientists surprisingly discovered that some of the interference activity remained in the fluid despite complete uptake of the virus by cells. They termed the interference factor "interferon" and proceeded to establish the kinetics of its release through an elegant set of experiments.

In short course, interferons were found to be produced by many cells and tissues in diverse animals and its initial classification was based on the type of cell that produced it—leukocyte, fibroblast, or lymphoblastoid cells. Then in the 1960s, Finnish scientist Kari Cantell succeeded in extracting large scale batches of interferon-α (IFN-α) from human leukocytes, which could be partially purified and used in clinical trials. However, these preparations consisted of crude purified extracts that contained IFN-α at levels of less than 1% of the total extract. Thus, it could not be established whether the effects of the extract in clinical trials were due to the interferons present or other contaminating proteins in the extract. Purification of interferons would not occur for at least another two decades until 1978, with the advent of reverse-phase and normal-phase high performance liquid chromatography. In the next few years, the laboratories of Alan Waldmann and Sidney Pestka spent considerable time and effort characterizing the chemical and immunological properties of IFN-α and interferon-β (IFN-β). They developed several techniques and cytopathic assays that confirmed the anti-viral effects of interferon and revealed the existence of a number of different interferons, establishing that IFN-α belonged to a family of interferon proteins. Simultaneously, Wellcome Pharmaceuticals in the UK developed novel ways of extracting large quantities of interferon from lymphoblastoid cell cultures for use in clinical trials as an anti-cancer agent. Finally, in 1980, the biotechnology company Genentech, in collaboration with Hoffman-LaRoche, announced the production of large-scale quantities of leukocyte and fibroblast interferon for use in clinical trials using recombinant DNA technology. Subsequently, they succeeded in cloning immune interferon or type II interferon (IFN-γ) using bacterial, yeast, and mammalian cell culture.

Today, at least seven interferon species are known to exist in humans. Six of these belong to the Type I interferon family, including IFN-α and IFN-β. Only IFN-γ is classified as a Type II interferon. Following their discovery, many of the cell surface receptors for interferons were also discovered, as well as the downstream JAK-STAT signaling pathway.

It is now known that the type I interferons have a breadth of biological activities, including the inhibitory anti-viral effects that were first demonstrated by Isaacs and Lindenmann. Other biological activities include the stimulation of cytotoxic T cells and natural killer cells, increased expression of tumor-associated antigens and MHC I, induction of pro-apoptotic genes (TRAIL, caspases), repression of anti-apoptotic genes (BCL2), and the inhibition of angiogenesis. The Food and Drug Administration (FDA) has approved several type I interferon formulations for a number of diseases and cancer. The first approval was for IFN-α2a and IFN-α2b (allelic versions of IFN-α2) in 1986 for the treatment of hairy cell leukemia. Ten years later, IFN-β1a and IFN-β1b were approved for treating relapsing-remitting multiple sclerosis. Additional diseases that IFN-α is approved for include malignant melanoma, follicular lymphoma, genital warts, AIDS-related Kaposi sarcoma, and chronic hepatitis B and C. IFN-γ is approved for chronic granulomatous disease and malignant osteopetrosis.

Hepatitis C virus (HCV) is an insidious chronic infection of the liver that has become a global public health concern and affects 2.7–4.0 million people in the United States. Initial infection with HCV is asymptomatic and 15–45% of patients are able to eliminate it. In the majority of infected patients, HCV infection becomes chronic, contributing to increasing rates of cirrhosis, hepatocellular carcinoma, and liver transplantations. HCV is a small RNA virus belonging to the family *Flaviviridae*. Seven genotypes are known to exist, along with 52 subtypes. Of these, genotype 1 is responsible for 70% of HCV infections in the U.S. Unfortunately, it is also the genotype that is most insensitive to treatment with IFN-α. Following HCV infections, type I interferons turn on a number of interferon-stimulated genes, leading to the inhibition of viral replication, activation of NK cells and increased viral resistance. HCV succeeds at establishing chronic infections by expressing NS3/4A, a non-structural serine protease that suppresses interferon signaling. Due to the high replication rates of HCV and lack of proofreading mechanisms for its viral RNA-dependent RNA polymerase (NS5B protein), the virus is able to mutate its antigens and escape the immune response, resulting in patients being infected with several quasi-species.

In the early 2000s, pegylated IFN-α was found to have a significantly increased half-life compared to recombinant IFN-α, extending its anti-viral activity. The purine analog ribavirin was also used to inhibit the replication of flaviviruses including HCV. The combination of ribavirin and pegylated IFN-α was successful at maintaining a sustained anti-viral response, improving survival, and lowering the risk of hepatocellular carcinoma in 75% of non-genotype 1-affected patients and 50% of genotype 1-infected patients. However, the enhanced half-life of IFN-α also contributed to serious side effects including fatigue, myalgia, fevers, and other symptoms associated with acute viral infections.

A number of HCV medications are currently available including inhibitors of the NS5A, NS5B, and NS3/4A proteins. These have substantially shortened the course of HCV therapy and resulted in 'cures' for many patients without the use of recombinant IFN-α and ribavirin. Although the continued need for IFN-α therapy during HCV infections has been questioned, studying the relationship between this highly subversive virus and IFN-α enabled us to appreciate the role of type I interferons in protecting against viruses.

Summary

The mucosal immune system of the GI tract plays a pivotal role in defending us from infectious pathogens and maintaining tolerance to ingested food and beneficial commensal bacteria. Abrogation of these tolerogenic mechanisms due to genetic, environmental, or immunologic factors can lead to abnormal proinflammatory immune responses that result in disease. These include inflammatory bowel diseases such as UC and CD, Celiac Disease, and food allergies. The goal of current research is to better understand the immune mechanisms involved in the pathogenesis of these diseases with the hope of developing novel therapeutic approaches for reversing inflammation. Approaches such as fecal microbial transfer or immunosuppressive cytokines have the potential to modulate the immune system by inducing regulatory T cells and suppressing the activation and proliferation of effector T cells.

Case Studies and Practice Questions

Provided by Charles Babcock, Pharm.D.

Case Study 1

Ethan Boyce is a 34 year-old male who was recently seen at a local urgent care clinic for a flare-up of his IBD. He stated that he has been suffering from IBD for several years, but is not sure if he has UC or CD. He has been taking two brown capsules called Delzicol® several times a day. However, during the last week he has had several bouts of diarrhea each day which has become unbearable. There does not appear to be visible blood in his stool. He states that he has not been able to eat much over the last few weeks due to intense pain every time he eats. Because of this, he has lost 6 lb over the last few weeks. Ethan does not have any family members with a history of IBD. He reports smoking about a pack a day for the last 10 years and has been taking Advil® liquid gels during the last few weeks for the pain in his stomach. He also states that he noticed some red scaly patches on his arms that he thinks started earlier this week. He can't think of any other changes in his diet or lifestyle that could have caused the sudden diarrhea and stomach pains.

1. Based on Ethan's prior history and current symptoms, which type of IBD is he most likely suffering from?
2. Which of Ethan's current medications medication is likely to cause a flare-up of his IBD?
3. A subsequent colonoscopy later revealed the presence of disease in several areas of the intestines. This included the small intestine, the ileocecal region, and the colon. These areas were interspersed by sections that otherwise appeared to be normal. What type of IBD is the colonoscopy indicative of?
4. The physician prescribes a corticosteroid product intended to reduce the inflammation in Ethan's intestines. Which of the following products is the best choice for Ethan?
   (a) Hydrocortisone enema
   (b) Hydrocortisone suppositories
   (c) Budesonide capsules
   (d) Budesonide rectal foam

5. Since the mesalamine that Ethan has been taking has not been extremely effective, the GI doctor would also like to initiate changes in his therapy. Which of the following drugs represent some therapeutic options for Ethan? Select all that apply.
   (a) Daily prednisone
   (b) Methotrexate
   (c) Adalimumab
   (d) Ustekinumab

Case Study 2

Brenda Rothchild is a 27 year-old female who presents to your clinic with severe abdominal cramping and diarrhea. She states that the pain appears to intensify when she has a bowel movement, which she has had a lot of lately. She reports 8–10 bowel movements in the last 2 days despite taking over-the-counter Imodium® and Motrin®. When asked, she mentions that her most recent stools have had some bright red material, which she thought might be blood. Her only other current complaint is the aphthous ulcer in her mouth that recently flared up. She does not have a family history of any gastrointestinal problems other than her mother having been treated for heartburn, and she has never smoked. A bowel perforation x-ray did not show a perforated colon.

6. Based on Brenda's presentation, can you determine the type of IBD she may have?
7. The results of a colonoscopy revealed continual inflammation and hemorrhage limited to the colon and rectum. Inflammation was not found in any other part of the gastrointestinal tract. A biopsy was taken and sent to the lab for pathological analysis. Based on the results from the colonoscopy, is it possible to determine the type of IBD that Brenda has?
8. The pathology report reveals the presence of numerous crypt abscesses without aphthoid ulcers. Does this determine the type of IBD Brenda has?
9. Further analysis of the pathology report revealed a depletion of goblet cells. However, no signs of mesenteric lymph node involvement, fistulas, or non-caseating granulomas were observed. Based on this information, is it possible to determine the type of IBD Brenda has?
10. Why did Brenda have aphthous ulcers in her mouth?
11. What is a good first line medication class to start Brenda on to induce remission?
12. What other class of drugs may be added to the treatment regimen to enhance the onset of remission and reduce flareups? Hint: This drug class should not be used long-term and can be given either orally or systemically.
13. If Brenda continues to have flareups after beginning treatment, what are some other types of drugs that could be considered?
14. Brenda has heard that some IBD drugs can cause a severe viral infection of the brain. She wants to avoid these drugs at all costs. What is the drug class and the drugs that Brenda wishes to avoid?

Suggested Reading

Ahnfelt-Rønne I, et al. Clinical evidence supporting the radical scavenger mechanism of 5-aminosalicylic acid. Gastroenterology. 1990;98:1162–9.

Blander JM, Longman RS, Iliev ID, Sonnenberg GF, Artis D. Regulation of inflammation by microbiota interactions with the host. Nat Immunol. 2017;18:851–60.

Boyce JA, et al. Guidelines for the diagnosis and management of food allergy in the United States: summary of the NIAID-sponsored expert panel report. J Allergy Clin Immunol. 2010;126:1105–18.

Bramuzzo M, Ventura A, Martelossi S, Lazzerini M. Thalidomide for inflammatory bowel disease. Medicine. 2016;95:e4239.

Bryce PJ. Balancing tolerance or allergy to food proteins. Trends Immunol. 2016;37:659–67.

Burks AW, Sampson HA, Plaut M, Lack G, Akdis CA. Treatment for food allergy. J Allergy Clin Immunol. 2018;141:1–9.

Carter MJ. Guidelines for the management of inflammatory bowel disease in adults. Gut. 2004;53:v1–v16.

Chang C, Lin H. Dysbiosis in gastrointestinal disorders. Best Pract Res Clin Gastroenterol. 2016;30:3–15.

Chehade M, et al. Phenotypic characterization of eosinophilic esophagitis in a large multicenter patient population from the consortium for food allergy research. J Allergy Clin Immunol Pract. 2018;6:1534–44.e1535.

DeRoche TC, Xiao SY, Liu X. Histological evaluation in ulcerative colitis. Gastroenterol Rep (Oxf). 2014;2:178–92.

Desreumaux P, et al. Safety and efficacy of antigen-specific regulatory T-cell therapy for patients with refractory Crohn's disease. Gastroenterology. 2012;143:1207–17.e1202.

Dotan I. New serologic markers for inflammatory bowel disease diagnosis. Dig Dis. 2010;28:418–23.

Du Toit G, et al. Randomized trial of peanut consumption in infants at risk for peanut allergy. N Engl J Med. 2015;372:803–13.

Du Toit G, et al. Food allergy: update on prevention and tolerance. J Allergy Clin Immunol. 2018;141:30–40.

Feagan BG, et al. Vedolizumab as induction and maintenance therapy for ulcerative colitis. N Engl J Med. 2013;369:699–710.

Fernández-Ramos AA, et al. 6-mercaptopurine promotes energetic failure in proliferating T cells. Oncotarget. 2017;8:43048–60.

Freeman HJ. Adult celiac disease and its malignant complications. Gut Liver. 2009;3:237–46.

Friedman RM, Contente S. Treatment of hepatitis C infections with interferon: a historical perspective. Hepat Res Treat. 2010;2010:323926.

Fuss IJ, Neurath MF, Boirivant M, Fiocchi C, Strober W. Disparate CD4+ lamina propria (LP) lymphokine secretion profiles in inflammatory bowel disease. Shock. 1997;7:130.

Gerner RR, Moschen AR, Tilg H. Targeting T and B lymphocytes in inflammatory bowel diseases: lessons from clinical trials. Dig Dis. 2013;31:328–35.

Gupta RS, et al. Hygiene factors associated with childhood food allergy and asthma. Allergy Asthma Proc. 2016;37:140–6.

Heim MH. Interferons and hepatitis C virus. Swiss Med Wkly. 2012;142:w13586.

Hendrickson BA, Gokhale R, Cho JH. Clinical aspects and pathophysiology of inflammatory bowel disease. Clin Microbiol Rev. 2002;15:79–94.

Hugot J-P, et al. Association of NOD2 leucine-rich repeat variants with susceptibility to Crohn's disease. Nature. 2001;411:599–603.

Isaacs A, Lindenmann J. Pillars article: virus interference. I. The interferon. Proc R Soc Lond B Biol Sci. 1957;147:258–67. J Immunol. 2015;195:1911–20.

Jabri B, Abadie V. IL-15 functions as a danger signal to regulate tissue-resident T cells and tissue destruction. Nat Rev Immunol. 2015;15:771–83.

Joyce MA, Tyrrell DL. The cell biology of hepatitis C virus. Microbes Infect. 2010;12:263–71.

Kaistha A, Levine J. Inflammatory bowel disease: the classic gastrointestinal autoimmune disease. Curr Probl Pediatr Adolesc Health Care. 2014;44:328–34.

Kalliolias GD, Ivashkiv LB. TNF biology, pathogenic mechanisms and emerging therapeutic strategies. Nat Rev Rheumatol. 2015;12:49–62.

Kamdar TA, et al. Prevalence and characteristics of adult-onset food allergy. J Allergy Clin Immunol Pract. 2015;3:114–5.e111.

Kaukinen K, Maki M. Coeliac disease in 2013: new insights in dietary-gluten-induced autoimmunity. Nat Rev Gastroenterol Hepatol. 2014;11:80–2.

Kaukinen K, Lindfors K, Maki M. Advances in the treatment of coeliac disease: an immunopathogenic perspective. Nat Rev Gastroenterol Hepatol. 2014;11:36–44.

Kinney SR, et al. Curcumin ingestion inhibits mastocytosis and suppresses intestinal anaphylaxis in a murine model of food allergy. PLoS One. 2015;10:e0132467.

Kobayashi T, et al. IL-10 regulates Il12b expression via histone deacetylation: implications for intestinal macrophage homeostasis. J Immunol. 2012;189:1792–9.

Koplin JJ, Perrett KP, Sampson HA. Diagnosing peanut allergy with fewer oral food challenges. J Allergy Clin Immunol Pract. 2019;7:375–80.

Kühn R, Löhler J, Rennick D, Rajewsky K, Müller W. Interleukin-10-deficient mice develop chronic enterocolitis. Cell. 1993;75:263–74.

Kuja-Halkola R, et al. Heritability of non-HLA genetics in coeliac disease: a population-based study in 107 000 twins. Gut. 2016;65:1793–8.

Larsen EP, Bayat A, Vyberg M. Small duct autoimmune sclerosing cholangitis and Crohn colitis in a 10-year-old child. A case report and review of the literature. Diagn Pathol. 2012;7:100.

Lebwohl B, Green PH, Genta RM. The coeliac stomach: gastritis in patients with coeliac disease. Aliment Pharmacol Ther. 2015;42:180–7.

Lebwohl B, Sanders DS, Green PHR. Coeliac disease. Lancet. 2018;391:70–81.

Leffler DA, Green PH, Fasano A. Extraintestinal manifestations of coeliac disease. Nat Rev Gastroenterol Hepatol. 2015;12:561–71.

Macpherson A, Khoo UY, Forgacs I, Philpott-Howard J, Bjarnason I. Mucosal antibodies in inflammatory bowel disease are directed against intestinal bacteria. Gut. 1996;38:365–75.

Maloy KJ, Powrie F. Intestinal homeostasis and its breakdown in inflammatory bowel disease. Nature. 2011;474:298–306.

Mantis NJ, Rol N, Corthésy B. Secretory IgA's complex roles in immunity and mucosal homeostasis in the gut. Mucosal Immunol. 2011;4:603–11.

Marild K, et al. Antibiotic exposure and the development of coeliac disease: a nationwide case-control study. BMC Gastroenterol. 2013;13:109.

Mbodji K, et al. Adjunct therapy of n-3 fatty acids to 5-ASA ameliorates inflammatory score and decreases NF-κB in rats with TNBS-induced colitis. J Nutr Biochem. 2013;24:700–5.

Millrine D, Kishimoto T. A brighter side to thalidomide: its potential use in immunological disorders. Trends Mol Med. 2017;23:348–61.

Murai M, et al. Interleukin 10 acts on regulatory T cells to maintain expression of the transcription factor Foxp3 and suppressive function in mice with colitis. Nat Immunol. 2009;10:1178–84.

Nagler-Anderson C. Man the barrier! Strategic defences in the intestinal mucosa. Nat Rev Immunol. 2001;1:59–67.

Naon H, Mcgilligan K, Reifen R, Sherman P, Sinatra F, Thomas D. Salivary secretory immunoglobulin A in pediatric patients with chronic idiopathic inflammatory bowel disease. Gastroenterology. 1995;108:A884.

Neurath MF. Current and emerging therapeutic targets for IBD. Nat Rev Gastroenterol Hepatol. 2017;14:269–78.

Nowak-Wegrzyn A, Szajewska H, Lack G. Food allergy and the gut. Nat Rev Gastroenterol Hepatol. 2016;14:241–57.

Oakley RH, Cidlowski JA. The biology of the glucocorticoid receptor: new signaling mechanisms in health and disease. J Allergy Clin Immunol. 2013;132:1033–44.

Odenwald MA, Turner JR. The intestinal epithelial barrier: a therapeutic target? Nat Rev Gastroenterol Hepatol. 2017;14:9–21.

Ogura Y, et al. A frameshift mutation in NOD2 associated with susceptibility to Crohn's disease. Nature. 2001;411:603–6.

O'Hara AM, Shanahan F. The gut flora as a forgotten organ. EMBO Rep. 2006;7:688–93.

Oyoshi MK, Oettgen HC, Chatila TA, Geha RS, Bryce PJ. Food allergy: insights into etiology, prevention, and treatment provided by murine models. J Allergy Clin Immunol. 2014;133:309–17.

Pamer EG. Immune responses to commensal and environmental microbes. Nat Immunol. 2007;8:1173–8.

Parzanese I, et al. Celiac disease: from pathophysiology to treatment. World J Gastrointest Pathophysiol. 2017;8:27–38.

Perkin MR, et al. Randomized trial of introduction of allergenic foods in breast-fed infants. N Engl J Med. 2016;374:1733–43.

Pestka S. The interferons: 50 years after their discovery, there is much more to learn. J Biol Chem. 2007;282:20047–51.

Plevy S, et al. Combined serological, genetic, and inflammatory markers differentiate non-IBD, Crohn's disease, and ulcerative colitis patients. Inflamm Bowel Dis. 2013;19:1139–48.

Polukort SH, et al. IL-10 enhances IgE-mediated mast cell responses and is essential for the development of experimental food allergy in IL-10-deficient mice. J Immunol. 2016;196:4865–76.

Prince BT, et al. Regulatory T-cell populations in children are affected by age and food allergy diagnosis. J Allergy Clin Immunol. 2017;140:1194–6.e1116.

Quinton JF, et al. Anti-Saccharomyces cerevisiae mannan antibodies combined with antineutrophil cytoplasmic autoantibodies in inflammatory bowel disease: prevalence and diagnostic role. Gut. 1998;42:788–91.

Rakoff-Nahoum S, Hao L, Medzhitov R. Role of toll-like receptors in spontaneous commensal-dependent colitis. Immunity. 2006;25:319–29.

Renz H, et al. Food allergy. Nat Rev Dis Primers. 2018;4:17098.

Roulis M, et al. Host and microbiota interactions are critical for development of murine Crohn's-like ileitis. Mucosal Immunol. 2015;9:787–97.

Sampson HA. Food allergy: past, present and future. Allergol Int. 2016;65:363–9.

Sandborn WJ, et al. Vedolizumab as induction and maintenance therapy for Crohn's disease. N Engl J Med. 2013;369:711–21.

See JA, Kaukinen K, Makharia GK, Gibson PR, Murray JA. Practical insights into gluten-free diets. Nat Rev Gastroenterol Hepatol. 2015;12:580–91.

Sicherer SH, Sampson HA. Food allergy: a review and update on epidemiology, pathogenesis, diagnosis, prevention, and management. J Allergy Clin Immunol. 2018;141:41–58.

Smith PK, Masilamani M, Li XM, Sampson HA. The false alarm hypothesis: food allergy is associated with high dietary advanced glycation end-products and proglycating dietary sugars that mimic alarmins. J Allergy Clin Immunol. 2017;139:429–37.

Soler D, et al. The binding specificity and selective antagonism of vedolizumab, an anti-α4β7 integrin therapeutic antibody in development for inflammatory bowel diseases. J Pharmacol Exp Ther. 2009;330:864–75.

Sollid LM, Jabri B. Triggers and drivers of autoimmunity: lessons from coeliac disease. Nat Rev Immunol. 2013;13:294–302.

Steinbach EC, Plevy SE. The role of macrophages and dendritic cells in the initiation of inflammation in IBD. Inflamm Bowel Dis. 2014;20:166–75.

Thaiss CA, Zmora N, Levy M, Elinav E. The microbiome and innate immunity. Nature. 2016;535:65–74.

Tokuhara D, et al. A comprehensive understanding of the gut mucosal immune system in allergic inflammation. Allergol Int. 2019;68:17–25.

Tordesillas L, Berin MC, Sampson HA. Immunology of food allergy. Immunity. 2017;47:32–50.

Tran-Minh M-L, Sousa P, Maillet M, Allez M, Gornet J-M. Hepatic complications induced by immunosuppressants and biologics in inflammatory bowel disease. World J Hepatol. 2017;9:613–26.

van Gils T, Nijeboer P, van Wanrooij RL, Bouma G, Mulder CJ. Mechanisms and management of refractory coeliac disease. Nat Rev Gastroenterol Hepatol. 2015;12:572–9.

Verdu EF, Galipeau HJ, Jabri B. Novel players in coeliac disease pathogenesis: role of the gut microbiota. Nat Rev Gastroenterol Hepatol. 2015;12:497–506.

Vilcek J. Fifty years of interferon research: aiming at a moving target. Immunity. 2006;25:343–8.

Volta U, De Giorgio R. New understanding of gluten sensitivity. Nat Rev Gastroenterol Hepatol. 2012;9:295–9.

Vriezinga SL, Schweizer JJ, Koning F, Mearin ML. Coeliac disease and gluten-related disorders in childhood. Nat Rev Gastroenterol Hepatol. 2015;12:527–36.

Wang J, Sampson HA. Safety and efficacy of epicutaneous immunotherapy for food allergy. Pediatr Allergy Immunol. 2018;29:341–9.

Zhang Y-Z. Inflammatory bowel disease: pathogenesis. World J Gastroenterol. 2014;20:91–9.

Mechanisms of Autoimmunity and Pharmacologic Treatments

7

Doreen E. Szollosi, Kirsten Hokeness, and Mohammed K. Manzoor

Learning Objectives

1. Discuss how autoimmunity develops, including the mechanisms leading to breach of self-tolerance.
2. Describe how a shift in the balance of regulatory T cells and T_H17 cells may contribute to the development of autoimmunity.
3. Explain basic mechanisms of autoimmune diseases including systemic lupus erythematosus, rheumatoid arthritis, multiple sclerosis, and other common autoimmune diseases.
4. Identify immune targets in the pathological mechanisms of the autoimmune diseases described, as well as the pharmacologic therapies which may be used.
5. Discuss the pharmacology of the immunosuppressant drugs used for autoimmunity, including mechanism of action, functional responses, clinical uses, and adverse effects.

Drugs discussed in this chapter

Drug	Classification
Abatacept (Orencia®)	Co-stimulation inhibitor
Adalimumab (Humira®)	Anti-TNF monoclonal antibody
Alemtuzumab (Lemtrada®)	Anti-CD52 monoclonal antibody
Anakinra (Kineret®)	IL-1 receptor antagonist
Atenolol (Tenormin®)	Beta blocker
Azathioprine (Imuran,® Azasan®)	Inhibitor of purine nucleic acid metabolism
Baricitinib (Olumiant®)	JAK/STAT signaling inhibitor
Belimumab (Benlysta®)	Anti-B lymphocyte stimulator (BLyS) monoclonal antibody
Brodalumab (Siliq™)	Anti-IL-17 monoclonal antibody
Canakinumab (Ilaris®)	Anti-IL-1β monoclonal antibody
Certolizumab pegol (Cimzia®)	Anti-TNF antibody fragment
Cyclophosphamide (Cytoxan®)	Alkylating agent
Cyclosporine (Neoral,® Sandimmune®)	Calcineurin inhibitor
Dimethyl fumarate (Tecfidera®)	Anti-inflammatory
Eltrombopag (Promacta®)	Thrombopoietin receptor agonist
Etanercept (Enbrel®)	Anti-TNF fusion protein
Fingolimod (Gilenya®)	Immunomodulator
Fluticasone	Glucocorticoid
Folic acid	Supplement
Glatiramer acetate (Copaxone®)	Immunomodulator
Golimumab (Simponi®)	TNF inhibitor

D. E. Szollosi (✉)
Department of Pharmaceutical Sciences,
School of Pharmacy and Physician Assistant Studies,
University of Saint Joseph, Hartford, CT, USA
e-mail: dszollosi@usj.edu

M. K. Manzoor
School of Pharmacy and Physician Assistant Studies,
University of Saint Joseph, Hartford, CT, USA

K. Hokeness
Bryant University, Smithfield, RI, USA

© Springer Nature Switzerland AG 2020
C. B. Mathias et al., *Pharmacology of Immunotherapeutic Drugs*,
https://doi.org/10.1007/978-3-030-19922-7_7

Drug	Classification
Guselkumab (Tremfya®)	Anti-IL-23 monoclonal antibody
Hydrocortisone	Glucocorticoid
Hydroxychloroquine (Plaquenil®)	Anti-protozoan agent + anti-rheumatic
Infliximab (Remicade®)	Anti-TNF monoclonal antibody
IFN-beta-1a (Avonex,® Rebif®) Pegylated (Plegridy®)	Interferon
IFN-beta-1b (Betaseron®)	Interferon
IVIG (Gammagard®), SCIG (Vivaglobin®)	Intravenous immunoglobulin, subcutaneous immunoglobulin
Ixekizumab (Taltz®)	Anti-IL-17 monoclonal antibody
Leflunomide (Arava®)	Pyrimidine synthesis inhibitor
Levothyroxine	Thyroid hormone
Methimazole (Tapazole®)	Antithyroid agent
Methotrexate (Rheumatrex®)	Purine and pyrimidine synthesis inhibitor
Methylprednisone	Glucocorticoid
Metoprolol (Lopressor,® Toprol-XL®)	Beta blocker
Mitoxantrone (Novantrone®)	Immunomodulator
Mycophenolate mofetil (CellCept®)	Inhibitor of inosine-5′-monophosphate dehydrogenase
Nadolol (Corgard®)	Beta blocker
Natalizumab (Tysabri®)	Anti-integrin monoclonal antibody
Ocrelizumab (Ocrevus®)	Anti-CD20 monoclonal antibody
Prednisone/prednisolone	Glucocorticoid/anti-inflammatory
Propranolol (Inderal®)	Beta blocker
Propylthiouracil	Antithyroid agent
Pyridostigmine	Acetylcholinesterase inhibitor
Rilonacept (Arcalyst®)	IL-1 antagonist
Rituximab (Rituxan®)	Anti-CD20 monoclonal antibody
Romiplostim (Nplate®)	Thrombopoietin receptor agonist
Sarilumab (Kevzara®)	Anti-IL-6 receptor monoclonal antibody
Secukinumab (Cosentyx®)	Anti-IL-17A monoclonal antibody

Drug	Classification
Siltuximab (Sylvant®)	Anti-IL-6 monoclonal antibody
Sulfasalazine (Azulfidine,® Sulfazine®)	5-Aminosalicylic acid derivative
Tacrolimus (Prograf,® Protopic®)	Calcineurin inhibitor
Teriflunomide (Aubagio®)	Immunomodulator
Tildrakizumab (Ilumya®)	Anti-IL-23 monoclonal antibody
Tocilizumab (Actemra®)	Anti-IL-6 receptor monoclonal antibody
Tofacitinib (Xeljanz®)	JAK/STAT signaling inhibitor
Ustekinumab (Stelara®)	Anti-IL-12/23 monoclonal antibody
Vedolizumab (Entyvio®)	Anti-integrin monoclonal antibody

Introduction

The term horror autotoxicus, or the horror of self-toxicity, was a term coined by the German immunologist Paul Ehrlich to describe the body's opposition to self-destruction by the immune system. Autoimmune disease is thought to affect more than 5% of the world's population, representing a significant healthcare burden. Simply put, autoimmunity describes an inappropriate immune response to self-antigens (also called **autoantigens**), resulting in inflammation and subsequent tissue damage. This destructive attack by the immune system can be organ-specific or systemic. Examples of organ-specific autoantigens include β cells of the pancreas (Type I diabetes) or acetylcholine receptors (Myasthenia gravis). An example of a systemic disease is systemic lupus erythematosus in which autoantibodies are created against various autoantigens including double-stranded DNA and nuclear proteins. Additional autoimmune diseases of organ-specific or systemic nature are described in Tables 7.1 and 7.2, respectively. In the sections below, we will consider the immunologic mechanisms underlying autoimmunity, discuss commonly utilized drugs in its treatment, and examine the immunopathogenesis and treatment of specific autoimmune diseases.

Table 7.1 Organ-specific autoimmune diseases

Organ/tissue	Disease	Mechanism/autoantigen
Red blood cells	Autoimmune hemolytic anemia	Autoantibodies against red blood cell membrane proteins
Platelets	Idiopathic thrombocytopenia purpura	Autoantibodies against platelet integrin $\alpha IIb\beta 3$
Thyroid	Hashimoto's	Autoantibodies against thyroid peroxidase and thyroglobulin
Thyroid	Grave's	Autoantibodies against thyroid-stimulating hormone receptor
Pancreas	Type I diabetes	Islet cell autoantibodies
Muscle	Myasthenia gravis	Autoantibodies against acetylcholine receptor
Small intestine	Crohn's	Multifactorial, intestinal influx of immune cells
Kidney	Goodpasture's	Non-collagenous domain of basement membrane collagen type IV
Adrenal cortex	Addison's	Autoantibodies against Cyp450 antigens
Heart	Acute rheumatic fever	Antibodies against streptococcal cell wall antigens cross-react with cardiac muscle

Table 7.2 Systemic autoimmune diseases

Disease	Mechanism/autoantigen
Multiple sclerosis	Myelin basic protein, proteolipid protein
Rheumatoid arthritis	Synovial joint antigen
Systemic lupus erythematosus	Autoantibodies against DNA, histones, ribosomes, ribonucleoprotein
Sjogren's syndrome	Antibodies against Ro52 involved in regulation of inflammation

Autoimmunity Correlates with Hypersensitivity Mechanisms

Autoimmunity is an adaptive response to autoantigens (self-antigens) when self-tolerance mechanisms fail. This is a type of **hypersensitivity**, defined as an inappropriate immune response to an antigen that should not normally trigger inflammation. In many cases, people with hypersensitivity can avoid the allergen/antigen; however, patients with autoimmunity cannot avoid their trigger antigen since it is derived from self-tissues. Mechanisms of autoimmunity can correspond to Hypersensitivities II, III, or IV. Conversely, type I hypersensitivity is mediated by IgE responses to foreign antigens (allergens) rather than autoantigens. Autoimmune type II hypersensitivity reactions are characterized by antibodies directed against cell surfaces or extracellular matrix (ECM). An example of this is autoimmune hemolytic anemia, in which IgG or IgM antibodies bind to markers on the surface of red blood cells and activate the classical complement cascade, resulting in inflammation and lysis of the targeted red blood cells and ultimately leading to anemia. Type III hypersensitivity is mediated by soluble immune complexes deposited in tissue. One of the prototype autoimmune disorders corresponding to Type III hypersensitivity is systemic lupus erythematosus (SLE), in which IgG antibodies target several surface and intracellular self-antigens, resulting in the formation of immune complexes. These immune complexes travel to and lodge themselves in various tissues where they induce inflammation and cause tissue damage. Common sites where immune complexes are deposited in SLE include the skin, kidneys, and joints. Type IV hypersensitivity reactions are mediated by effector T cells rather than antibodies. One example of an autoimmune disorder mediated by T cells is multiple sclerosis (MS), in which the myelin sheath or neurons are attacked by self-reactive CD8 T cells, leading to macrophage activation, tissue damage, and resultant demyelination.

Development of Autoimmunity

The development of autoimmune diseases is still not well understood and thus continues to be a major area of ongoing studies. Several themes which emerge include genetics, environmental factors, as well as failure of immune regulation. In combination, several of these factors regulating susceptibility can tip the scales towards the immune system initiating an attack against self-tissues. Another hypothesis, also known as the Hygiene Hypothesis, is that the development of compounding autoimmune disorders may be linked to the notion that an overly hygienic environment has shifted the focus of immunity away from pathogenic invaders and towards the development of autoimmune and hypersensitivity disorders.

Mechanisms Underlying Autoimmunity

Loss of Tolerance to Self

Humans are capable of generating as many as 10^7 unique lymphocytes that can recognize epitopes of foreign antigens. During immune cell development, checkpoints are in place to essentially "delete" self-reactive lymphocytes. Thus, autoimmunity can be thought of as a failure of immune tolerance. If **self-tolerance** checkpoints are breached, self-reactive T cells or B cells can initiate an abnormal immune response, create inflammation, and cause tissue damage. The role of positive and negative selection in lymphocyte development and repertoire diversity is described in Chap. 3. Some hypotheses for the failure of immune checkpoints during immune cell development include genetic defects such as those described below, which may lead to tissue damaging events that release self-antigens not normally detected in healthy tissue. Prolonged expression of these self-antigens may then contribute to checkpoint failure and loss of self-tolerance.

As mentioned in Chap. 3, the protein **autoimmune regulator (AIRE)** is a transcription factor expressed in the medulla of the thymus and is important for the negative selection (deletion) of early T cells (thymocytes) that bind to certain self-antigens. AIRE allows for a wide variety of organ-specific antigens, such as those found in endocrine glands, to be expressed in the thymus where T cells are developing and undergoing the selection process. Thus, T cells with TCRs that bind strongly to these antigens receive a signal to undergo apoptosis and are eliminated from the repertoire. Loss of function mutations in AIRE are found in a condition called **autoimmune polyendocrinopathy-candidiasis-ectodermal dystrophy (APECED)**, characterized by abnormalities in hair, fingernails, and teeth. APECED tends to be more common in Sardinian, Iranian Jewish, and Finnish patients. Additional manifestations of the disease include chronic Candida infection, hypoparathyroidism, adrenal insufficiency, fulminant autoimmune hepatitis, and squamous cell carcinoma.

The active suppression of autoreactive T cells by **regulatory T cells** is also important for protecting individuals from autoimmune diseases (Fig. 7.1). As discussed in Chap. 3, T_{reg} cells are a subset of CD4 T cells and uniquely utilize the transcription factor Foxp3. Tregs have been identified in the past by assessing the expression of CD4 and CD25 and intracellular FoxP3. Growing evidence suggests that these markers may not exclusively be expressed in T_{regs}, but they are useful for identifying the ratio of T_{reg}:effector TH subsets in experimental studies.

Mutations in the X-linked gene encoding for Foxp3 lead to a severe autoimmune disorder called **immune dysregulation, polyendocrinopathy, enteropathy, and X-linked syndrome (IPEX)**. This disease primarily affects boys due to its X-linked nature and is characterized by enteritis, type I diabetes, eczema, and infections in the first few months of life. Over time other organs such as the thyroid and GI tract are attacked. To cure IPEX and survive, infants need a stem cell transplantation from an HLA-identical sibling without disease in order to provide a source of Foxp3-expressing T_{regs}. The lack of functional regulatory T cells in IPEX leads to higher than normal levels of T_H17 cells, eosinophils, and IgE, signifying that T_{regs} are necessary for limiting pro-inflammatory responses and preventing autoimmunity. In support, experimental models have demonstrated that mice with T cells deficient in Foxp3 exhibit a lymphoproliferative autoimmune syndrome. Additional and potentially lethal lymphoproliferative disorders occur due to loss of function

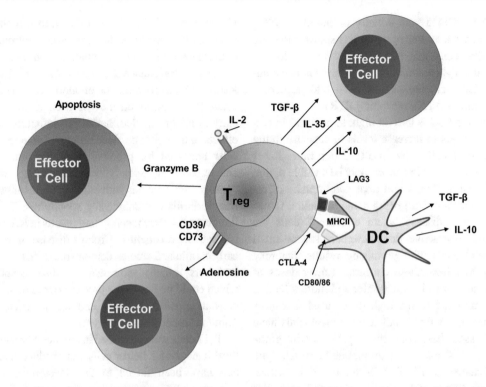

Fig. 7.1 Normal regulatory T cell function. T_{regs} may downregulate the immune system via several mechanisms, including inhibition of APC stimulation, apoptosis of effector T cells, and the release of anti-inflammatory mediators. Expression of CD39 and CD73 on T_{reg} cells contribute to local accumulation of adenosine which may mediate an anti-inflammatory function

mutations in CTLA-4 (which blocks co-stimulation) or the anti-inflammatory cytokine TGF-β.

Some autoimmune diseases are described as "B cell diseases" due to the development of autoantibodies generated by autoreactive B cells. These **autoantibodies** can mimic natural agonists and cause activation of a signal that should not normally occur, act as an antagonist or competitive inhibitor for a natural ligand, prevent a process from occurring, or bind to a fixed target and stimulate inflammation.

Striking a Balance Between T_{reg} and T_H17 Cells

Autoimmune diseases such as systemic lupus erythematosus (SLE), rheumatoid arthritis (RA), and multiple sclerosis (MS), among others, affect a staggering 23.5 million Americans. No cure currently exists to curb the immune system from attacking the body's own tissues, however, three of the five best selling drugs in the U.S. in 2017 (Humira,® Rituxan,® and Enbrel®) are prescribed

for symptomatic relief of autoimmunity.

Basic science research in the last few decades has elucidated the role of two critical immune cells, Tregs and T_H17 cells in regulating the development of autoimmunity. While Tregs are important for the suppression of autoimmune responses, T_H17 cells have been found to be critical for their progression in many autoimmune diseases. In this section, we will examine some of the current strategies being used to either boost Treg responses or inhibit T_H17-mediated autoimmune responses. Many recent research efforts have been focused on boosting immune suppressing T cells (T_{regs}) to help dampen the supercharged immune response that results in tissue damage in autoimmune disorders. Research has shown that patients suffering with autoimmunity tend to have fewer than normal levels of T_{regs}. Commitment of CD4 T cells to the T_{reg} lineage is regulated by expression of the Foxp3 transcription factor, of which continued expression maintains mature T_{regs}. Mutations in Foxp3 result in multi-organ autoimmunity

(IPEX). CD25 was initially proposed as a T_{reg} marker, but newer research has shown there are CD25+ cells that lack suppressive activity. To identify T_{regs}, a combination of markers is recommended, including CTLA4, PD-1, and glucocorticoid induced TNF receptor (GITR).

While IL-2 is used at high, toxic doses in certain cancers to increase levels of cancer-fighting effector T cells, low-dose IL-2 (ten times lower than doses used in cancer) may be a viable option to boost T_{reg} cells and treat autoimmune disorders. Despite there being some hesitation to use IL-2 in a disease where effector T cells are already overactive, there have been several small clinical trials with promising results that may help to relieve these concerns. Lower doses of IL-2 appear to be much safer and more tolerable as compared to the high doses used in cancer treatment. A few small-scale clinical trials have addressed these concerns in patients with graft-versus-host disease, autoimmune hepatitis, Type 1 Diabetes, and SLE. Still, the possibility exists for binding to and activating effector T cells. For this reason, a couple biotech companies have taken up the task of engineering a chemically-modified IL-2 which has a lower affinity for binding to effector T cells. Another therapeutic approach is to exploit the patient's own T_{regs} to suppress inflammation. Towards this, biotech companies are currently developing approaches that isolate T_{regs} from the patient's blood, expand them and expose them to an antigen such as ovalbumin in culture, then infuse them back into the patient. Because ovalbumin is present in the gut, these T_{regs} will migrate naturally to the gut and begin releasing anti-inflammatory mediators, making this approach a potential therapy in Crohn's disease. Another possible therapy is similar to the CAR-T cell approach but would instead be a CAR-T_{reg} therapy which would engineer T_{regs} to target certain areas of inflammation.

While promoting anti-inflammatory T cell functions is a potential therapeutic option, IL-17-producing cells (T_H17 cells) may also pose a novel target in treating autoimmune diseases. New monoclonal antibodies against IL-17 such as secukinumab, brodalumab, and ixekizumab have already shown efficacy in certain disease states like psoriasis. IL-17 has been shown to stimulate inflammatory responses by promoting neutrophil recruitment during chronic inflammation. In addition, IL-17 can induce the expression of CCL20, leading to the recruitment of more T_H17 cells. Thus, IL-17 inhibition may be used therapeutically to inhibit the detrimental pro-inflammatory effects of the cytokine. Secukinumab was specifically approved for psoriasis, psoriatic arthritis, and ankylosing spondylitis. Ixekizumab was approved for psoriasis with ongoing trials for psoriatic arthritis and ankylosing spondylitis. IL-17 inhibition has shown conflicting results in RA and has shown no benefit in Crohn's disease. In fact, early-terminated studies demonstrated that IL-17 inhibitors actually worsened the disease state, which could be due to the protective role of T_H17 cells at mucosal surfaces and maintenance of immune homeostasis in the gut.

T_H17 cells were described in the late 2000s as a third lineage of T helper cells that produce IL-17 and have been linked to the development of asthma, COPD, and even certain cancers. T_H17 cell differentiation is induced by TGF-β and IL-6, with studies showing that blocking TGF-β decreases T_H17 cells in a mouse model of experimental autoimmune encephalomyelitis (EAE). IL-6 supports the induction of T_H17 cells by activating the STAT3 transcription factor. Additionally, the IL-23 receptor is expressed on differentiated T17 cells and has been shown to upregulate TGF-β3 as part of a positive feedback loop to maintain T_H17 cell function. The differentiation of T_H17 cells requires the transcription factor retinoic acid related orphan receptor (RORγt), distinguishing this subset from T_{regs} expressing Foxp3 (Fig. 7.2). The inflammatory/tissue damaging potential of T_H17 cells appears to depend on the cytokine milieu. TGF-β dominant environments may allow T_H17 cells to be more "regulatory" while inflammation including IL-22 and IFN-γ dominant conditions may favor a more "pathogenic" T_H17 cell. Yet another layer of complexity in the behavior of T_H17 cells is the microbiota present in the gut mucosa, as certain bacterial species can support the generation of these tissue-damaging T_H17 cells. Thus, the microbiome may be another therapeutic target for modulating inflammation.

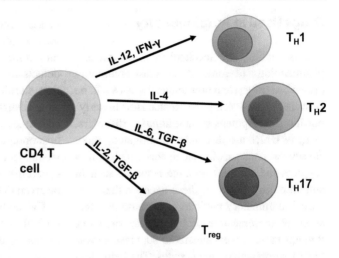

Fig. 7.2 CD4 T cells can differentiate into T_H17 or T_{reg} cells, in addition to effector T_H1 or T_H2. T_H17 cell differentiation is induced by TGF-β and IL-6, while T_{reg} cells are often promoted by IL-2 and TGF-β

Table 7.3 Drugs that inhibit T_H17 function

IL-6 inhibitors	IL-6R inhibitors	IL-23 inhibitors	IL-17 inhibitors	STAT3 inhibitors	RORγt inhibitors
Siltuximab	Tocilizumab	Ustekinumab	Secukinumab	Tofacitinib	VTP-43742[a]
Olokizumab[a]	Sarilumab	Guselkumab	Ixekizumab	Baricitinib	GSK2981278[a]
Clazakizumab[a]		Tildrakizumab	Brodalumab		

[a]Not yet approved

More recently, research has suggested that a disruption in the balance of T_{regs} and T_H17 cells is correlated with development of autoimmune diseases such as RA, psoriatic arthritis, inflammatory bowel disease (IBD) and Crohn's disease, MS, and SLE. Several drugs are already on the market or are in development that inhibit cytokines produced by T_H17 cells or signals needed for their differentiation (Table 7.3).

Maintaining the T_{reg}/T_H17 balance may be possible by affecting their respective transcription factors. After RORγt was discovered as a transcription factor specific for T_H17 cells, research has focused in on this as a potential drug target. Interestingly, the cardiac drug digoxin has been reported to inhibit RORγt's transcriptional activity, inhibiting IL-17 levels and attenuate markers of EAE activity in preclinical studies. Other small molecules that are under investigation target post-translational modifications of RORγt that inhibit its function and are currently in clinical trials for psoriasis.

Targeting Foxp3 may also be a potential method of promoting T_{reg}/T_H17 balance. Gene therapy to increase Foxp3 expression or the transfer of T_{reg}-like cells have suppressed markers of arthritis in a mouse mode. Foxp3 may also be

inadvertently targeted by drugs that are already available. Cytokine inhibitors such as tocilizumab and etanercept have been suggested to increase the Foxp3/RORγt ratio in RA and psoriasis patients, respectively. Adalimumab also appears to promote function of Foxp3+ T_{regs}. B-cell depletion by rituximab may also increase Foxp3 levels in patients with SLE. This may be due to a concurrent increase in TGF-β production.

While autoimmunity appears to result from a shift in the balance of T_{regs} and T_H17 cells towards T_H17 and inflammation, there have been quite a few advances made in identification of possible drugs targets to maintain a proper balance. Since T_H17 cells and their signature cytokines, including IL-17, contribute to host defense on mucosal surfaces, more must be understood about how and why these cells drive a "pathogenic" state of autoimmunity leading to tissue damage in susceptible individuals. While mouse models have shown promise in novel compounds which may help to maintain a T_{reg}/T_H17 balance towards protection, some of these still present safety/toxicity challenges in humans and must undergo more trials to identify possible candidates.

Drugs Used in Autoimmunity

In this section, the mechanism of action and pharmacology of some of the most commonly prescribed drugs for autoimmune diseases will be described. Considering the mechanisms underlying the development of autoimmune disorders, many of which are still under investigation, there are several pharmacological agents which aim to suppress the aberrant immune response seen in autoimmunity. Many of these agents either suppress inflammatory mediators, decrease proliferation of autoreactive lymphocytes, or work through various mechanisms to suppress activation of autoreactive lymphocytes. The individual uses of these drugs will be discussed in detail in the latter sections related to immune mechanisms involved in specific autoimmune diseases.

Glucocorticoids

Glucocorticoids, or corticosteroids, are hormonal drugs with anti-inflammatory properties and generally suppress the functions of immune cells. When glucocorticoids cross the cell membrane they bind to the glucocorticoid receptor (GR) to form a glucocorticoid/GR complex. At this point, the complex binds to activator protein-1 (AP-1), which is one of the mechanisms which inhibits the cellular response to proinflammatory cytokines. Upon activation, the glucocorticoid/GR complex translocates from the cytoplasm to the nucleus where it binds to glucocorticoid response elements and exerts its effects through a variety of mechanisms. This includes the *de novo* synthesis of the glucocorticoid-induced leucine zipper (GILZ), IκB (an NF-κB antagonist) and lipocortin-1. These molecules are responsible for preventing the transcription of pro-inflammatory cytokines (including IL-1, IL-2, TNF-α) and lipid mediators (prostaglandins, leukotrienes). Glucocorticoids have also been shown to degrade mRNA encoding for pro-inflammatory cytokines. In addition, glucocorticoids have been shown to upregulate the transcription of anti-inflammatory mediators. Proposed mechanisms

of glucocorticoid resistance in patients include the abnormal expression of glucocorticoid receptors (GRs), increases in kinase activity, and defects in transcription factor activity. In addition, steroids often come with a long list of possible adverse effects including but not limited to an increased risk for infections caused by immunosuppression, osteoporosis, hyperglycemia, weight gain, fluid retention, iatrogenic Cushing's syndrome and insomnia. Glucocorticoids may be given PO, IV, or injected locally into the joint.

Currently, several glucocorticoids are prescribed for their anti-inflammatory properties. Choice of the agent may depend on the desired dosage form, potency, duration of action, and receptor selectivity. Many glucocorticoids also bind the mineralocorticoid receptor (MR), leading to sodium and fluid retaining effects. Perhaps the most commonly prescribed systemic oral agent is prednisone, whereas hydrocortisone is the most widely used topical agent, and fluticasone is the most popular inhaled corticosteroid.

Cytotoxic Drugs (Antiproliferative Agents)

Methotrexate (MTX, Rheumatrex®)

Methotrexate was first used for rheumatoid arthritis (RA) in 1951, around the same time as glucocorticoids, but it wasn't until the mid-1980s that studies began to show efficacy and superiority over placebo in treating RA. Methotrexate (MTX) is a competitive inhibitor of folate, suppressing the function of dihydrofolate reductase and levels of tetrahydrofolate, a folic acid derivative required for purine and pyrimidine synthesis. In this manner, MTX suppresses the proliferation of activated lymphocytes. Methotrexate may be used in combination with other **disease-modifying anti-rheumatic drugs (DMARDs)**, but care should be taken when administering MTX with other folate-depleting drugs such as trimethoprim-sulfamethoxazole. Taking folic acid supplements along with MTX appears to reduce two of its main side effects: gastrointestinal toxicity and liver enzyme elevation. Adverse effects include leukopenia, increased risk of infection, nausea, fatigue, and fever. Due to this drug being highly teratogenic it should not be given to women who are pregnant. Additionally, because MTX is cleared via the kidneys (80–90% is excreted unchanged in the urine), dose adjustments may need to be made for patients with a decreased **glomerular filtration rate (GFR)**. For treating RA, MTX is usually taken orally once per week, and should not be given more frequently due to its toxicity. If oral MTX is not producing a desired response, a subcutaneous autoinjector may be used.

Leflunomide (Arava®)

Leflunomide is a prodrug inhibitor of pyrimidine synthesis. Following its conversion to the active form teriflunomide, the clonal expansion of autoimmune lymphocytes is inhibited during their cell cycle progression from G1 to S phase. More specifically, leflunomide is thought to inhibit a mitochondrial enzyme that produces ribonucleotide uridine monophosphate (rUMP). By initiating the apoptosis/cell cycle arrest of activated lymphocytes, several of the effector responses contributing to autoimmune inflammation are dampened. Common adverse effects of leflunomide include hypertension, nausea, diarrhea, increased liver enzymes (which should be monitored), skin rash, leukopenia, and teratogenic effects (do not use while pregnant). While some suggest that using a loading dose may achieve a quicker therapeutic effect, higher doses may also increase the likelihood of gastrointestinal side effects in patients.

Azathioprine (Imuran®)

Azathioprine is a prodrug of mercaptopurine (Fig. 7.3) and is well-absorbed from the gastrointestinal tract. While 45% of the drug is excreted in the urine unchanged, the rest is metabolized to 6-mercaptopurine. Azathioprine is a purine analog which interferes with the purine biosynthesis required for lymphoid cell proliferation, thus decreasing circulating B and T cells. Due to its mechanism of action, azathioprine can cause bone marrow suppression in addition to skin rash, fever, and GI upset (which may be reduced by taking azathioprine with food). Since the xanthine oxidase inhibitors used to treat gout,

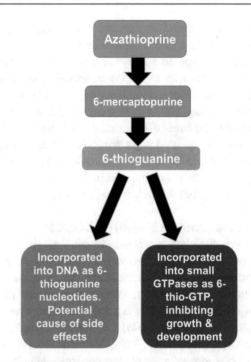

Fig. 7.3 Azathioprine is a prodrug of mercaptopurine. Azathioprine interferes in purine nucleic acid metabolism in rapidly proliferating lymphoid cells, resulting in fewer lymphocytes

including allopurinol and febuxostat, can slow the elimination of **6-mercaptopurine**, this drug combination should be avoided. Additionally, azathioprine can cause fetal harm and should not be taken during pregnancy. In addition to its use in RA, azathioprine is also indicated for transplantation procedures (Chap. 8).

Cyclophosphamide (Cytoxan®)

This drug is an alkylating agent which crosslinks DNA, RNA, and proteins, thus impairing replication, leading to cell death or dysfunction. This makes it a potent immunosuppressive drug which has been used in various autoimmune disease states including SLE. **Cyclophosphamide** is a prodrug and must be converted in the liver into its active form, phosphoramide mustard and acrolein. Because its active and inactive metabolites are excreted unchanged in the urine, cyclophosphamide must be dose-adjusted based on renal dysfunction and creatinine clearance. Oral doses are usually taken daily. It also comes as an IV formulation that is normally given every 2–4 weeks. Despite its efficacy, cyclophosphamide is very toxic and thus reserved for patients with severe disease to control and limit the degree of organ damage. Its adverse effects, which can be more severe with higher doses, include pancytopenia, bone marrow suppression, alopecia, nausea/vomiting, and discoloration of skin or nails. Cyclophosphamide can cause fetal harm and should not be used in pregnant women. It is also excreted into breast milk and could cause leukopenia and thrombocytopenia in the infant; thus it should not be used in lactating mothers.

Mycophenolate Mofetil (CellCept®)

Mycophenolate is a semisynthetic derivative of mycophenolic acid, isolated from the microorganism *Penicillium glaucus* and has been used since the early 1990s to prevent acute transplant rejection. The pro-drug is administered as **mycophenolate mofetil (MMF)** and is hydrolyzed to mycophenolic acid (MPA), which reversibly inhibits inosine monophosphate (IMP) dehydrogenase, an enzyme used for the *de novo* production of guanosine-5′-monophosphate. Since T and B lymphocytes are heavily dependent on *de novo* purine synthesis for their proliferation, MMF therapy aids in reducing actively replicating autoreactive lymphocytes. CellCept® can be used for rheumatic diseases, including SLE, systemic sclerosis, and inflammatory myopathies. The most common adverse effects involve the GI tract, accounting for about 30% of drug discontinuations, with other adverse effects including hypertension and neutropenia. In comparison to cyclophosphamide, MMF is generally considered to be less toxic. To monitor for possible cytopenia following MMF therapy, complete blood cell counts can be performed within the first 2 weeks, followed by every 6–8 weeks thereafter. Importantly, MMF is a teratogen and should not be used during pregnancy since it is known to cross the placenta. Due to its immunosuppressive effects, MMF should not be used while the patient has an active or life-threatening infection. While it is not known if MMF passes into breast milk, it is recommended for this drug to be avoided while breastfeeding. Prior to initiating therapy, tests for latent TB, HBV and HCV should be performed.

Immunomodulatory Drugs

Hydroxychloroquine (HCQ, Plaquenil®)

While chloroquine and its analog **hydroxychloroquine** are typically considered to be antimalarial agents, they do have utility in RA as well. These agents may inhibit immune responses to autoantigens in both RA and SLE through several mechanisms. One theory is that they may interfere with antigen processing in macrophages and other APCs, resulting in decreased expression of MHC:peptide complexes on the cell surface. In the absence of self-antigen presentation, autoreactive CD4 T cell responses are downregulated. Other mechanisms may include interference with TLR activation and signaling as well as decreased production of pro-inflammatory cytokines by APCs. While these are amongst the safest of the DMARDs, adverse effects include gastrointestinal disturbances (the biggest reason for discontinuation), skin rash, skin hyperpigmentation, and retinal damage with long-term use. While retinal toxicity seems to be less of a concern with lower doses, patients on these drugs are usually monitored by their ophthalmologist every 6 months. Like most of the DMARDs, response to treatment is fairly slow, and symptom relief may require treatment for 1–3 months, or even up to 6 months.

Sulfasalazine (Azulfidine®)

Sulfasalazine is a drug that is reduced chemically in the gut by coliform bacteria to **5-aminosalicylic acid (5-ASA or mesalamine)** and **sulfapyridine** (Fig. 7.4). While its role in RA

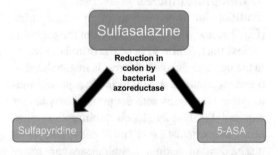

Fig. 7.4 Chemical reduction of sulfasalazine in the colon by bacterial azoreductase to 5-amino salicylic acid and sulfapyridine. The 5-ASA component stays in the colon and is useful in treating inflammation in the colon

is unclear, it is thought to decrease erythrocyte sedimentation rate, C-reactive protein levels, and cytokines, making it anti-inflammatory. Following the chemical reduction of sulfasalazine in the colon, sulfapyridine is largely absorbed while the 5-ASA component is primarily excreted in feces, making it a useful treatment for IBD (Chap. 6). Adverse effects include GI upset which tends to improve over time, skin rash, hemolytic anemia, and liver function abnormalities which should be monitored, as well as photosensitivity. To prevent GI upset, patients can take sulfasalazine with food and a full glass of water. Headaches are also a common complaint, especially with higher doses. Enteric coated preparations are available and should not be chewed or crushed. In men, sulfasalazine may cause a decreased sperm count, which is reversible upon discontinuation of the drug. Lastly, sulfasalazine may cause patients to notice a yellow-orange tinge in their sweat, tears, or urine.

Calcineurin Inhibitors: Cyclosporine (Neoral®, Sandimmune®) and Tacrolimus (Prograf®, Protopic®)

Both **cyclosporine** and **tacrolimus** can be used in autoimmunity as well as for the prevention of transplant rejection. Cyclosporine is a cyclic peptide consisting of 11 amino acids isolated from the fungus *Tolypocladium inflatum,* while tacrolimus is a macrolide antibiotic isolated from *Streptomyces tsukubaensis.* Both of these drugs block the function of **calcineurin** in T cells by binding to cyclophilin (Fig. 7.5). This inhibits activation of the transcription factor NFAT, and subsequent production of cytokines including IL-2, TNF-α, IL-4, IL-3, GM-CSF, and IFN-γ, suppressing the activation of autoreactive T cells. While calcineurin inhibitors primarily suppress T helper cells, regulatory T cells and cytotoxic cells may also be affected. Cyclosporine has also been shown to increase levels of the anti-inflammatory cytokine TGF-β.

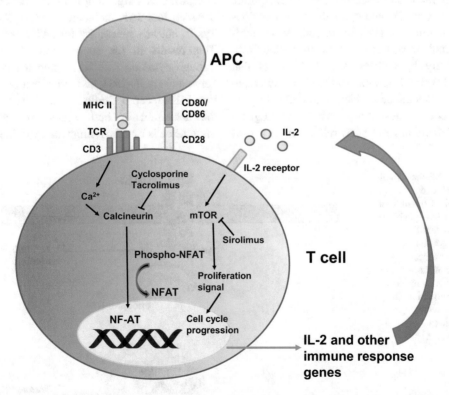

Fig. 7.5 Cyclosporine & Tacrolimus in T cell signaling. Sirolimus is a proliferation signal inhibitor which inhibits mammalian target of rapamycin (MTOR) and in turn inhibits propagation of the proliferation signal initiated by IL-2

Adverse effects tend to be more common in transplant patients rather than patients taking these drugs for autoimmunity due to lower doses used for treating autoimmunity. Acute nephrotoxicity manifests as an increase in plasma creatinine, which patients should be monitored for while on these drugs and can be reversed by decreasing the dose. Long-term nephrotoxicity can be a significant concern with the use of both cyclosporine and tacrolimus, and chronic renal disease is usually irreversible. For this reason, other drugs known to possibly be nephrotoxic should be avoided while using cyclosporine or tacrolimus. Hypertension due to renal vasoconstriction and sodium retention may develop in the first few weeks on therapy. Possible gastrointestinal adverse effects include nausea, vomiting, diarrhea, and abdominal discomfort, with patients on tacrolimus being more likely to encounter these effects. Additional adverse effects can include increased risk of infection, increased risk of malignancy, neurotoxicity, altered mental state, or metabolic abnormalities. Cyclosporine comes in oral, IV, and ophthalmic formulations while tacrolimus is available in oral, IV, and topical formulations. Because they are metabolized extensively by CyP450 CYP3A4, drugs that inhibit CYP3A4, as well as grapefruit and grapefruit juice should be avoided concomitantly.

For both of these drugs, a risk of teratogenic birth defects has not been ruled out. If use of cyclosporine during pregnancy is absolutely necessary to the extent that the mother's health is threatened by her inflammatory disease, the smallest possible dose should be used, and the mother's renal function should be monitored closely. Tacrolimus has been safely used in pregnancy as an alternative to more cytotoxic drugs, but a potential risk for fetal harm still has not been 100% ruled out. Both of these medications seem to be compatible with breastfeeding.

Tofacitinib (Xeljanz®) and Baricitinib (Olumiant®)

The JAK/STAT pathway in cytokine receptor signaling has been shown to play an important role in several inflammatory conditions including RA and psoriatic arthritis. JAK is a tyrosine kinase which phosphorylates **signal transducers and activators of transcription (STAT)** proteins needed for the transcription of several inflammatory cytokines (Fig. 7.6). **Tofacitinib (Xeljanz®)** is a signaling inhibitor that can suppress all four JAK molecules (JAK 1, 2, 3, and Tyk2), but has specificity for JAK1 and JAK3. This results in the suppression of signaling through cytokine receptors using the common gamma chain IL-2RG, and to a lesser extent, the type I IFN receptor family. Because it can inhibit the activation of both innate and adaptive immune cells by interfering with cytokine recep-

Fig. 7.6 Mechanism of tofacitinib and baricitinib. Both of these drugs are JAK inhibitors which prevent the phosphorylation of signal transducer and activator of transcription (STAT) which results in transcription of more cytokines which contribute to inflammation

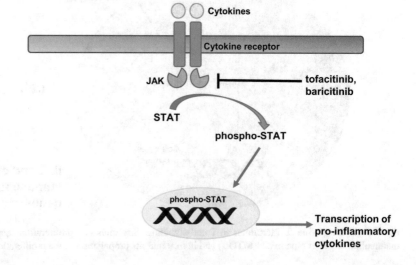

tor signaling, it is used for various autoimmune disease states. Tofacitinib comes with an increased risk of infection, changes in WBC counts, increased risk of cancer (lymphoma), and tears in stomach or intestines (in people taking NSAIDs, corticosteroids, or methotrexate). Tofacitinib has boxed warnings for risk of serious infections and malignancy. Many of the patients who developed serious infections were taking concomitant immunosuppressive agents such as steroids or methotrexate, and patients should be closely monitored for signs of infection. Tofacitinib is a substrate of CYP3A4 and should thus be avoided with drugs that inhibit or induce CYP3A4, as this could affect the serum concentration of tofacitinib. Tofacitinib should be avoided during pregnancy, and some guidelines recommend avoiding during lactation due to uncertain exposure to the infant.

Baricitinib (Olumiant®) was approved in 2018 for treating RA at the 2 mg dose. While similar in its mechanism to tofacitinib, it has specificity for JAK 1 and 2. Adverse effects include upper respiratory infection, nausea, cold sores, and reactivation of VZV in the form of shingles. Since they come with an increased risk of infection on their own, JAK inhibitors should not be combined with any biological DMARDs or other potent immunosuppressants, as the combination would result in severe immunosuppression.

Co-stimulation Inhibition

Abatacept (Orencia®)

Abatacept, like tofacitinib, is used for psoriatic arthritis and RA. Abatacept is a fusion protein made up of the extracellular portion of human CTLA-4 (CD152) and the Fc region of human IgG1. **CTLA-4**, also known as cytotoxic T-lymphocyte associated protein 4, is a natural inhibitor of costimulation and is expressed on all T cells. It is constitutively expressed on regulatory T cells. By binding to CD80 and CD86 on the APC, abatacept prevents the CD28 costimulatory receptor from becoming activated in the presence of an antigen. This interaction mimics the natural "off" switch that is provided by endogenous CTLA-4 (Fig. 7.7). The most common adverse reactions include headache and nausea, as well as increased risk of infection. Since data for use in pregnancy is limited, it is often recommended to avoid abatacept during gestation. Risks to the infant during breastfeeding are not known; thus, it is also recommended to avoid during lactation.

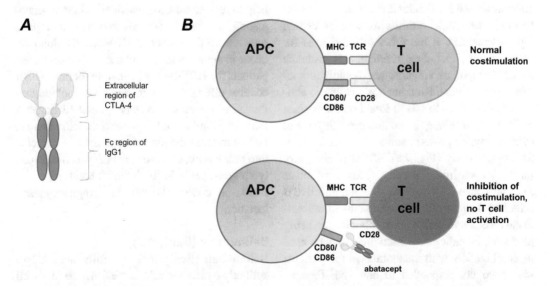

Fig. 7.7 (**a**) Structure of the human recombinant fusion protein abatacept. (**b**) Mechanism of action of abatacept. Abatacept binds to CD80/CD86 on the APC, preventing costimulation which results in T cell anergy

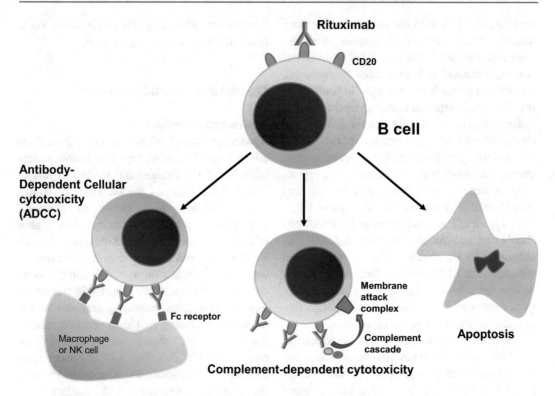

Fig. 7.8 Rituximab binds to CD20 on mature B cells. This can lead to three scenarios: ADCC, complement-dependent cytotoxicity, and apoptosis, all of which can lead to B cell death

Targeted Therapies/Biologics

Rituximab (Rituxan®)

Rituximab is a B cell inhibitor which can be used to treat rheumatoid arthritis as well as certain types of cancers. It has other off-label uses for autoimmunity including refractory Myasthenia gravis, Pemphigus vulgaris, and hemolytic anemia, among others. Rituximab is a chimeric antibody which binds to **CD20** found on the surface of B cells, resulting in complement-dependent cytotoxicity, apoptosis or antibody-dependent cellular cytotoxicity (Fig. 7.8). CD20 is necessary for B cell cycle initiation and may also function as a calcium channel. The removal of autoreactive B cells may help to alleviate symptoms of autoimmune diseases in which autoantibodies are being produced, including RA. Rituximab may be used in combination with methotrexate for patients who have not responded to anti-TNF therapy. Rituximab is given as an IV infusion and can sometimes cause a serious infusion reaction

which can be fatal. For this reason, patients should be monitored closely, especially during the first infusion. Gradually increasing the dosing may help to prevent infusion reactions, while pre-medicating with antihistamines and acetaminophen may reduce their severity. HBV reactivation may occur in some patients, and it is important to test patients for HBV before beginning therapy. Other adverse effects seen with rituximab include cardiovascular events such as peripheral edema, cardiac arrhythmias, and hypertension. Rituximab is known to cross the placenta and may be excreted into breast milk, which can possibly lead to B-cell lymphocytopenia in the infant. Therefore, rituximab is contraindicated in pregnancy and lactation.

Belimumab (Benlysta®)

Belimumab (Benlysta®) is a fully human IgG antibody which neutralizes the function of B-cell activating factor (BAFF), also known as B lymphocyte stimulator (BLyS), and is used to induce

B cell death in patients with active systemic lupus erythematosus (SLE). In 2011, it became the first drug approved for SLE in more than 50 years and is currently the only Food and Drug Administration (FDA)-approved biologic therapy for treating SLE. BAFF/BLyS is a part of the TNF superfamily and is expressed as inactive membrane-bound or biologically active soluble forms. B-cells express three types of BLyS receptors (BR3, TACI, and B-cell maturation antigen). The activation of BR3 (also known as BAFF receptor) by BLyS promotes the survival of B-cells by preventing them from undergoing apoptosis. BLyS that is bound to belimumab is unable to bind to BR3, thus causing autoantibody-producing B cells to undergo negative selection and apoptosis. The BLISS trials were two multicenter trials that assessed efficacy of IV belimumab, as measured by the Systemic Lupus Erythematosus Responder Index (SRI), as compared to placebo. Both trials met their primary endpoints in finding SRI improvement in SLE patients taking belimumab and also demonstrated the rates of adverse effects from belimumab were similar to placebo. While it was fairly well-tolerated in the trials, some post-trial adverse effects have been reported including arthralgia, rash, diarrhea, nausea, and increased risk of infection. Other effects may include urticaria, infusion reactions, and neutropenia and thrombocytopenia. Psychiatric events, including depression appear to occur more often with belimumab than with placebo.

TNF Inhibitors

TNF-α is a major proinflammatory cytokine that initiates many biological functions including the upregulation of immune responses during bacterial encounters in response to TLR signaling. TNF-α is predominantly secreted by macrophages and monocytes, but also by neutrophils, mast cells, T cells, and B cells. Altered expression and production of TNF-α may play a role in several autoimmune disorders including Rheumatoid Arthritis, Multiple Sclerosis, and Crohn's disease. As introduced in Chap. 2, several TNF antibodies are used for their neutralizing function. **Adalimumab (Humira®)** is a humanized anti-TNF-α monoclonal antibody that is among the most widely used, with others including another fully human antibody (**golimumab, Simponi®**), the chimeric mouse/human monoclonal antibody **infliximab (Remicade®)**, and the humanized Fab anti-TNF fragment **certolizumab (Cimzia®)**. A TNF receptor fusion protein with a similar function, named **etanercept (Enbrel®)**, is also used. Compared to traditional drug molecules, the structures of biologics such as antibodies are generally much larger and complex. Producing these agents can take a significant amount of time and effort, resulting in high sale prices. Monoclonal antibodies must be given via injection (IV or SC). Due to the increased risk of infection resulting from anti-TNF therapy, it is important to test patients for latent TB before beginning therapy. An FDA black box warning also indicates increased risk of lymphoproliferative disorders and other cancers, especially in children and adolescents. Patients with chronic heart failure should not take TNF inhibitors. Due to a widespread role for TNF in autoimmunity, TNF inhibitors have been shown to be useful in RA, psoriatic arthritis, Crohn's disease, among several other diseases.

IL-1/IL-6 Inhibitors

As discussed earlier, the IL-1 family is a group of pro-inflammatory cytokines involved in the pathogenesis of several diseases. Natural antagonists for IL-1 are produced as well, such as the IL-1 receptor antagonist (IL-1Ra). Since the IL-1 family represents a promising therapeutic target, there are a number of IL-1 inhibitors currently on the market or in development. **Rilonacept (Arcalyst®)** is approved for the treatment of **Cryopyrin Associated Periodic Syndromes (CAPS)**, a group of rare, inherited autoinflammatory diseases in which the proinflammatory cytokine IL-1β is overproduced. Rilonacept is a dimeric fusion protein that binds to and inhibits the actions of IL-1β and has been shown to decrease the severity of symptoms associated with CAPS. This protective effect correlates with decreased levels of Serum Amyloid A (SAA) and C-Reactive Protein (CRP), inflammatory markers that are generally elevated in patients with CAPS.

Canakinumab (Ilaris®) is a human monoclonal IL-1β neutralizing antibody and is indicated for the treatment of **Systemic Juvenile Idiopathic Arthritis (SJIA)** (rheumatic disease of unknown etiology affecting children 5 and younger) and **Periodic Fever Syndrome** (group of autoinflammatory diseases including CAPS characterized by cyclical fevers). Since IL-1β is overproduced in Periodic Fever Syndrome and SJIA, canakinumab has been shown to improve symptoms of both of these conditions, correlating with decreases in CRP and SAA levels.

Anakinra (Kineret®) is a recombinant IL-1 receptor antagonist that competitively inhibits IL-1α and IL-1β and is used for treating RA in patients who have failed one or more DMARDs. It is also approved for the treatment of **Neonatal Onset Multisystem Inflammatory Disease (NOMID)**, a type of CAPS. RA patients who take anakinra experience a delayed progression of their physical symptoms, and those with NOMID experience improvement in symptoms and reductions in SAA and CRP levels.

Overproduction of IL-6 is also implicated in the pathogenesis of many autoimmune diseases RA, (Castleman's disease, SJIA), with anti-IL-6 treatments demonstrating efficacy. One medication indicated in the US for treating severe RA is **tocilizumab (Actemra®)**, a humanized antagonistic monoclonal against the IL-6 receptor. The IL-6 receptor can be membrane-bound or soluble, and the ligation of either form with IL-6 results in the complex associating with a membrane-bound glycoprotein named gp130 on responsive cells. This leads to the activation of signaling pathways consisting of JAK/STAT, SHP-2, ERK, and MAPK molecules, resulting in the transcription of inflammatory mediators. Another IL-6 receptor inhibitor, **sarilumab (Kevzara®)** was approved in 2017 for the treatment of moderate to severe RA. **Siltuximab (Sylvant®)** is a chimeric monoclonal antibody which binds to IL-6 itself and is used for treating multicentric Castleman's disease (MCD). Several other IL-6 inhibitors are currently being studied in clinical trials, including clazakizumab, olokizumab, and sirukumab.

Adhesion Molecule Inhibitors

Cell adhesion molecules (CAMs) are another target for suppressing aberrant inflammation due to their specific interactions with ligands involved in cell-to-cell interactions or migration. For instance, some CAMs allow leukocytes to migrate out of the circulation, slowly roll along the surface of vessels, strongly attach to endothelium and permeate through to reach inflamed tissues. Leukocytes expressing a type of CAM named $\alpha_4\beta_7$ integrin have been implicated in the pathogenesis of inflammatory bowel diseases (ulcerative colitis, Crohn's disease; described in Chap. 6). Cells expressing $\alpha_4\beta_7$ integrin have been shown to exhibit preferential binding to endothelial surfaces of the GI tract. **Vedolizumab (Entyvio®)** is a monoclonal antibody targeting $\alpha_4\beta_7$ integrin (Figs. 6.6 and 7.9) and is approved for adult ulcerative colitis and Crohn's disease. Thus, vedolizumab significantly decreases the symptoms of IBD by inhibiting leukocyte binding to the GI tract. Adverse effects of vedolizumab include infusion-related reactions, nasopharyngitis, headache, arthralgia, and upper respiratory tract infection. A related drug, **natalizumab (Tysabri®)** is a monoclonal antibody which targets $\alpha_4\beta_1$ integrin. This is used for Crohn's disease and multiple sclerosis. Due to a possible risk for a severe brain disease named **progressive multifocal leukencephalopathy (PML)**, natalizumab must be prescribed strictly under the Tysabri Outreach: Unified Commitment to Health (TOUCH) program. This program provides information on monitoring patients for PML. Before beginning natalizumab therapy, patients should be tested for JC virus, a brain infection which many adults are exposed to and does not normally pose a problem in immunocompetent individuals. It has been hypothesized that blocking the $\alpha_4\beta_1$ integrin renders patients unable to suppress viral replication, leading to the more serious PML.

Intravenous Immune Globulin (IVIG)

Intravenous immune globulin (IVIG) consists of IgG antibodies pooled from thousands of healthy donors and can be given to patients with

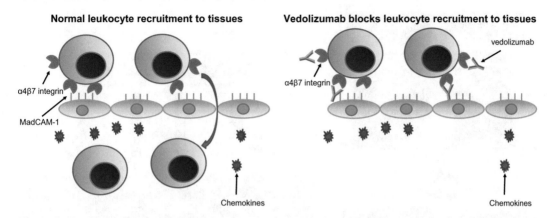

Fig. 7.9 Vedolizumab and natalizumab block integrins and leukocyte recruitment. Vedolizumab binds to $\alpha_4\beta_7$ integrin on leukocytes. This prevents $\alpha_4\beta_7$ integrin from binding to the adhesion molecule MAdCAM-1 on the surface of endothelial cells, which in turn, prevents them from rolling and entering the inflamed tissue

certain immunodeficiencies as well as autoimmunity. These pooled antibodies have no specific antigen target and are thought to have a normalizing effect on the patient's immune networks. Hyperimmune globulin consists of antibodies taken from the plasma of people with high titers of antibodies to specific pathogens or antigens, acting as a form of passive immunity. The exact mechanism by which IVIG works is largely unknown but there are several proposed mechanisms, including the inhibition of phagocytosis by the Fc regions of given antibodies, antibody-dependent cellular cytotoxicity, prevention of immune complexes binding to FcRs, and the deposition of activated complement, as described in Chap. 1 and Chap. 6. Immune globulins given subcutaneously are referred to as **SCIG** and are given in smaller amounts. The Fab arm of the antibodies may have effects on cellular adhesion, suppression of proliferation, decreased levels of biologically active cytokines, or the induction of leukocyte apoptosis. Adverse effects of IVIG include local injection site reactions, itching, low grade fever, muscle and joint aches, headache, hives, chest tightening, or wheezing. Some of these effects may be ameliorated by slowing the infusion rate, giving IV saline pre-infusion, or pre-medicating with ibuprofen. While SCIG is associated with fewer systemic side effects, frequent injections may need to be administered if large volumes are needed.

Mechanisms of Selected Autoimmune Disorders

Systemic Lupus Erythematosus

Mechanisms

Systemic lupus erythematosus (SLE) correlates with Type III hypersensitivity due to the presence of self-reactive IgG antibodies that form immune complexes with antigens derived from cell surface and intracellular proteins. These immune complexes can deposit at various locations, but most commonly in the joints, kidneys or blood vessels, causing arthritis, glomerulonephritis or vasculitis, respectively. Patients with SLE often exhibit a characteristic butterfly rash on their face. This disease is more common in women of African or Asian background (1/500 people). Diagnoses are made from clinical findings characteristic of SLE that manifest in the joints, kidneys, nervous system, and skin. Early symptoms include fever, fatigue, arthralgia, the characteristic facial "butterfly rash" and joint swelling. Laboratory tests that identify SLE include high erythrocyte sedimentation rate, elevated CRP, presence of **anti-nuclear antibodies (ANA)**, or autoantibodies against other self-antigens including double-stranded DNA (dsDNA) or Smith antigens. Anti-Smith (anti-Sm) antibodies are a specific marker given that they are absent in 99% of people who do not have

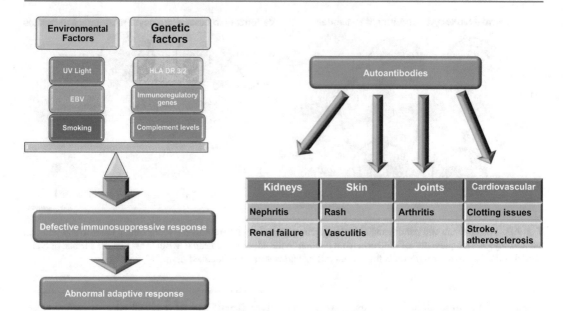

Fig. 7.10 Genetic and environmental factors contribute to the pathophysiology of SLE. Autoantibodies produced have an impact on the joints, kidneys, skin, and cardiovascular system resulting in signs and symptoms including joint pain, kidney failure, skin rashes, and clotting issues

SLE; however, they are only present in approximately 15–30% of patients with SLE. **Anti-Smith antibodies** target seven proteins that constitute the common core of small nuclear ribonuclear protein particles. The degree of renal involvement can be assessed with tests that include serum creatinine and urinary sediment.

Risk factors leading to SLE most likely include both genetic and environmental factors (Fig. 7.10). Genetic susceptibility is due to several malfunctioning intracellular signaling pathways, with over 30 genetic loci thought to be involved including STAT4, IRF-5, and IRAK-1. Data suggests that increased activity of interleukin-1 receptor associated kinase (IRAK-1) may lead to hyperresponsiveness of B and T cells through the overproduction of type I IFNs. Additionally, hyperreactive B cell responses against self-antigens may result from defective TCR/CD3 expression and impaired CTL activity through a lack of IL-2 production. Another potential gene encodes for mammalian target of rapamycin (mTOR), which plays a role in T cell activation and may promote recycling of the TCR/CD3 chain into the endosome. It may also suppress the expression of Foxp3, leading to the

decreased numbers of regulatory T cells seen in SLE patients. Lastly, mTOR may promote the activation of B cells and DCs. Data shows that inhibition of Syk, downstream of mTOR, does not affect production of autoantibodies but does decrease numbers of activated CD4 T cells since it is found to be abnormally increased on the T cells of SLE patients. mTOR seems to play a broad role in SLE and may become activated in response to metabolic stress. Because it is activated in several different cell types, not just T cells, but also B cells, macrophages, and non-immune organs including the liver and the kidney, it is an attractive target for therapy.

SLE, like other autoimmune diseases, represents a loss of self-tolerance of T and B lymphocytes, leading to the production of autoantibodies that form immune complexes with self-antigens and cause inflammation and tissue injury when deposited in certain tissues. Ultimately, increases in BCR, BLyS (also known as BAFF), and TLR signaling allows for the survival of autoreactive B cells. For this to occur, a subset of autoreactive CD4 T cells also must have evaded tolerance checkpoints during development. Studies have suggested that activated follicular T helper cells

(T_{FH}) cells in the germinal centers of lymph nodes provide the CD40L signals necessary for the maturation of these B cells in lupus. For this reason, molecular interactions between T_{FH} cells and B cells may represent novel therapeutic targets.

Nephritis in the kidney results from a deposition of immune complexes in the glomerulus, leading to complement fixation and the engagement of FcRs. This results in macrophage infiltration, perpetuating the inflammatory response and tissue damage. T_H17 cells may also infiltrate the kidneys as well as the skin. Increased levels of IL-17 from T_H17 cells and some innate cell types has been found in injured tissues as well as the circulation in SLE and may play a role in autoantibody production. Further research on these possible correlations is particularly important given that there are approved biologic treatments against IL-17, which may represent another novel target in lupus.

Treatment

Lifestyle changes are often recommended as a part of managing SLE. Patients should be instructed to quit/avoid smoking as this can trigger inflammation as well as put extra stress on the lungs, heart, and kidneys, exacerbating the condition. Because SLE patients are photosensitive and more likely to develop sunburn and exacerbate skin rashes, UV light should be avoided. Patients should avoid direct exposure to the sun or wear SPF 30 or higher sunscreen. Because commonly prescribed medications for SLE cause the patient to be immunosuppressed, they should attempt to prevent infection by staying up-to-date on vaccines, including the yearly influenza vaccine, be diligent about handwashing, and try to avoid contact with persons who are ill. Eating a healthy diet including omega-3 fatty acids can be beneficial in patients with SLE, and exercise can improve strength and well-being. Conversely, stress can have a deleterious effect on the immune system and should be avoided in patients. Lastly, medications that might trigger lupus-like symptoms, such as procainamide and hydralazine, should not be used in patients with SLE.

Antimalarials have been used for many years and are often recommended for treating SLE, cases with musculoskeletal and cutaneous involvement. Hydroxychloroquine (HCQ) and chloroquine are immunomodulatory drugs used to maintain remission and decrease flares. A proposed mechanism by which HCQ suppresses inflammation in SLE is through the inhibition of TLRs, in particular TLR9 which appears to play a role in rheumatic diseases. Other mechanisms include interfering with antigen presentation and inhibiting phospholipase A2. These effects would result in decreased levels of proinflammatory cytokines including TNF-α, IL-1β, IFN-γ, and IL-6. More recently, HCQ was proposed to decrease production of proinflammatory T_H17-type cytokines including IL6, IL-17, and IL-22. This may occur due to HCQ's ability to interfere with antigen presentation. In those SLE patients who are pregnant or breastfeeding, HCQ can often be continued. The time to achieve its desired effect can be 1–3 months or as long as 3–6 months, with skin lesions sometimes responding quicker at 4–6 weeks. Patients should be advised not to smoke while taking antimalarials, as this can decrease their efficacy. Doses may need to be adjusted for renal insufficiency. Patients should also be advised these drugs (particularly chloroquine) may cause GI upset, although this can be decreased if taken with food. Other adverse effects include skin rash or pigment changes, as well as damage to the retina with long-term use. For this reason, possible retinopathy should be monitored with an ophthalmologist.

Glucocorticoids may be used topically for SLE skin lesions, particularly on the scalp, palms of hands, or soles of feet. These should not be used long term for many reasons, including immunosuppression and prolonged adverse effects which may include hypertension, bone fracture, as well as metabolic issues (Type 2 diabetes, weight gain, hyperglycemia). Topical calcineurin inhibitors such as tacrolimus and pimecrolimus are sometimes used off-label and can be taken for longer spans than the glucocorticoids. Compared to antimalarials and traditional DMARDs which may take months to provide relief, glucocorticoids including prednisolone or NSAIDs may be used to achieve a faster onset of relief.

Immunosuppressive treatments, including DMARDs may be used in patients with organ involvement such as the kidneys or CNS. Such treatments may include Mycophenolate mofetil (MMF), azathioprine, cyclosporine, or cyclophosphamide. MMF is used off-label for SLE with good efficacy and relatively low toxicity. These drugs reduce the levels of autoreactive lymphocytes; however, due to their cytotoxicity, they should be avoided during pregnancy.

Belimumab, a B cell inhibitor which binds to B lymphocyte stimulator (BLyS), was approved in 2011 as an add-on to standard therapy for SLE in autoantibody-positive patients. It is a fully humanized IgG1 antibody, and the only biological agent approved for SLE. BLyS may also be referred to as B cell-activating factor (BAFF) and is necessary for B cell survival and function, including the production of antibodies. The neutralization of BLyS with belimumab results in B-cell apoptosis. Circulating levels of BLyS are found to be increased in SLE and has also been found to correlate with disease activity. Belimumab most likely affects newly formed autoreactive B cells as opposed to memory or plasma cells. Thus, B cell suppression occurs about 8 weeks after the initiation of therapy, with symptoms improving within 16 weeks. In general, belimumab is well-tolerated but comes with an increased risk of infection, infusion-related reactions, and hypersensitivity. There is a paucity of information on potential risks of belimumab to fetuses during pregnancy, and more data is being collected from pregnant women exposed to this drug to better evaluate pregnancy outcomes and potential birth defects.

Rituximab is sometimes used by physicians off-label due to the generous amount of anecdotal clinical evidence for its efficacy in lupus. The use of rituximab is based on the same hypothesis as the use of belimumab: that B cell depletion will lead to decreases in autoantibodies and improvement of symptoms. Despite what is seen in clinical practice, two randomized trials utilizing rituximab (EXPLORER and LUNAR) failed to meet their primary endpoints and did not show improvement in lupus over placebo. Post-trial discussions among the medical community suggest that poor study design contributed to the failures. Still, physicians sometimes turn to rituximab as an alternative to steroids and for treating refractory SLE.

Patients with SLE may also require treatment for comorbidities including but not limited to hypertension, infection, dyslipidemia, diabetes, or osteoporosis.

Rheumatoid Arthritis

Mechanisms

Aberrant innate and adaptive immune responses resulting in release of proinflammatory cytokines are also associated with the pathogenesis of **rheumatoid arthritis (RA)**. Genetic predisposition appears to be linked to certain MHC molecules, particularly HLA-DR4 and HLA-DR1 on T lymphocytes. Environmental factors play a role as well, including smoking and pulmonary disease. Certain infections may increase the risk for RA, including EBV, *E. coli*, and those from periodontal disease. In the past, RA was thought to be a B cell-mediated disease due to pathogenic roles for autoantibodies including **Rheumatoid factor (RF)** and **anti-cyclic citrullinated protein (anti-CCP)** antibodies. RF is an autoantibody which is detectable in the blood of approximately 80% of adults with RA. RF binds to the Fc region of IgG antibodies, forming immune complexes that can become deposited in the joint, leading to inflammation. While RF often exists as IgM, it can exist as any of the antibody isotypes. Anti-CCP is also present in many RA patients (approximately 60–70%), and its presence can indicate severity of disease. Patients who are positive for anti-CCP are referred to as having seropositive RA, and may have a more aggressive development of disease, including more frequent flareups and more damage to the affected joints. Anti-CCP antibodies bind to proteins which are citrullinated, a process that converts arginine residues to citrulline residues during inflammation. Certain proteins which may become enzymatically citrullinated during inflammation include fibrin and vimentin. Vimentin is an intermediate filament protein

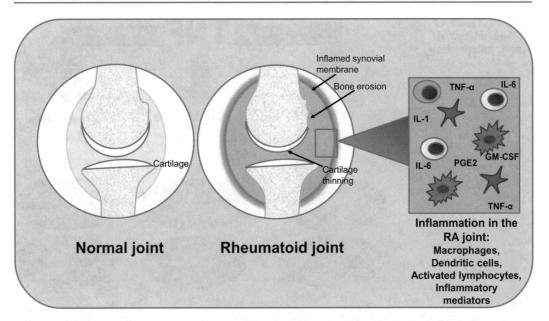

Fig. 7.11 In rheumatoid arthritis, joint inflammation is a result of infiltration of immune cells, including macrophages, dendritic cells, and activated B and T lymphocytes. Inflammatory mediators released contribute to the infiltration of more leukocytes, resulting in bone erosion, cartilage thinning, and pannus formation

which is a part of the cell cytoskeleton. Studies suggest that macrophages secrete and citrullinate vimentin in response to apoptosis, and that citrullinated vimentin is an important autoantigen in RA. While the formation of these autoantibodies often classifies RA as a B cell disease, recent evidence suggests a critical role for T cells too. Other autoantigens targeted include cartilaginous components, enzymes, and nuclear proteins. Both genetic and environmental factors contribute to the formation of autoantibodies, which can be found in the serum and synovial fluid of the joint. These can usually be detected before the symptoms of RA appear, suggesting that it takes time for synovial inflammation to set in prior to the joint damage and erosion of bone characteristic of RA (Fig. 7.11).

Prior to the activation of autoreactive B cells, APCs present self-antigens in the joint to T cells on MHC II molecules. The subsequent activation and differentiation of B cells into plasma cells leads to autoantibody accumulation in the joints and activation of the classical complement cascade. This in turn results in the chemotaxis of leukocytes to the synovium and joint space, causing synovitis. Some of these leukocytes are

neutrophils that release hydroxyl and oxygen free radicals that damage the synovium. Studies have suggested that several ligands for chemokine receptors expressed by neutrophils are present in RA-damaged joints. Chronic inflammation (Fig. 7.11), including increases in TNF-α, IL-1, and IL-6, seems to promote articular damage, resulting in the further release of self-antigens and propagation of the autoimmune attack. In addition to proinflammatory cytokines, growth factors including GM-CSF are present in the synovium of RA patients and appear to play a pathophysiological role. GM-CSF augments the function of innate immune cells present in the joint (neutrophils, macrophages, and dendritic cells), resulting in the continued release proinflammatory cytokines (IL-1, IL-6, TNF) as well as autoantigen presentation on MHC II molecules.

Pannus is an abnormal layer of tissue found in RA that results from the inflammatory response and contributes to joint pain when it invades the joint space. Osteoclasts, cells that normally break down bone during the remodeling process are often found at the pannus-bone junction in arthritic joints. Osteoclasts are stimulated to

Fig. 7.12 The role of
TNF-α in rheumatoid
arthritis pathophysiology

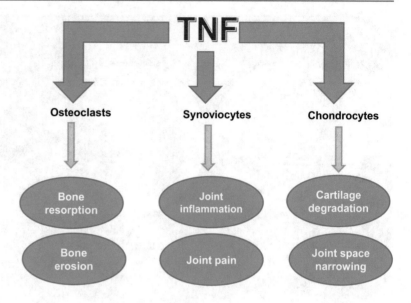

resorb bone by **receptor activator of nuclear factor κB (NF-κB) ligand (RANKL)**, which also promotes osteoclast survival. IL-17 produced by T_H17 cells can stimulate the production RANKL in osteoblasts and mesenchymal stem cells. RANKL is a member of the TNF superfamily of cytokines and binds to its receptor, RANK. RANK is expressed on monocyte-lineage osteoclast precursor cells, mature osteoclasts and DCs, and when bound to RANKL, an intracellular signaling pathway is initiated which results in NF-κB activation. This in turn promotes osteoclast development and activation. Osteoclasts may also be affected by TNF-α which has degradative and inflammatory effects on other several cell types in the joint, including chondrocytes and synoviocytes (Fig. 7.12). TNF-α and IL-6 released by macrophages also stimulate fibroblasts to release matrix metalloproteinases (MMPs) which aid in bone degradation, as well.

Treatment

Achieving remission is the goal of the RA patient. While the initial drug of choice for RA continues to be methotrexate, there are several DMARDs, as well as biologic therapies, which can be utilized if there is an inadequate response with methotrexate. While about two-thirds of patients have good responses (and a quicker relief of symptoms) with biologic therapies, these are costly and require parenteral administration. Small-molecule DMARDs are more economical but can also take several months to begin providing symptom relief. All these agents help slow RA progression.

NSAIDs or corticosteroids (prednisone, prednisolone) may be used for quicker symptom relief, although neither are used as monotherapies. While NSAIDs may relieve pain and reduce stiffness, they do not have any effect on disease progression. Corticosteroids are not an attractive choice for long-term use due to many adverse effects, although their anti-inflammatory effects are conducive for use alongside DMARD therapy. Corticosteroids can inhibit cellular migration, reduce proinflammatory cytokines including IL-1, IL-2, IL-3, TNF-α and IFN-γ, as well as enzymes such as collagenase, elastase, and COX-2, and reduce numbers of T cells.

The most commonly used DMARDs are methotrexate, sulfasalazine, hydroxychloroquine, and leflunomide. Methotrexate is most commonly used for initial therapy and may be combined with other medications if monotherapy does not produce an adequate response. By inhibiting the conversion of folic acid into tetrahydrofolate, methotrexate blocks purine synthesis. Supplementation with folic acid may help to reduce some of the adverse effects associated with methotrexate. In addition, this medication has also been shown to suppress pro-inflammatory cytokine production. For long-term treatment in RA, leflunomide has similar clinical efficacy to methotrexate. It is an inhibitor of pyrimidine synthesis, resulting in decreased proliferation of activated lymphocytes. Hydroxychloroquine may be used in mild disease or in combination with another DMARD. While its mechanism of action in autoimmune diseases is not entirely understood, hydroxychloroquine may interfere with antigen processing, resulting in decreased presentation of self-antigens to autoreactive T cells. Because it is not myelosuppressive like some of the other DMARDs, it results in less toxicity to the kidneys and liver. On the other hand, antimalarial agents can cause retinal toxicity. Following hydroxychloroquine treatment, the incidence of preretinopathy is 2.7%, and usually does not progress. Patients on antimalarials should follow up with an ophthalmologist, especially if vision changes occur. The mechanism of action of sulfasalazine for treating RA is largely undetermined, but has been shown to reduce inflammation, pain and joint stiffness. A meta-analysis of 15 randomized controlled trials found that sulfasalazine was superior to hydroxychloroquine at alleviating symptoms. Most patients experience few adverse effects with sulfasalazine, with the most common being nausea and abdominal discomfort. This can be ameliorated by taking an enteric-coated tablet or by starting with a low dose which increases over time to a maintenance dose.

Five TNF inhibitors (etanercept, adalimumab, certolizumab, golimumab, infliximab) are approved to treat RA. Due to elevated levels of TNF-α in RA joints, these biologic agents can slow or stop joint damage by significantly decreasing inflammation. TNF inhibitors may be used as a monotherapy or in combination with methotrexate. The onset of relief is usually quicker than DMARDs, with improvement of symptoms as early as 2–4 weeks. Patients may also experience additional improvement over the next 3–6 months. However, since TNF-α is a key mediator in propagating immune responses, inhibition results in an increased risk for infection or lymphoma.

The IL-6 receptor inhibitor tocilizumab is approved for use in RA in patients who have not had a response to TNF inhibitors. IL-6 is a pro-inflammatory cytokine produced by synovial and joint endothelial cells, among other cells, and promotes T cell activation as well as autoantibody production. Studies have shown that blocking IL-6 results in decreased RA symptoms including joint pain and inflammation, with radiographs showing decreased/slowed joint damage. Tocilizumab inhibits IL-6-mediated effects by antagonizing the function of soluble and membrane-bound IL-6 receptors. Patients on tocilizumab may begin to experience symptom relief within 4–8 weeks, and this medication can be used as a monotherapy or in combination with a traditional DMARD. It is usually recommended to begin with a lower dose and gradually increase to the maintenance dose. Like the TNF inhibitors, IL-6 receptor inhibition comes with a risk of serious infection. Patients with diverticulitis should not receive this medication, as it increases the risk of GI perforation. Monitoring for other adverse effects, including thrombocytopenia, neutropenia, and elevated liver enzymes, should occur every 4–8 weeks while the patient is on the therapy.

If the standard treatments do not yield an adequate response, IL-1 inhibition may be utilized. Anakinra is a peptidomimetic of naturally occurring IL-1ra, differing by the addition of an N-terminal methionine. Because anakinra is taken daily by subcutaneous injection, common adverse effects are injection site reactions including redness and itching. Compared to other treatments, anakinra comes with a modest increased risk of infection, with fewer opportunistic infections occurring compared to TNF inhibitors. Patients can expect to see relief of symptoms within 2–4 weeks.

Tofacitinib is a Janus kinase (JAK) inhibitor which decreases signaling through cytokine receptors utilizing the JAK/STAT pathway. JAK is a tyrosine kinase which phosphorylates STAT proteins involved in the transcription of several inflammatory cytokines. Tofacitinib is used for moderate-to-severe RA, particularly in patients who have failed MTX therapy. Seven ORAL

(Oral Rheumatoid Arthritis triaL) trials included patients who had failed methotrexate therapies and were subsequently given tofacitinib, adalimumab, or placebo (including background MTX). Patients on tofacitinib or adalimumab were found to have achieved higher ACR20 response rates at 6 months based on reduction of RA symptoms, using criteria set forth by the American College of Rheumatology. A newer drug, baricitinib (Olumiant®), inhibits JAK1 and JAK2-mediated signaling and has been shown to significantly improve responses in RA patients who had failed MTX therapy. The RA-BEAM trial was another phase III trial using baricitinib, and demonstrated improved responses compared to adalimumab or placebo in patients who were refractory to MTX. At 12 weeks, baricitinib was determined to be superior to adalimumab based on ACR20 criteria. In both the adalimumab and baricitinib groups, infections were more frequent at week 24 and neutrophils were often found to be decreased as compared to placebo. Despite success in phase III trials and its approval in Europe, the FDA did not approve baricitinib in April 2017, citing the need for more clinical data on dosing. In 2018, the baricitinib 2 mg dose was approved by the FDA for moderate-to-severe RA.

The JAK inhibitors tofacitinib and baricitinib are formulated as oral tablets whereas the biologic agents for treating RA are injectable solutions. Therefore, oral JAK inhibitors may be more attractive for patients who cannot tolerate injections and injection related reactions. A caveat is that JAK inhibitors need to be taken every day whereas most biologic agents are injected at weekly or monthly intervals. Therefore, patients with adherence issues may benefit from injectable formulations.

As described above, the costimulation inhibitor abatacept (Orencia®) blocks the function of CD80/CD86 on APCs, preventing ligation with the costimulatory receptor CD28 on autoreactive T cells. Abatacept has demonstrated efficacy in RA, associated with decreased production of T cell-derived cytokines including TNF-alpha. Abatacept is given either IV or subcutaneously, with responses occurring within 3 months.

Like SLE, B cell depletion appears to also be beneficial in the treatment of RA. Rituximab is often the biologic chosen for this strategy. While rituximab treatment does not necessarily reduce autoantibody levels, it aids in the suppression of cytokines produced by autoreactive B cells. While a single course of treatment can result in a rapid reduction of B cells, clinical effects may not occur for 3 months. In general, responses to rituximab may last 6–12 months, or even longer. Rituximab is given intravenously, with the most common adverse event being infusion-related reactions.

One of the most important nonpharmacologic treatments is rest of the inflamed joints. This can help to alleviate pain and prevent additional joint damage. Weight loss is another option to help relieve the stress on inflamed joints. Other nonpharmacologic treatments include occupational and physical therapy to help retain mobility and prevent muscle atrophy, and the use of supportive walking devices. Viable surgical options include tendon repair or joint replacement.

Multiple Sclerosis

Mechanisms
Multiple sclerosis (MS, which means "many scars") is an autoimmune disorder mediated by CD4 T cells which cause damage to the myelin sheath of neurons, resulting in sclerotic plaques. MS affects approximately 2.5 million people around the world, and patients usually begin experiencing symptoms between the ages of 20–40 years. While genetic factors such as major histocompatibility complex polymorphisms (the HLA-DRB1*1501 haplotype represents an increased risk) play a role in the development of MS, environmental factors also contribute to disease. Interestingly, the prevalence of MS tends to be higher in Scotland, parts of Scandinavia, and Canada. Studies show that people who migrate from a region of low MS incidence to one of these regions have a higher likelihood of developing MS. Other environmental factors may include infection with Epstein Barr virus (EBV), low exposure to sunlight/UV radiation or Vitamin

D deficiency. Development of MS is likely resultant of a complex interplay between genetic factors, the immune system, and environmental factors. Patients with MS typically exhibit muscle weakness, lack of coordination (ataxia), excessive contraction of muscles, vertigo, as well as impaired vision. T_H1 CD4 T cells acting in response to myelin basic protein (MBP) and proteolipid proteins of the myelin sheath release IFN-γ which activates macrophages. These activated macrophages release cytokines and proteases which cause damage at the site of inflammation. The plaques resulting from destruction of myelin can be classified according to the stage of lesion formation. Acute plaques generally have the most inflammatory cells including T cells, monocytes, and macrophages, as well as poorly-defined margins of myelin destruction. Chronic active plaques tend to have not only loss of myelin with clearly-defined margins but also glial scarring. The borders of the chronic plaque may contain activated microglia and macrophages, as well as complement and antibodies. Chronic silent lesions, on the other hand, do not have as much inflammation on the border, and also have less axonal density with no oligodendrocytes. The progression of the MS plaque from acute to chronic active to chronic silent demonstrates the role of inflammation in demyelination, and eventually leads to a largely scarred lesion resulting in impaired neuronal messaging.

Studies evaluating the roles of lymphocytes have confirmed that CD4 T cells and B cells recognizing antigens derived from **myelin basic protein (MBP)** are elevated in MS patients, indicating that MBP may be a potential therapeutic drug target. Some studies are searching for molecules to "protect" MBP from autoimmune attack by competitively inhibiting its binding to autoantibodies. Other CNS antigens targeted by autoimmune T cells including proteolipid proteins, αB-crystallin, phosphodiesterases, myelin oligodendrocyte glycoprotein, and myelin-associated oligodendrocytic basic protein, among others. It is still not clear how CD4 T cells become activated towards these autoantigens. Some postulate that there may be an infectious trigger, such as

EBV, containing similar epitopes to the ones derived from myelin, resulting in cross-reactive responses towards myelin. Antigen presentation of these epitopes to CD4 T cells in the periphery results in their activation and differentiation into T_H1 and T_H17 subsets. These cells migrate to the central nervous system where they interact with adhesion molecules on the endothelium of blood vessels and cross the blood-brain-barrier (BBB) with the help of chemokines and proteases. These T helper cells continue to proliferate as well as activate B cells to mature and produce antibodies against these targets. The infiltration of lymphocytes and macrophages, accompanied with the release of cytokines such as IL-12, IFN-γ, IL-23, and TNF-α, leads to the demyelination of sheath surrounding axons and the loss of oligodendrocytes. T_H17 cells are induced by IL-6, IL-1, and TGF-β and are maintained by IL-23 secreted by DCs. This cell type has been shown to kill human neurons *in vitro*, and to cross the blood brain barrier more efficiently than T_H1 cells. Damage to the BBB may lead to the infiltration of other immune cells into the CNS. T_H17 cells are also found on the borders of active lesions, suggesting they are recruited there, while IL-17 is also found to be increased in these lesions. Studies suggest that serum levels of IL-17 are elevated in relapsing MS patients. This may be due to memory CD4 T cells that produce IL-17 becoming elevated in the peripheral blood. These studies suggest T_H17 cells may have a larger role in demyelination and destruction of axons than once thought, making them a potential novel therapeutic target in MS.

Treatment

In early 2018, The European Committee for Treatment and Research in Multiple Sclerosis and the European Academy of Neurology (ECTRIMS/EAN) released new clinical guidelines for the treatment of MS. Several recommendations for treatment were made based on patients' disease progression. Additionally, interferon or Copaxone® were recommended for patients who did not meet the 2010 diagnostic criteria for MS who have experienced CIS (clinical isolation syndrome, first episode of neurological symptoms lasting at least 24 h caused by inflammation/demyelination) and have MRI lesions suggestive of MS.

There are four major clinical phases of MS. The first phase called relapse-remitting is characterized by clearly defined episodes of decreasing neurologic function intermixed with varying phases of stability and recovery. The secondary-progressive phase follows with increased neurologic decline and very few relapse or recovery phases. In primary-progressive disease there are no recovery phases and almost no relapses, only a gradual, continual decline in functioning. There is also a phase called progressive relapsing in which there is an overall progressive decline in neurologic function from onset with short lived or acute relapse phases intertwined.

Early treatment with disease-modifying therapy including interferon beta-1b, interferon beta-1a, peginterferon beta-1a, glatiramer acetate, teriflunomide, dimethyl fumarate, cladribine, fingolimod, natalizumab, ocrelizumab, or alemtuzumab is strongly recommended for patients with active relapse remitting MS. As the medications have distinct side effects and contraindications, they may be selected based on the patient's comorbidities and characteristics. There is some evidence that IFN-beta-1a or 1b, mitoxantrone, ocrelizumab or cladribine are more effective for patients with active secondary-progressive MS and ocrelizumab for patients with primary-progressive MS.

Treatment of Exacerbations

The American Academy of Neurology recommends treating MS exacerbations, especially those that affect functional ability, with high dose corticosteroids such as IV **methylprednisone**. Steroids are used to reduce inflammation and edema at the areas of demyelination, decreasing exacerbations; however, they do not slow disease progression. Oral **prednisone** may, in some cases, be used instead of IV methylprednisone. Symptom improvement generally occurs within 3–5 days. Severe attacks that are characterized by varying degrees of paralysis that do not improve with steroid therapy may be treated with plasma exchange or IVIG.

Disease-Modifying Therapies (DMTs)

IFN-β is FDA-approved to treat MS, although its exact mechanism of action is not well understood for this disease. It is thought that IFN-β helps to improve the integrity of the blood-brain-barrier by downregulating matrix metalloproteinases, reducing the number of myelin-attacking lymphocytes which can cross the barrier. IFN-β may also decrease IFN-γ release by activated lymphocytes as well as enhance the activity of anti-inflammatory cells including T_{regs} and C56 bright NK cells. **IFN-beta-1b (Betaseron®)** is a synthetic analog of recombinant IFN-β and is given at home by subcutaneous injection to the patient every other day. **IFN-beta-1a (Avonex®,Rebif®)** is a glycosylated, natural sequence IFN. While Avonex® is given IM once a week, Rebif® is given subcutaneously three times a week. A pegylated form of **IFN-beta-1a (Plegridy®)**, consists of polyethylene glycol polymers attached to interferon, increasing its half-life and resulting in the less-frequent dosing of once every 2 weeks. Typical adverse effects associated with the IFNs include transient elevation of liver enzymes, redness and swelling at the injection site, and flu-like symptoms which generally decrease 1–3 months after the beginning of therapy.

Glatiramer acetate (Copaxone®) is a mixture of synthetic polypeptides containing four amino acids (L-glutamic acid, L-alanine, L-tyrosine, L-lysine). Antigens from glatiramer acetate can compete with myelin antigens for binding to MHC class II molecules, which may inhibit the activation of MBP-specific T cells. In addition, glatiramer acetate may induce T_{reg} differentiation through Foxp3 expression, reducing T cell-mediated damage against myelin. Common side effects include injection site reactions, flushing, chest tightness, palpitations, anxiety and shortness of breath.

Fingolimod (Gilenya®) is an oral agent that modulates sphingosine 1-phosphate receptor (S1P-R), blocking the capacity of lymphocytes to egress from lymph nodes and reducing lymphocyte numbers in peripheral blood. Fingolimod treatment induces a rapid and transient decrease in blood lymphocyte counts. As such, this decreases their ability to enter the CNS. Bradycardia is a major side effect of this drug, and it is recommended to obtain electrocardiogram (ECG) readings before and after taking the first dose due to potential atrioventricular conduction delays. It is contraindicated for patients with cardiac issues such as a history of myocardial infarction, stroke, or arrythmias. Other adverse effects include increased liver enzymes, macular edema, decreased respiratory capacity, increased risk of infection, and hypertension. Fingolimod should not be combined with ketoconazole, as ketoconazole will increase its blood levels. Another side effect is that fingolimod reduces the immune response to vaccination.

As mentioned previously, natalizumab (Tysabri®) is a monoclonal antibody raised against α_4 integrin, an adhesion molecule that facilitates the recruitment of immune cells into the CNS. The binding of natalizumab to these adhesion molecules therefore blocks immune cells from entering the CNS. This injectable drug is given once a month and has a black box warning for progressive multifocal leukoencephalopathy (PML), a progressive viral infection of the brain caused by the John Cunningham Virus (JCV). As mentioned previously, the TOUCH program ensures safe prescribing and dispensing of this medication. Other side effects include hypersensitivity reactions such as itchiness, dizziness, fever, rash, hypotension and anaphylaxis as well as liver injury and increased risk for infection.

Mitoxantrone (Novantrone®) is an anticancer drug that intercalates DNA, causing strand crosslinks and breaks. It also inhibits topoisomerase II which is responsible for uncoiling and repairing DNA. By suppressing the activity of all immune cells, mitoxantrone decreases myelin damage. Its drawback, however, is its many adverse effects which include GI side effects, heavy menstrual bleeding or secondary amenorrhea, hair loss, blue-green colored urine, or a blue tinge to the whites of the eyes. Cladribine is another anti-cancer drug that has shown efficacy in reducing MS relapses, specifically when combined with IFN-β therapy, but may come with a higher risk of developing lymphopenia.

An immunomodulatory drug known as **teriflunomide (Aubagio®)** reversibly inhibits dihydroorotate dehydrogenase, an enzyme responsible for the *de novo* synthesis of pyrimidines. In this manner, teriflunomide helps to reduce the number and activation of lymphocytes which may be propagating autoimmune responses. Teriflunomide is an active metabolite of leflunomide, which is used for treating RA. Following oral ingestion, leflunomide is converted to teriflunomide and has shown promise in the treatment of MS. In general, teriflunomide is well-tolerated and the most common adverse effects include nausea, diarrhea, alopecia, liver enzyme increase, paresthesia, and arthralgia.

Dimethyl fumarate (Tecfidera®), whose mechanism of action is largely unknown, is also used in MS due to evidence that it protects neural stem cells from oxidative damage via the Nrf2-ERK1/2 MAPK pathway. In addition, it promotes anti-inflammatory functions in immune cells. Adverse effects usually improve within a month and include increased liver enzymes, lymphocytopenia, GI effects, and flushing. These adverse effects can also be mitigated by taking Tecfidera® with a meal.

Alemtuzumab (Lemtrada®) is a humanized anti-CD52 monoclonal antibody for treatment of relapsing-remitting MS. CD52 is highly expressed on both T and B cells, and infusion of alemtuzumab results in the depletion of CD52+ lymphocytes through complement-mediated lysis and antibody-dependent cell-mediated cytotoxicity. When compared to IFN-β in phase III trials, alemtuzumab resulted in a significant reduction in MS relapses. While alemtuzumab has proven to be efficacious, it does come with significant risks. Infections of the respiratory tract and urinary tract are common, including herpes, spirochetal gingivitis, tuberculosis and esophageal candidiasis. Infusion-related reactions also occur in many patients, which are mitigated by concomitant administration with corticosteroids and antihistamines. Some patients also experience secondary autoimmunity, particularly in the thyroid (both hyperthyroidism and hypothyroidism).

Daclizumab (Zinbryta®) is a monoclonal antibody that binds to the alpha subunit of the IL-2 receptor, CD25, and was used as a treatment for relapsing MS. However, it was announced in early March 2018 that it would be withdrawn from the market after reported cases of serious inflammatory brain disorders in Europe including meningoencephalitis and encephalitis, with three of the cases ending in patient death.

Ocrelizumab (Ocrevus®) is a humanized monoclonal antibody against CD20 and is approved for treating relapsing or primary-progressive MS. In controlled trials, ocrelizumab treatment resulted in lower MS relapse rates compared to subcutaneous IFN-β. Depending on the symptoms of MS, symptomatic therapies may also be prescribed for sensory issues, tremors, fatigue, depression, or bladder issues.

Grave's Disease

Mechanisms

Graves' disease is an autoimmune disorder that affects thyroid function and is the most common cause of hyperthyroidism in the United States. The thyroid produces thyroxine (T4) and triiodothyronine (T3), hormones which regulate metabolism in several cell types through the induction of gene expression. The production of thyroid hormones is regulated by the hypothalamus producing thyrotropin-releasing hormone (TRH), which subsequently activates the anterior pituitary gland to secrete thyroid-stimulating hormone (TSH). Activation of the TSH receptor on thyroid follicular cells results in the production and iodination of thyroglobulin, the thyroid hormone precursor, as well as the release of free T4 and T3 molecules (Fig. 7.13). The TSH receptor is expressed also on adipocytes, fibroblasts and bone cells, although its primary physiological function is to stimulate thyroid hormone production and release. The maintenance of homeostatic

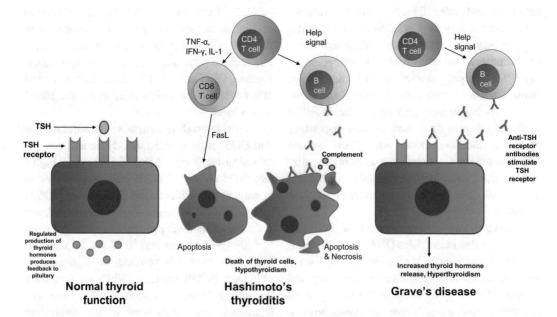

Fig. 7.13 Mechanisms of Hashimoto's and Grave's disease. In Hashimoto's thyroiditis, CD4 T cells which recognize thyroid cell antigens activate B cells to make antibodies resulting in thyroid cell apoptosis or necrosis. Similarly, CD8 T cells are aimed to induce apoptosis of thyroid cells via Fas-FasL signaling. In either situation, death of thyroid cells results in decreased thyroid hormones and hypothyroidism. In Grave's disease, CD4 T cells activate B cells to create antibodies against TSH receptor which stimulates the receptor signaling to increase release of thyroid hormone, resulting in hyperthyroidism

concentrations of thyroid hormones (T4 and T3) is regulated by negative feedback, as elevated levels are normally detected by the hypothalamus, resulting in decreased production of TRH. This, in turn, leads to decreased TSH release from the pituitary. Dysregulation of this hormonal pathway can lead to thyroid disorders including Grave's disease.

In Graves' disease, breakdowns in central and peripheral tolerance during B cell development results in the production of several autoantibodies. First, thyroid-stimulating immunoglobulins (TSI) bind to the TSHR, causing the thyroid to produce high levels of T3 and T4 hormones even in the absence of endogenous TSH. Second, thyroid growth immunoglobulins (TGI) can induce the growth of thyroid follicles by also binding to the TSHR. Lastly, thyrotropin binding-inhibiting immunoglobulins (TBII) block TSH from engaging with the TSHR. Due to elevated levels of thyroid hormones in the circulation, TSH production is shut down in the pituitary. The continued stimulation of thyroid gland growth and hormone release by autoantibodies leads to hyperthyroidism and the characteristic diffuse goiter presentation in patients. In addition to an enlarged thyroid gland, the disease is also characterized by a lymphocytic infiltration of the thyroid parenchyma and infiltration of retro-orbital and dermal tissues which can result in eye disease (Graves' ophthalmopathy), and occasionally pretibial myxedema or thickening of the skin, most often seen on the shins and tops of the feet.

Susceptibility to Graves' disease has been associated with several risk factors including certain HLA alleles, CD40 and the TSHR. In addition, multiple environmental factors have been suggested to contribute to the development of the disease including sex hormones, pregnancy, stress, other autoimmune disorders and previous infection. As with most autoimmune diseases, susceptibility is increased in females with onset typically occurring between 20 and 40 years of age.

Diagnostic blood tests in patients with Grave's disease typically show elevated levels of T3 and T4, low TSH levels, increased radioiodine uptake by the thyroid, and the presence of TSI

antibodies. Pathology shows lymphocytic infiltration in target organs along with the presence of antigen-reactive T and B cells. If left untreated, Graves' disease can cause severe thyrotoxicosis which could potentially lead to a life-threatening thyroid storm. Sustained severe thyrotoxicosis can cause substantial weight loss with possible catabolism of bone and muscle, resulting in brittle bones and muscle weakness. An increased heart rate is often observed, which may lead to additional heart complications.

Treatment

There are several treatment options for patients with Graves' disease including radioactive iodine therapy, anti-thyroid medications, beta blockers and surgical intervention. The most common treatment modality is radioactive iodine (RAI) which is given in capsule or water-based form and concentrates in the thyroid gland and destroys thyroid tissue. This treatment can lead to hypothyroidism as the tissue is destroyed and replacement thyroid hormone must be administered.

Anti-thyroid medications including **propylthiouracil (PTU)** and **methimazole (Tapazole®)** suppress thyroid hormone production by blocking the iodination of thyroglobulin by an enzyme named thyroperoxidase. PTU and methimazole inhibit the function of thyroperoxidase, resulting in decreased production of thyroid hormones. Side effects of both drugs include rash, joint pain, liver failure or a decrease in disease-fighting white blood cells. Relapse of hyperthyroidism may occur upon cessation of therapy.

Beta-blockers such as **atenolol (Tenormin®)**, **propranolol (Inderal®)**, **nadolol (Corgard®)** and **metoprolol (Lopressor®, Toprol-XL®)**, are often prescribed to alleviate the heart irregularities that often characterize Graves' disease.

Surgery can be performed to remove all or part of the thyroid (thyroidectomy or subtotal thyroidectomy). Thyroid hormone therapy is administered following the surgery. Risks of this surgery include potential damage to the nerve that controls your vocal cords and the parathyroid glands which assist in regulating calcium levels in the blood.

Hashimoto's Thyroiditis

Mechanisms

Hashimoto's disease is an autoimmune disorder that results in hypothyroidism or an underactive thyroid due to damage and inflammation caused by autoreactive immune cells (Fig. 7.13). This disease is also known clinically as Hashimoto's thyroiditis, chronic lymphocytic thyroiditis, or autoimmune thyroiditis. It is the most common cause of hypothyroidism in the United States, and women are 7–8 times more likely to get the disorder than men. Pregnancy also appears to play a role in development. Typically, patients present with symptoms between the ages of 30 and 60, although they can emerge at any age. In addition to gender being a risk factor, there is also a strong genetic predisposition to developing the disease, as individuals with a family history of the disease are far more likely to get the disease. Also, several immune-related and thyroid-specific genes have been linked to the development of Hashimoto's disease, including human leukocyte antigen (HLA), cytotoxic T lymphocyte antigen-4 (CTLA-4), protein tyrosine phosphatase nonreceptor-type 22 (PTPN22), thyroglobulin (Tg), vitamin D receptor (VDR), and several cytokines. It has been suggested that having a pre-existing autoimmune disorder such as celiac disease, Type 1 diabetes, Rheumatoid arthritis and vitiligo could enhance an individual's risk for developing Hashimoto's. Lastly, there have been several indications that environmental factors can also enhance an individual's risk for developing the disease such as previous viral infections, drug use including cytokines for the treatment of cancer along with excessive exposure to radiation, selenium deficiency and high iodine intake.

Both cellular and humoral arms of the immune system are implicated in the pathogenesis of Hashimoto's disease. Infiltration of both T and B cells has been noted as hallmarks of the thyroiditis pathology preceding the gradual destruction of thyroid parenchymal tissue. Some patients may also develop goiter as a result of the massive infiltration of T cells to the area. The sera from patients typically show thyroid autoantibodies (TAbs) against thyroperoxidase (TPO) and thyroglobulin (Tg). TPO is an enzyme required for thyroid hormone synthesis while Tg is a glycoprotein precursor that serves as a reservoir that can be processed into thyroid hormones for future use. The presence of autoantibodies alone is not sufficient to induce disease; however, they serve as diagnostic markers for patients with disease.

The precise mechanism for the development of the disease is not completely understood but it appears that individuals with the previously described genetic, endogenous and environmental triggers have greatly enhanced rates of autoantigen presentation by dendritic cells, macrophages and thyroid follicular cells to T and B cells. The resulting cytokines produced, (TNF-α, IFN-γ, IL-1) tip immunity towards a T_H1 response along with the activation of cytotoxic CD8 T cells. The cytotoxic actions of the T cells along with the autoantibody production by B cells and complement activation leads to the destruction of thyroid cells by apoptosis.

In addition to the goiter presentation, diagnosis is made by detecting levels of autoantibodies in the patient's serum and by measuring hormone levels. Although prognosis is good with treatment, an underactive thyroid gland (hypothyroidism) left untreated can lead to a number of health problems. The goiter can result in difficulty swallowing and breathing. Heart disease can develop due to heightened levels of LDL cholesterol. Mental health issues have been associated with the disease including depression and decrease in libido. Birth defects have been seen in women who are not treated and become pregnant. A life-threatening myxedema coma characterized by hypothermia, decreased mental status, and loss of organ function may also occur.

Treatment

Treatment for Hashimoto's disease typically includes thyroid hormone replacement for T4 and/or T3, with the treatment of choice a synthetic form of T4 or **thyroxine (levothyroxine)**. This medication is taken indefinitely, and in many cases for the life of the individual, in order to alleviate signs and symptoms of the disease. Dosages may be adjusted following close monitoring of the patient's TSH levels, which inversely correlate with serum concentrations of thyroid hormones.

Myasthenia Gravis

Mechanisms

The term **myasthenia gravis** refers to severe muscle weakness (i.e. myo = muscle, asthenia = weakness, gravis = severe), and is thus characterized by a progressive weakening of the muscles. Antibodies produced in patients with MG attack the postsynaptic membrane of the neuromuscular junction (NMJ). Muscle weakening may be generalized or localized; muscle weakness of the respiratory muscles can pose a life-threatening situation. Antibodies produced in MG patients are generally IgG1 and/or IgG3 against the **acetylcholine receptor (AChR)**. When these antibodies bind to the AChR and stimulate the complement system, damage ensues on the postsynaptic membrane of the receptor (Fig. 7.14). This impairs neuromuscular transmission, resulting in progressive muscle weakness and fatigue. A small percentage of patients exhibit autoantibodies against another target, the muscle-specific kinase (MUSK), which is a transmembrane tyrosine receptor necessary for the maintenance of AChR clusters at the NMJ. This alternative mechanism through which disease occurs has only begun to be elucidated. Studies of the genome have looked at predisposing factors and have suggested that among others, defects in the CTLA4 gene may be associated with the development of certain types of MG.

Treatment

The goal of therapy for Myasthenia gravis is to achieve sustained remission. Treatment strategies may depend on patient age and disease severity. Acetylcholinesterase inhibitors are often used as first-line agents for symptoms associated with Myasthenia gravis, the main medication being **pyridostigmine bromide**. Acetylcholinesterase inhibitors slow down the degradation of acetylcholine (ACh) that occurs at the neuromuscular junction, prolonging the activity of ACh and providing a significant improvement in many patients.

Immunosuppressant agents used as second-line therapies in MG include azathioprine, mycophenolate mofetil, and cyclosporine.

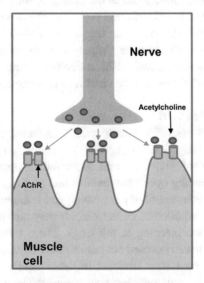

Normal muscle activation

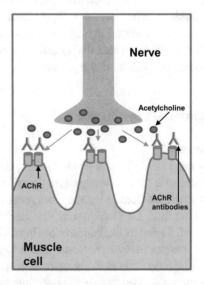

Impaired muscle activation

Fig. 7.14 The neurotransmitter acetylcholine is normally involved in communication between nerves and muscles at the neuromuscular junction. In Myasthenia gravis, acetylcholine receptor antibodies block acetylcholine from binding to its receptor on the muscle cell, resulting in impaired muscle activation and muscle weakness. Credit: CDC/Dr. J. Lieberman; Dr. Freideen Farzin, Univ. of Tehran

Glucocorticoids provide remission for approximately 30% of patients. Roughly half of patients on glucocorticoids experience at least a significant improvement in their symptoms. Relief of symptoms can take 2–3 weeks, unless high-dose glucocorticoids are initiated (usually only in the hospital setting). High-dose glucocorticoids are associated with a transient deterioration in about half of MG patients 5–10 days after initiation. This transient worsening only lasts for approximately 5–6 days.

Rapid immunomodulating agents are used because they begin to provide relief in just a few days. Intravenous immune globulin (IVIG) is immunoglobulin pooled from thousands of healthy donors. While the mechanism is unclear in MG, patients treated with IVIG experience improvement in their symptoms.

Plasmapheresis, or plasma exchange to remove autoantibodies, is another treatment that has a quicker onset of relief. This treatment consists of 5 exchanges of plasma over 1–2 weeks to remove anti-ACh antibodies. Improvement in symptoms correlates with a reduction in antibody levels. Combining this treatment with prednisone and azathioprine has been suggested to produce clinical improvement (sustained decrease in AChR titers) in refractory MG. While improvement can be experienced in only a few days, this benefit only last 3–6 weeks due to anti-ACh antibodies building back up in the plasma.

Goodpasture's Syndrome

Mechanisms

During the 1919 influenza pandemic, physician and pathologist Ernest Goodpasture described a patient who died from pulmonary and renal disease. At the time, Dr. Goodpasture was studying the Spanish flu and its likelihood of having a viral etiology, despite many hypotheses that it was a bacterial infection due to many cases of secondary pneumonia. He presented two influenza patients in his 1919 paper who tested negative for bacteria. One of these patients had exhibited pulmonary hemorrhage consistent with the flu, but also glomerular inflammation. While it cannot be verified that this patient had this pulmonary/renal

syndrome, the association between Goodpasture and this disease persists (even with the suggestion that Dr. Goodpasture did not approve of this association). **Goodpasture's syndrome** is characterized by autoantibodies produced against extracellular matrix, specifically the $\alpha 3$ chain of type IV collagen, mainly found in the basement membranes of the lungs and kidneys. IgG in particular binds in the basement membrane of renal glomeruli. For this reason, these antibodies are often referred to as **anti-glomerular basement membrane (anti-GBM)** antibodies. Because these antibodies bind in the renal glomeruli as well as the renal tubules, resultant inflammation causes renal impairment. It is not known if the 1919 patient had anti-GBM, thus the possible misnomer.

Studied risk factors include smoking, hair dying, exposure to metallic dust, and cocaine use, as well as genetic factors. General symptoms of Goodpasture's syndrome include fatigue, nausea, vomiting, and weakness. Symptoms indicating inflammation in the lungs include shortness of breath and coughing with or without blood. Renal symptoms include bloody or foamy urine, swelling of the legs, and high blood pressure. Goodpasture's can be diagnosed by the presence of red blood cells and protein in the urine, anti-GBM antibodies in the blood, and a kidney biopsy to visualize glomerular changes and the presence of anti-GBM antibodies. Lung abnormalities may also be visualized on a chest X-Ray.

Treatment

Treatment for Goodpasture's includes plasma exchange (plasmapheresis) to remove offending autoantibodies as well as immunosuppressants including cyclophosphamide and corticosteroids to reduce antibody formation and inflammation. The addition of corticosteroids may also help to reduce bleeding in the lungs. These treatments are usually carried out until anti-GBM antibodies are no longer detected in the patient's serum. While rituximab has been suggested as a possibility because it results in B cell depletion, it would need to be initiated very early due to the fact that this disease can progress rapidly. Thus, it is not an ideal option for primary induction therapy.

Pemphigus Vulgaris

Mechanisms

Pemphigus is a group of potentially life-threatening autoimmune diseases characterized by epithelial blistering affecting the cutaneous and mucosal lining. Pemphigus affects the skin and has also been seen to affect the mouth (Fig. 7.15), nose, conjunctivae, genitals, esophagus, pharynx and larynx. **Pemphigus vulgaris** is the most common variant and most often affects the mouth. This disorder mainly targets middle-aged and elderly patient populations, and once again, as in other autoimmune disorders, there has been a higher incidence in women. Genetics also certainly plays a role as there is a fairly strong linkage to developing the disease in certain ethnic groups including Ashkenazi Jews and those of Mediterranean descent. Other factors which can predispose individuals to develop the disorder can include prior infections with viruses including herpesviruses, the existence of additional autoimmune disorders such as myasthenia gravis, rheumatoid arthritis and lupus, and the use of some pharmaceutical drugs containing either sulfhydryl radicals or nonthiol drugs.

The symptoms of pemphigus vulgaris include the presentation of blisters that start in the mouth or skin areas. These blisters appear near the surface of the skin and can come and go and can be itchy or painful. The blisters often test positive for Nikolsky's sign in which the skin shears off at the touch. A punch biopsy of the lesion is done followed by immunofluorescent staining to look for the presences of autoantibodies to ultimately confirm diagnosis.

The epithelium, which is grossly affected by this disease, is a complex structure made of many cell types including keratinocytes, which adhere to each other by desmosomes. These desmosomes, or adhesive proteins, provide the architectural support and integrity the epithelial layer requires given its function in the body. Pemphigus vulgaris is initiated by the production of autoantibodies against epithelial intercellular adhesion components, including cadherins, and desmogleins 1 and 3 (Dsg1 and Dsg3). The production of these autoantibodies damages the desmosomes and cell-cell adhesion in the epithelial layer is often lost leading to intra-epithelial vesiculation and the presentation of the characteristic sores and blisters. The presentation of the disease can be attributed to the presence of these autoantibodies as seen by transfer experiments in mice with these circulating IgG antibodies.

The role of cellular immunity is unclear despite the moderate infiltration of CD4 T cells that are reactive to Dsg3. In addition, there is a strong association between certain human leukocyte antigen (HLA) class II alleles and susceptibility to pemphigus vulgaris. The autoreactive CD4 T cells predominantly produce T_H2 cytokines including IL-4, IL-6 and IL-10. Studies are currently being done to investigate the role of

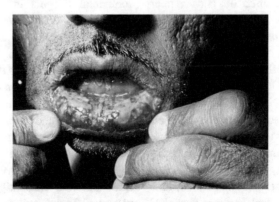

Fig. 7.15 This photo depicts intraoral lesions on the lower lip of a patient diagnosed with pemphigus vulgaris. These painful lesions, upon presentation, had been present for 3 years and were covered with grayish-white membranes. Underneath the membranes were red sores. Credit: CDC/Dr. J. Lieberman; Dr. Freideen Farzin, Univ. of Tehran, https://phil.cdc.gov/

cellular immunity despite the clarity that the humoral response directly leads to the presentation of the disease.

Treatment

Corticosteroids including prednisone have been effective in the treatment of pemphigus vulgaris and are given both systemically and locally. In addition to limiting inflammation, it is thought that these corticosteroids perhaps increase the production of desmogleins and help to restore adhesion despite the continual production of antibodies to Dsg3 and Dsg1. General immunosuppressants such as such as azathioprine and mycophenolate mofetil are also given to patients to minimize immune responses.

Rituximab administration is also commonly used for treatment and leads to a depletion of CD20+ peripheral B cells and a concurrent decrease in Dsg1 and Dsg3 antibodies in the serum of patients. Once used as a second-line treatment, anti-CD20 therapy is now often considered for first-line therapy since it is more successful if initiated early in the course of disease, perhaps even at diagnosis. Remission is often seen after administration of one round of treatment in a number of patients.

Acute Rheumatic Fever

Mechanisms

Acute rheumatic fever (ARF) occurs secondary to Group A streptococcal infections and can manifest as carditis, arthritis, involuntary movements (chorea), red pink rings on the skin known as erythema marginatum, or subcutaneous nodules. Due to effective antibiotic treatments and improved sanitation, ARF is less common in developed countries. It is uncertain why some individuals are more susceptible than others, but genetics, including class II HLA antigens may play a role. Certain immune genes for chemotaxis and apoptosis may also be associated. In order to resolve a streptococcal infection, antibodies against streptococcal antigens including M proteins are produced. It is thought that these antibodies, based on molecular mimicry, may

also be capable of binding to certain autoantigens including those in the brain and the heart, resulting in inflammation.

Treatment

Patients presenting with symptoms of ARF are usually hospitalized for observation and further investigation of symptoms. Antibiotics against *Streptococcus pyogenes* are administered to eradicate any persistent infection. Patients are also treated for arthritis and/or carditis, as well as other symptoms.

Type I Diabetes Mellitus

Mechanisms

While **Type 1 diabetes mellitus (T1D)** is normally diagnosed in childhood, it can occur at any age. Type 1 diabetes, as opposed to Type 2, is classified as an autoimmune disease in which T cells destroy pancreatic insulin-producing β cells in the islets of Langerhans. It is thought that the underlying mechanisms are not only genetic but also environmental. Expression of HLA DR3/DQ2 and DR4/DQ8 have been found to be highly correlated with Type 1 diabetes. Non-HLA genes that are associated with higher T1D risk often include genes encoding for insulin, CTLA-4 and FOXP3. These genes may have variable numbers of tandem nucleotide repeats in their coding region, resulting in decreased expression. Some evidence suggests that environmental triggers in genetically-predisposed individuals, such as infections with enteroviruses (Coxsackie B4) and congenital rubella, precipitate the disease. Viruses may promote damage to the pancreas through direct infection resulting in immune attack, molecular mimicry (cross-reactivity of lymphocytes to viral and autoantigens) and enhancing the function of APCs presenting autoantigens. Individuals who develop T1D as a result of breaches in tolerance to islet antigens may have autoantibodies against three possible autoantigens expressed in the pancreas. These include insulin, glutamic acid decarboxylase (GAD), or islet-associated antigen (IA-2).

Studies in both humans and mice suggest autoreactive lymphocytes, specifically CD8 T cells, are responsible for the destruction of β cells, likely through a Fas-FasL apoptotic pathway. Evidence suggests that CD8 T cells also utilize perforin for β-cell killing and release large amounts of pro-inflammatory cytokines including IFN-γ. While it is clear that T cells play a role in T1D, evidence also suggests there is a humoral component. Islet-specific autoantibodies are a hallmark of T1D and are detectable in the prediabetic stage in approximately 90% of affected individuals.

Treatment

Like Type 2 Diabetes, treatment of Type 1 Diabetes aims to manage blood sugar levels through diet, exercise, and insulin therapy. Despite the mechanism being autoimmune in nature, the immune system is generally not a target of therapy when treating T1D since the pancreatic β cells that are destroyed cannot be replenished. Pharmacological therapies can include various types of insulin.

Autoimmune Hemolytic Anemia

Mechanisms

Autoimmune hemolytic anemia (AIHA) is a relatively uncommon disorder which corresponds to Type II hypersensitivity where either IgG or IgM antibodies bind to the surface of red blood cells. This binding activates the classical complement cascade and membrane attack complex (C5-9), causing red blood cells to lyse. Additionally, this may result in the coating of red blood cells by complement C3 and antibodies, resulting in their opsonization and clearance by phagocytes whose Fc receptors recognize these red blood cells as being tagged for removal. Both of these mechanisms result in a decrease in red blood cell counts, resulting in anemia. Diagnosis can be made based on the presence of anti-erythrocyte antibodies as detected by a direct antiglobulin test (DAT). AIHA can be furthered classified into warm antibody AIHA (which accounts for approximately 80–90% of adult cases), and cold-reactive (cryopathic hemolytic syndrome). These two classifications are based on the temperature at which the autoantibodies bind to RBCs. In warm AIHA, optimal binding and resultant hemolysis occurs at 37 °C (98.6 °F, or normal body temperature). DAT is usually positive for IgG antisera, and sometimes anti-C3d. In cryopathic hemolytic syndrome, also known as cold hemagglutinin disease, antibody binding (usually IgM) occurs below normal body temperature. Children may be more likely to experience cold antibody binding of the IgG isotype. Patients with mixed warm and cold AIHA are rare. In approximately half of all cases AIHA is idiopathic in nature but it can also be secondary to lymphoproliferative syndromes or other autoimmune diseases, or even infection.

Treatment

Corticosteroids such as prednisone or prednisolone are first-line treatments for warm AIHA, with 70–85% of patients achieving a response. Corticosteroids should be tapered over 6–12 months, with a minimum of 3–4 months. Relapse seems to occur less frequently in patients who have received low dose prednisone for longer than 6 months, and when steroid therapy is started early. Long-term remission after discontinuing the steroid occurs in approximately 1 out of 3 patients.

Rituximab has been used with good results in warm antibody AIHA, especially when used in combination with prednisolone. This combination yielded a good response after 12 months in 75% of the patients, with 70% of patients still in remission 36 months later. Cyclosporine and azathioprine have also been used with good results, albeit in small groups of patients. Additionally, while IVIG has been used in AIHA patients, only a handful have had a response to this treatment.

Folic acid may be used as a supplement in AIHA since active hemolysis consumes folic acid, resulting in megaloblastosis (anemia resulting from folate and vitamin B12 deficiency). Supportive therapy, including blood transfusions to maintain hemoglobin levels may be required, and may be based on the patient's symptoms and severity of anemia/hemolysis.

In refractory AIHA, splenectomy is a second-line treatment for patients with warm AIHA. While some patients have obtained partial or complete remission, it is difficult to predict outcomes for every patient.

While treatment for AIHA is still not evidence-based, some immunomodulatory drugs have been used as last resort treatments with mixed results. High dose cyclophosphamide is one of these last resort treatments, as is alemtuzumab and ofatumumab. Similarly, as there are no true evidence-based recommendations for cold AIHA, treatment of the underlying disease is common, including protection of the patient against cold temperatures, or transfusion(s) during the winter months. Steroid use in cold AIHA is still controversial as this practice hasn't been supported with systematic evidence. The decision to treat will likely be based on symptoms of anemia or other circulatory symptoms.

Immune Thrombocytopenia Purpura

Mechanisms

Immune thrombocytopenia purpura (ITP) is a disorder characterized by excessive bleeding or bruising due to low levels of platelets. Purpura are small bruises caused by bleeding of small blood vessels under the skin. These can also be seen in the mouth. Some patients with ITP may also exhibit small red dots on the skin resembling a rash. These are known as petechiae. There are two types of ITP, acute and chronic. Acute ITP primarily affects children and generally lasts for less than 6 months. It is the most common type of ITP and often occurs after a viral infection. Mild cases generally do not require treatment, and platelet levels go back up on their own within a few months. If treatment is warranted, the type of treatment depends on platelet count and severity of bleeding. Chronic ITP generally affects adults and lasts for more than 6 months. It has been found that women are 2–3 times more likely to have ITP than men. Causes often point to an autoimmune response leading to destruction of platelets. Some cases have been linked to HIV,

Hepatitis C, or *Helicobacter pylori* infection, suggesting that the immune response triggered by infection may continue and attack self-antigens due to cross-reactivity to antigens through molecular mimicry. Successful treatment of these infections often correlates with increasing platelets and a decreasing severity of bleeding. It is thought that the autoimmune response mounted against platelets is both antibody and T-cell mediated. With regard to antibody-mediated destruction, IgGs targeting glycoproteins on the surfaces of platelets and megakaryocytes will bind to the surfaces of these cells, and upon recognition by Fc receptors on phagocytes, will ultimately undergo phagocytosis. This destruction of platelets and megakaryocytes by phagocytes appears to occur mainly in the spleen. Interestingly, 30–40% of patients with ITP do not exhibit detectable levels of autoantibodies against platelets, suggesting a T-cell mediated mechanism. In this case, antigen presenting cells would degrade platelets and present their antigens to T cells. In accordance with this, some ITP patients exhibit higher levels of reactive T helper cells (which may release IL-2), higher levels of CD8 T cells (which can directly lyse platelets), or even lower levels of CD25+ Foxp3+ regulatory T cells. Lower levels of T_{regs} that can interact with APCs and inhibit the activities of B cells as well as CD8 T cells can contribute to a decrease in self-tolerance seen in ITP.

Treatment

Treatment is determined based on severity of bleeding and platelet count. Mild cases may not need treatment. Since it is thought that destruction of platelets is a result of autoimmune attack, prednisone to decrease inflammation is often the first line for children and adults requiring treatment. Prednisone may be given with or without IVIG or Anti-Rh (D) immunoglobulin. Although IVIG mechanisms are not well understood, it is thought that IVIG saturates Fc receptor on phagocytes, thus decreasing the phagocytosis of platelets. IVIG treatment may also decrease C-reactive protein, which appears to exacerbate antibody-mediated platelet destruction. Thus, IVIG can help to increase platelet levels and decrease bleeding. Rituximab may be considered as a second-line immunosuppressive agent for depleting B cells that are producing autoantibodies against platelets.

Since antibodies are made in the spleen which may mistakenly destroy platelets, splenectomy is another option to treat ITP, especially if the disorder has not responded to pharmacological treatment. The downside to removing the spleen is that it raises the patient's risk of infection.

Thrombopoietin receptor agonists including **eltrombopag** or **romiplostim** to increase the numbers of circulating platelets are considered third-line treatments.

Platelet transfusions may be given to patients with severe bleeding or for patients who are having surgery, temporarily raising platelet counts. Patients with ITP should avoid taking medications that raise the risk of bleeding or lower platelet counts, including aspirin and ibuprofen.

From Bench to Bedside: Development of Methotrexate Therapy

Methotrexate is considered to be a landmark drug—one that evolved from a cancer treatment to a treatment for autoimmune diseases including Rheumatoid arthritis. Methotrexate was discovered in the late 1940s and pursued for its folate-reducing properties. At the time, research had shown that folic acid deficiency decreased the synthesis of purines and pyrimidines in actively dividing cells and resulted in a decrease in leukemia cells. As such, drugs such as aminopterin, a dihydrofolate reductase inhibitor, showed promise in acute lymphoblastic leukemia. A 1951 study conducted in RA, psoriasis, and psoriatic arthritis patients showed rapid improvements in symptoms in response to aminopterin. Major drawbacks to aminopterin were its toxicity and difficulty in being manufactured. For these reasons, researchers at Lederle laboratories continued their search for folate analogues which would reduce folic acid, and thus cancer cells, with fewer toxic effects. Aminopterin was subsequently modified to a compound that was easier to synthesize, named methotrexate. Corticosteroids were studied in RA patients at the same time as folate-reducing drugs, and the enthusiasm of rheumatologists for corticosteroids was far greater than their interest in aminopterin and methotrexate. It wasn't until 1962 that positive results for methotrexate were reported in an NIH study for RA and psoriatic arthritis. In the 1960s, methotrexate was also becoming a popular choice for cancer treatments including advanced breast, lymphoma, and bladder cancer. At that time, the combination of cyclophosphamide, methotrexate, and fluorouracil (CMF) was considered a breakthrough adjuvant treatment in operable breast cancers.

Ten years later, a rheumatologist named Rex Hoffmeister studied 10–15 mg/week doses of methotrexate in 29 of his RA patients. Out of the 29 patients in this study, 14 had moderate clinical improvements in their RA symptoms, and 11 had major improvements. Unfortunately, this study was never published due to negative feedback at the National American Rheumatism Association meeting, as rheumatologists were very much against using a cancer drug in RA. Dr. Hoffmeister expanded his study to 78 patients, however, and finally published his results in 1983, noting that 58% of his patients exhibited a significant improvement in their RA symptoms, with 36% in complete remission. This published report led to other rheumatologists using MTX in their RA patients and generating positive results. Most of these treatments were reserved for patients who had failed the commonly used DMARDs at the time (sulfasalazine, gold, and penicillamine).

In the mid-1980s, placebo-controlled trials in RA were finally performed with positive results over placebo. Based on data obtained from these studies, the FDA approved MTX to be used as therapy for RA in 1988. Follow-up comparator studies and long-term experiences led

MTX to become the standard of care in RA in the early 1990s. It was reasonably tolerated, clinically effective in reducing symptoms, and was shown to slow the progression of joint damage seen on radiograph. The most notable adverse effects included GI upset, fatigue, and dizziness. Folic acid supplementation aided in diminishing some of these adverse effects.

Subsequent studies of methotrexate included combination therapies with cyclosporine, sulfasalazine, or hydroxychloroquine, and concluded that combinations tended to be more efficacious than MTX monotherapy. With the arrival of biologic treatments in the mid-1990s, head-to-head studies compared the efficacy of TNF inhibitors to methotrexate- the first being the Early Rheumatoid Arthritis study which evaluated 632 patients using either subcutaneous etanercept or oral methotrexate. Unsurprisingly, etanercept was able to yield a faster clinical response and an even better effect on radiographic joint progression. Further combination studies demonstrated that a TNF inhibitor plus methotrexate yielded better responses than MTX monotherapy. Because of the high cost of biologics, patients may only receive the addition of a biologic to their initial MTX treatment if they do not achieve enough of a clinical response on the much less expensive MTX monotherapy. This tends to be true in approximately two-thirds of patients who have started MTX. While methotrexate has essentially been replaced by newer therapies in cancer treatment, it is still a mainstay of therapy for patients with RA.

Summary

Autoimmunity can occur due to a lack of tolerance to self during immune cell development. Regulatory T cells (T_{regs}) appear to be critical in the maintenance of self-tolerance, and thus autoimmunity may be more likely to occur due to a shift in the balance of T_H17/T_{regs}. Some autoimmune disorders result from the generation of autoreactive T cells, autoantibodies from autoreactive B cells, or a combination of both. Many of these correspond to hypersensitivities II, III, and IV, depending on the mechanisms involved. SLE, for example, is an autoimmune disorder that corresponds to Hypersensitivity type III due to the formation of immune complexes that deposit in the kidneys, skin, or joints. Type I diabetes mellitus, on the other hand, is an example of an autoimmune disorder in which autoreactive T cells attack pancreatic insulin-producing beta cells in the islets of Langerhans. Most treatment strategies for autoimmunity are aimed at suppressing the immune response and may be T cell specific, B cell specific or global immunosuppressants, while some therapies treat the symptoms associated with the disorder. When the goal is to suppress the immune system, some immunomodulatory drugs may suppress the actions of both actively dividing B and T cells. As expected, many of these treatments come with increased risk of infection to the patient. Since many of the immunomodulatory drugs are cytotoxic in nature for suppressing rapidly dividing lymphocytes, they are also considered to be teratogenic in nature and should not be used during pregnancy.

Case Study: Myasthenia Gravis

Provided by Michele Riccardi, PharmD, BCPS

Samantha Moore is a 32-year-old woman who works as a data analyst at a big corporation. She was diagnosed with myasthenia gravis 2 years ago. Over the past 2 years, Samantha was treated for myasthenia gravis with various medications but developed medication allergies to mycophenolate, corticosteroids and pyridostigmine. She had been treated with IVIG for the past year, with a good response. Today Samantha presents to the emergency department complaining of exhaustion, shortness of breath, difficulty walking, and cramping of her muscles for the past week. She has a history of droopy eyelids, double vision and heavy limbs.

Her past medical history includes, Myasthenia Gravis, dysphagia, chronic pain, neck pain and occipital neuralgia. **Her medication allergies include**: Mycophenolate (rash), corticosteroids (anaphylaxis), pyridostigmine (reaction unknown). Her hemoglobin was 12.5 g/dL, and her hematocrit was 36.1%. Her WBC count was 4800 cells/uL, platelets 210,000. Electrolytes are normal.

Medications:	Alprazolam 0.25 mg tid prn
	Neurontin 600 mg tid
	Percocet 1 tablet q4h prn pain
	IVIG (last dose over a month ago received as an outpatient)
Family history:	Sister has Myasthenia Gravis
Social history:	Lives at home married has one child
	Occasional alcohol use
	No tobacco use
Physical Exam:	Positive for shortness of breath and feeling tired
	Blood pressure: 106/51
	Pulse 75
	Temp 97
	Respirations 19
	Weight: 115 lb
	Height: 5′4″

Questions

1. Based on this patient's presenting symptoms in the emergency room, are they related to her myasthenia gravis?
2. How should this patient's MG deterioration be treated?
3. The hospital neurologist decided to initiate IVIG for this patient. How might IVIG work in this case?
4. What are the side effects of IVIG, and should patients receive premedication?
5. How should this patient be monitored?
6. Prior to discharge Samantha's medications for MG are evaluated. Several medication allergies are noted. Would IVIG be appropriate for chronic treatment of MG?
7. Can immunoglobulin be administered by another route (other than IV) for MG?
8. What other clinical information would be helpful in evaluating this patient's MG?

Case Study: Rheumatoid Arthritis

Provided by Michele Riccardi, PharmD, BCPS

First Visit

Rebecca Price is a 35-year-old patient with a history of rheumatoid arthritis for the past 2 years. Today she presents for a follow up visit with her rheumatologist Dr. Sampson. Upon examination the patient's temperature, blood pressure and pulse were normal. Her review of systems is normal with the exception of musculoskeletal findings. There is joint pain located in the wrists and ankles the left and her morning stiffness is reported to be about 5 min. Swelling of her fingers have gone down since her last visit. Motor strength of all extremities is noted to be equal. Her complete blood count and electrolytes were normal as well as her calcium, magnesium and phosphorus levels. She is positive for anti-cyclic citrullinated peptide (CCP) antibodies and rheumatoid factor. Her labs include a complete blood count, electrolytes and glucose which are all normal. Hair pull test is negative. She drinks alcohol rarely and does not smoke. She is allergic to "sulfa" drugs. Due to continuing symptoms of morning stiffness, joint pain and swelling she was initiated on subcutaneous golimumab 3 weeks ago. Recently she was able to decrease her prednisone to 5 mg daily. Her current medications include golimumab 50 mg subcutaneous once monthly, prednisone 5 mg orally once daily, duloxetine 30 mg orally once daily, diclofenac 75 mg orally once daily, protonix 40 mg orally once daily, methotrexate 12.5 mg orally once a week and sulfasalazine 500 mg orally 2 tablets twice daily.

Questions

This patient is positive for anti-cyclic citrullinated peptide (CCP) antibodies and rheumatoid factor, what does this indicate?

This patient is receiving methotrexate; should a folic acid supplement be prescribed? Why or why not?

Despite being on two DMARD medications, is the initiation of golimumab appropriate?

How should this patient be monitored while receiving DMARD medications and golimumab?

Should this patient's "sulfa" allergy be further clarified?

Second Visit-2 Months Later

Rebecca Price presents for a follow up visit for RA. Her complete blood count and electrolytes are normal. Rebecca requests to discontinue golimumab treatment because of increased RA symptoms. She reports that she needs a least 20 mg of prednisone to be comfortable. Her morning stiffness is 10 min and she has joint pain in her wrists ankles and hands. Her exam is normal with the exception of the musculoskeletal findings.

Can this patient's golimumab be discontinued? Can another TNF-α inhibitor or a non-TNF biologic be trialed?

Rebecca's golimumab was discontinued and she was prescribed tocilizumab. What is the mechanism of action of tocilizumab and how is it administered?

What are the side effects of tocilizumab and how should this patient be monitored?

Practice Questions

1. Which of the following is a JAK-STAT signaling inhibitor?
   (a) Tofacitinib
   (b) Abatacept
   (c) Ustekinumab
   (d) Rituximab
2. Side effects of methotrexate may be alleviated by which of the following?
   (a) Supplementation with vitamin D
   (b) Supplementation with folic acid
   (c) Supplementation with vitamin C
   (d) By adding a biologic to the therapy
3. SLE is characterized by immune complexes and correlates with Hypersensitivity Type ____.
   (a) I
   (b) II
   (c) III
   (d) IV
4. All of the following are correct statements about rheumatoid arthritis except:
   (a) Osteoclasts may be activated by IL-17 to break down bone.
   (b) Smoking is an environmental factor which may increase a person's risk of RA.
   (c) RA antibodies are found only in the synovium of the joint.
   (d) RA is mainly considered to be a B cell disease which produces antibodies against joint components.
5. Loss of Foxp3 function is associated with which of the following disorders?
   (a) IPEX
   (b) APECED
   (c) AIHA
6. Which of the following statements is true concerning Grave's disease?
   (a) Autoantibodies bind to and stimulate TSH receptor.
   (b) Autoantibodies block thyroid hormone resulting in underactive thyroid.
   (c) Autoantibodies bind to AchR resulting in muscle weakening and fatigue.
   (d) Autoantibodies bind to red blood cells resulting in fatigue and malaise.

7. Which of the following is NOT an IL-17 inhibitor?
   (a) Brodalumab
   (b) Secukinumab
   (c) Ixekizumab
   (d) Guselkumab
8. Anti-CCP antibodies are associated with which autoimmune disease?
   (a) Rheumatoid arthritis
   (b) Psoriasis
   (c) Systemic lupus erythematosus
   (d) Hashimoto's
9. This monoclonal antibody can be used for B-cell depletion but may also cause a severe infusion reaction:
   (a) Siltuximab
   (b) Infliximab
   (c) Rituximab
   (d) Tocilizumab
10. Which of the following disease modifying therapies may be indicated for treatment of MS? (Select all that apply)
    (a) Teriflunomide
    (b) Adalimumab
    (c) Natalizumab
    (d) Alemtuzumab
    (e) IFN-β
11. This drug is considered to be one of the safest DMARDs and is thought to affect antigen processing in APCs.
    (a) Sulfasalazine
    (b) Methotrexate
    (c) Cyclophosphamide
    (d) Hydroxychloroquine
12. Sulfasalazine is reduced in the gut to sulfapyridine and _____, which stays in the colon and doesn't enter the bloodstream.
    (a) 6-Mercaptopurine
    (b) Azathioprine
    (c) 5-Aminosalicylic acid
    (d) Sirolimus
13. This drug is currently the only biologic FDA-approved for SLE.
    (a) Tocilizumab
    (b) Belimumab
    (c) Rituximab
    (d) Ustekinumab

14. Which of the following autoimmune disorders is caused by autoantibodies against the acetylcholine receptor, resulting in progressive muscle weakening?
    (a) Grave's disease
    (b) Pemphigus vulgaris
    (c) Hashimoto's
    (d) Myasthenia gravis
15. Which of the following autoimmune diseases affect the thyroid? (Select all that apply)
    (a) Grave's disease
    (b) Hashimoto's
    (c) Goodpasture's
    (d) Myasthenia gravis

Suggested Reading

Amano Y, Lee SW, Allison AC. Inhibition by glucocorticoids of the formation of interleukin-1 alpha, interleukin-1 beta, and interleukin 6: mediation by decreased mRNA stability. Mol Pharmacol. 1993;43:176–82.

Barnes PJ, Adock IM. Glucocorticoid resistance in inflammatory diseases. Lancet. 2009;373:1905–17.

Berrebi D, Bruscoli S, Cohen N, Foussat A, Migliorati G, Bouchet-Delbos L, Maillot MC, Portier A, Couderc J, Galanaud P, Peuchmaur M, Riccardi C, Emilie D. Synthesis of glucocorticoid-induced leucine zipper (GILZ) by macrophages: an anti-inflammatory and immunosuppressive mechanism shared by glucocorticoids and IL-10. Blood. 2003;101:729–38.

Boyapati R, Satsangi J, Ho GT. Pathogenesis of Crohn's disease. F1000 Prime Rep. 2015;7:44.

Bresson D, von Herrath M. Mechanisms underlying type 1 diabetes. Drug Discovery Today Dis Mech. 2004;1(4):321–7.

Brian J. From cancer to rheumatoid arthritis treatment: the story of methotrexate. Pharm J. 2012.

Cheung TT, McInnes IB. Future therapeutic targets in rheumatoid arthritis? Semin Immunopathol. 2017;39(4):487–500.

Choi J, Kim ST, Craft J. The pathogenesis of systemic lupus erythematosus-an update. Curr Opin Immunol. 2012;24(6):651–7.

Corthay A. How do regulatory T cells work? Scan J Immunol. 2009;70(4):326–36.

Couser WG. Pathogenesis and treatment of glomerulonephritis—an update. J Bras Nefrol. 2016;38(1):107–22.

Cruz da Silva J, Mariz HA, da Rocha LF, de Oliveira PS, Dantas AT, Duarte AL, et al. Hydroxychloroquine decreased Th17-related cytokines in systemic lupus erythematosus and rheumatoid arthritis patients. Clinics (Sao Paulo). 2013;68(6):766–71.

Dierickx D, Kentos A, Delannoy A. The role of rituximab in adults with warm antibody autoimmune hemolytic anemia. Blood. 2015;15:3223–9.

Dong C. Targeting Th17 cells in immune disease. Cell Res. 2014;24:901–3.

Farrell RJ, Kelleher D. Glucocorticoid resistance in inflammatory bowel disease. J Endocrinol. 2003;178:339–46.

Fasching P, Stradner M, Graninger W, Dejaco C, Fessler J. Therapeutic potential of targeting the Th17/Treg axis in autoimmune disorders. Molecules. 2017;22(1):E134.

Fox R. Mechanism of action of hydroxychloroquine as an antirheumatic drug. Semin Arthritis Rheum. 1993;2(1):82–91.

Ge WS, Fan JG. Integrin antagonists are effective and safe for Crohn's disease: a meta-analysis. World J Gastroenterol. 2015;21(15):4744–9.

Gracia-Tello B, Ezeonyeji A, Isenberg D. The use of rituximab in newly-diagnosed patients with systemic lupus erythematosus: long-term steroid-saving capacity and clinical effectiveness. Lupus Sci Med. 2017;4(1):e000182.

Haanstra KG, Hofman SO, Lopes Estêvão DM, Blezer EL, Bauer J, Yang LL, et al. Antagonizing the α4β1 integrin, but not α4β7, inhibits leukocytic infiltration of the central nervous system in rhesus monkey experimental autoimmune encephalomyelitis. J Immunol. 2013;190(5):1961–73.

Howard JF. Myasthenia gravis: a manual for the health care provider. St. Paul, MN: Myasthenia Gravis Foundation of America; 2008.

Huennekens FM. The methotrexate story: a paradigm for development of chemotherapeutic agents. Adv Enzym Regul. 1994;34:397–419.

Kuhn A, Bonsmann G, Anders HJ, Herzer P, Tenbrock K, Schneider M. The diagnosis and treatment of systemic lupus erythematosus. Dtsch Arztebl Int. 2015;112:423–32.

Ledford H. Drug companies flock to supercharged T-cells in fight against autoimmune disease. Nature. 2017.

Mclean LP, Shea-Donohue T, Cross RK. Vedolizumab for the treatment of ulcerative colitis and Crohn's disease. Immunotherapy. 2012;4(9):883–98.

Mihara M, Hashizume M, Yoshida H, Suzuki M, Shiina M. IL-6/IL-6 receptor system and its role in physiological and pathological conditions. Clin Sci (Lond). 2012;122(4):143–59.

Mittelstadt PR, Ashwell JF. Inhibition of AP-1 by the glucocorticoid-inducible protein GILZ. J Biol Chem. 2001;276:29603–10.

Montalban X, Gold R, Thompson AJ, Otero-Romero S, Amato MP, Chandraratna D, et al. ECTRIMS/EAN guideline on the pharmacological treatment of people with multiple sclerosis. Mult Scler. 2018;24(2):96–120.

Neurath M. Thiopurines in IBD. Gastroenterol Hepatol (NY). 2010;6(7):435–6.

Packman CH. The clinical pictures of autoimmune hemolytic anemia. Transfus Med Hemother. 2015;42:317–24.

Pedersen J, Coskun M, Soendergaard C, Salem M, Nielsen OH. Inflammatory pathways of importance for management of inflammatory bowel disease. World J Gastroenterol. 2014;20(1):64–77.

Phillips WD, Vincent A. Pathogenesis of myasthenia gravis: update on disease types, models, and mechanisms. F1000Res. 2016;5:F1000 Faculty Rev-1513.

Ray S, Santhalia N, Kundu S, Ganguly S. Autoimmune disorders: an overview of molecular and cellular basis in today's perspective. J Clin Cell Immunol. 2012;S10:003.

Sanders DB, Wolfe GI, Narayanaswami P. Author response: international consensus guidance for management of myasthenia gravis: executive summary. Neurology. 2017;88(5):505–6.

Singh N, Rieder MJ, Tucker MJ. Mechanisms of glucocorticoid-mediated anti-inflammatory and immunosuppressive action. Pediatr Perinat Drug Therapy. 2004;6:107–15.

Singh JA, Saag KG, Bridges SL, Akl EA, Bannuru RR, Sullivan MC, et al. 2015 American College of Rheumatology guideline for the treatment of rheumatoid arthritis. Arthr Rheumatol. 2015; 68(1):1–26.

Song YW, Kang EH. Autoantibodies in rheumatoid arthritis: rheumatoid factors and anticitrullinated protein antibodies. QJM. 2010;103(3):139–46.

Srivastava A. Belimumab in SLE. Indian J Dermatol. 2016;61(5):550–3.

Sussman J, Farrugia ME, Maddison P, Hill M, Leite MI, Hilton-Jones D. Myasthenia gravis: Association of British Neurologists' management guidelines. Pract Neurol. 2015;15(3):199–206.

Szollosi DE, Manzoor MK, Aquilato A, Jackson PB, Ghoneim O, Edafiogho IO. Current and novel anti-inflammatory drug targets for inhibition of cytokines and leucocyte recruitment in rheumatic diseases. J Pharm Pharmacol. 2018;70(1):18–26.

Taylor PC, Keystone EC, van der Heijde D, Weinblatt ME, del Carmen Morales L, Gonzaga JR, et al. Baricitinib versus placebo or adalimumab in rheumatoid arthritis. N Engl J Med. 2017;376:652–62.

Tobler A, Meier R, Seitz M, Dewald B, Baggiolini M, Fey M. Glucocorticoids downregulate gene expression of GM-CSF NAP1/IL-8, and IL-6, but no M-CSF in human fibroblasts. Blood. 1992;79:45–51.

Tullman MJ. Overview of the epidemiology, diagnosis, and disease progression associated with multiple sclerosis. Am J Manag Care. 2013;19(2 Suppl):S15–20.

Wahl K, Schuna A. Chapter 91. Rheumatoid arthritis. In: Pharmacotherapy: a pathophysiologic approach. 10th ed. New York: McGraw Hill Education; 2017.

Wajant H, Pfizenmaier K, Scheurich P. Tumor necrosis factor signaling. Cell Death Differ. 2003;10(1):45–65.

Weinblatt ME. Methotrexate in rheumatoid arthritis: a quarter century of development. Trans Am Clin Climatol Assoc. 2013;124:16–25.

Whittle SL, Hughes RA. Folate supplementation and methotrexate treatment in rheumatoid arthritis: a review. Rheumatology. 2004;43(3):267–71.

Wu GF, Alvarez E. The immuno-pathophysiology of multiple sclerosis. Neurol Clin. 2011;29(2):257–78.

Zenella A, Barcellini W. Treatment of autoimmune hemolytic anemias. Haematologica. 2014;99(10): 1547–54.

Zhang J-M, An J. Cytokines, inflammation and pain. Int Anesthesiol Clin. 2007;45(2):27–37.

Zufferey A, Kapur R, Semple JW. Pathogenesis and therapeutic mechanisms in immune thrombocytopenia (ITP). J Clin Med. 2017;6(2):E16.

Transplantation: Immunologic Principles and Pharmacologic Agents

8

Clinton B. Mathias and Jeremy P. McAleer

Learning Objectives

1. Identify and describe the terms used to describe solid organ transplants and hematopoietic stem cell transplantation.
2. Explain the immunological principles that are responsible for donor/recipient compatibility in organ transplantation.
3. Explain the immunological mechanisms governing blood transfusions and their role in hemolytic anemia of the newborn.
4. Describe the different types of graft rejection and the immune mechanisms involved.
5. Explain the principles underlying hematopoietic stem cell transplantation.
6. Discuss the mechanisms involved in graft versus host disease and its treatment.
7. Describe and explain the immunopharmacology of medications used for both induction and maintenance therapy in transplantation.

Drugs discussed in this chapter

Drug	Classification
Alemtuzumab (Lemtrada®, Campath®)	Anti-CD52 monoclonal antibody
Anti-thymocyte globulin (thymoglobulin®)	T cell-depleting polyclonal antibody
Azathioprine (Imura®)	Anti-proliferative, purine analog
Basiliximab (Simulect®)	Anti-CD25 monoclonal antibody
Belatacept (Nulojix®)	Fusion protein, CTLA-4/IgG1 Fc
Cyclophosphamide (Cytoxa®)	Anti-proliferative, DNA alkylating
Cyclosporine (Sandimmune®)	Calcineurin inhibitor
Daclizumab (Zenapax®) *discontinued	Anti-CD25 monoclonal antibody
Everolimus (Afinitor®)	Anti-proliferative, mTOR inhibitor
Etanercept (Enbrel®)	Fusion protein, anti-TNF
Glucocorticoids	Global immunosuppressive agents
Intravenous immunoglobulin	Polyclonal antibody, total IgG
Muromonab-CD3 (Orthoclone OKT3®)	Anti-CD3 monoclonal antibody,
Mycophenolate Mofetil (CellCept®)	Anti-proliferative, purine synthesis inhibitor
Pentostatin (Nipent®)	Anti-proliferative, adenosine deaminase inhibitor
Rapamycin, Sirolimus (Rapamune®)	Anti-proliferative, mTOR inhibitor
RhoGAM®	Polyclonal antibody, anti-Rh D
Rituximab (Rituxan®)	Anti-CD20 monoclonal antibody

C. B. Mathias (✉)
Department of Pharmaceutical and Administrative Sciences, College of Pharmacy and Health Sciences, Western New England University, Springfield, MA, USA
e-mail: clinton.mathias@wne.edu

J. P. McAleer
Pharmaceutical Science and Research, Marshall University School of Pharmacy, Huntington, WV, USA
e-mail: mcaleer@marshall.edu

© Springer Nature Switzerland AG 2020
C. B. Mathias et al., *Pharmacology of Immunotherapeutic Drugs*,
https://doi.org/10.1007/978-3-030-19922-7_8

Drug	Classification
Tacrolimus, FK506 (Prograf®)	Calcineurin inhibitor
Tocilizumab (Actemra®)	Anti-IL-6 receptor monoclonal antibody

Introduction

The ability to cure individuals of disease or disability by replacing organs or other damaged tissues has always been something to which humans have aspired. Ancient writers envisioned the possibility of replacing entire limbs in injured individuals and throughout the centuries physicians have attempted to restore bodily function by transplanting tissue from one area to another in both animals and humans. Major efforts at understanding the mechanisms underlying successful transplantation began to be pioneered by several physicians and scientists in the early part of the twentieth century. For example, it was not clear why autografts (tissues transplanted from one area of the body to another) tended to result in successful outcomes, while allografts (transplants between different individuals of the same species) always failed. Transplantation research during these decades led to the uncovering of several pivotal concepts including the role of lymphocytes and major histocompatibility genes in determining the outcome of procedures. These pioneering studies by several researchers culminated in the first successful solid organ transplant in humans: a kidney transplant between identical twins in 1954. Thereafter, breakthroughs occurred in transplanting other organ systems such as the liver and heart. The use of radiation and chemotherapy to suppress immune responses against transplanted grafts became common and the discovery and use of cyclosporine revolutionized the trajectory of the entire field, making the ancient dream of replacing damaged organs a present reality. In this chapter, we provide a brief overview of the immune mechanisms involved in solid organ and hematopoietic stem cell transplantation and discuss the drugs used to induce immunosuppression, graft tolerance and maintenance.

Types of Transplantation

Transplantation refers to the transfer of an organ, tissue, or cells from one body to another, or from one site to another location on the patient's own body in order to replace damaged or missing organs, tissues or cells. In order for a transplant to be successful, it is necessary to overcome several challenges. The transplanted tissue or organ must retain its capacity to perform normal bodily functions in the recipient, both the donor and recipient's health must be cared for throughout the process, and immune responses must be suppressed in order to prevent rejection of the graft or **graft versus host disease (GVHD)**. Transplantation is categorized into four types: **autograft** (donor and recipient are the same person), **allograft** (donor and recipient are different individuals of the same species), **isograft** (donor and recipient are identical twins) or **xenograft** (donor and recipient are different species), described in Table 8.1. Successful long-term engraftment of solid organs is challenging due to adaptive immune responses against donor- or recipient-derived antigens, especially nonidentical MHC proteins expressed by the donor and recipient. Complications from transplanted tissues include the rejection of transplanted tissue (manifested as hyperacute, acute, or chronic rejection) or GVHD. Since organ availability is limited, compatibility between the donor and recipient is rarely at or above 90%.

Table 8.1 Types of transplants routinely performed at medical facilities

Transplant type	Donor/recipient	Example(s)	Graft survival rate (%)
Autograft	Same person	Skin, bone reconstruction, blood	80–97
Allograft	Same species	Kidney, liver, heart	30–90
Isograft	Identical twins	Kidney, liver, heart	~100
Xenograft	Different species	Heart	50

Xenotransplantion is an avenue to counteract the limited organ availability, although this is met with challenges including the expression of non-human antigens by the donor tissue, increasing the likelihood of acute rejection. Additionally, infectious complications including retroviruses transferred from the donor to recipient may result in chronic diseases. As such, allotransplantation has remained the mainstay of procedures, with human leukocyte antigen (HLA) matching and immunosuppressive regimens significantly increasing the likelihood of long-term engraftment. Kidneys are the most commonly transplanted organ, with over 30,000 procedures performed in the United States in 2015, and also have the highest likelihood of engraftment survival after 1 year.

Blood Transfusions

Blood transfusions are the most common type of transplanted tissue in clinical medicine. One in four individuals receives a blood transfusion during their lifetimes in order to replace and replenish red blood cells, proteins, and fluids that are lost as a result of trauma, disease, childbirth or surgery. The concept of blood transfusion is simple, requiring only an intravenous liquid allograft, and no extensive surgery on the part of the donor or recipient. Moreover, in most cases blood donations are readily available, precluding the necessity of finding a suitable match, and saving considerable effort and time. Lastly, since the infused blood is only necessary for replenishment and not long-term engraftment, maintenance of the transfused blood is not required. One reason for the widespread success of blood transfusions is due to the lack of MHC class I or II expression on the surface of red blood cells, which are common targets for immune responses during allotransplantation.

The success of blood transfusions is determined by matching different polymorphic antigens between the donor and the recipient. The ABO system of compatibility testing classifies people as having type A, B, AB or O blood based on their expression of the oligosaccharide antigens named A and B. The type A and type B antigens are enzymatic modifications of the type O antigen, which is a glycolipid consisting of a lipid ceramide and an oligosaccharide. Since these antigens resemble common oligosaccharides found in food or microorganisms, individuals produce natural antibodies (IgG, IgM) recognizing the erythrocyte antigens they do not express. For instance, someone with type A blood is tolerized to the A antigen but produces antibodies that can target the B antigen. Therefore, type B blood that is transfused into a patient with type A blood will likely be rejected. Antibodies binding to the surface of RBCs induce a type II hypersensitivity reaction, leading to the activation of the classical complement cascade, and resulting in intravascular hemolysis. People with type AB blood are tolerized to both antigens and are referred to as universal recipients, capable of receiving transfusions from donors having any of the major blood types. People with type O blood do not express the A or B antigen, and are referred to as universal donors. On the other hand, type O patients can only receive transfusions from type O donors since they produce antibodies recognizing both A and B antigens. Minor reactions from incompatible blood transfusions, including hives and itching, are treated with antihistamines and acetaminophen. Major transfusion reactions can be life threatening, including intravascular coagulation, acute kidney failure, acute lung injury and shock.

Compatibility between the donor and recipient blood cells is determined by performing agglutination or cross-match tests. The recipient's serum is tested for reactivity against red blood cells from various donors. Incompatibility is determined by the presence of blood clotting or agglutination, which occurs when antibodies in the recipient's serum recognize antigens on the surface of donor RBCs.

Hemolytic Anemia of the Newborn
In addition to the ABO antigens, the rhesus (Rh) system of antigens, particularly rhesus factor D (RhD) also presents a problem with incompatibility during blood transfusion. Transfusion of a RhD$^-$ individual with RhD$^+$ blood makes successive transfusions with RhD$^+$ blood extremely

dangerous for the recipient. This is especially of concern in RhD⁻ pregnant women married to RhD⁺ fathers. As such, during pregnancy, couples are routinely tested for RhD on their red blood cells. As discussed in Chap. 3, the birth of an RhD⁺ child to a RhD⁻ mother will result in the recognition of RhD by the mother's immune system as a non-self antigen, resulting in an antibody response. The initial exposure of the mother to RhD is termed as sensitization and results in the production of low-affinity IgM antibodies that do not cross the placenta. As such, the fetus is not normally harmed during the first pregnancy. Sensitization may occur when a small amount of fetal blood enters the maternal circulation during delivery, or as a result of a previous blood transfusion from an RhD⁺ donor. However, subsequent pregnancies involving RhD⁺ babies inevitably result in a secondary immune response, eliciting IgG antibodies that cross the placenta and attack fetal RBCs during the third trimester, causing hemolysis. This condition is termed **hemolytic disease of the newborn** and can be mild, moderate or severe, resulting in anemia, jaundice or *hydrops fetalis*. Although most cases are due to antibodies attacking the RhD antigen, mild hemolytic disease of the newborn can also occur when a woman with type O blood carries a fetus with type A or B blood.

Prophylaxis for hemolytic disease of the newborn involves injecting RhD⁻ women with anti-RhD IgG antibodies (**RhoGAM®**) during the last trimester of pregnancy. RhoGAM prevents sensitization of the mother's immune system to RhD by binding fetal RBCs and blocking their recognition by maternal B cells. RhoGAM® is concentrated IgG from human plasma containing anti-RhD antibodies, and given at 26–28 weeks of pregnancy, and within 72 h of delivery. Anti-RhD antibodies are also indicated for the transfusion of Rh-incompatible blood. Adverse reactions to RhoGAM® are rare, including a skin rash and elevated temperature. Since antibody injections can impair the efficacy of live vaccines, vaccination should be delayed until 12 weeks after the final dose of RhoGAM®.

Solid Organ Transplantation

Solid organ transplantation of the kidney, liver, lung, and heart has become a routine medical procedure that is commonly performed at hospitals throughout the world. Kidney transplants account for greater than 80,000 cases each year worldwide, with thousands of patients on waiting lists. Compared to other types of solid organ transplants, kidney transplants are relatively easier to perform since the patients can be maintained on dialysis for extended periods of time. Furthermore, since only one kidney is needed for survival and maintaining quality of life, organs can be procured from both living donors (especially family members) and cadavers, thereby significantly increasing the number of potential matches available.

The successful outcome of a transplantation procedure depends on a number of factors. Since it is necessary that the transplanted organ be able to perform normal physiological functions in the recipient's body, the health of both the donor and the recipient must be considered. Further, the immune status of the patient and his or her ability to respond to immunosuppressive drugs must be considered. This is especially important considering that the initial processes leading to organ damage may have involved an autoimmune reaction or other type of inflammation. In the case of donated organs, it is important to preserve them in a manner that reduces their damage and prevents the development of ischemia (loss of blood) prior to the transplantation procedure or during its transport. Ischemia can induce an inflammatory reaction that involves the activation of endothelium and complement, followed by the recruitment of leukocytes and cytokine secretion in the donor organ, causing tissue damage. For organs donated from cadavers, especially individuals who may have died as a result of trauma or other stress, care must be taken to limit the damage caused by ischemia. In the case of patients receiving organs from living donors, the development of ischemia can be significantly minimized by performing surgery on the donor and recipient at the same time in the same room. Obtaining a donor match is pivotal to minimizing immune rejection and ensuring successful transplantation outcomes.

Donor Matching

The most important factor that determines long-term organ survival following transplantation is HLA matching between the donor and recipient. Immune rejection of transplanted organs is directly caused by antigenic differences between the highly polymorphic MHC Class I and II antigens. As such, these are also referred to as **transplantation antigens** or alloantigens. The HLA gene complex is located on chromosome 6 and encodes MHC genes. One HLA set is inherited from each parent and siblings have a 25% chance of being HLA-matched (Fig. 8.1). The function of MHC class I and MHC class II in adaptive immunity is described in Chap. 3. Three separate genes encode MHC class I molecules (HLA-A, -B, -C), and MHC class II genes (HLA-DR, -DQ, -DP). These genes are inherited as a single unit from chromosome 6. Each gene has several

alleles due to polymorphisms in their sequence. These polymorphisms are responsible for allograft rejections when an organ recipient's immune system recognizes the donor MHC alleles as non-self. Children inherit one MHC haplotype from each parent, resulting in their expression of six different alleles for MHC class I and six alleles for MHC class II. Combined, the 12 HLA genes expressed by people constitute their **haplotype**. Thousands of haplotypes have been identified, although the prevalence of certain haplotypes can differ by geographic regions.

Laboratory screening for donor and recipient compatibility involves HLA typing, mixed lymphocyte reactions and cross-matching. Techniques used for **HLA typing** include flow cytometry or lymphocytotoxicity assays to measure surface MHC expression, or DNA sequencing. **Mixed lymphocyte reactions** measure cytotoxic activity from cell cultures containing lymphocytes from both the donor and recipient. In this assay, tolerance is indicated by nonresponsiveness between the donor and recipient lymphocytes that are co-cultured, whereas

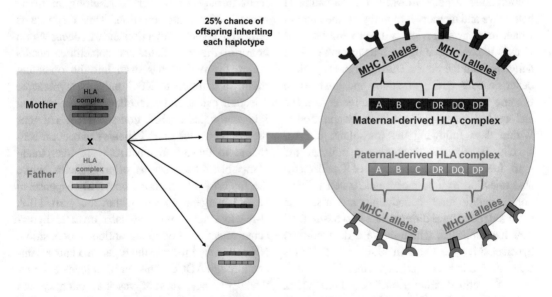

Fig. 8.1 HLA inheritance. The genes encoding MHC class I (A, B, C) and class II (DR, DQ, DP) molecules are inherited together due to their proximity on chromosome 6, and are expressed in a codominant manner. Several polymorphisms exist for each gene, and the entire set of MHC molecules expressed in an individual is termed a haplotype. Since offspring from parents may inherit one of four possible HLA combinations, siblings have a 25% chance of being MHC-matched. This is an important consideration for organ transplantation

cytotoxic reactions resulting in cell death indicate that the donor and recipient may be incompatible. **Cross-match testing** determines if the recipient has pre-existing antibodies against HLA (MHC class I or class II) antigens from the donor. The presence of complement fixing IgG antibodies against donor antigens is a contraindication for transplantation. To assess the degree of HLA compatibility between the donor and the recipient, the **panel-reactive antibody (PRA)** test is performed. This is done by adding the recipient's serum to leukocytes from a panel of individuals representing the population. The total number of positive reactions determines the percentage of the population to which the recipient's serum is reactive. This value is called the **PRA** and expressed as a percentage. The higher the PRA for a given individual, the more difficult it is to find a suitable, compatible donor.

Mechanisms of Solid Organ Transplant Rejection

Alloimmune responses involve the activation of both naïve and memory lymphocytes, the latter of which may have previously been stimulated by viruses expressing antigens that resemble HLA antigens from the donor. During organ rejection, dendritic cells (DCs) of donor and host origin become activated and present antigens to naïve and central memory T cells in lymph nodes. Within days following the transplant, effector T cells, B cells and macrophages infiltrate the graft. Lesions that are indicative of T cell-mediated rejection include mononuclear cell infiltration, tubulitis and endothelial arteritis. The recruited monocytes differentiate into tissue-resident macrophages, which cause a delayed-type hypersensitivity reaction. In addition, activated B cells can produce antibodies against donor HLA antigens, termed **alloantibodies**, which attack the capillary endothelium and activate the complement cascade. As a result, the transplanted tissue has altered capillary permeability, extracellular matrix deposition and deterioration of parenchymal function. Immunosuppressive regimens are necessary to prevent transplant rejection by inducing **adaptation**, resulting in the patient's immune system becoming tolerant to alloantigens over time. Organ rejection can be classified as hyperacute, acute or chronic.

Hyperacute Rejection

Hyperacute rejection is mediated by pre-existing recipient antibodies that recognize donor-derived blood group antigens or non-self HLA I and HLA II antigens. This type of rejection often occurs during or soon after the transplantation procedure has been performed and can be best avoided by performing cross-matching prior to the onset of the transplantation procedure.

The polymorphic ABO antigens present on erythrocytes and blood vessels within organs can be a major source of rejection during the transplantation of solid organs, especially when transplanting highly vascularized organs such as the kidney. IgG antibodies against the donor-derived AB antigens can rapidly activate and fix complement throughout the graft, resulting in tissue necrosis and graft rejection. This response is termed hyperacute rejection and can occur within hours of the transplant, and sometimes occurs before the patient has even left the operating room. In addition to RBC antigens, hyperacute rejection can also be mediated by pre-existing IgG antibodies against non-self HLA antigens present within the graft. Patients can become sensitized to these antigens from previous transplants, blood transfusions, or pregnancies. While the majority of reactions occur in response to HLA I antigens present within the graft, HLA II-reactive antibodies can also mediate hyperacute rejection. Following antibody deposition, NK cells may infiltrate the organ and cause damage through ADCC. This reaction leads to endothelial damage, loss of vascular integrity and increased coagulation in the transplant. While hyperacute rejection is predominantly IgG-mediated, naturally occurring IgM antibodies can also be involved. Cross-match testing is necessary to detect the presence of donor-specific antibodies in patients prior to transplantation.

Acute Rejection

Acute rejection, also referred to as the direct pathway of allorecognition, occurs days to weeks following transplantation and is mediated by effector T cells reacting to mismatched HLA antigens. In the absence of a rare complete donor match, most solid organ transplants are performed with some HLA I or HLA II allelic differences between the donor and recipient. This results in the activation of naïve T cells in the recipient that recognize donor-derived HLA antigens. During acute rejection, DCs from the transplanted organ can migrate to secondary lymphoid organs within the recipient where they present donor-derived peptides to alloreactive T cells (Fig. 8.2). Some of these T cells may have developed in response to structurally similar antigens expressed by viruses or other pathogens. CD8 T cells can become activated to non-self HLA I-derived peptides, resulting in their recruitment to the graft where they mediate its killing through cytotoxicity. Correspondingly, CD4 T cells can become activated against non-self HLA II-derived antigens, resulting in their T_H1 cell differentiation and secretion of cytokines that recruit monocytes and neutrophils to the organ, leading to endotheliitis and damage. Lastly, graft-specific antibodies produced by B cells can fix complement on blood vessels, promoting coagulation. The risk of acute rejection is significantly reduced or prevented through the use of immunosuppressive therapy before, during, and after transplantation. Following the procedure, the patient is carefully monitored for early signs of rejection and treated with additional drugs to minimize rejection if necessary.

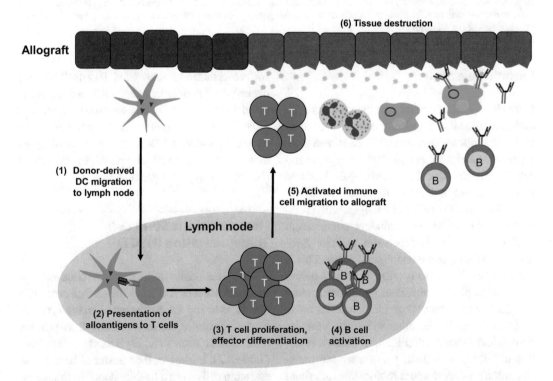

Fig. 8.2 Acute rejection of allografts. Immune cells from organ donors are often transplanted into recipients. Dendritic cells from the graft can initiate acute rejection by activating T cells recognizing mismatched MHC alleles. This can result in T cell effector differentiation and the production of antibodies against alloantigens by B cells. Allograft destruction is caused by the infiltration of activated immune cells, including T cells, monocytes/macrophages, neutrophils and antibody-producing B cells

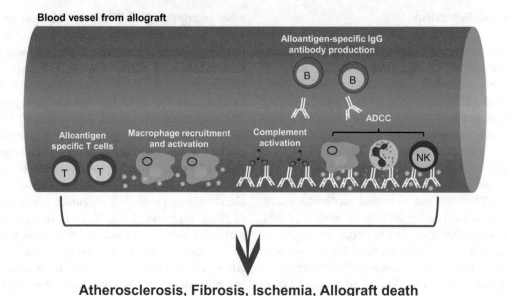

Fig. 8.3 Cellular causes of vascular damage during chronic allograft rejection. Organ recipient-derived lymphocytes contribute to chronic allograft rejection through vascular injury. T cells recognizing alloantigens can have direct cytotoxic effects on vessels as well as recruit macrophages and neutrophils. Antibodies produced by B cells promote vascular injury through complement activation and ADCC. Chronic inflammation over the course of years leads to vascular smooth muscle cell proliferation, extracellular matrix deposition, fibrosis, atherosclerosis, organ ischemia and ultimately death of the allograft

Chronic Rejection

Chronic rejection occurs months to years after transplantation due to vascular damage caused by antibodies, alloantigen-specific T cells, and macrophages. Cycles of endothelial damage, extracellular matrix deposition and repair leads to vascular smooth muscle proliferation and thickening. The blood vessel wall enlarges, with HLA-specific IgG antibodies mediating complement fixation and antibody-dependent cellular cytotoxicity (ADCC) in the endothelial tissue. This is accompanied by CD40-positive B cells, T helper cells, macrophages and neutrophils infiltrating the graft where they promote tissue damage, resulting in ischemia, atherosclerosis, vascular fibrosis and tissue death (Fig. 8.3). Chronic rejection usually occurs 5–10 years after the transplantation procedure and is responsible for failure in more than half of all kidney and heart transplants. This process is termed the indirect pathway of allorecognition since recipient DCs acquire donor-derived HLA-associated antigens

for presentation to naive CD4 T cells. This may occur when apoptotic donor DCs are phagocytosed by recipient DCs in secondary lymphoid organs. Since the target antigens are not produced by recipient-derived DCs, this process of rejection is more gradual compared to the direct (acute) pathway of organ rejection.

Hematopoietic Stem Cell Transplantation (HSCT)

HSCT, previously referred to as bone-marrow transplantation or BMT, is a life-saving procedure that is used for the treatment of many types of cancers involving leukocytes as well as primary immunodeficiencies and erythrocyte deficiencies (Table 8.2). It involves the transfer of hematopoietic stem cells from a healthy donor to the recipient with the aim of replacing his or her hematopoietic system. As such, the HSCT recipient is a chimera comprised of hematopoietic cells that have originated from the donor, while the

Table 8.2 List of genetic deficiencies, primary immune deficiencies, and cancers for which HSCT has been proven to be effective

Primary immune deficiencies	Defect
Severe combined immune deficiency	Cytokine receptor chain (common γ chain/IL2Rγ chain) JAK3 IL-7R Rag1/Rag2 CD45 Adenosine deaminase TCR subunits
Omenn syndrome	Rag1/Rag2
DNA ligase IV deficiency	Lymphocyte deficiency
Purine nucleoside phosphorylase (PNP) deficiency	PNP
Bare lymphocyte syndrome	MHC II
Store-operated calcium channel deficiency	STIM1 and ORAI1; T cell lymphopenia
DiGeorge syndrome	Incomplete thymic development
Zeta-chain-associated protein-70 (ZAP-70) deficiency	ZAP70; defective T cell function
Hyper IgM syndrome	CD40L; defective antibody class-switching and neutropenia
Wiskott–Aldrich syndrome	Defect in T cell function and platelets
X-linked lymphoproliferative disease	T and NK cell lymphoproliferative disorder
Immunodysregulation, polyendocrinopathy, and enteropathy X-linked (IPEX)	FoxP3; deficiency in Tregs
NF-κB essential modulator (NEMO) deficiency	IκB kinase; immunological (inactive NF-κB) and developmental defects
CD25 deficiency	IL-2Rα; deficiency in Tregs
Autoimmune lymphoproliferative syndrome (ALPS)	Fas; autoimmunity
Chronic granulomatous disease	Phagocyte deficiency
Leukocyte adhesion deficiency	Phagocyte deficiency
Kostmann syndrome	Low neutrophil count (neutropenia)
Chédiak-Higashi syndrome	Phagocyte and natural killer cell deficiency
IFN-γ receptor deficiencies	Susceptibility to mycobacteria
Cartilage–hair hypoplasia	Short limbs, fine sparse hair; immunodeficiency
Hemoglobinopathies	**Defect**
Thalassemia major	Hemoglobin; impaired erythrocyte function
Sickle-cell anemia	Hemoglobin; impaired erythrocyte function
Bone marrow failures	**Defect**
Aplastic anemia	Defect in blood cell production
Fanconi anemia	Decreased production of blood cells
Myelodysplastic syndrome	Deformed, underdeveloped blood cell production
Infantile malignant osteopetrosis	Defective osteoclast function; incomplete bone modeling and remodeling
Inherited metabolic disorders (lysosomal and peroxisomal storage disorders)	**Defect**
Mucopolysaccharidosis and mucolipidosis	Deficiencies of lysosomal enzymes
Gaucher's syndrome	Deficiency of the lysosomal enzyme glucocerebrosidase
Malignancies	**Type of cancer**
Acute myelogenous leukemia (AML)	Cancer of white blood cells
Acute lymphocytic leukemia (ALL)	Cancer of white blood cells
Chronic myelogenous leukemia (CML)	Cancer of white blood cells
Multiple myeloma	Cancer of plasma cells
Non-Hodgkin's lymphoma	Cancer involving lymphocytes
Hodgkin's lymphoma	Cancer involving lymphocytes

non-hematopoietic cellular compartment is endogenously-derived. It is therefore extremely important that the recipient is conditioned prior to the transplantation procedure in order to limit the activation of donor-derived lymphocytes. In previous years, HSCT was exclusively performed using bone marrow; however, it is now routinely performed by isolating and culturing CD34+ hematopoietic stem cells from donors, followed by intravenous transfusion into recipients. These pluripotent cells then go on to reconstitute the entire hematopoietic system within the recipient.

Prior to undergoing HSCT, it is important that patients are conditioned with radiation and chemotherapy to destroy the patient's hematopoietic system including any malignant cells. This process is termed as myeloablative therapy and uses high doses of drugs, resulting in the death of hematopoietic stem cells. As a result, the transplanted cells are protected from attack by the patient's lymphocytes, and there is space available for the new hematopoietic cells to interact with stromal cells and flourish in the bone marrow. This is termed **allogeneic** transplantation since the patient receives bone marrow from another individual. In some cases, non-myeloablative therapy may be employed, in which lower doses of radiation and chemotherapy are used in order to preserve some hematopoietic function within the recipient prior to the injection of blood or bone marrow cells from a donor. A variation of this is called **autologous** transplantation, in which stem cells are collected from the patient prior to conditioning and then reinfused to re-establish the hematopoietic compartment after cancerous cells have been ablated.

Once HSCT is complete, the donor-derived stem cells begin to reconstitute the recipient's hematopoietic system. Initially, innate immune cells reconstitute the individual, followed by adaptive immune cells. Complete restoration of the hematopoietic compartment can take approximately 1 year. During this time, thymic selection ensures that donor-derived T cells develop the ability to recognize antigens presented by HLA molecules from both the donor and recipient, shaping the T cell repertoire. In order for HSCT to be successful, it is crucial for both the donor and recipient to share some HLA molecules, and the number of shared alleles directly correlates to transplantation success and survival of the recipient. If cells from the original transplant are rejected, an additional infusion may be necessary. Due to myeloablative and immunosuppressive therapies, the HSCT procedure increases a patient's risk for infections.

Graft-Versus-Host Disease

Graft-versus-host disease (GVHD) is a common but potentially life-threatening complication in patients undergoing HSCT, and can be classified as acute or chronic. GVHD occurs when donor-derived T cells and B cells attack tissues in the recipient including the skin, liver or intestine. In order for GVHD reactions to occur, the graft must contain immunologically competent cells, the recipient must express antigens not present in the donor, and the recipient must be incapable of mounting a response to destroy the transplanted cells. The inability to destroy transplanted cells is often the result of immunosuppression, which also increases susceptibility to opportunistic infections. The incidence of acute GVHD is 10–80%, with symptoms such as a skin rash, severe diarrhea, or hepatotoxicity developing 2–3 weeks post-transplant. The targets in GVHD are primarily epithelial cells of the epidermis, bile ducts and intestinal crypts. Chronic GVHD occurs approximately 100 days following transplantation in 30–60% of patients, correlating with risk factors such as patients receiving HLA-non-identical transplants containing mature T cells.

Immunosuppressive drugs are required to decrease the risk of GVHD, but cannot always prevent its occurrence. The pathophysiology of GVHD occurs in sequential phases including APC activation, antigen presentation, effector cell proliferation, differentiation, migration, and target tissue destruction.

The activation of recipient and donor-derived APCs is the first phase of a GVHD reaction. This may occur following transplantation or prior to it as a result of conditioning regimens. Irradiation and chemotherapy can damage host tissues including the intestinal mucosa, resulting in microbial translocation into the circulation and inflammatory cytokine release from macrophages. These cytokines, including IL-1 and TNF-α, activate DCs to increase their expression of MHC class I and class II, costimulatory molecules, and adhesion molecules. Donor-derived DCs can present **alloantigens** to donor T cells, resulting in their activation and differentiation into T_H1, T_H2, T_H17 or cytotoxic effector cells. In general, CD8 T cells recognize alloantigens from donor MHC class I proteins, while CD4 T cells recognize alloantigens from donor MHC class II proteins. As described in Chap. 3, T_H1 cells activate macrophages, T_{FH} and T_H2 cells promote B cell antibody production and isotype switching, and T_H17 cells facilitate neutrophil recruitment to the site of inflammation. Tissues expressing the alloantigens recognized by donor-derived T cells will be attacked, with the mechanism of tissue destruction similar to that observed for allograft rejections (Fig. 8.2). TNF-α is involved in all three phases of GVHD pathophysiology, and the GI tract is susceptible to damage from TNF-mediated inflammation. Acute GVHD is preceded by high levels of CD4 and CD8 T cells in the blood while chronic GVHD is often antibody-mediated with the reaction resembling autoimmunity. Extended immunosuppression may be required for treating chronic GVHD, and B cell depletion with rituximab has shown efficacy. Most stem cell transplant patients are able to eventually discontinue immunosuppressive drugs within 1–2 years of the transplant.

Post Transplantation Lymphoproliferative Disorders (PTLDS)

Post transplantation lymphoproliferative disorders (PTLDs) are a complication that can occur following transplantation, resulting in lymphomas. Recipients of solid-organ or allogeneic hematopoietic stem-cell transplants have increased risks of cancers related to immunosuppression and Epstein-Barr virus (EBV) infection. The overall incidence is 3%, although patients with multi-organ or intestinal transplants have a 20% incidence of PTLDs. Most cases are thought to be caused by reactivation of a latent EBV infection in B cells, leading to their proliferation and transformation. While EBV infection normally elicits a T cell response, lymphomas are more likely to occur in immunosuppressed patients. Treatments for PTLDs include reducing doses of immunosuppressive drugs, radiotherapy, chemotherapy, adoptive transfer of EBV-specific cytotoxic T cells, B cell depletion, antiviral therapy, and autologous HSCT from EBV-negative donors.

Xenotransplantation

Xenotransplantation is the transfer of cells, tissues and organs from one species into another to replace damaged or missing components. Xenotransplantation has increasingly been studied and is being considered as an avenue to increase organ availability. Pigs are the most likely donor species for xenotransplantation due to their physiological similarity to humans, short reproduction time, large number of progeny, and ability to be genetically modified. Towards this, pigs have been engineered to lack expression of β-1,3-galactosyltransferase, a target of antibody-mediated hyperacute and acute rejection. Aside from the human rejection of transplanted porcine tissue, other risks associated with xenotransplantation include physiological incompatibility and the transmission of porcine retroviruses and hepatitis E virus. Clinical safety trials for islet cell transplantation have demonstrated the possibility of transplanting pathogen-free cells from pigs to humans. Treatments that reduce the risk of virus transmission include performing embryo transfer, cesarean delivery of pigs followed by gnotobiotic isolation, colostrum deviation, early weaning, vaccination, and the use of antiviral drugs.

Immunosuppressive Treatment in Transplantation Therapy

Immunosuppressive drugs are the mainstay of transplantation therapy and are required for inducing tolerance to transplanted organs in the initial days following transplantation (**induction**), maintaining tolerance long-term (**maintenance**) and for treating episodes of **acute organ rejection**. Induction drugs used at the time of transplantation include monoclonal and polyclonal antibodies that target lymphocytes. Maintenance drugs used for long-term prevention of graft rejection include calcineurin inhibitors, anti-proliferative agents, mTOR inhibitors and glucocorticoids. In the months following a transplant, immunosuppressive therapy facilitates adaptation, or decreased responsiveness, of a patient's immune system to the organ. During the adaptation phase, donor antigen presenting cells are depleted as T cells become less responsive to donor-derived antigens. The mechanisms by which immunosuppressive treatments promote transplant tolerance include lymphocyte depletion, suppression of lymphocyte trafficking, and inhibition of lymphocyte activation. Side effects from these treatments are correlated with the intensity of immunosuppression, and include increased susceptibility to infections and cancer as well as organ toxicity.

Induction Drugs

Prior to transplantation and soon after, monoclonal antibodies can be used to induce a generalized suppression of the immune system. These antibodies typically target a wide variety of immune cells; however, specific antibodies that deplete T cells may also be used. **Alemtuzumab** is a humanized monoclonal IgG antibody that recognizes CD52, a marker expressed by several cell types including T cells, B cells, NK cells, and macrophages and is used before transplantation to weaken the recipient's immune system. The physiological function of CD52 is not well understood; however, due to its wide range of expression, the use of alemtuzumab is associated with severe lymphopenia, neutropenia, anemia and thrombocytopenia. Similarly, purified rabbit **antithymocyte globulins (rATG)** may also be given as a means of inducing generalized immunosuppression. This polyclonal mixture is prepared by immunizing horses or rabbits with

lymphoid tissue or cells from humans, followed by collecting the immune serum. When given to humans, antithymocyte globulins deplete lymphocytes, DCs, macrophages and other cells through opsonization/phagocytosis, complement-mediated lysis, or ADCC. In addition to depletion, this treatment can suppress antigen-dependent T cell proliferation. Adverse reactions include serum sickness, urinary tract infection and impaired kidney function if antibody complexes localize to glomeruli. Since anti-thymocyte globulin is produced in horses and rabbits, patients may develop humoral immunity against these therapeutic antibodies. Anaphylactic reactions are a rare but serious side effect of antithymocyte globulin use.

T cell-depleting antibodies are often given to prevent episodes of acute rejection, but may be accompanied by the release of cytokines which produce severe systemic symptoms. An example is **muromonab-CD3 (OKT3)**, which targets the CD3 receptor expressed on T cell surfaces. This was the first monoclonal antibody to be approved for clinical use in humans, and was approved by the FDA for treating acute, glucocorticoid-resistant rejection of allogeneic renal, cardiac, and hepatic transplants. Treatment with the antibody results in the initial activation and subsequent apoptosis of T cells, thereby having beneficial effects during T cell-mediated acute rejection. Due to the initial activation CD3-mediated signaling, first-time treatment with muromonab-CD3 is often associated with cytokine release syndrome (CRS), a condition in which T cells secrete IL-2, IFN-γ, and TNF-α. This results in fever, fatigue, chills, skin reactions, diarrhea with the potential of developing life-threatening conditions such as cardiac arrest and flash pulmonary edema. Also, since the antibody was developed in mice, muromonab-CD3 is often associated with serum sickness, a type III hypersensitivity reaction in which the patient makes antibodies against the mouse antibody. Due to the adverse reactions, treatment with muromonab-CD3 fell out of favor, resulting in its discontinuation in 2008.

While depleting antibodies reduce the risk of early rejection, they significantly increase the

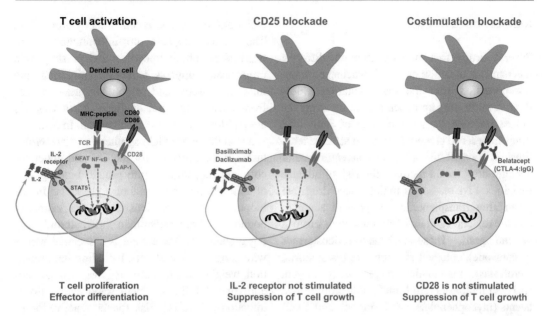

Fig. 8.4 Suppression of T cell activation. T cell activation by MHC:peptide complexes and costimulatory molecules (CD80, CD86) on DCs leads to the nuclear translocation of transcription factors (NFAT, NF-κB, AP-1) that are essential for T cell proliferation and effector differentiation (left panel). This leads to the production of IL-2, an autocrine cytokine that promotes T cell growth by activating a heterotrimeric complex of CD25 (IL-2Rα chain), CD122 (IL-2Rβ chain) and IL2Rγ chain. Blockade of CD25 using basiliximab or daclizumab prevents IL-2 receptor activation, STAT5 nuclear translocation, proliferation and effector cell differentiation (middle panel). Blockade of the costimulatory ligands CD80 and CD86 with belatacept prevents CD28 activation on T cells (right panel). Through these mechanisms, CD25 or costimulation blockade can prevent the activation of T cells recognizing transplantation-associated antigens

risk of infection and post-transplantation lymphoproliferative disorders including malignancies. Following immune depletion, it may take several months or years for the patient's immune system to fully recover. In contrast to T cell-depleting antibodies, B cell depletion is usually not accompanied by significant side effects and antibody titers are maintained due to the resistance of plasma cells to treatment. **Rituximab** is a humanized antibody targeting the CD20 antigen on mature B cells, and labels B cells for complement-mediated lysis, macrophage-mediated phagocytosis, and NK cell-dependent lysis via ADCC. Possible uses of rituximab include the prevention of hyperacute rejection, acute rejection in which B cells present antigens to T cells, and chronic antibody-mediated rejection. Other uses of rituximab include ABO blood group incompatible transplantation, post-

transplantation lymphoproliferative disorders, and HLA-incompatible renal transplantation.

Non-depleting therapeutic antibodies are used to block T cell costimulation or growth factor signaling, reducing proliferation, effector cell differentiation and cytokine production. **Basiliximab** and **daclizumab** are humanized anti-CD25 antibodies that prevent IL-2 from binding to its receptor on T cells (Fig. 8.4). In the absence of growth signals from IL-2, T cell activation and proliferation are suppressed. Compared to depleting antibodies, non-depleting antibodies do not cause profound immune suppression and have fewer side effects such as malignancies or a systemic cytokine release storm. These antibodies are typically used in patients with a lower risk for rejection. Daclizumab was voluntarily withdrawn from the market in March 2018 due to reports of encephalitis associated with its use in Europe.

Maintenance Drugs

Several drugs that operate through different mechanisms of action are used to achieve immunosuppression after the transplantation procedure. A multi-drug approach allows for using the lowest possible therapeutic dose of individual drugs in order to prevent long-term adverse reactions. In contrast, using higher concentrations of a single drug would increase the risk of adverse toxicities. Five classes of maintenance drugs are given after transplantation to prevent acute or chronic rejection and maintain long-term survival of the graft. These include corticosteroids (prednisone), calcineurin inhibitors (calcineurin, tacrolimus), mammalian target of rapamycin (mTOR) inhibitors (sirolimus), anti-proliferative agents (mycophenolate, azathioprine), and T cell co-stimulation blockers (Belatacept). High concentrations are initially used to induce immunosuppression during induction therapy, with doses becoming tapered over time for long-term maintenance. This is important since long-term immunosuppression is associated with increased susceptibilities to infections and cancers. It is therefore crucial to find the right balance between preventing organ rejection and minimizing the risk of developing infections and cancer.

Corticosteroids

Glucocorticoids (GCs) such as prednisone are the most extensively used drug to prevent organ rejection during and after transplantation. Prednisone is a synthetic derivative of hydrocortisone (cortisol), the principal steroid made by the adrenal cortex. It is four times more potent than hydrocortisone and is a pro-drug which is converted *in vivo* to prednisolone, the active form of the drug. The mechanism of action of prednisone is described in detail in Chaps. 4, 5, and 6. Glucocorticoids such as prednisone have a wide range of effects on the immune system and are a first line therapy for solid organ transplantation and HSCT. By themselves, GCs are insufficient to prevent graft rejection, but are often used in combination with other immunosuppressive drugs. In the context of transplant rejection, GCs can inhibit antigen presentation, T cell activation and proliferation, and B cell antibody production. They also suppress pro-inflammatory gene expression, inhibit lipocortin and prostaglandin production, suppress leukocyte migration into inflamed tissues, and inhibit histamine release from mast cells. Oral synthetic corticosteroids are rapidly and completely absorbed. In comparison to endogenous GCs, synthetic corticosteroids differ in their affinity for the GC and mineralocorticoid receptors, serum protein binding, rate of elimination and metabolic products. In the blood, synthetic corticosteroids are primarily bound to albumin rather than corticosteroid binding globulin. GC treatment is associated with a wide range of side effects, including fluid retention, weight gain, diabetes and loss of bone mineral. Since GC therapy increases susceptibility to infections, there is a risk for the reactivation of dormant tuberculosis during prolonged therapy. Several of the undesirable effects of GCs are caused by their hormonal actions, leading to iatrogenic Cushing syndrome following long-term use (>2 weeks). Peptic ulcers can be a potentially severe adverse effect of GC use. Long-term use results in adrenal gland atrophy due to the suppression of pituitary ACTH release; thus, dose tapering is necessary when removing these patients from therapeutic GCs.

Calcineurin Inhibitors

Calcineurin inhibitors are used to selectively inhibit T cell activation and are hailed as having the most impact on successful transplantation outcomes during the 1980s and 1990s. Their use resulted in significantly improved graft survival, with transplantation becoming the recommended treatment for several diseases. Both cyclosporine and tacrolimus block T cell proliferation by inhibiting the activation of the NFAT transcription factor. This prevents the production of IL-2 and the subsequent expansion of alloreactive T cells. The mechanism of action of calcineurin inhibitors is described in detail in Chaps. 5 and 6.

Cyclosporine is a cyclic decapeptide derived from the soil fungus *Tolypocladium inflatum*. It is a potent immunosuppressant used in maintenance therapy for most types of organs transplants. Cyclosporine binds to intracellular cyclophilins and inhibits the calcineurin-mediated dephosphorylation of NFAT following T cell receptor (TCR) stimulation, thereby preventing its nuclear translocation. As a result, antigen-specific T cells do not produce cytokines such as IL-2 and IFN-γ in the presence of cyclosporine. In addition, cyclosporine blocks the activation of MAP kinases JNK and p38 following TCR stimulation, but does not affect signaling through CD28. The adverse effects of cyclosporine are related to its concentration, including nephrotoxicity, neurotoxicity, hepatotoxicity and hypertension. Due to its distinct mechanism of action, cyclosporine can be used in combination with GCs or methotrexate. **Tacrolimus (FK 506)** is a macrolide antibiotic produced by *Streptomyces tsukabaensis* and binds to cytoplasmic FK506-binding protein 12 (FKBP12), creating a complex that inhibits calcineurin activity. By weight, tacrolimus is 10–100 times more potent than cyclosporine and is primarily used for organ and stem cell transplantation. Tacrolimus is a standard prophylactic agent against GVHD in combination with methotrexate or mycophenolate mofetil. Adverse effects from tacrolimus include nephrotoxicity and hemolytic-uremic syndrome. However, compared to cyclosporine, it is considered to have fewer nephrotoxic effects. It is also less likely to cause hyperlipidemia and hypertension, although more likely to induce post-transplantation diabetes. Therefore, patients with hypertension, hyperlipidemia and increased risk for rejection are more likely to receive tacrolimus, whereas patients at risk for diabetes (old age, obesity) are more likely to be treated with cyclosporine. Both types of calcineurin inhibitors are metabolized by the cytochrome P450 (CYP 3A4) enzyme system, thereby posing a risk for severe drug interactions in the presence of CYP 3A4 inhibitors including calcium channel blockers, macrolide antibiotics (erythromycin), triazole antifungals (ketoconazole), amiodarone, cimetidine, omeprazole, and protease inhibitors. These treatments, along with grapefruit and grapefruit juice increase systemic concentrations of calcineurin inhibitors. In contrast, treatment with anticonvulsants, rifampin, and St. John's Wort, decreases the concentration of calcineurin inhibitors. Additional medications such as aminoglycosides, amphotericin B, diuretics, and non-steroidal anti-inflammatory drugs (NSAIDs) can increase the renal toxicity associated with these drugs. Due to the narrow therapeutic index of calcineurin inhibitors and the plethora of drugs interactions affecting their bioavailability, therapeutic drug monitoring is required.

Mammalian Target of Rapamycin (mTOR) Inhibitors

mTOR inhibitors are used as either alternative drugs to replace calcineurin inhibitors or in conjunction with variable or lower doses of calcineurin inhibitors. **Rapamycin** is a natural anti-fungal metabolite produced by *Streptomyces hygroscopicus*. In humans, rapamycin (sirolimus) and its derivative **everolimus** form a complex with FKBP12 that acts as an allosteric inhibitor of mTOR. By integrating multiple signals from growth factors, nutrients, energy and oxygen status, the mTOR pathway is an important regulator of cell growth, proliferation, angiogenesis and metabolism. Stimulation of the T cell receptor and costimulatory receptors CD28, ICOS, and OX40 lead to activation of the mTOR pathway and induction of aerobic glycolysis in T cells (Fig. 8.5). This metabolic shift is required for their growth, proliferation, and effector differentiation. Blocking mTOR with rapamycin or everolimus inhibits the shift from fatty acid oxidation in resting T cells to glycolytic metabolism in activated T cells. Thus, mTOR inhibitors suppress T cell proliferation and effector differentiation. In addition, they have suppressive effects on B cell activation, proliferation, and antibody production. Due to their unique mechanism of action, rapamycin and its analogs have been used in combination with corticosteroids, cyclosporine, tacrolimus, or mycophenolate mofetil to prevent rejection of solid organ allografts. They may also be used for steroid refractory-GVHD in HSCT recipients. Both drugs come with black box warnings for increased risks of developing infections and malignancies. Other adverse reactions include myelosuppression and hepatotoxicity. Everolimus also has a black box warning for an increased risk of kidney thrombosis, followed

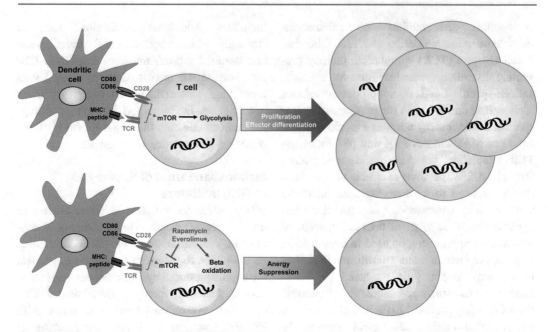

Fig. 8.5 Mechanism of action for mTOR inhibitors. Signaling through the T cell receptor (TCR) and costimulatory receptor (CD28) activates mTOR, resulting in a shift in cellular metabolism from beta oxidation to aerobic glycolysis. This metabolic shift in activated T cells is required for their proliferation and effector differentiation. Treatment with mTOR inhibitors (rapamycin, everolimus) prevents the glycolytic shift, with fatty acid oxidation providing the primary source of cellular energy. This is associated with suppression of T cell proliferation and non-responsiveness (anergy) in the presence of mTOR inhibitors

by loss of the graft, within the first 30 days after transplantation. It should also be avoided during heart transplantation due to increased risk of infections and mortality within the first 3 months after transplantation. Both drugs are metabolized via the CYP3A4 system and therefore drug interactions must be taken into account as described above for calcineurin inhibitors. Finally, therapeutic drug monitoring is required for both drugs due to their narrow therapeutic index.

Anti-proliferative Agents

Azathioprine is a purine analog with anti-proliferative properties that suppresses DNA and RNA synthesis, resulting in the apoptosis of proliferating cells, including T cells (Fig. 8.6). Its mechanism of action is described in detail in Chaps. 6 and 7. In the body, azathioprine is converted into 6-mercaptopurine (6-MP), which is subsequently converted to 6-thioinosonic acid. The latter compound inhibits an enzyme (amido-phosphoribosyltransferase; ATase) required for purine synthesis, thus inhibiting the replication of

T cells and other leukocytes. For transplantation, azathioprine is a second line drug to cyclosporine. Like all anti-proliferative drugs, azathioprine has no selectivity, targeting all replicating cells. Thus, its use can lead to the development of severe side effects, including damage to the bone marrow (anemia, thrombocytopenia, leukopenia), intestinal epithelium, and hair follicles (hair loss). Azathioprine concentrations are increased with the concomitant use of allopurinol. Conversely, treatment with azathioprine is also known to inhibit the anticoagulant effects of warfarin through an unknown mechanism.

Mycophenolic acid was first isolated from *Penicillium breviocompactum*, and was found to have antibacterial as well as anti-tumor activity. It was later discovered that mycophenolic acid suppresses guanine synthesis and hence proliferation of lymphocytes by inhibiting inosine monophosphate dehydrogenase. **Mycophenolate mofetil** (a pro-drug) is widely used in transplantation and is rapidly metabolized into mycophenolic acid following administration, but has

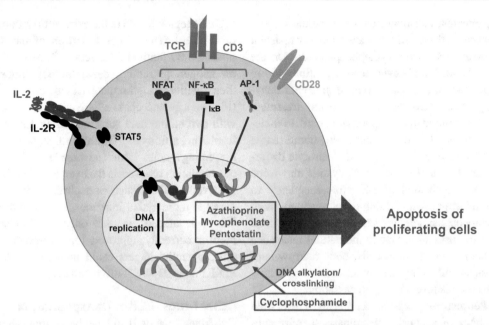

Fig. 8.6 Anti-proliferative agents impair DNA replication or stability. These drugs include nucleoside analogs that prevent DNA synthesis (azathioprine, mycophenolate mofetil, pentostatin) and an alkylating agent that induces DNA crosslinking (cyclophosphamide). Proliferating cells undergo apoptosis in the presence of these drugs

better bioavailability than mycophenolic acid after oral dosing. It is used in combination with calcineurin inhibitors to provide a sparing effect, decreasing side effects such as nephrotoxicity, diabetes, and PTLDs. The most common adverse effects with mycophenolate mofetil are diarrhea, abdominal pain and nausea, which may necessitate a dose reduction. These side effects may be due to the localization of mycophenolate mofetil to epithelial cells in the gastrointestinal tract. Mycophenolate concentrations are decreased with the use of drugs such as antacids, iron, and rifamycins. Medications that increase concentrations include antivirals such as acyclovir and uric acid reducers such as probenecid. Treatment with mycophenolate can also interfere with the efficacy of other drugs such as oral contraceptives and phenytoin by decreasing their concentrations after dosing. Lastly, the drug should be avoided during pregnancy due to the risk of first trimester-associated congenital malformations and/or loss of pregnancy.

Cyclophosphamide is a DNA alkylating agent that was originally designed to destroy cancerous cells. It is widely used in HSCT to prevent GVHD due to its cytotoxic effects on proliferating lymphocytes. It has also been used as a replacement for total body irradiation in HSCT due to its anticancer and immunosuppressive properties. Cyclophosphamide is a pro-drug that requires enzymatic and chemical activation to release the active phosphoramide mustard moiety and acrolein. Phosphoramide induces DNA crosslinking, causing cytotoxicity, while acrolein is responsible for hemorrhagic cystitis, a major side effect of treatment. In the body, oral cyclophosphamide is rapidly absorbed and then converted into active metabolites by the CYP450 system into 4-hydroxycyclophosphamide or 4-hydroxyifosfamide that equilibrate with their aldo tautomers, aldocyclophosphamide or aldoifosfamide. The aldophosphamides freely diffuse into cells where they are further metabolized into the active moieties, phosphoramide mustard and acrolein. These metabolites are highly protein bound and distributed to all tissues. They are also known to cross the placenta and are present in breast milk. Aldophosphamides are oxidized by aldehyde dehydrogenases and cells expressing high levels of aldehyde dehydrogenase, such as hepatocytes, intestinal mucosa or hematopoietic stem cells; these cell types are relatively resistant to cytotoxicity from cyclophosphamide. On the other hand, lymphocytes are susceptible due to their lower expression levels of aldehyde dehydrogenase. Adverse effects from treatment include bone marrow suppression, cardiac toxicity, gonadal failure (amenorrhea), hemorrhagic cystitis, nausea, vomiting, and electrolyte disturbances. Cases of hemorrhagic cystitis may to be due to reactivation of BK virus secondary to immunosuppression. Long-term treatment with cyclophosphamide is significantly associated with malignancies. Due to the natural resistance of hematopoietic stem cells, bone marrow suppression following treatment with cyclophosphamide is reversible upon cessation.

Pentostatin is a purine analog and a reversible inhibitor of adenosine deaminase, thereby suppressing DNA synthesis. Lymphocytes express high levels of adenosine deaminase and are a major target of pentostatin, resulting in prolonged and profound T cell depletion. Pentostatin is commonly used in the treatment of steroid-refractory acute or chronic GVHD after allogeneic HSCT in patients with hematologic disorders including hairy cell leukemia. It has also been found to be useful in preventing allogeneic reactions with nonmyeloablative or less intensive conditioning regimens during HSCT. These regimens have been found to facilitate alloreactive responses in favor of graft-versus-leukemia effects while minimizing GVHD in certain types of patients. In combination with cyclosporine A and mycophenolate mofetil, pentostatin significantly decreases blood levels of T cells, B cells and NK cells. However, its toxic effects on non-lymphocyte populations are minimal.

Costimulation Blockade

Belatacept (Nulojix®) is a selective T cell costimulation blocker that is used to prevent the activation of T cells during transplantation. It is approved for use in renal transplantation and is often used in combination with basiliximab, mycophenolate, or glucocorticoids. Its use is also being examined for hepatic and cardiac transplants. Belatacept is a fusion protein of the human IgG1 Fc region linked to the extracellular domain of CTLA-4. The CTLA-4 portion of the drug binds the B7 family of molecules (CD80, CD86) on antigen presenting cells, thereby blocking their ability to stimulate CD28 on T cells (Fig. 8.4). Belatacept is a derivative of abatacept with two amino acid substitutions that increase its binding affinity to CD80 and CD86 on antigen presenting cells. An advantage of using costimulation blockers is the decreased incidence of adverse effects, such as nephrotoxicity, compared to more global immunosuppressive drugs. While belatacept is the only costimulation blocker currently approved for transplantation, other potential targets could include the PD-1/PD-L1 and CD40/CD40L pathways.

Other Drugs Used in Transplantation

Cytokines such as IL-6 have been implicated in GVHD and the antibody-mediated rejection of renal transplants. IL-6 has many pro-inflammatory functions in the immune system, including the stimulation of antibody production from B cells and induction of acute phase proteins from the liver. **Tocilizumab** is a humanized monoclonal antibody against the IL-6 receptor. As an adjunctive treatment, tocilizumab has shown efficacy against GVHD, donor-specific anti-HLA antibody production, and the systemic cytokine-release syndrome during GVHD. **Etanercept,** a TNF-α inhibitor, is also used for similar purposes. It is a fusion protein consisting of the extracellular domain of the TNF receptor fused to the constant region of IgG. The pharmacology of TNF inhibitors is described in detail in other chapters (Chaps. 2, 5, and 7).

Intravenous immunoglobulin (IVIG) is often used to treat patients with pre-existing antibodies against donor-derived HLA antigens. IVIG can reduce the levels of anti-HLA antibodies, thereby decreasing the risk of antibody-mediated hyperacute rejection in these patients. IVIG consists of immunoglobulin that has been pooled from the plasma of thousands of healthy blood donors. Thus patients receiving IVIG treatment are infused with a broad repertoire of antibodies that recognize pathogens as well as self-antigens and other antibodies. Several mechanisms have been proposed to explain how the variable and constant regions of IVIG antibodies suppress allo-antibody responses. These include the saturation of Fc receptors (preventing Fc receptor-mediated phagocytosis), the saturation of the FcRn Brambell receptor (decreasing the half-life of IgG), upregulation of the inhibitory FcγRIIB receptor on antigen-presenting cells, neutralization of allogeneic antibodies by anti-idiotypic antibodies, attenuation of complement activity, and the downregulation of antigen presentation and lymphocyte activation. Commercial preparations of IVIG contain IgG subclasses with the same distribution as that observed in normal human serum. Following infusion, the half-life of IVIG is 3 weeks. Adverse reactions occur in less than 5% of patients, such as headache, chills, nausea and fatigue. Severe anaphylaxis reactions are rare and may occur within the first hour following infusion. Patients with impaired renal function are at increased risk for acute renal failure following IVIG administration. In addition to being a valuable immunosuppressive treatment for sensitized transplant recipients and patients with autoimmune disorders, IVIG can also be used to provide passive immunity to patients with immune deficiencies. In these cases, IVIG is used for its antimicrobial functions.

From Bench to Bedside: Cyclosporine, the Life-Saving Drug That Almost Never Was...

Commentary by Kaitlin Armstrong and Charles Babcock

The discovery of cyclosporine A revolutionized the course of transplantation therapy, giving rise to the modern era of organ transplantation. Until its discovery, the prevention and treatment of graft rejection relied on pan-immunosuppressive drugs that could induce global immunosuppression in transplant recipients. With the advent of cyclosporine, the selective suppression of immune cells soon became a reality, resulting in the widespread success of renal, hepatic, and cardiac grafts. It has now truly become an essential drug and is widely used to induce immunosuppression in a variety of diseases and conditions, including post-operative rejection prophylaxis in transplant patients.

Cyclosporine suppresses T cell proliferation and activation, thus inhibiting the activity of the principal cell type involved in transplant rejection. In response to T cell receptor stimulation and calcium mobilization, calcineurin dephosphorylates NFAT, resulting in its nuclear translocation and the induction of the genes encoding IL-2, CD40L, IFN-γ, and Fas ligand. Cyclosporine exerts its effects by binding to cyclophilin molecules in lymphocytes, forming a drug-cyclophilin complex that inhibits intracellular calcineurin. Inhibition of this calcineurin/NFAT/IL-2 pathway using cyclosporine thus prevents the expression of genes necessary for T cell activation and proliferation.

Despite its widespread use in transplantation, the therapeutic value of cyclosporine was not immediately evident and was nearly dismissed. In 1958, the drug manufacturer Sandoz®, now a part of Novartis, started an antibiotic and antifungal screening program, testing soil samples for compounds containing antimicrobial activity. It became commonplace for employees who went on vacation to return with samples from their destination. In 1969, a soil specimen from Hardanger Vidda, Norway began a journey that changed the life trajectory for many people. In a microbiology laboratory, B. Thiele isolated *Tolypocladium inflatum* from these samples, a fungus that produces metabolites named cyclosporins. While metabolites containing cyclosporine were found to have weak antifungal activity, they were noted to have low toxicity in mammalian cells. In subsequent studies, cyclosporine was found to selectively inhibit the proliferation of lymphocytes *in vitro*, without affecting somatic cells. This was important considering that Sandoz® had previously tested another drug in 1962 that had greater potency than cyclosporine, but a high degree of toxic effects, leadings to a cessation of research on that medication. Similarly, other non-selective immunosuppressive drugs used at this time (azathioprine, methotrexate) were known to be cytostatic, blocking all rapidly-dividing cells in mitosis and causing severe and life threatening drug limiting adverse events such as anemias and diarrhea.

By 1973, it was determined that a large sum of investment (over $250 Million) would be required to develop cyclosporine for organ transplantation. At this time, transplantation drugs were a small market, since most of the available drugs were inexpensive and solid organ transplants were primarily restricted to kidney allografts. While Sandoz® management proposed abandoning the project, cyclosporine continued to be studied as a treatment for chronic inflammation. Several findings were published in a seminal 1976 paper by Borel et al., demonstrating the antilymphocytic properties of cyclosporine A in rodent models of haemagglutinin formation, skin graft rejection, allergic encephalomyelitis, and arthritis. Parallel studies continued to assess the efficacy of cyclosporine in preventing transplantation rejection. Cyclosporine was found to be effective in all the animal models studied, including mice, rats, pigs and monkeys. Importantly, in comparison to pan-cytostatic drugs, only weak myelotoxicity was observed with the more selective cyclosporine. A follow-up paper in 1978 by Calne et al. demonstrated an improved median survival time of 22 days versus 6 days in pig heart allograft recipients that were treated with cyclosporine. Promising results from these animal studies cleared the way for human clinical trials to proceed.

Around the time that the first cyclosporine trials in humans were underway, researchers in the realm of biochemistry were simultaneously isolating and characterizing calcineurin, the molecular target of cyclosporine. In 1978, Klee and Krinks were the first to purify the protein through affinity chromatography. Further insight into the involvement of calcineurin in the cyclosporine-mediated inhibition of T cells would come much later. In 1990, Matilla et al. demonstrated that the inhibition of T cell activation by cyclosporine and tacrolimus, another calcineurin inhibitor, occurred *via* NFAT and hypothesized that the effects of these drugs were mediated through a calcium-dependent pathway. Then in 1991, Liu et al. discovered that the target of cyclosporine and tacrolimus was calcineurin. By 1992, several other research laboratories confirmed the importance of calcineurin as an integral component of T cell activation.

Back in the late 1970s, initial human testing found that cyclosporine powder was poorly absorbed from gelatin capsules, and a better vehicle for oral delivery was required. Such a setback could have prevented further research on cyclosporine. Following the development of a technique to measure blood concentrations of the drug, it was discovered that an aqueous solution of Tween 80® was the best vehicle for oral absorption. In 1978, the first human kidney transplant recipients to receive cyclosporine were part of a study in the United Kingdom. Although cyclosporine was effective at inhibiting rejection, there was evidence of both nephrotoxicity and hepatotoxicity. Additional studies demonstrated a high incidence of lymphomas, impaired kidney function, and mortality.

Two main reasons have been identified for the limited success of early clinical trials with cyclosporine. First, patients were only treated with cyclosporine and given no other synergistic immunosuppressive drugs. Second, the dose of cyclosporine used was extremely high leading to misinterpretation of the renal dysfunction observed as a consequence of transplant rejection rather than cyclosporine-induced nephrotoxicity. This misinterpretation caused clinical researchers to give prednisolone (a steroid) and a cyclophosphamide derivative, causing further damage to the kidney. In spite of these early setbacks, cyclosporine drastically reduced the number of adverse events compared to azathioprine and methotrexate, allowing the treatment of some patients who previously had severe adverse events from pan-cytostatic drugs.

In 1981, Starzl et al. demonstrated that lower doses of cyclosporine in conjunction with a corticosteroid yielded much better results and fewer mortalities. In light of this, over the next few years, the dose of cyclosporine was reduced and a corticosteroid was added to therapeutic regimens. By 1983, cyclosporine and prednisone were shown to produce a survival rate of 72% in kidney transplants compared to the current standard drug regimen consisting of azathioprine and prednisone. This was followed by additional successes in liver, heart, and bone marrow transplants. Overall, titrating an individual patient's dose and monitoring blood cyclosporine levels has made the adverse event profile much easier to manage.

In 1983, the United States Food and Drug Administration (FDA) initially approved cyclosporine for transplant rejection under the brand name Sandimmune® (cyclosporine A). Over a decade later in 1995, a new, modified formulation that had more predictable pharmacokinetics and a greater bioavailability than the oil-based formulation was also approved. According to Eisen et al. this product, known by the name Neoral® (Cyclosporin A MODIFIED), significantly prevented graft rejection compared to the original drug formulation and allowed lower doses of corticosteroid to be used. Although cyclosporine is a substrate of CYP3A4 and has concerning drug interactions, it is still accepted as a first-line treatment in many solid organ transplants for both initial transplant rejection and prophylaxis of rejection. In addition, cyclosporine A is now approved for a number of diseases including severe plaque psoriasis, chronic dry eye, severe atopic dermatitis, Crohn's Disease, and severe rheumatoid arthritis in patients who do not respond to methotrexate.

Summary

The transplantation of solid organs as well as hematopoietic stem cell transplantation have revolutionized the course of medicine and given hope to countless individuals suffering from various diseases, immune deficiencies, and cancers. Solid organ transplantation includes the transplantation of kidney, liver, heart, and several other organs. HSCT involves the transplantation of hematopoietic stem cells in recipients whose hematopoietic system has been conditioned using myeloablative therapy. The major cause of adverse immune reactions during transplantation are due to HLA-derived differences across donors and recipients. The greater the HLA match between the donor and the recipient, the higher the success rate of transplantation. Solid organ rejection can occur due to immune mechanisms involved in hyperacute, acute, and chronic rejection. On the other hand, GVHD occurs in HSCT recipients, when the donor's immune cells attack the recipient's body.

The understanding of the mechanisms by which the immune system mediates organ rejection and the discovery of a wide spectrum of immunosuppressive agents has turned the ancient dream of organ replacement into a modern-day reality. Transplantation is now a routine medical procedure that is used to save lives throughout the world. A number of drugs are utilized to prevent the development of transplant rejection and GVHD, significantly improving the success of transplantation. These include immunosuppressive agents such as glucocorticoids, calcineurin inhibitors, anti-proliferative agents, and T cell blockers. Furthermore, recent advances in transplantation research have opened the possibility for breakthroughs in several areas including both autologous transplantation and xenotransplantation. Advances in other areas such as stem cell engineering and gene editing further raise the possibility of generating organs for transplantation outside the human body, thus circumventing the need for histocompatibility and human donors. All of these developments have only been possible because of the pioneering work of many transplant physicians and scientists over the centuries as well as countless immunologists who have transformed our understanding of how the immune system works. Conversely, transplantation research itself has directly contributed to our understanding of how the immune system works, leading to the discovery of the MHC genes and molecules, and further insights into T cell function and immunity.

Case Study

Provided by Elizabeth Cohen, PharmD, BCPS

George Johnson is a 45-year-old African American male with chronic kidney disease secondary to diabetes and hypertension. His past medical history is also significant for hyperlipidemia, previous myocardial infarction, arthritis, and GERD. Patient reports getting a rash when taking sulfa antibiotics. He has a calculated panel reactive antibody (cPRA) of 87%. He has just received a deceased donor kidney transplant after being on dialysis for 5 years.

George's medications taken prior to transplant include:

- Amlodipine 5 mg by mouth daily
- Losartan 100 mg by mouth daily
- Metoprolol ER 100 mg by mouth daily
- Omeprazole 20 mg by mouth daily
- Aspirin 81 mg by mouth daily
- Insulin glargine 20 units subcutaneously at bedtime
- Insulin lispro 9 units subcutaneously three times daily before meals
- Atorvastatin 40 mg by mouth daily
- Sevelamer 800 mg TID with meals
- Sodium bicarbonate 650 mg BID
- OTC: naproxen 220–440 mg by mouth as needed for knee pain

1. Given the patient's cPRA of 87%, relatively younger age, African American and deceased donor transplant, the transplant team decides to use antithymocyte globulin. How does antithymocyte globulin exert its immunosuppressive effects as an induction agent?
2. For maintenance immunosuppression, the team decides on a three drug regimen with tacrolimus, mycophenolate mofetil and prednisone. What class of medication is tacrolimus? Where does it act on the immune cascade?
3. Omeprazole, one of George's home medications can affect the drug levels of tacrolimus. Which system does it interact with?
4. Six weeks after transplant, George is admitted with an increasing serum creatinine to 4.7 mg/dL after a period of admitted nonadherence to his immunosuppressive medications. A renal biopsy is performed and he is found to have acute cellular rejection (ACR), Banff grade IIA and antibody-mediated rejection (AMR). The team decides to treat the ACR with methylprednisolone pulse and antithymocyte globulin due to the severity of the rejection. For the AMR, the team decides to use rituximab. What is the mechanism of action for rituximab for AMR?

Practice Questions

1. Describe the terms listed below and provide an example of each: autograft, isograft, allograft, xenograft, alloantigens.
2. Explain the causative mechanisms involved in the hyperacute rejection of solid organ transplants.
3. Explain the immunological principles underlying successful blood transfusions.
4. A cross-match test is one in which:
   (a) the recipient's antibodies are tested for reactivity against donor blood antigens
   (b) the donor's antibodies are tested for reactivity against recipient blood antigens
   (c) the recipient's antibodies are tested for reactivity against donor HLA antigens
   (d) the donor's antibodies are tested for reactivity against recipient HLA antigens
5. Which of the following is false regarding hyperacute rejection?
   (a) It is mediated by pre-existing antibodies against blood group antigens
   (b) It can be treated by immunosuppressive drugs
   (c) It occurs within minutes to hours of transplantation
   (d) Intravenous immunoglobulin may be used to prevent it
6. Compare and contrast the mechanisms involved in acute and chronic rejection of solid organ transplants.
7. Identify three general classes of drug that are used to suppress acute transplant rejection, and provide examples of each class. What are some side-effects and toxic effects that are associated with each class of drug?
8. Jonathan, a 52-year-old construction worker, recently received a renal transplant for immune complex-mediated nephropathy. Maintenance therapy involved treatment with cyclosporine, mycophenolate, and prednisone. A few weeks post-transplantation, Jonathan began to present with deteriorating renal function. He was treated with basiliximab and the doses of his other medications were also increased. His symptoms subsided and his condition improved significantly. Which of the following represents a likely cause of the symptoms being experienced by Jonathan?
   (a) Hyperacute rejection
   (b) Acute rejection
   (c) Chronic rejection
   (d) None of the above
9. The success of solid organ transplantation is directly correlated with:
   (a) ABO compatibility
   (b) the degree of HLA matching
   (c) expression of minor histocompatibility antigens
   (d) immune status of the recipient
10. Which of the following describes the mechanism of action of cyclosporine?
    (a) It is an inhibitor of T cell costimulation
    (b) It prevents the activation of NFAT by binding cyclophilins
    (c) It inhibits DNA replication in T cells
    (d) It is a prodrug that is converted to an active phospharamide moiety *in vivo*
11. Which of the following is a potential concern when treating with cyclosporine?
    (a) Nephrotoxicity
    (b) Leukopenia
    (c) Myelosuppression
    (d) Damage to hair follicles
12. Which of the following best describes the mechanism of action of basiliximab?
    (a) It inhibits mTOR
    (b) It blocks T cell proliferation by inhibiting IL-2 signaling
    (c) It blocks T cell costimulation
    (d) It inhibits calcineurin
13. In 1985, OKT3 was the first monoclonal antibody to be approved for clinical use in humans. Despite its efficacy in transplantation, it was eventually taken off the market in 2008. Which of the following represent concerns associated with OKT3? Select all that apply.
    (a) It caused the systemic release of cytokines by T cells soon after treatment had started
    (b) It was not effective at depleting T cells and so could only be used during the induction phase
    (c) It could only be used once, since subsequent treatments caused the development of serum sickness

(d) It only depleted T cells and therefore was not effective at inducing immunosuppression

14. Jonathan returned to his physician and complained that he was feeling very depressed and sometimes felt like he was day-dreaming. Which of the following drugs may be a cause of his symptoms?
    (a) Cyclosporine
    (b) Basiliximab
    (c) Prednisone
    (d) Mycophenolate

15. Mycophenolate is an example of a cytotoxic drug. What is the mechanism of action of this drug?
    (a) It inhibits NF-κB
    (b) It is converted in vivo to 6-MP and thioinosonic acid which inhibits T cell proliferation
    (c) It suppresses lymphocyte proliferation by inhibiting guanine synthesis
    (d) It is converted to aldophosphamides which block T cell function

16. Mouse monoclonal antibodies are extremely effective during transplantation therapy. Provide an example of a depleting and a nondepleting antibody used to suppress graft rejection. Describe its use in transplantation therapy.

17. Select all that apply. Myeloablative therapy is given to transplant patients to:
    (a) destroy the patient's immune system in preparation for hematopoietic cell transplantation
    (b) increase the patient's capacity to fight cancers
    (c) prevent the development of graft versus host disease
    (d) provide space for the flourishing of the donor's hematopoietic system

18. Which of the following organs are associated with severe adverse reactions during graft versus host disease? Select all that apply.
    (a) Skin
    (b) Liver
    (c) Heart
    (d) Intestine

19. Belatacept is a novel immunomodulator used for the treatment of graft rejection. What is its mechanism of action?:
    (a) It inhibits the IL-2 receptor
    (b) It inhibits activation via CD28
    (c) It suppresses mTOR
    (d) It inhibits CD52

20. Which of the following drugs is associated with impaired metabolism of azathioprine?
    (a) Tacrolimus
    (b) St John's wort
    (c) Allopurinol
    (d) Rifampin

Suggested Reading

Almeida CC, et al. Safety of immunosuppressive drugs used as maintenance therapy in kidney transplantation: a systematic review and meta-analysis. Pharmaceuticals (Basel). 2013;6:1170–94.

Appelbaum FR. Hematopoietic cell transplantation as immunotherapy. Nature. 2001;411:385–9.

Armitage JO. Bone marrow transplantation. N Engl J Med. 1994;330:827–38.

Barker CF, Markmann JF. Historical overview of transplantation. Cold Spring Harb Perspect Med. 2013;3:a014977.

Barnett ANR, Hadjianastassiou VG, Mamode N. Rituximab in renal transplantation. Transpl Int. 2013;26:563–75.

Bohmig GA, Farkas AM, Eskandary F, Wekerle T. Strategies to overcome the ABO barrier in kidney transplantation. Nat Rev Nephrol. 2015;11:732–47.

Borel JF, Feurer C, Gubler HU, Stahelin H. Biological effects of cyclosporin A: a new antilymphocytic agent. Agents Actions. 1976;6:468–75.

Borel JF, Feurer C, Gubler HU, Stahelin H. Biological effects of cyclosporin A: a new antilymphocytic agent. 1976. Agents Actions. 1994;43:179–86.

Calne RY, White DJ, Rolles K, Smith DP, Herbertson BM. Prolonged survival of pig orthotopic heart grafts treated with cyclosporin A. Lancet. 1978;1:1183–5.

Calne RY, et al. Cyclosporin A initially as the only immunosuppressant in 34 recipients of cadaveric organs: 32 kidneys, 2 pancreases, and 2 livers. Lancet. 1979;2:1033–6.

Chang YJ, Zhao XY, Huang XJ. Strategies for enhancing and preserving anti-leukemia effects without aggravating graft-versus-host disease. Front Immunol. 2018;9:3041.

Choi J, et al. Assessment of tocilizumab (anti-interleukin-6 receptor monoclonal) as a potential treatment for chronic antibody-mediated rejection and transplant glomerulopathy in HLA-sensitized renal allograft recipients. Am J Transplant. 2017;17:2381–9.

Chong AS, Alegre ML. The impact of infection and tissue damage in solid-organ transplantation. Nat Rev Immunol. 2012;12:459–71.

Clipstone NA, Crabtree GR. Identification of calcineurin as a key signalling enzyme in T-lymphocyte activation. Nature. 1992;357:695–7.

Colombo D, Ammirati E. Cyclosporine in transplantation—a history of converging timelines. J Biol Regul Homeost Agents. 2011;25:493–504.

Copelan EA. Hematopoietic stem-cell transplantation. N Engl J Med. 2006;354:1813–26.

Cyclosporin in cadaveric renal transplantation: one-year follow-up of a multicentre trial. Lancet. 1983;2:986–9.

Dean L, National Center for Biotechnology Information (U.S.). Blood groups and red cell antigens. Bethesda: NCBI; 2005.

Dierickx D, Habermann TM. Post-transplantation lymphoproliferative disorders in adults. N Engl J Med. 2018;378:549–62.

Durrbach A, Francois H, Beaudreuil S, Jacquet A, Charpentier B. Advances in immunosuppression for renal transplantation. Nat Rev Nephrol. 2010;6:160–7.

Eisen HJ, et al. Safety, tolerability, and efficacy of cyclosporine microemulsion in heart transplant recipients: a randomized, multicenter, double-blind comparison with the oil-based formulation of cyclosporine—results at 24 months after transplantation. Transplantation. 2001;71:70–8.

Enderby C, Keller CA. An overview of immunosuppression in solid organ transplantation. Am J Manag Care. 2015;21:s12–23.

Epstein FH, Ferrara JLM, Deeg HJ. Graft-versus-host disease. N Engl J Med. 1991;324:667–74.

Fantus D, Rogers NM, Grahammer F, Huber TB, Thomson AW. Roles of mTOR complexes in the kidney: implications for renal disease and transplantation. Nat Rev Nephrol. 2016;12:587–609.

Ford ML, Larsen CP. Translating costimulation blockade to the clinic: lessons learned from three pathways. Immunol Rev. 2009;229:294–306.

Ford ML, Adams AB, Pearson TC. Targeting co-stimulatory pathways: transplantation and autoimmunity. Nat Rev Nephrol. 2014;10:14–24.

Gabardi S, Martin ST, Roberts KL, Grafals M. Induction immunosuppressive therapies in renal transplantation. Am J Health Syst Pharm. 2011;68:211–8.

Ganetsky A, et al. Tocilizumab for the treatment of severe steroid-refractory acute graft-versus-host disease of the lower gastrointestinal tract. Bone Marrow Transplant. 2019;54(2):212–7.

Halloran PF. Immunosuppressive drugs for kidney transplantation. N Engl J Med. 2004;351:2715–29.

Harousseau JL, Moreau P. Autologous hematopoietic stem-cell transplantation for multiple myeloma. N Engl J Med. 2009;360:2645–54.

Jenq RR, van den Brink MR. Allogeneic haematopoietic stem cell transplantation: individualized stem cell and immune therapy of cancer. Nat Rev Cancer. 2010;10:213–21.

Johnston JB. Mechanism of action of pentostatin and cladribine in hairy cell leukemia. Leuk Lymphoma. 2011;52:43–5.

Jordan SC, Vo AA, Peng A, Toyoda M, Tyan D. Intravenous gammaglobulin (IVIG): a novel approach to improve transplant rates and outcomes in highly HLA-sensitized patients. Am J Transplant. 2006;6:459–66.

Jordan SC, et al. Interleukin-6, a cytokine critical to mediation of inflammation, autoimmunity and allograft rejection. Transplantation. 2017;101:32–44.

Jorgensen KA, Koefoed-Nielsen PB, Karamperis N. Calcineurin phosphatase activity and immunosuppression. A review on the role of calcineurin phosphatase activity and the immunosuppressive effect of cyclosporin A and tacrolimus. Scand J Immunol. 2003;57:93–8.

Kanakry CG, Fuchs EJ, Luznik L. Modern approaches to HLA-haploidentical blood or marrow transplantation. Nat Rev Clin Oncol. 2016;13:10–24.

Kazatchkine MD, Kaveri SV. Immunomodulation of autoimmune and inflammatory diseases with intravenous immune globulin. N Engl J Med. 2001;345:747–55.

Klee CB, Krinks MH. Purification of cyclic 3′,5′-nucleotide phosphodiesterase inhibitory protein by affinity chromatography on activator protein coupled to Sepharose. Biochemistry. 1978;17:120–6.

Kuba A, Raida L. Graft versus host disease: from basic pathogenic principles to DNA damage response and cellular senescence. Mediat Inflamm. 2018;2018:9451950.

Li HW, Sykes M. Emerging concepts in haematopoietic cell transplantation. Nat Rev Immunol. 2012;12:403–16.

Liu J, et al. Calcineurin is a common target of cyclophilin-cyclosporin A and FKBP-FK506 complexes. Cell. 1991;66:807–15.

Liu J, et al. Inhibition of T cell signaling by immunophilin-ligand complexes correlates with loss of calcineurin phosphatase activity. Biochemistry. 1992;31:3896–901.

Lutz HU. Intravenously applied IgG stimulates complement attenuation in a complement-dependent autoimmune disease at the amplifying C3 convertase level. Blood. 2004;103:465–72.

MacDonald KPA, Betts BC, Couriel D. Reprint of: emerging therapeutics for the control of chronic graft-versus-host disease. Biol Blood Marrow Transplant. 2018;24:S7–S14.

Malvezzi P, Jouve T, Rostaing L. Costimulation blockade in kidney transplantation. Transplantation. 2016;100:2315–23.

Mancusi A, Piccinelli S, Velardi A, Pierini A. The effect of TNF-alpha on regulatory T cell function in graft-versus-host disease. Front Immunol. 2018;9:356.

Marcen R. Immunosuppressive drugs in kidney transplantation: impact on patient survival, and incidence of cardiovascular disease, malignancy and infection. Drugs. 2009;69:2227–43.

Mattila PS, et al. The actions of cyclosporin A and FK506 suggest a novel step in the activation of T lymphocytes. EMBO J. 1990;9:4425–33.

Metalidis C, Kuypers DR. Emerging immunosuppressive drugs in kidney transplantation. Curr Clin Pharmacol. 2011;6:130–6.

Montgomery RA, Tatapudi VS, Leffell MS, Zachary AA. HLA in transplantation. Nat Rev Nephrol. 2018;14:558–70.

Pascual M, Theruvath T, Kawai T, Tolkoff-Rubin N, Cosimi AB. Strategies to improve long-term outcomes after renal transplantation. N Engl J Med. 2002;346:580–90.

Pavletic SZ, et al. Lymphodepleting effects and safety of pentostatin for nonmyeloablative allogeneic stem-cell transplantation1. Transplantation. 2003;76: 877–81.

Santos ESP, Bennett CL, Chakraverty R. Unraveling the mechanisms of cutaneous graft-versus-host disease. Front Immunol. 2018;9:963.

Scandling JD, et al. Chimerism, graft survival, and withdrawal of immunosuppressive drugs in HLA matched and mismatched patients after living donor kidney and hematopoietic cell transplantation. Am J Transplant. 2015;15:695–704.

Schrem H. Mycophenolate mofetil in liver transplantation: a review. Ann Transplant. 2013;18: 685–96.

Sheilagh B. Red blood cell antigens and human blood groups. In: Handbook of pediatric transfusion medicine. Elsevier; 2004. p. 45–61.

Srinivas TR, Kaplan B. Transplantation in 2011: new agents, new ideas and new hope. Nat Rev Nephrol. 2011;8:74–5.

Starzl TE, et al. Cyclosporin A and steroid therapy in sixty-six cadaver kidney recipients. Surg Gynecol Obstet. 1981;153:486–94.

Suthanthiran M, Strom TB. Renal transplantation. N Engl J Med. 1994;331:365–76.

Taylor AL, Watson CJE, Bradley JA. Immunosuppressive agents in solid organ transplantation: mechanisms of action and therapeutic efficacy. Crit Rev Oncol Hematol. 2005;56:23–46.

Ureshino H, et al. Tocilizumab for severe cytokine-release syndrome after haploidentical donor transplantation in a patient with refractory Epstein-Barr virus-positive diffuse large B-cell lymphoma. Hematol Oncol. 2017;36:324–7.

van Gelder T, van Schaik RH, Hesselink DA. Pharmacogenetics and immunosuppressive drugs in solid organ transplantation. Nat Rev Nephrol. 2014;10: 725–31.

Wang J. CYP3A polymorphisms and immunosuppressive drugs in solid-organ transplantation. Expert Rev Mol Diagn. 2009;9:383–90.

Zeiser R, Blazar BR. Pathophysiology of chronic graft-versus-host disease and therapeutic targets. N Engl J Med. 2017;377:2565–79.

Zhang L, Chu J, Yu J, Wei W. Cellular and molecular mechanisms in graft-versus-host disease. J Leukoc Biol. 2015;99:279–87.

Zwang NA, Turka LA. Transplantation immunology in 2013: New approaches to diagnosis of rejection. Nat Rev Nephrol. 2014;10:72–4.

Immunopathogenesis, Immunization, and Treatment of Infectious Diseases

9

Doreen E. Szollosi, Clinton B. Mathias,
Victoria Lucero, Sunna Ahmad,
and Jennifer Donato

Learning Objectives

1. Describe the principles of vaccination and discuss the immune mechanisms involved
2. Discuss the role of adjuvants and vaccine additives in vaccines
3. Given a vaccine, discuss the type of vaccine, its mechanism of action, functional responses, and adverse effects.
4. Explain the immune mechanisms involved in the pathogenesis of HIV infection and the development of AIDS
5. Explain the role of the immune system in protection from AIDS-related opportunistic infections

6. Explain the immune mechanisms involved in the development of sepsis and septic shock
7. Discuss the pathogenesis, diagnosis, and treatment of tuberculosis
8. Explain the immune mechanisms involved in the pathogenesis of leprosy
9. Explain the immune mechanisms involved in the pathogenesis of Toxic Shock Syndrome

Vaccines discussed in this chapter

Vaccine	Classification
DTaP (Daptacel,® Infanrix®)	Inactivated
Herpes zoster (Zostavax,® Shingrix®)	Live attenuated, recombinant
Hepatitis A (Havrix,® Vaqta®)	Inactivated
Hepatitis B (Recombivax HB,® Engerix-B®, Heplisav-B®)	Recombinant, subunit
Hepatitis A, Hepatitis B combo (Twinrix®)	Inactivated
Human papillomavirus (Gardasil-9®)	Recombinant, subunit
Influenza (Afluria,® Fluad,® Fluarix,® Flublok,® Flucelvax,® FluLaval,® FluMist,® Fluvirin,® Fluzone,® Fluzone®-High Dose, Fluzone®-Intradermal)	Inactivated, recombinant (Flublok®), live (FluMist®)
Measles, Mumps, Rubella (M-M-R®II)	Live attenuated
Measles, Mumps, Rubella, Varicella (ProQuad®)	Live attenuated
Meningococcal ACWY (Menactra,® Menveo®)	Conjugate
Meningococcal ACWY (Menomune®)	Polysaccharide
Meningococcal serogroup B (Bexsero,® Trumenba®)	Protein

D. E. Szollosi (✉)
Department of Pharmaceutical Sciences,
School of Pharmacy and Physician Assistant Studies,
University of Saint Joseph, Hartford, CT, USA
e-mail: dszollosi@usj.edu

S. Ahmad
School of Pharmacy and Physician Assistant Studies,
University of Saint Joseph, Hartford, CT, USA

C. B. Mathias
Department of Pharmaceutical and Administrative
Sciences, College of Pharmacy and Health Sciences,
Western New England University, Springfield, MA,
USA
e-mail: clinton.mathias@wne.edu

V. Lucero
Yale New Haven Hospital, New Haven, CT, USA

J. Donato
St. Vincent's Medical Center, Bridgeport, CT, USA

© Springer Nature Switzerland AG 2020
C. B. Mathias et al., *Pharmacology of Immunotherapeutic Drugs*,
https://doi.org/10.1007/978-3-030-19922-7_9

Vaccine	Classification
Pneumococcal (Prevnar13,® Pneumovax23®)	Conjugate, polysaccharide
Tdap (Boostrix,® Adacel®)	Toxoid, acellular pertussis
Varicella zoster (Varivax®)	Live attenuated

Drugs discussed in this chapter

Drug	Classification
Baloxavir marboxil (Xofluza®)	Influenza antiviral
Bezlotoxumab (Zinplava®)	Anti-*C.diff* toxin B monoclonal antibody
Drotrecogin alfa (Xigris®) *discontinued	Recombinant human activated protein C
Ethambutol	TB antibiotic
Isoniazid (INH)	TB antibiotic
Oseltamivir (Tamiflu®)	Influenza antiviral
Peramivir (Rapivab®)	Influenza antiviral
Pyrazinamide	TB antibiotic
Rifampin	TB antibiotic
Zanamivir (Relenza®)	Influenza antiviral
Zidovudine (AZT)	Antiretroviral therapy

Introduction

Human beings have been plagued by infectious diseases since the beginning of their existence. At various points throughout history, human encounter with infectious organisms has not only resulted in disease and death, but has played a major role in the rise or fall of individuals and nations, the persistence of poverty, and the inability to thrive as a society. In the past, entire populations have been wiped out by diseases such as the plague, black death, and small pox. Other diseases such as leprosy and syphilis sealed the fate of those who succumbed to them, leading to being associated with stigma, and exclusion from society. In our own day, diseases such as malaria and Acquired Immune Deficiency Syndrome (AIDS) have had a tremendous impact on the health and the well-being of nations. Furthermore, the threat of pandemics posed by diseases such as influenza, the emergence of novel infectious organisms, and the development of antibiotic resistance are pressing health concerns for the medical community throughout the world.

During the last two centuries, the knowledge of microbial structure, life cycle, and pathogenesis, as well as the mechanisms of immunity, have significantly advanced our ability to fight the scourge of infectious disease. The advent of vaccination was a major force in the battle against infectious disease and paved the way for pioneering research into the mechanisms by which the immune system fights infectious organisms. This knowledge has led to improvements in public health, hygiene, the provision of safe food and drinking water, and many other sanitary practices that have resulted in either the eradication or the prevention of once feared diseases such as small pox, tuberculosis (TB), and cholera. Similarly, government-mandated vaccination programs throughout the world have succeeded in limiting the spread of many infectious diseases including poliomyelitis, measles, and pertussis among others. Lastly, knowledge of the pathogenesis of various pathogens, and the immune mechanisms involved in their destruction, has allowed the development of many novel drugs that have improved the lives of people throughout the world.

In this chapter, we will consider various immunological approaches towards the elimination of infectious diseases. In the first part of the chapter, we will discuss the mechanisms of vaccination and currently approved vaccines for various diseases. In the second part, we will discuss the immune mechanisms involved in the pathogenesis and control of diseases such as AIDS and TB, as well as examine the role of the immune system in mediating the symptoms associated with sepsis and toxic shock syndrome.

Mechanisms of Vaccination

The modern era of vaccination began in the late 1700s, when Dr. Edward Jenner, a doctor in his native town of Berkeley, England, first demonstrated that exposure to the cowpox virus could protect from subsequent infection with the smallpox virus. Jenner's method of exposing an individual to a weakened version of a pathogen to create protection against the more virulent

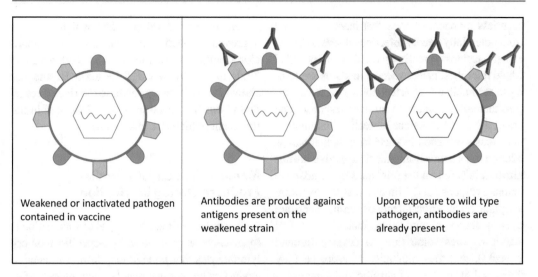

Fig. 9.1 Antigens on a weakened strain of the microbe can stimulate the immune response to create antibodies that will also recognize antigens on a pathogenic strain, creating a memory response

version of that pathogen came to be known as **vaccination**, after the vaccinia virus, which is the causative agent of cowpox. What is now known about the surface antigens of vaccinia virus and the smallpox virus is that they are closely related and share some of the same antigens (Fig. 9.1). Subsequent vaccines in the 1800s that were created by Pasteur included cholera, anthrax, and rabies. Due to an intense vaccination program, smallpox was officially declared eradicated by the World Health Organization (WHO) in 1980. Vaccination programs in the late 1900s have also led to a significant reduction in cases of infectious diseases such as polio, measles, mumps, and rubella. Currently, there are also vaccines against chickenpox, Hepatitis A, Hepatitis B, rotavirus, influenza, and pneumonia.

Production of Adaptive Immunity and Memory

As discussed in detail in Chap. 3, the goal of immunization or vaccination is to induce an adaptive immune response that confers immunological memory to the specific pathogen for which protection is being sought. This established adaptive immune response allows the vaccinated individual to mount a quicker, more efficient fight against the pathogen once it has breached the barriers of the innate immune sys-

tem. Vaccination allows the immune system to encounter the pathogenic organism in the context of a 'non-infectious' environment. Thus, individuals are typically immunized with weakened or inactivated strains of pathogens that allow the immune system to "see" potential pathogens as a non-harmful first exposure in order to determine how to react upon subsequent exposure(s) (Fig. 9.1). Initial exposure to the strain in the vaccine initiates the development of a primary immune response, with the activation of effector T and B cells and the production of antibodies. As the primary immune response wanes, antigen-specific memory T and B cells are generated with the potential to confer life-long immunity against the weakened pathogenic strain in the vaccine. When the vaccinated individual is re-exposed to the offending pathogen in the context of an infectious setting, a rapid and powerful secondary immune response is mediated resulting in destruction of the pathogen and termination of the infection. In an ideal vaccine, the effectiveness of the secondary response which has been built from immunization should allow rapid clearance of the infection before symptoms develop. As such, the quality and quantity of the secondary response may be significantly improved with successive immunizations or booster doses of the vaccine.

Immunization programs have been the most successful medical procedure used, simply by the countless numbers of lives that have been saved from potentially deadly infectious diseases. While earlier vaccines typically used either live or killed whole microbes, newer vaccine methods are turning to recombinant DNA technology to create antigens that will stimulate an immune response. The use of a vaccine to induce protective immunity to infectious organisms in vaccinated individuals is referred to as active immunization. **Active immunization** is based on the principles of the adaptive immune response and mimics a real-life exposure to a pathogen in a non-infectious setting. There are cons to active immunization, including the fact that it requires some time to develop (around 2 weeks), and thus immunity may not be fully developed at the time of specific antigenic exposure. But, active immunity is still preferable to passive, since it allows the individual to develop immunity against the pathogen, thereby conferring life-long protection. This immunity is mediated through the development of highly effective neutralizing antibodies and antigen-specific T and B cells that can be sustained for long periods of time. An ideal immunogen to include in a vaccine to promote an active, adaptive immune response should have several properties which facilitate complete prevention of disease, inhibit transmission of the disease through individuals who serve as carriers, produce prolonged immunity with a minimum of immunizations, lack toxicity, and be suitable for mass immunization.

Passive immunization on the other hand, is when a susceptible individual acquires temporary immunity through the transfer of antibodies formed by other individuals or animals. Examples of this include a newborn receiving IgA antibodies through its mother's breast milk, or anti-venom IgG antibodies being administered to the victim of a snakebite. Passive immunization is useful for patients who are unable to generate antibodies on their own (such as those with agammaglobulinemia), to prevent disease when time does not permit active immunization (post-exposure prophylaxis), or for treatment of diseases normally prevented by immunization, such as tetanus. IgG antibodies have a long half-life and can last a number of months before degrading in recipients of passive immunization, thus providing limited time protection to susceptible individuals.

One recently-developed drug which has been approved for passive immunization is the monoclonal antibody **bezlotoxumab**. Bezlotoxumab binds to *Clostridium difficile* toxin B, and has shown to significantly decrease the risk of recurrent *C. difficile* infection within 12 week of initial treatment in high risk individuals.

Memory Cells and Antibodies Produced During Vaccination

As discussed in Chap. 3, the goal of vaccination is to generate a pool of antigen-specific memory lymphocytes that provide long-lasting protection against pathogens that may be encountered. After clonal selection of B and T lymphocytes whose BCR and TCR match the antigen contained in the vaccine, activated T helper cells help differentiate B cells into plasma cells which secrete high amounts of antibodies. Memory B cells resulting from this clonal expansion phase persist for several years. Upon re-exposure to the antigen that was contained in the vaccine, memory B cells rapidly differentiate into antibody-secreting plasma cells which help to clear the pathogen efficiently.

Types of Vaccines

The currently available vaccines for bacterial infections are outlined in Table 9.1. Most vaccines for viruses are made from attenuated or inactivated viruses, but newer methods include making vaccines using recombinant DNA technology (Table 9.2). The success of the first viral vaccine, the smallpox vaccine, was greatly facilitated by the incorporation of safe non-human counterparts which shared epitopes with the original virus and allowed the generation of cross-reactive neutralizing antibodies. Thus, the smallpox vaccine consisting of vaccinia virus which caused cowpox infection in cattle, also conferred immunity to variola virus, the causative agent of smallpox. However, unlike the smallpox/cowpox relation, most pathogenic viruses that infect humans do not have a non-virulent relative, thus creating the need to alter the actual virus or use parts of the virus for the

Table 9.1 Available bacterial vaccines and type

Bacterial diseases	Vaccine type	Recommended for
Anthrax (*Bacillus anthracis*)	Subunit	PEP, Military personnel, laboratory personnel who work with *B. anthracis*
Cholera (*Vibrio cholerae*)	Inactivated	Travelers to areas where cholera is endemic (age range 18–64)
Diphtheria (*Corynebacterium diphtheriae*)	Toxoid	Children and adults as part of DTaP or Tdap according to immunization schedule
Meningitis (*Hemophilus influenzae* type b, Hib)	Conjugate	Children younger than 5 years old
Meningitis (*Neisseria meningitidis*)	Conjugate or polysaccharide	Pre-teens and teens/young adults. Younger children at increased risk
Pertussis (*Bordetella pertussis*)	Inactivated	Children and adults as part of DTaP or TDaP according to immunization schedule
Pneumonia (*Streptococcus pneumoniae*)	Conjugate, polysaccharide	Babies and children younger than 2 years old, adults 65 years and older, people ages 2–64 with higher risk/certain medical conditions, ages 19–64 who smoke
Tetanus (*Clostridium tetani*)	Toxoid	Children and adults as part of DTaP or Tdap according to immunization schedule
Tuberculosis (*Mycobacterium*)	Attenuated *Bacille Calmette-Guerin* (BCG)	Rarely used in the U.S.A.
Typhoid fever (*Salmonella typhi*)	Inactivated, polysaccharide	Travelers to countries where typhoid is common

PEP Post-exposure prophylaxis

Table 9.2 Available viral vaccines and type

Viral diseases	Vaccine type	Recommended for
Adenovirus	Attenuated	Military personnel
Hepatitis A	Inactivated	Those at increased risk for Hep A (see text)
Hepatitis B	Subunit, recombinant Hep B sAg	Usually within 24 h of birth
HPV	Subunit, VLPs	Adults through age 26
Japanese encephalitis	Attenuated	Travelers to Asia, specifically areas where JE occurs, laboratory workers who work with JE virus
Measles	Attenuated	Babies and kids through age 6, teens and adults booster as part of MMR vaccine
Mumps	Attenuated	Babies and kids through age 6, teens and adults booster as part of MMR vaccine
Polio	Inactivated	Babies and children up to age 6
Rabies	Inactivated	PEP, veterinary staff, rabies researchers, wildlife workers
Rotavirus	Attenuated	Babies younger than 8 months old
Rubella	Attenuated	Babies and kids through age 6, teens and adults booster as part of MMR vaccine
Seasonal influenza	Inactivated, attenuated, or recombinant, depending on brand	Yearly-everyone
Vaccinia (Smallpox)	Live vaccinia virus	Lab workers who work with smallpox or viruses similar to smallpox. Vaccine stockpiles exist in the U.S. in the event of outbreak
Varicella zoster (chickenpox, shingles)	Attenuated	Children, teens, and adults (chickenpox) Adults 60 years and older (shingles)
Yellow fever	Attenuated	Travelers to yellow fever endemic regions

PEP Post-exposure prophylaxis, *MMR* Measles, mumps, rubella vaccine

vaccine. The components of the vaccine however, should not be capable of causing disease.

Attenuated (Live) vaccines contain a live pathogen with reduced virulence. In the case of most viral vaccines, this is achieved by growing viruses in cells of non-human primates or other animals until they are unable to grow well in human cells and as a result are unable to produce disease in humans. The attenuation of the virus occurs as a result of successive mutations that have occurred that facilitate its growth in the new species but prevents its replication in human cells. When individuals receive the vaccine, this allows the immune system sufficient time to generate a primary immune response against the weakened viral strain. For vaccines against pathogenic bacteria, the particular bacterium can be grown in cell culture and genetically manipulated to reduce virulence. Because attenuated vaccines are modified live pathogens, they may produce a small infection, which triggers a true adaptive immune response. Due to this small infection, live vaccines may be dangerous for immunocompromised patients as well as pregnant women. The possibility of genetic reversion in humans also exists and has been noted in the case of the Sabin vaccine, the oral vaccine for poliomyelitis. This vaccine consists of three strains of the polio virus, one of which requires only a few mutations for reversion to occur. While the oral vaccine is highly effective at preventing the epidemic spread of polio, in many countries such as the U.S., where the disease is no longer endemic, the Salk vaccine, which is the heat-killed polio vaccine, is preferred.

Inactivated (killed) vaccines contain whole pathogens which have been deactivated with formalin, physical heat, or irradiation. As such, they are unable to mutate, revert to virulence, or replicate. While this makes them safer than live attenuated vaccines, they are not as effective when given by themselves, since they are unable to stimulate toll-like receptors and antigen presenting cells, as a live, replicating organism. For this reason, inactivated vaccines are often given with adjuvants to increase the efficacy of the vaccine. The adjuvants act by stimulating local antigen-presenting cells and inducing the development of inflammation.

Toxoid vaccines use chemically or thermally modified toxins from bacteria to stimulate antibody-mediated immunity. Examples of toxoid vaccines include the diphtheria and tetanus vaccines. Because the toxoids by themselves, as in the case of inactivated vaccines, are unable to stimulate potent immune responses, they are given in combination with heat-killed or acellular vaccine components to increase their potency. The DTP vaccine, which was used in the U.S. until the 1980s consisted of the diphtheria and tetanus toxoids and heat-killed *pertussis* bacteria. The present vaccine, the Tdap vaccine consists of acellular *pertussis* components that have been deemed to be safer than the DTP vaccine.

Subunit vaccines contain a protein, usually the most antigenic component, which has been isolated from the pathogen. Thus, the vaccine consists of purified antigens for the immune system to recognize without infectious particles that could potentially cause disease. One of the most common examples of a subunit vaccine is the HBV vaccine which at first was composed of the **hepatitis B surface antigen (Hep B sAg)** that had been purified from the plasma of people infected with the Hepatitis B virus. To mitigate the possibility of infectious particles making it into the vaccine along with the surface antigen, recombinant DNA technology was used to generate Hep B sAg by inserting the gene for the antigen into a yeast genome. The Hep B sAg-producing yeast can be grown in culture and the antigen can be purified in large quantities.

Recombinant vaccines Since Louis Pasteur's first vaccine manufacturing methods of isolating a pathogenic microorganism, inactivating it, and injecting it into animals and people to elicit an immune response, other methods have been developed that may prove more useful in creating new vaccines. Recombinant vaccines are produced utilizing DNA technology (Fig. 9.2). When an antigen is identified that can elicit an immune response from the host, the DNA encoding that antigen is cloned and inserted into a cell line, which in turn starts expressing that antigen. The antigen can then be purified from the cell line and used in the vaccine. Examples of commonly-used recombinant protein vaccines are HBV in which

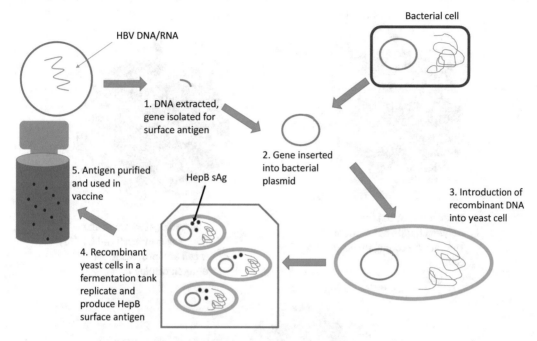

Fig. 9.2 Recombinant DNA vaccines are made by extracting the gene for the antigen of interest and inserting it into a vector. The recombinant DNA is introduced into a host cell (yeast, or another cell line) which begins transcribing the introduced DNA and producing the protein of interest

the immunogenic antigen HBsAg is expressed in yeast cells. Thus, it is considered a recombinant subunit vaccine. Another example is the Human Papilloma Virus (HPV) vaccine which is composed of virus-like particles (VLPs) expressed in either yeast or insect cells. Because the antigen is oftentimes a stand-alone protein (not expressed in a whole microbe), these types of vaccines often require an adjuvant to aid in producing a protective immune response.

Many pathogenic bacteria such as *Staphylococcus, Pneumococcus, Haemophilus,* and *Neisseria* are covered by a polysaccharide shell. The best defense against such encapsulated organisms is the elicitation of neutralizing antibodies that prevent the bacterium from initiating infection. However, polysaccharide antigens by themselves are unable to stimulate an effector helper T cell response, since antigen-presenting cells are unable to present the polysaccharide antigens on MHC II molecules to naïve helper CD4 T cells. As such, polysaccharide antigens are termed as poor antigens, and when used alone in vaccines, they have not been found to yield robust

immune responses. To mitigate this, polysaccharides are conjugated to carrier proteins forming molecular complexes that can be recognized by T cells. **Conjugate vaccines** contain a poor polysaccharide antigen which is covalently attached to a carrier protein such as the tetanus or diphtheria toxin to generate a more robust T and B cell response. This allows antigen-presenting cells (APCs) to present antigens from the protein subcomponent of the molecular complex to helper T cells, which can now activate B cells to produce high-affinity antibodies against the polysaccharide antigens. A common conjugate vaccine is the pneumococcal conjugate, or PCV13, which protects against 13 serotypes of *Streptococcus pneumoniae*. In this vaccine, the capsular polysaccharides of 13 pneumococcal serotypes are conjugated to the diphtheria CRM197 protein. Given that B cell receptors will recognize the polysaccharides on the conjugated antigen cluster, they will internalize the whole molecular complex, followed by the presentation of diphtheria toxin antigens on the surface of MHC II molecules to naïve CD4 T cells (Fig. 9.3).

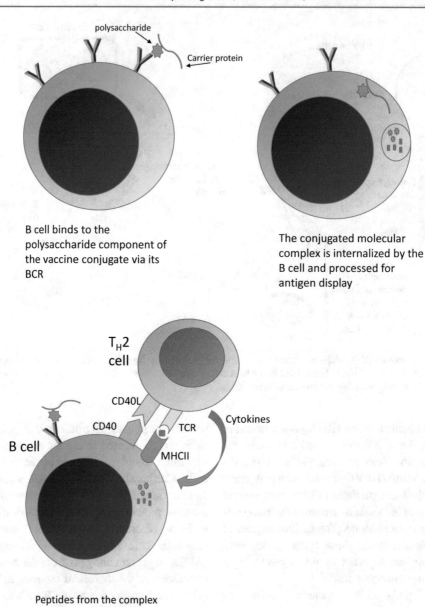

B cell binds to the polysaccharide component of the vaccine conjugate via its BCR

The conjugated molecular complex is internalized by the B cell and processed for antigen display

Peptides from the complex are presented on MHCII to a T cell, which activates the B cell via CD40/CD40L

Fig. 9.3 Conjugate vaccines use a carrier protein covalently attached to a polysaccharide antigen. When the polysaccharide bind to the BCR, the conjugate complex is internalized and processed by the B cell. Peptides from the conjugate complex are then presented by the B cell on MHC II to a T cell which activates it via CD40/CD40L binding

Examples of Commonly Used Vaccines

Pneumococcal

Streptococcus pneumoniae (pneumococcus) can cause a variety of life-threatening illnesses including meningitis, and pneumonia, and is considered to be one of the most common causes of serious illness in the United States. There are two Food and Drug Administration (FDA)-approved vaccinations for use against pneumococcal infections: PCV13 and PPSV23. PCV13 is also known as Prevnar13®, and is a conjugate vaccine that protects against 13 serotypes of *Streptococcus pneumoniae*. PPSV23 is commonly known as Pneumovax23®, a polysaccharide vaccination that contains antigens from 23 different pneumococcal bacteria. Twelve of these are also found in the PCV13 vaccination.

As mentioned, **Prevnar13® (pneumococcal conjugate vaccine [PCV13])** protects against 13 strains of pneumococcus, and is usually the first pneumococcal vaccine given to children. It can also be given to those ages 2–64 who have increased risk of pneumococcal disease due to certain health conditions. Adults 65 and older who have no prior history of pneumococcal vaccination will generally receive a single dose of PCV13 first, followed by PPSV23 a year later.

Pneumovax® (pneumococcal polysaccharide vaccine [PPSV23]) is a 23-valent vaccine that is FDA-approved for the prevention of pneumococcal infections in adults over the age of 50 and children 2 years or older with increased risk for developing pneumococcal infections. The 23-valent vaccine is scheduled to be given 8 weeks to 1 year after the 13-valent vaccine in patients where the 13-valent vaccine is indicated. Pneumovax® is not routinely scheduled for administration before the age of 65, but can be administered to adults age 19 and older with certain qualifying medical conditions that put them at higher risk of complications from pneumococcal infection. These include chronic heart, liver and lung diseases, and diabetes mellitus. People who smoke also fall into this high risk category. Patients who are immunocompromised, are asplenic, and patients with cerebral spinal fluid leaks or cochlear implants also qualify for vaccination with PPSV23 prior to the age of 65.

Re-vaccination with PPSV23 is indicated in some patients to boost the effect of the vaccine due to declining antibody levels within the decade following original administration. Re-vaccination is only indicated for patients with anatomic or functional asplenia, or immunocompromising conditions including HIV infection, chronic renal failure, blood cancers, or patients using immunosuppressive therapies like chemotherapy and long-term corticosteroid use. In this population revaccination is recommended 5 years following the original PPSV23 administration.

Meningococcal

Neisseria meningitidis is one of the most prevalent causes of bacterial meningitis in the world, and is able to cause large epidemics of meningitis with rates of incidence up to 1000 cases per 100,000 people in sub-Saharan Africa. In the United States during the period of 2006–2011, the incidence rate was approximately 0.3 cases per 100,000 people, which represented a decrease since the 1990s, likely a result of vaccination practices. *N. meningitidis* is a Gram-negative encapsulated cocci bacteria transmitted via direct contact or aerosol droplets, of which there are at least 12 serotypes characterized. The various serotypes have differences in the polysaccharide capsule. Serogroups A, B, and C are responsible for roughly 90% of diseases caused by meningococcus. However, groups Y and W135 strains are causing more and more cases.

There are three types of meningococcal vaccines against *Neisseria meningitidis*. These are purified capsular polysaccharide or conjugate vaccines which offer protection against the five most common serogroups of meningococcus. For children ages 2 months-10 years at increased risk of meningococcal disease due to certain medical conditions or travel, there are two meningococcal conjugate vaccines against serotypes MenACWY (Menactra and Menveo). **Menomune®** also covers MenACWY but is an unconjugated polysaccharide vaccine (MPSV4). Hib-MenCY-TT [**Menhibrix®**] was a conjugated polysaccharide vaccine also covering MenACWY, as well as *H. influenzae b*. It was introduced in 2012 but discontinued in the U.S. in 2016 due to low demand. The MenACWY quadrivalent vaccine is also recommended for 11–18 year olds, and for adults with certain medical conditions including asplenia and complement deficiency. Other individuals with increased risk such as military recruits, college freshman living in dormitories, individuals traveling to a region where meningococcal disease is common, or laboratory personnel working with this organism should also receive the quadrivalent vaccine. It is important to note that the quadrivalent vaccines do not cover for serogroup B. Serogroup B vaccines have only been available since late 2014.

Trumenba® (approved 2014) and **Bexsero®** (approved 2015) are two brands of the serogroup B meningococcal vaccine composed of proteins found on the surface of meningococcus. Individuals at risk of meningitis B due to certain medical conditions, taking certain medication, or at high risk because of a recent outbreak may consider vaccination. Both brands are given in a two-dose series and should not be used interchangeably (i.e. one brand should be used for the whole series).

DTaP, Tdap

DTAP stands for diphtheria, tetanus, and acellular pertussis. Generally, children under the age of 7 receive the **DTaP (Daptacel,® Infanrix®)** or DT vaccine, while those over the age of 7 receive **Tdap (Boostrix,® Adacel®)** or Td. Adolescents will usually receive Tdap at around age 11 or 12 before entering middle school. Adults should receive a Td booster every 10 years and pregnant women should receive a single dose during each pregnancy. Adults over the age of 65 should receive Tdap. **Diphtheria** is caused by the microbe *Corynebacterium diphtheriae.* Due to widespread use of vaccination, diphtheria rates dropped in the U.S. in the 1920s. Diptheria is usually spread via the airborne route and infects the respiratory system leading to sore throat, fever, weakness, and swollen lymph nodes in the neck. *C. diphtheriae* produces a toxin which destroys healthy tissue, and can get into the bloodstream leading to other complications including damage to the heart muscle, nerve damage, pneumonia, and paralysis. Mortality is approximately 10% with treatment and 50% without treatment. As mentioned earlier, the vaccine against diphtheria is an example of a toxoid vaccine, and as such uses modified diphtheria toxin that results in production of IgG antibodies that recognize the toxin. Similarly, inactivated tetanus toxin is also a component of this vaccine in order to afford protect against **tetanus**, an infection caused by *Clostridium tetani* and is commonly known as "lockjaw." *C. tetani* spores are present in many locations in the environment including the soil and manure, so wounds that are contaminated with soil, are caused by a puncture, burns, or crash injuries are at risk of being infected with these spores which develop into bacteria after entering the body. Tetanus can lead to jaw cramping (hence the term lockjaw), muscle spasms or stiffness, seizures, trouble swallowing, and fever. Complications can be severe and can include bone fractures, difficulty breathing, uncontrolled tightening of the vocal cords, pneumonia, or pulmonary embolism. Vaccine boosters for tetanus as well as proper wound care are the best methods of preventing tetanus infection. The **pertussis** component of the DTaP or Tdap vaccine is comprised of acellular pertussis, or purified components of the bacteria including inactivated pertussis toxin, filamentous hemagglutinin, or other antigens. Pertussis, also known as whooping cough, is caused by a Gram-negative coccobacillus known as *Bordetella pertussis* which infects the mucosal layers of the respiratory tract. It is transmitted via the airborne route and leads to sore throat and cough that develops into worse coughing spasms that end in a "whoop" sound, hence its name. Coughing can be so severe that it can result in vomiting or cracked ribs. Pertussis is particularly dangerous for infants who can have trouble breathing and thus need to be hospitalized. Protecting all ages against whooping cough can protect babies who may be too young to be vaccinated and are at increased risk of complications.

Hepatitis A Vaccine

The Hepatitis A vaccine (**Havrix®, Vaqta®**) is a killed, inactivated vaccine given in two doses at least 6 months apart. Children, especially those in daycare settings are recommended to receive this vaccine between the ages of 12 and 23 months, however, older children and adults can also receive the vaccine if they want protection or are in a higher risk group for Hepatitis A. Those with a higher risk for Hepatitis A are people traveling to or adopting a child from countries where hepatitis A is common, are a man who has sex with other men, illegal drug users, those with chronic liver diseases (Hep B or C), patients being treated with clotting-factor concentrates, work in a hepatitis A virus research laboratory or work with hepatitis A-infected animals. As with most vaccines, patients who have experienced anaphylaxis in the past as a result of this vaccine or who have allergies to any of the vaccine components (especially neomycin) should not receive this vaccine. Additionally, patients who have a fever or are moderately to severely ill should wait to receive the vaccine. Common vaccine reactions include low-grade fever, soreness or redness at the injection site, headache, or fatigue.

Hepatitis B

As discussed earlier, the hepatitis B vaccine is a subunit vaccine composed of recombinant hepatitis B surface antigen (sAg) produced in yeast using recombinant DNA technology. It is estimated that 5% of the world's population is living with chronic Hepatitis B infection. Approximately a quarter of those people with chronic hepatitis will have their infection progress to cirrhosis, or hepatocellular carcinoma. The progression to these complications seem to occur more rapidly in HIV co-infected individuals. Thus, the HBV vaccination is recommended for children, adolescents, and healthy adults. Additionally, the WHO recommends universal vaccination for newborns within 24 h after birth. It has been found that a protective antibody response (anti-HBs >10 mIU/mL) occurs in 90% of individuals after three vaccinations, with immune memory lasting for at least 20 years or more.

In addition to prevention of infection before exposure, the HBV vaccines can also be used for post-exposure prophylaxis. This is sometimes given at the same time as HB immunoglobulin which can be administered as passive immunity at the same time as the HBV vaccine, but at different injection sites.

Those individuals who have had a life-threatening reaction to this vaccine in the past, or any of its components, including yeast, should not receive this vaccine. Additionally, those who are moderately to severely ill should wait to receive the vaccine. Common adverse effects include soreness at the injection site, fever, or a feeling of faintness. In addition to the two brand names **Recombivax HB®** and **Engerix B®**, the Hepatitis B vaccine can be administered together with Hepatitis A vaccine in a combination called **Twinrix®**. More recently, an adjuvanted version of the Hepatitis B vaccine was approved **(Heplisav-B®)**.

HPV Vaccine

The vaccine which protects against human papillomavirus (**Gardasil-9®**) is considered subunit vaccines in that they contain **virus-like particles (VLPs)**, which are capsid proteins from several strains of the virus. Earlier versions of the vaccine were bivalent (protein against two strains, 2vHPV) and quadrivalent (protect against four strains, 4vHPV). The newest version of the vaccine approved in 2014 (Gardasil-9®) is nine-valent (nine strain protection, 9vHPV). All of these vaccines protect against HPV-16 and -18 which are thought to cause two-thirds of the cases of cervical cancer. The nine-valent vaccine also protects against HPV types 6, 11, 31, 33, 45, 52, and 58. The CDC recommends boys and girls get the vaccine at ages 11 or 12 to yield the most protection before the initiation of sexual activity. While originally the vaccine was approved for adults up until age 26, the FDA expanded its approval in October 2018 to include adults ages 27–45.

Some vaccines can cause allergic reactions related to the manufacturing process or the packaging. The 4vHPV and 9vHPV vaccines may contain traces of yeast because the manufacturing process uses yeast to produce the viral capsid proteins. Thus, patients with hypersensitivity to yeast should avoid these two vaccines. Both of these vaccines also contain alum adjuvant to aid the uptake of viral proteins by immune cells. The most common adverse reaction from the vaccine itself is pain and redness at the injection site.

Varicella Zoster; Herpes Zoster

The varicella zoster vaccine was introduced in 1995 and has significantly decreased the number of zoster infections, preventing approximately 70–90% of cases. There is currently one vaccine against varicella zoster (**Varivax®**), but it can also be combined with the MMR vaccine as one combination vaccine (**MMRV, ProQuad®**). Chickenpox is a primary infection that occurs in non-immune individuals and is characterized by a skin rash of itchy blisters that eventually scab over. Herpes zoster/shingles is a reactivation of latent virus, usually later in life as memory immunity to the zoster virus wanes. Because

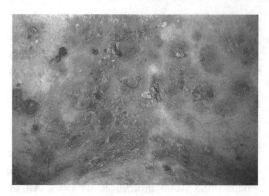

Fig. 9.4 Shingles outbreak caused by herpes zoster. Credit: CDC, Dr. Dancewiez

varicella zoster stays latent in the nervous system, shingles usually presents as a painful rash (Fig. 9.4) which occurs typically on one side of the torso in the distribution of a spinal nerve (a dermatome). The **Zostavax®** vaccine is aimed at boosting immunity to varicella zoster to prevent a possible outbreak of shingles.

Initial infection with varicella zoster usually results in chickenpox during childhood. Varicella zoster virus (VZV) can be transmitted through direct contact with an infected person's secretions as well as through aerosolized droplets. The virus infects immune cells such as dendritic cells in the nasal pharyngeal region and Langerhans cells in the skin and respiratory mucosa. These cells normally migrate to draining lymph nodes and so spread the virus to CD4 T cells. These T cells home to the skin where dermal fibroblasts and keratinocytes become infected resulting in proinflammatory cytokine release and the itchy rash characteristic of chickenpox. Varicella zoster is a member of the Herpes virus family; a commonality among the viruses in this family is their ability to establish latent infection. As the varicella infection progresses, VZV gains access to nerve ganglia from the peripheral lesions and establishes latent infection for life.

Reactivation from latency may be in part due to immunosenescence, or the natural decline in T cell function with age. This may be due to repeated stimulation of VZV-specific T cells over a long period of time as well as just a general decrease in these cell numbers as a person gets older.

Both vaccines are live, attenuated vaccines containing the Oka strain of varicella zoster. To prevent chickenpox, children are usually immunized at the age of 12 months with a booster between 4 and 6 years of age. Zostavax® is recommended for adults 60 years of age and older. Recently, the FDA has approved a recombinant vaccine for herpes zoster (**Shingrix®**) which is given as two IM injections, and has shown an efficacy of over 90% in the prevention of shingles in Phase III clinical trials.

Shingrix® is composed of zoster glycoprotein E antigen, and AS01B adjuvant to generate protective immunity against herpes zoster in people 50 years of age and older. While Shingrix® is more likely to cause significant short term adverse effects (headaches, arm pain, and diarrhea that can affect day-to-day activities) than Zostavax®, Shingrix® has been shown to be more effective in preventing shingles. The ZOE-50 and ZOE-70 trials analyzed efficacy rates of Shingrix.® In the 60–69 age group Shingrix® is approximately 97% effective, while Zostavax® is 64% effective. Additionally, Shingrix® yields a higher efficacy in the above 70 and 80 age groups whereas Zostavax® efficacy wanes over time. The current recommendation is to use Shingrix® initially and patients who have received Zostavax in the past can also opt to receive Shingrix® as well. Since Shingrix® needs to be given in two doses and can have significant short term adverse effects, patients should be counseled ahead of time to manage expectations and increase the likelihood that they will get the second dose.

Seasonal Influenza

Influenza is a single strand RNA enveloped virus from the orthomyxovirus family, expressing the viral glycoproteins **Hemagglutinin (HA)** and **Neuraminidase (NA)** on the surface (Fig. 9.5). These antigens are recognized by the immune system, serving as the basis for immunity against influenza. Seasonal or pandemic influenza outbreaks usually result due to genetic changes in the influenza virus, with HA and NA being frequent sites of mutation. Influenza A and B strains are typically associated with seasonal outbreaks, whereas strain C causes milder symptoms.

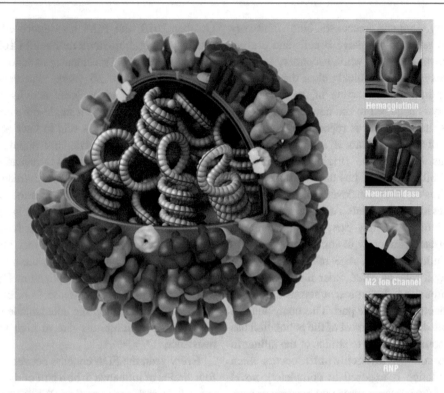

Fig. 9.5 Structure of the influenza virus. Hemagglutinin and neuraminidase glycoproteins are expressed on the surface. A portion of the outer protein coat has been cut away to show the ribonucleoproteins present inside. M2 ion channels in the viral envelope of the virus promotes uncoating of the virus after entering a host cell. Credit: CDC, Doug Jordan, M.A.

Several subtypes of influenza A have been identified based on mutations in the HA and NA antigens, including at least 15 HA antigens and 9 NA antigens. However during any given flu season, only a few strains are usually in circulation and can cause disease. Influenza B viruses are not classified according to subtypes, but by lineages including the Yamagata and Victoria lineages.

Immune responses to mutating viruses such as influenza are constrained by exposure to the first antigenic strain encountered. As mutating viruses acquire new epitopes, the development of immunity to the new antigens is suppressed by the original antigen, significantly weakening the immune response to mutated strains. This phenomenon is termed as **original antigenic sin**, which is described below, and is the reason why influenza infections often present as either milder seasonal epidemics or worldwide pandemics. When an individual is first exposed to a novel influenza strain, a powerful primary immune response is produced, which is accompanied by severe symptoms including fever, chills, muscle aches and other respiratory or neurological manifestations. Because all the epitopes in the infecting strain are new, no memory response exists, and the infection is not cleared until adaptive immunity has peaked about 1 or 2 weeks after the onset of infection. If re-exposed to the same strain, secondary immune responses against the original antigens are rapidly able to clear the infection. However, re-exposure to a mutated strain of the virus that has retained most of the epitopes of the original virus, but has acquired some new epitopes, only induces secondary immune response to the original epitopes. Furthermore, these secondary responses also suppress the development of primary immune responses to the new antigenic epitopes, thus leaving the individual vulnerable during future infections comprising these epitopes. Any IgG antibodies that have been produced during the secondary immune response bind inhibitory FcγRIIB receptors on naive B cells and prevent their activation. Thus, while secondary immune responses are able to quickly clear the infection, resulting in a milder version of the disease, no immunity is acquired to the new epitopes. Over time, as the individual is repeatedly exposed to variants of the same strain, all immunity is lost as the virus loses all the original epitopes and acquires all new ones. Thus the original epitopes of the virus constrain the development of immune responses to novel variants. At any given moment, several individuals may exist within a community that have immunity to some of the epitopes of the influenza virus. Age related differences also play a role, as some older individuals may have immunity to both present strains as well as those encountered in the past. This contributes to **antigenic drift**, where most of the population has at least some immunity to strains of the influenza virus. In contrast, **antigenic shift**, occurs when the population is exposed to completely novel strains of the influenza virus that have never been encountered before. This can happen when influenza A infects another species (usually bird or pig) and recombines with another strain of the influenza virus predominant in that species. The resultant novel strain is typically termed as a type of bird flu or swine flu virus. All of the global influenza pandemics within the last 100 years have occurred due to antigenic shifts, including the deadly Spanish Influenza of 1918, which killed over 18 million people. An example of an antigenic shift occurred in 2009 when the H1N1 strain emerged that spread quickly because most people did not have protection against the new strain.

Currently, two main types of drugs are available to treat influenza. These include neuraminidase inhibitors and a recently approved endonuclease inhibitor. Neuraminidase is an enzyme that cleaves the budding influenza virions from the host cells. The neuraminidase inhibitor prevents the release of new virions from host cells and curtails the infection. **Zanamivir (Relenza®), oseltamivir (Tamiflu®)**, and the newer IV formulation **peramivir (Rapivab®)** are FDA-approved neuraminidase inhibitors. In October 2018, the FDA also approved a new influenza drug, **baloxavir marboxil (Xofluza®)**, the first with a novel mechanism of action against influenza in almost 20 years. Baloxavir is an inhibitor of the endonuclease activity of viral polymerase. Baloxavir is a single-dose oral treatment for influenza that is said to have about the same efficacy as oseltamivir. Until about a decade ago, M2 inhibitors such as amantadine and rimantadine were also used in the treatment of influenza. Viral replication requires the viral M2 protein to be modified in the trans-golgi network in order to help in maintaining effective hemagglutinin configuration. M2 inhibitors block the transport of M2 proteins through the trans-golgi network and so disrupt viral replication. However, in 2009, the Center for Disease Control (CDC) stopped recommending the adamantane class of viral uncoating inhibitors due to high levels of resistance.

Every year, the FDA chooses between three to four strains of influenza to be a part of the upcoming year's influenza vaccine. While the WHO makes a recommendation of strains to include based on patient samples surveyed from the previous influenza season all over the world, the FDA has the final say in the vaccine that is sold in the United States. The trivalent vaccine normally contains two influenza A strains and one influenza B strain, while the quadrivalent vaccine contains an extra influenza B strain.

It is recommended that everyone 6 months and older receive an annual influenza vaccine. Because there are several different formulations (Table 9.3), choosing the right one may happen on a case-by-case basis. Most will receive the standard dose of the trivalent or quadrivalent vaccine.

Older individuals are at higher risk of morbidity from the flu, and may be less able to produce an adequate adaptive immune response from the vaccine. For this reason, there are two vaccines that are specifically recommended for people 65 years and older. The high dose trivalent Fluzone® vaccine contains four times the amount of antigen than the standard-dose vaccine, and is intended to produce a more robust immune response for individuals 65 years and older.

Table 9.3 Brands and formulations of available influenza vaccines

Brands	Ages	Formulation	Route
Fluzone®, Fluvirin®, Fluarix®, Afluria®, FluLaval® (standard dose)	6 months and older	IIV3 or IIV4	IM
Fluzone® (high dose)	65 years and older	IIV3	IM
Fluzone®	18–64 years old	IIV4	ID
Afluria®	18–64 years old	IIV3	Jet injector IM
Fluad™ (adjuvanted)	65 years and older	aIIV3	IM
Flucelvax®	4 years and older	ccIIV4	IM
Flublok®	18 years and older	RIV3	IM
FluMist®a	2–49 years old	LAIV4	Intranasal

aWas not recommended by the CDC for flu seasons 2016–2017 and 2017–2018

Clinical trials have shown higher influenza antibody titers after the high-dose versus the standard dose. Additionally, high-dose Fluzone® appears to be approximately 24% more effective at preventing flu in adults 65 years and older versus the standard dose. Similarly, the adjuvanted vaccine Fluad™ is also designed to enhance the protective immune response to influenza in individuals 65 years and older. It is the standard-dose inactivated egg-based influenza vaccine but contains the MF59 adjuvant oil-in-water immersion to enhance the immune response. Currently, there are no trials that have compared Fluad™ to the high-dose Fluzone®.

Egg-based influenza vaccines The majority of the flu vaccines on the market are grown in eggs, a method that is over 70 years old. The process involves several steps and begins with **candidate vaccine viruses (CVVs)** which are injected into fertilized chicken eggs. The eggs are incubated over several days, allowing the viruses to replicate. The fluid containing the viruses is subsequently removed from the eggs. The viruses are then killed (inactivated), purified, and tested.

Cell-based influenza vaccine For individuals allergic to eggs, there is a method which does not use chicken eggs as the host cell source. The cell-based method was approved in 2012 by the FDA, and in August 2016 the FDA approved the manufacturer Seqirus to begin this process. First, CVVs are inoculated into a cultured Madin-Darby Canine Kidney (MDCK) cell line. For several days, the viruses are allowed to replicate in the cell culture. The viruses are then harvested from the cell culture, purified, and tested. While this method removes the possibility of egg proteins being present in the final vaccine, there is another benefit to using cell-based vaccine production. It has been shown that viruses grown in eggs change/mutate slightly to adapt themselves to the egg environment, possibly producing less of an accurate immune response to the initially targeted wild-type viruses. Thus, mammalian cell-based vaccine production may help in maintaining the effectiveness of the flu vaccine. Currently, this cell-based influenza vaccine is marketed as **Flucelvax®**.

Recombinant influenza vaccine Another process that does not involve chicken eggs to produce influenza antigens is the recombinant DNA method. This method was approved in 2013 and uses a protein from a recommended influenza virus. This protein is usually hemagglutinin (HA), an antigen from the virus that usually produces an immune response in people. The gene for this protein is inserted in a viral vector (baculovirus) which is then grown in insect cells (Fig. 9.6). The insect cells subsequently begin producing the influenza protein, which can be isolated, purified, and used in the vaccine. Currently, the vaccine on the market utilizing this technology is **FluBlok®**.

Adjuvants
The word adjuvant comes from the Latin word *adjuvare*, which means help or aid. Several

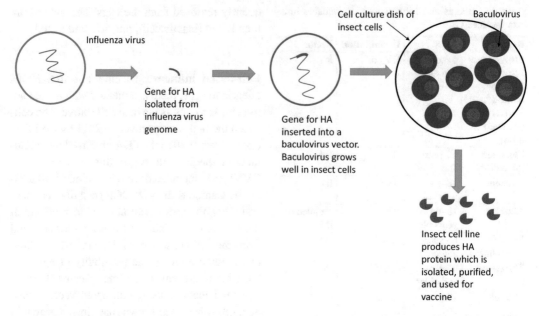

Fig. 9.6 FluBlok® is made by isolating the gene for influenza hemagglutinin, inserting it into a viral vector and introducing it into an insect cell line which begins producing the HA protein

vaccines which are not live attenuated may have antigens that need help being recognized by the immune system. Subunit or conjugate vaccines which contain stand-alone antigens do not have other components (specifically, pathogen-associated molecular patterns, or PAMPs as described in Chap. 2) from the whole microbe that would be recognized by Toll-like receptors of the innate immune response.

Adjuvants do not induce an immune response against themselves, but are substances that enhance immune responses by inducing inflammation and uptake of antigen by an APC, such as dendritic cells. Adjuvants are thought to have several possible mechanisms of action, the first being a depot effect, which results in sustained release of the antigen at the site of injection. A second effect is the increased induction of cytokines and chemokines by localized immune cells such as macrophages. When the antigen plus the adjuvant is taken up by phagocytes, NF-κB is activated which induces a state of inflammation, and enhances the secretion of cytokines such as IL-1 and IL-12 by macrophages. Neutrophils and eosinophils may also be recruited to the injection site. One of the biggest effects is likely the effects of the adjuvant on the antigen presenting cell. It is thought that adjuvants increase uptake of antigen by the APC and promote their maturation, the expression of MHC II, and co-stimulatory molecule expression. APCs also migrate to the draining lymph nodes which kick start the adaptive response to the antigen. Lastly, adjuvants appear to activate inflammasomes, which are innate system components that contain receptors that induce inflammation.

While there are various types of adjuvants, the most common adjuvants used in human vaccines are alum, MF59, and MPL.

Aluminum salts include aluminum hydroxide, aluminum phosphate, alum (potassium aluminum sulfate), or mixed aluminum salts. Alum was approved in 1924 for use in human vaccines, and was the only adjuvant for 73 years. Among the adjuvants, it is probably the least powerful.

MF59® was approved in 1997. It is a squalene oil-in-water emulsion which elicits both cellular (T_H1) and humoral (T_H2) immune responses through the recruitment and activation of APCs and the stimulation of cytokine production by macrophages.

MPL, also known as monophosphoryl lipid A, is a purified fat-like substance.

CpG 1018, or cytosine phophoguanine is synthetic DNA that simulates bacterial or viral DNA to induce an immune response through TLR9.

Several combinations of adjuvants also exist, these are denoted as AS, or adjuvant system. For example, $AS01_B$ is an adjuvant system consisting of MPL and QS-21, a natural compound from the Chilean soapbark tree together in a liposomal formulation. AS04 contains MPL and an aluminum salt; this was the adjuvant contained in the former Cervarix® vaccine. Newer adjuvants that contain PAMPs such as PolyIC and flagellin are in development, with the goal of initiating inflammation through TLR signaling. Currently used vaccine adjuvants are outline in Table 9.4.

Possible Vaccine Additives

Thimerosal is an organic compound that contains mercury, and may be found in some vaccines. Because of its antimicrobial properties, it is used as a preservative in multi-dose vials. It is metabolized to ethylmercury and thiosalicylate. Ethylmercury is related but different than methylmercury, which is the type of mercury that at high exposure levels can be toxic to humans. Thimerosal has been used in many studies, and has been found to be safe and effective at preventing contamination in vaccine vials. Over the years, the use of thimerosal as a preservative has declined, partially due to the development of vaccines that are dispensed in single-dose vials. All U.S. pediatric vaccines recommended for children under 6 years old are available in thimerosal-free vials. Similarly, vaccines for adults can also be formulated as thimerosal-free in single-dose vials. Some vaccines may still have trace amounts from the manufacturing process. If that is the case, trace amounts of thimerosal contain 1 μg or less of mercury per dose.

Antibiotics such as neomycin, polymixin B, streptomycin, or gentamicin may be present in small quantities in vaccines to prevent bacterial contamination during the manufacturing process. While many people are concerned with possible hypersensitivity, the antibiotics most likely to lead to hypersensitivity (e.g. penicillins,

Table 9.4 Currently used vaccine adjuvants

Adjuvant	Mechanism of action	Vaccines found in
Alum	Inflammasome NLRP3 activation Increase in cytokines, chemokines Recruitment of eosinophils, monocytes, macrophages Increased antigen presentation Primarily T_H2/ antibody response	Hepatitis A, Hepatitis B, DTaP/IPV, Tdap, HIB, HPV, pneumococcal, meningococcal B, anthrax, Japanese encephalitis
MPL	Signals through TLR4 for APC activation Increase in cytokines, chemokines Recruitment of dendritic cells, macrophages Increase in antibody response Increase in T_H1 response	HPV (Cervarix®) [discontinued] Shingrix®
MF59	Increase in cytokines, chemokines Recruitment of neutrophils, monocytes, macrophages Increase in antigen uptake Balanced T_H1/T_H2 response	Influenza (Fluad™)
CpG 1018	Activation of TLR9 on dendritic cells Triggers B cell activation and a T_H1 response	Hepatitis B (Heplisav-B®)

cephalosporins, or sulfonamides) are not used in vaccine manufacturing. The antibiotics that are utilized usually end up being decreased to trace or undetectable amounts during the purification process.

Formaldehyde may also be found in some vaccines from the manufacturing process. Formaldehyde is used to inactivate viruses (as is the case with poliovirus vaccine), and detoxify bacteria toxins (such as diphtheria toxin). The formaldehyde present usually becomes diluted after several steps of the purification process, but may be present in trace amounts. While some may worry that formaldehyde in vaccines is harmful, humans are exposed to formaldehyde more commonly in the environment, and from the production of it in the body itself. Formaldehyde is produced during energy and amino acid production. Thus, the body is able to process what it produces on its own as well as what is gathered from the environment. There has been no scientific evidence linking the small amount exposed from a vaccine and a higher risk of cancer.

Other possible vaccine ingredients include sugars such as sucrose and lactose, amino acids like glycine, or proteins such as human serum albumin or gelatin. These are frequently used as vaccine stabilizers, and help protect it from adverse conditions. Fetal calf/bovine serum may also be found in trace amounts in viral vaccines. This is used as a source of nutrition for cells that are used to culture the virus during manufacturing.

Contraindications

While vaccines can be life-saving, there are several reasons why a person cannot be vaccinated, cannot receive a particular vaccine, or who should simply wait to receive a vaccine. These instances include:

- People who are currently experiencing moderate to severe illness should avoid getting a new vaccine until they recover. People who are mildly ill may receive certain vaccines, but also may be advised to wait until they recover.
- People who have had a serious allergic reaction, such as anaphylaxis to a certain vaccine or any of its components in the past, should avoid getting that vaccine again.
- People who have had Guillain Barré syndrome may avoid vaccines such as anthrax, influenza, and Tdap.
- People who have experienced coma, nervous system disease, or repeated seizures within 7 days of DTP or DTaP should not receive DTaP again, or Tdap.
- Women who are currently pregnant can usually safely receive inactivated or subunit vaccines but should avoid lives vaccines such as

varicella zoster, adenovirus, live influenza, Japanese Encephalitis, and MMR. The HPV vaccine is also not recommended for pregnant women. Since little information exists concerning the meningococcal ACWY and MenB vaccines during pregnancy or lactation, it should be reserved only if needed.
- People with a weakened immune system due to HIV/AIDs, genetic immunodeficiency, immunosuppressants including steroids, cancer, or cancer treatments may also be advised to avoid live vaccines.

Concerns About Vaccines

During the last few decades, an increasing number of parents have refrained from vaccinating their children due to concerns about the development of autism. Others believe that vaccines damage the immune system and the best means of offering protection against infection is to acquire the infection through natural causes.

Much of the concern about autism stemmed from a study published in the *Lancet* in 1998, by Andrew Wakefield and 12 of his colleagues, that suggested that the measles-mumps-rubella (MMR) vaccine contributes to the development of autism. Although this study lacked any definitive conclusions, had a small sample size of 12 children, and was conducted using an uncontrolled design, it was still published, receiving much publicity and creating lots of distrust and concern amongst parents worldwide. In light of the increasing diagnoses of autism, from 1 in every 150 children in 2006, to 1 in every 68 children in the U.S. according to a 2016 study using 2012 data, a number of concerned parents who are fearful of vaccinations have chosen not to vaccinate their children out of the fear of risk of autism. Ironically, following immediate epidemiological studies and retraction of the interpretation of the original data, it was found that there was no link between the MMR vaccine and autism, citing the data as being insufficient. Today, the 1998 Lancet study is regarded as "one of the most serious frauds in medical history", which resulted in hundreds of parents refusing to vaccinate their children and exposing them to the risk of disease and several other complications.

Another autism-related concern expressed by many parents is that the preservative thimerosal contained in many vaccines is toxic to the central nervous system. In 1997, the United States Food and Drug Administration Modernization Act required all foods and drugs to be accompanied with the identification and quantification of mercury. Two years later, the American Academy of Pediatrics and the Public Health Service made a conservative precautionary recommendation that mercury be removed immediately from all vaccines administered to young infants. As such, in addition to the already established concern of risk of autism with the MMR vaccine, parental concern again increased. However, as in the case of the MMR vaccine, the likelihood that mercury can be a cause of autism has not been borne out by the evidence. The symptoms of autism and mercury poisoning are completely different from each other and a study conducted years later by the Centers for Disease Control and Prevention showed that mercury in vaccines does not cause signs or symptoms of mercury poisoning. Similarly, several other studies demonstrated that thimerosal in vaccines does not contribute to autism development.

Lastly, some individuals have proposed that injecting a child with multiple vaccines can weaken their immune system, leading to the development of autoimmune effects that mediate autism. In this context, it is important to note that autism is not an immune-mediated disease like multiple sclerosis. Therefore, it does not make sense to propose that vaccination precipitates autism following an inappropriate immune response. Furthermore, although immature, an infant's immune system is immediately capable of a variety of protective responses. Some researchers have predicted the ability of a child's immune system to respond to up to 1000 simultaneous vaccines. Vaccinations should not be dismissed due to fear of the possible risks. Parents must be advised of the risks involved in not vaccinating their children and exposing them to the risk of dangerous diseases and complications.

Immunizations in the Geriatric Population: A Case Study

Provided by Andrea L. Leschak, Pharm.D., BCGP

Gerald is a 67 year old man recently admitted to a skilled nursing facility (SNF) for wound care and disease state management. He has a past medical history of long term uncontrolled type II diabetes. He is self-employed and for the past 7 years has been unable to afford consistent medical care. Lapses in insurance resulted in a number of emergency department visits for diabetic related complications. Over time he found it difficult to pay for the complex insulin and drug therapy required to manage his condition. Five months ago while working in his yard he stepped on a stone resulting in a bruised heel. He assumed the discomfort would resolve and the severity of the injury went unnoticed. Unfortunately the affected area became increasingly painful and he is now unable to walk or perform daily activities. Upon arrival to the emergency department it was decided Gerald would need extensive wound management. He has been admitted to the SNF for treatment.

Social history:
- Divorced
- Two children and four grandchildren (both children live out of state and are unable to assist with care)

Work history: General contractor, masonry, welder

Past medical history:
- Type II Diabetes Mellitus
- Bilateral peripheral neuropathy (feet)
- Pre-glaucoma

Immunization history: Unknown other than basic childhood immunizations required to attend school and a tetanus booster 8 years ago after a work-related injury

Objective:
- Ht: 6′1″
- Wt.: 213 lb
- BP: 143/79
- P: 68
- Temp: 98.7

Assessment Questions

1. Considering his age, what immunizations would be most appropriate for Gerald?
2. Which pneumococcal immunization should Gerald receive first?
3. What is the recommended pneumococcal immunization schedule for adults 65 years and old with no history of receiving a pneumococcal vaccine?
4. What is the difference between PCV13 and PPSV23?
5. Does Gerald have any contraindications to being immunized?
6. You suggest that Gerald also receive a flu vaccine. What flu vaccines could Gerald possibly receive?

Infectious Diseases Which Affect the Immune System

In the next section, some of the ways in which infectious organisms interact with the immune system will be considered. Some of these result in immunosuppression, as is the case with HIV and AIDS. Sepsis, on the other hand, is often due to an overwhelming immune response to infection which can lead to tissue injury, multiple organ failure, and even death. The complex interplay between timing of sepsis, the early inflammatory phase as well as the later immunosuppressive phase and the mediators involved will be explored. Lastly, three other infections that affect the immune system including tuberculosis, leprosy, and toxic shock syndrome will be discussed.

Acquired Immune Deficiency Syndrome

Acquired Immune Deficiency Syndrome (AIDS) is a disease that is characterized by a dramatic reduction in the numbers of helper CD4 T cells, resulting in the development of severe secondary infections and cancers, that eventually lead to the death of the AIDS patient. The disease was first described by physicians in the early 1980s, who were unable to explain the presence of infections in many patients that were normally controlled by the immune system by otherwise healthy individuals. Since then, the disease has reached pandemic proportions, with many countries in Africa and South East Asia exhibit widespread prevalence of the disease. The implementation of public health measures and the development of many

AIDS-targeting drugs have curbed the spread of the disease in North America and many countries in Europe. However, the prohibitive cost of these drugs, as well as other factors including poverty, illiteracy, and superstition among others, has contributed to its persistence in endemic countries.

AIDS is caused by the RNA retrovirus, the human immunodeficiency virus (HIV). Two main strains of HIV exist, HIV-1 and HIV-2. While both can progress to AIDS, there are large genetic differences between the two strains. HIV-1 is most widespread around the world, while HIV-2 is less common and mostly confined to West Africa. While there are diagnostic tests that can detect both, tests designed specifically for one will likely not detect the other. While HIV-1 is more likely to progress through the stages of HIV infection and to AIDS, HIV-2 tends to progress at a slower rate, and progresses amidst higher CD4 counts and lower viral load. This seems to be because of a more protective immune response to HIV-2. Transmission of both occurs via blood and bodily fluids, primarily through sexual contact, from mother to fetus during birth, blood transfusions, or the sharing of needles.

HIV targets the body's immune system directly, specifically the body's CD4 T cells. CD4 cells, otherwise known as T helper cells, play a critical role in the body's ability to fight infections. As such, once infected, it becomes difficult for the immune system to mount a response to protect itself against the virus. AIDS is a progressive disease that can be classified by stage. Initial symptoms can include fever, malaise, rash, and swollen lymph nodes. The viral load is an important diagnostic measure of the amount of virus present per mm^3 of plasma. Ideally treatment goals aim to decrease the viral load to an undetectable level or less than 50 copies/μL.

Table 9.5 highlights the stages of HIV infection. The first stage, **acute infection** usually begins 2–4 weeks after infection. The infected individual will usually experience flu-like symptoms, the body's normal response to a viral infection. Typical symptoms include muscle aches, fever, swollen lymph nodes, and malaise. At this point in time, the individual will have a high viral load and is easily able to transmit the virus to

Table 9.5 Stages of HIV infection

HIV stages		
Stage I	Acute	Symptomatic early infection, active viral replication
Stage II	Clinical latency	Viral DNA is integrated into host genome, but it not actively being transcribed
Stage III/ AIDS	Acquired immunodeficiency syndrome	<200 CD4 T cells/mm^3 in blood

another person. In this stage, the individual will also likely be unaware of his or her HIV status. Additionally, during this time seroconversion takes place, in which antibodies to HIV develop and become detectable. After several weeks, the infection will progress to **clinical latency**. During this stage, the individual is asymptomatic; the virus is present, but replicating at low levels. Even for those not on **anti-retroviral therapies (ART)** this stage could last from 1 to 10 or more years. Those who are taking ART and who are adherent to their medications may be in this stage for several decades. Even though these individuals may be virally suppressed, they are still able to transmit the virus, though the risk of transmission may be lower than for those with a higher viral load. It is important to note that AIDS is not a separate disease state (Table 9.5), but can be thought of as end stage HIV. Once the CD4 T cell count has decreased to less than 200 cells/mm^3 of blood, the patient is classified as having AIDS (Fig. 9.7). With a severely compromised immune system, patients with AIDS have an increased chance of contracting more severe infections (opportunistic infections). Patients with AIDS have a high viral load and are easily able to transmit the virus to another person. The typical amount of time patients live with AIDS with no treatment is approximately 3 years.

With ART, the progression rates from clinical latency to AIDS has decreased. In 1993, the approximate number of people receiving a stage 3 HIV (AIDS) diagnosis was almost 45,000. In the year 2015, that number decreased to 18,303. This decrease can be attributed to not only availability

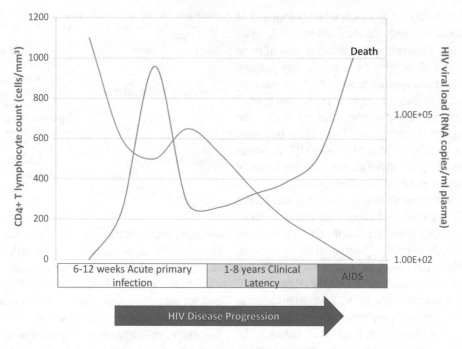

Fig. 9.7   Progression of HIV based on CD4 T cell count and HIV viral load

of efficacious antiretroviral drugs, but also a decrease in the number of new infections. The CD4 T cell count is one way to monitor ART efficacy, as well as act as a predictor of disease progression.

HIV Pathogenesis

HIV is an RNA retrovirus belonging to the lentivirus family. The structure of the virus was uncovered between 1983 and 1984 by two independent labs (Luc Montagnier in France and Robert Gallo in the US). The virus contains a RNA nucleoprotein core or capsid surrounded by a lipid envelope. The spikes in the lipid envelope represent glycoproteins that are involved in initiating infection. Nine viral genes have been identified. The *gag* or group-specific antigen genes give rise to the core or matrix proteins. The *pol* or polymerase genes encode for the reverse transcriptase, protease and integrase enzymes. The *env* or envelope genes encode for the envelope proteins gp160, gp120, and gp41.

HIV infection is initiated by the two envelope proteins gp120 and gp41. These proteins are synthesized as a single polypeptide, gp160, which is

then cleaved by host proteases to give the individual proteins. Viral entry begins when gp120 binds to the human cellular receptor CD4 on the surface of macrophages, dendritic cells, or CD4 T helper cells (Fig. 9.8). This results in a conformational change in gp120 which allows it to bind to a second receptor, C-C chemokine receptor 5 (CCR5) or C-X-C chemokine receptor 4 (CXCR4). After the successful binding of both receptors, gp41 initiates fusion of the viral membrane with the host cell membrane resulting in the viral RNA being injected into the host cell's cytoplasm. Once viral RNA has been released into the host cell, RNA reverse transcription occurs. The enzyme reverse transcriptase converts viral RNA into a single stranded DNA. Reverse transcription by reverse transcriptase acting as DNA polymerase occurs a second time to produce a complementary strand of DNA. Next, retroviral integrase, which is an enzyme produced by the virus, binds the newly formed double stranded DNA molecule and carries it through a pore into the nucleus of the cell. Here, the integrase makes a cut in the host chromosome allowing the viral DNA to integrate

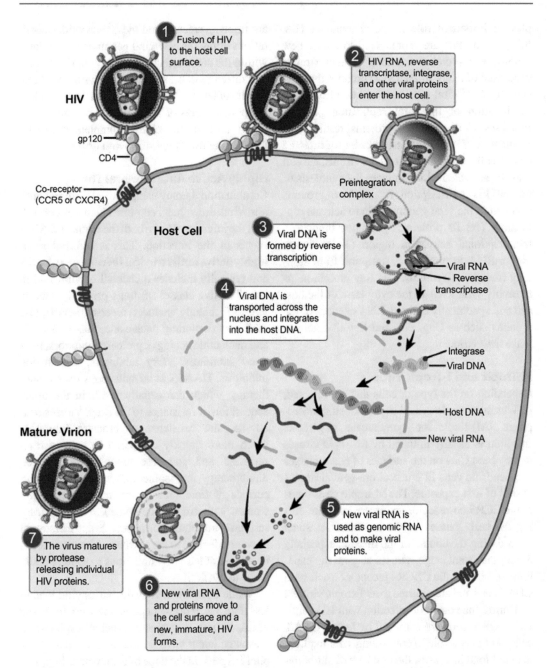

Fig. 9.8 HIV life cycle Credit: National Institute of Allergy and Infectious Diseases (NIAID)

itself and become a part of the host's DNA. Once the viral DNA has been integrated it can actively be transcribed by the host cell enzyme, RNA polymerase, into mRNA. This integration of viral DNA is what makes HIV a **provirus**; every daughter cell now expresses viral DNA and can produce infectious virions. Once the viral mRNA leaves the nucleus it will begin to make proteins with the assistance of ribosomes. Key viral proteins include envelope proteins and viral polyproteins. The envelope proteins relocate to the cell surface and display themselves as new gp120 receptors that can bind to new CD4 cells, aiding in the progression of the disease. Viral proteases play an important role in the cleaving of HIV polyproteins that are reorganized to create new virions. Polyproteins are long protein strands composed of many smaller viral proteins that will code for HIV viral enzymes, and be utilized for continuation of the viral replication process. Proteases cleave the polyproteins resulting in production of viral proteins. In order for infected CD4 T cells to produce infectious virions, the cell must be activated which induces the synthesis of the NF-kB transcription factor. Two proteins encoded in the viral genome help to activate replication. The Tat protein in particular binds to a transcriptional activation region (TAR) in the viral mRNA to prevent transcription from stopping (thus amplifying it). The Rev protein helps to supply viral RNA to the cytoplasm of the host cell and specifically delivers RNA needed for the proteins such as Gag, Pol, and Env that help to make new virions.

M-Tropic and T-Tropic Viruses

Depending on the type of cells that are infected, HIV viruses are described as either being macrophage (M)-tropic or lymphocyte (T)-tropic. Infection is usually initiated by M-tropic viruses as they bind CD4 on the surfaces of macrophages and dendritic cells in mucosal ora-genital tissues at sites of first exposure. The M-tropic virus binds to the CCR5 co-receptor and is predominant during the early phases of the infection. At some point during the course of the disease, especially during the latent stage, viruses acquire the capability of binding the CXCR4 receptor on activated CD4 T cells and are referred to as T-tropic viruses.

During the course of infection with HIV, anti-HIV CD8 T cells are activated by helper CD4 T cells, and play a role in controlling viral load. As the viral load increases, the numbers of antibody-producing B cells also increases. However, the combination of all of these adaptive responses is not sufficient to eliminate the virus. This is because as the virus replicates in new cells, it undergoes constant mutations, which occur due to reverse transcriptase's lack of proofreading ability. This allows the virus to escape immune responses and evade total elimination by the immune system. Errors made during replication

are rarely corrected, and these nucleotide substitutions allow for new viral genomes and variants within the same infected host, giving rise to several different quasi species of the virus. Vast reservoirs of latent virus also persist in the secondary lymphoid organs of HIV-infected patients, making it difficult to achieve complete remission through the use of anti-retroviral drugs.

Highly Active Antiretroviral Therapy

Combination therapy using several different antiretroviral drugs has been efficacious in controlling the infection during both the latent and AIDS stages of the infection. This is referred to as **highly active antiretroviral therapy or HAART** and typically includes a cocktail of viral inhibitors. The five classes of drugs presently used in HAART therapy include: reverse transcriptase inhibitors (including nucleoside, non-nucleoside and nucleotide analogs), protease inhibitors, integrase inhibitors, entry inhibitors, and fusion inhibitors. HAART is advantageous over monotherapy, which can usually result in the quick acquisition of resistance to the drug. Viruses usually acquire resistance to protease inhibitors much more quickly compared to reverse transcriptase and integrase inhibitors. However, monotherapy may sometimes be used for short periods of time such as treatment of pregnant women with zidovudine (AZT), a reverse transcriptase inhibitor, during the last trimester to prevent infection to the newborn. The virus needs to acquire at least 3–4 mutations to acquire resistance to AZT.

While HAART therapy decreases viral load to less than 5%, it does not completely eradicate the virus. Newer strategies are being explored to reawaken latent virus within the secondary lymphoid organs, in the hope of achieving a complete cure.

Opportunistic Infections

Death of an HIV-infected CD4 T cell usually occurs within a few days. Not only are these virally-infected cells susceptible to apoptosis, but they are subject to cytotoxic killing from CD8 T cells specific for the viral peptides displayed on the surface of the infected CD4 T cell.

Additionally, binding of virions to cell surface receptors is also thought to contribute to CD4 T cell death in a direct way. During the clinical latency stage, CD4 T cell numbers steadily decrease. Towards the end of this stage, their numbers are so low that the patient is extremely susceptible to opportunistic infections, especially from organisms that are normally controlled by immunocompetent individuals. There does appear to be an approximate "order" of opportunistic pathogens that cause infection depending on which stage of AIDS and immune breakdown the person is experiencing. CD4 T_H1 response is lost first. This can result in the reactivation of infections such as latent TB or susceptibility to infection with active TB or *Mycobacterium avium complex*. T_H17 responses are also compromised giving rise to infections with extracellular bacteria and fungi. A common opportunistic fungal infection that tends to occur first is *Candida*, manifesting as oral thrush. Similarly, loss of T_{FH} and T_H2 responses results in defective humoral immunity and the attenuation of antibody responses to various infections that aren't commensal in nature, including *Toxoplasma* and *Cryptosporidium*. Lastly, as CD8 T cell function is lost, latent viruses such as herpes zoster, or CMV can reactivate. Viral-related tumors can also progress. EBV can cause Burkitt's lymphoma while herpesvirus HHV8 can lead to Kaposi's sarcoma. As AIDS progresses, patients become even more susceptible to fungi such as *Pneumocystis jirovecii*, *Cryptococcus neoformans, Histoplasma capsulatum*, and *Coccidioides* species. Death is usually a result of a combination of immune system damage from the virus and the microbial infections themselves.

Currently there is no vaccine to prevent HIV, but with early detection and the advent of HAART treatment in 1996, it can be managed as a chronic condition allowing people to live for many years although mortality rates remain higher than the general population. Newer research and evidence has shown that mutations in the genes encoding CCR5 are likely associated with a decreased susceptibility to HIV infections. Ten-percent of the Caucasian population is heterozygous and one percent is homozygous for a mutation in CCR5 encoding for a 32 nucleotide deletion that results in a non-functional protein. The one-percent cannot be infected with the M-tropic strain of the virus, although infection with the T-tropic strain is theoretically possible. This is well-illustrated by the case of HIV patient, Timothy Brown, also called the "Berlin" patient, who was given hematopoietic stem cell transplantation to treat HIV-associated cancer during AIDS. Doctors used bone marrow from a homozygous CCR5 mutation donor and it resulted in complete eradication of the virus, representing the only known cure for HIV/AIDS. More recently, another patient, referred to as the "London" patient, has also been reported to be cured of HIV infection, using the same procedure.

Other genetic variants of the host immune system have an effect on HIV infection. Certain HLA allotypes, including *HLA-B*27* and *HLA-B*57* seem to slow the progression to AIDS. This may be related to their ability to induce stronger CD8 T cell responses to presented antigens. Both of these allotypes also have the Bw4 epitope which is a ligand for an NK cell receptor known as KIR3DL1/S1, thereby having the potential to also stimulate NK cell responses against the virus.

Some people are also able to control the infection in their blood to undetectable viral loads. These people, about 1 in 300 HIV-infected people are considered to be elite controllers. Others are able to maintain a low viral load of at least 2000 copies/μL or less. These are known as viremic controllers. Being able to "control" viral load appears to be associated with the HLA-B type.

Additionally, around 1 in 500 HIV-infected patients make antibodies after 2 or more years of infection that are able to neutralize many HIV-1 strains. These people are known as elite neutralizers. Subsequently, techniques have been developed to isolate the B cells that are able to produce broadly neutralizing antibodies, and then clone the heavy and light chains of these antibodies to further analyze them. Broadly neutralizing antibodies are able to recognize at least one of the four epitopes of the envelope glycoprotein, in particular the binding site on gp120 for CD4, a highly conserved and important binding region for the virus. It is thought that due to exposure to different strains and several antigen-mediated somatic mutations in the framework as well as in the CDR loops, this gives them the ability to neutralize and gain access to the gp120 binding site. They are also thought to be polyreactive and have the ability to react with a variety of different antigens. Continued research with broadly neutralizing antibodies to HIV may at some point lead to the design of a useful vaccine, or even passive immunity in infected or exposed individuals.

Sepsis/Septic Shock

The effect of sepsis in the United States is a relatively large one: approximately 750,000 new cases are reported every year, with approximately 15–30% of hospitalizations resulting in mortality. Annual costs associated with sepsis are estimated at more than $20 billion. Sepsis, which is the 11th leading cause of death in the U.S., is a complex, overwhelming immune system response to infection, and for that reason, can be difficult to diagnose and treat. Common causes of sepsis include systemic severe bacterial infection, severe burns, and traumatic injury. Studies that have analyzed specific causes of hospitalizations from sepsis have identified respiratory infections as the leading cause in approximately 44% of cases, with genitourinary, abdominal, and soft tissues infections also contributing. The aberrant immune response produced during sepsis can lead to tissue damage, multiple organ failure, or death. Of note, while sepsis can affect any individual, there is increased risk in critically ill patients, elderly or very young patients, and post-surgical patients.

Many studies have indicated a major role for the immune system in the pathogenesis of sepsis, with two major events taking place: the early pro-inflammatory phase and the later anti-inflammatory phase. The early phase, also known as the systemic inflammatory response syndrome (SIRS). The later stage is characterized by a shift to an anti-inflammatory phase, compensatory anti-inflammatory response syndrome (CARS).

SIRS, which was replaced by a new definition of sepsis in 2016 (Sepsis-3) was previously defined with the following criteria in an adult patient:

1. Temperature >38 °C or <36 °C
2. Heart rate >90 beats per minute
3. Respiratory rate >20 breaths per minute or $PaCO_2$ <32 mmHg
4. White blood cell count >12,000/cu mm, <4000/cu mm, or >10% immature (band) forms.

Two or more of these criteria in response to an infection would be considered sepsis. The addition of organ dysfunction, hypoperfusion abnormalities (including lactic acidosis, oliguria, or altered mental status), or hypotension would fall into the category of severe sepsis. The addition of hypotension induced by sepsis despite fluid resuscitation would classify as septic shock.

For sepsis, diagnostic criteria included documented or suspected infection and some of a list of general parameters including fever, hypothermia, heart rate >90 bpm, tachypnea, altered mental status, significant edema or positive fluid balance (fluid gain exceeds fluid loss), or hyperglycemia in the absence of diabetes. The newer definition of sepsis, Sepsis-3, includes scoring using the Sequential (Sepsis-related) Organ Failure Assessment (SOFA), which has higher predictive validity for in-hospital mortality than SIRS. Sepsis can be life-threatening due to the organ dysfunction caused by a dysregulated host response to infection. Despite definitions, the fact remains that sepsis is not well defined, and there is no definitive laboratory test for it.

Treatment regimens continue to be geared towards supportive therapy to maintain blood pressure and early initiation of appropriate antibiotic therapy. The Surviving Sepsis Campaign prepares guidelines for healthcare professionals to follow for the management of sepsis and septic shock. Septic shock is a subgroup of sepsis with circulatory and cellular/metabolic dysfunction. Septic shock tends to be associated with an increased risk of mortality. When a patient is diagnosed with sepsis, he or she needs to be started on fluid resuscitation within the first 3 h. The Surviving Sepsis Campaign recommends patients to be resuscitated with 30 mL/kg of intravenous (IV) crystalloid fluids, typically normal saline or lactated ringers. Fluid resuscitation is used immediately for the stabilization of sepsis-induced tissue hypoperfusion or septic shock. Sepsis-induced hypoperfusion exhibits as acute organ dysfunction and/or decreased blood pressure and increased lactate. Healthcare professionals measure the success of fluid resuscitation by utilizing physiologic variables like blood pressure, mean arterial pressure (MAP), urine output, heart rate, and many more. MAP is an important factor since it is the pressure that best represents tissue perfusion. The goal for MAP is to have it be at least 65 mmHg or greater. If this goal is not reached with initial fluid resuscitation, then vasopressors, drugs that constrict blood vessels and thus increase blood pressure are added to help increase MAP. Currently, the Surviving Sepsis Campaign suggests the use of hydrocortisone in septic shock when a patient remains hemodynamically unstable despite adequate resuscitation and vasopressor therapy. The use of hydrocortisone is optional and remains controversial. Clinical trials demonstrate that corticosteroids consistently lead to a faster resolution of shock. However, they do not consistently demonstrate a reduction in mortality and many patients develop hypoglycemia. At this point, many targeted measures, included activated protein C (Xigris®), anti-endotoxin antibodies (i.e. anti-CD14, anti-LPS-binding protein), anti-IL-1, as well as TNF inhibitors have failed clinically.

Microbiology

For patients both inside and outside the ICU, the respiratory tract is the most common source of bacteria and appears to be increasing in incidence. Intra-abdominal infections are also common sources of microbes as well as the urinary tract. It is important to note that one-third to one-half of sepsis cases may be culture-negative, meaning that bacteria are not found in the patient's blood. Culture-negative and culture-positive cases of sepsis, however, seem to exhibit similar morbidity and mortality rates, in addition to similar clinical features. Among culture-positive patients, studies suggest different cytokine profiles exist between Gram-positive and Gram-negative sepsis, with higher TNF, IL-1β, and IL-6 in Gram-negative sepsis, and higher IL-18 in Gram-positive patients. It is possible that in the future these specific molecular features can help guide diagnosis and therapeutic options.

Gram-Positive Sepsis

Gram-positive bacteria are responsible for slightly more than half of all sepsis cases. Common causative agents include *Staphylococcus aureus, Streptococcus pneumoniae,* and *Enterococci* species. While Gram-positive cocci are often associated with skin and skin structure infections, they are also causative agents of respiratory infections, and may be found on intravascular devices and long-term indwelling catheters. Gram-positive organisms are capable of producing exotoxins that act as superantigens which bind to MHC class II on APCs and in doing so stimulate T cells to produce proinflammatory cytokines. Gram-positive organisms may also initiate immune responses through TLR2 binding to bacterial products on Gram-positive cell walls, including peptidoglycan and lipoteichoic acid.

Gram-Negative Sepsis

Gram-negative sepsis is mainly caused by Gram-negative bacilli including *Escherichia coli*, *Klebsiella* species, and *Pseudomonas aeruginosa* in the lungs, GI tract as a result of intestinal injury or perforation, bloodstream, or urinary tract. As a component of the outer membrane of the Gram-negative cell wall, LPS (bound to CD14 and TLR4 on the surfaces of immune cells) plays a major role in initiating Gram-negative sepsis. Among the critically ill, Gram-negative bacteremia often stems from the respiratory tract or a central venous catheter. Elderly patients admitted to the hospital from a nursing home may have Gram-negative bacteremia which has originated at the urinary tract, with *E. coli* being the most common organism found. Patients with Gram-negative bacteremia are more likely to become septic and even progress to septic shock as opposed to patients with Gram-positive bacteremia. This may be due to the immune system's stronger response to endotoxin (as opposed to peptidoglycan) in the blood. Patients with Gram-negative sepsis who also have a co-morbidity such as leukemia, cirrhosis, or HIV will have a higher mortality rate than those without these underlying conditions.

Fungal Sepsis

Sepsis caused by a fungus, most often *Candida albicans* accounts for approximately 4–5% of all sepsis cases. *Candida* normally colonizes the skin as well as the gastrointestinal tract as a commensalistic organism. While non-albicans *Candida* species do account for some isolated cases, other fungal causes of sepsis include *Fusarium, Aspergillus, Coccidioides*, and *Cryptococcus.* While many of these begin as skin infections, fungal spores can also be inhaled and can lead to lung infections in some immunocompromised individuals. Invasive fungal infections are usually associated with risk factors such as poorly controlled diabetes mellitus, HIV, immunosuppressive treatments, total parenteral nutrition (TPN, IV nutrition in patients that can't take food by mouth), prolonged time in the hospital, living in a nursing home, central venous

catheters, or indwelling Foley catheters. Retrospective studies analyzing mortality from Candidemia have found rates as high as 49%. Rates are even higher with underlying comorbidities. Thus, early recognition of fungal sepsis and proper antifungal treatments are key to improving therapeutic outcomes.

Hemostasis and Hypercoagulation

Under normal conditions, blood flows freely within the blood vessels and relies on the complex clotting cascade to control bleeding when appropriate. Oftentimes the heightened inflammatory response which occurs during sepsis alters various points within this cascade, resulting in consumption of platelets and more frequent blood clotting and disseminated intravascular coagulation (DIC) (Fig. 9.9). This excessive clotting results in microclots that clog blood vessels, reducing blood flow, leading to multiple organ failure (MOF). The underlying pathobiology of this process is multifactorial, due to multiple interactions between the clotting cascade, the endothelium, platelets, and circulating leukocytes. As mentioned, a drug that attempted to mitigate this was approved by the FDA in 2001 based on the results from a large phase III clinical trial called the PROWESS study. Protein C is a

Fig. 9.9 Sepsis can lead to DIC which results in microvascular thrombosis and decreased tissue perfusion leading to multiple organ failure

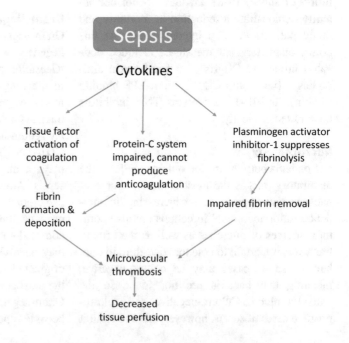

vitamin K-dependent plasma protein which has been shown to be decreased in patients with sepsis and inactivates factors Va and VIIIa which in turn decreases release of thrombin. Besides anticoagulant properties, it is hypothesized to have anti-inflammatory and anti-apoptotic properties. Drotrecogin alfa (Xigris®) consisted of recombinant human Activated Protein C. It was withdrawn from the market by Lilly in 2011 due to its inability to produce a statistically significant reduction in 28-day all-cause mortality in patients with septic shock in the PROWESS-SHOCK study. Prior to this, the treatment also did not have a statistically significant effect on patients with severe sepsis in the ADDRESS trial.

Hyperinflammation

Research of both animal models and humans with sepsis indicate that many of the manifestations of sepsis are likely due to a complex pro-inflammatory cascade which may or may not be counterbalanced by appropriate anti-inflammatory mediators. Proinflammatory cytokines released into the circulation during sepsis include TNF-α, IL-1β, IL-6, and IL-8. IL-10 is an anti-inflammatory cytokine that is also released and can block the production of the aforementioned pro-inflammatory cytokines. Additionally, there are naturally occurring inhibitors, including sTNFr and IL-1ra, but in the case of lethal sepsis these may not be present in adequate enough concentrations to block inappropriate hyperinflammation effectively. Pro-inflammatory cytokines can be categorized based on where they have their effect. TNF-α and IL-1β are referred to as proximal cytokines due to their more immediate and local effects. In contrast, IL-6 and IL-8 may be referred to as distal cytokines.

TNF

In sepsis, studies in both clinically-relevant animal models as well as humans suggest that increases in pro-inflammatory cytokines correlate with a higher likelihood of mortality. In humans, studies revealed that septic patients with increased level of TNF-α in particular had a higher mortality rate. This observation was reproducible in animal models upon injection of high doses of TNF-α as well as lethal doses of endotoxin leading to increased release of TNF-α and IL-1.

Upon bacterial encounter, activated macrophages release TNF-α to initiate an immune response. As mentioned in Chap. 2, TNF is an endogenous pyrogen (fever-inducer), a pro-apoptotic factor, and an inducer of other inflammatory pathways. With regard to sepsis, Tracey and Cerami described TNF's role as a key mediator in lethal septic shock in the late 1980s. In 1990 another study helped confirm this by reporting that patients with sepsis had extremely elevated levels of TNF-α, and those patients whose elevated TNF levels persisted past Day 3 postonset had 100% mortality. While under normal conditions, the production of other cytokines or regulatory molecules are aimed at balancing produced of proinflammatory mediators, it is hypothesized that exaggerated TNF released during sepsis and septic shock may be too much to control by endogenous regulatory factors.

Several attempted TNF inhibitors have failed as significantly effective therapeutic options for sepsis due to the fact that they just simply cannot be given early enough. With animal models of sepsis suggesting efficacy with the use of anti-TNF treatments, several clinical trials were conducted in the 1990s and 2000s utilizing TNF inhibitors, including monoclonal antibodies against TNF, in an attempt to control aberrant TNF release with the hypothesis that this would decrease septic mortality. Individually, the trials did not indicate a significant improvement, yet meta-analyses did show some improvement overall. Part of the issue may be that earlier on in sepsis, cytokines may be acting at the local level even when not detected yet in the plasma.

IL-1β

In addition to TNF, IL-1β appears to play a role in the pathophysiological characteristics associated with sepsis. Studies have shown that injection of both of these cytokines in experimental animals mimics a sepsis state while blocking them reduces the morbidity seen in clinical sepsis. IL-1β is not normally present in human plasma but is produced by monocytes in response to endotoxin. Like TNF, IL-1β is a pyrogen and can cause not only fever, but also hemodynamic dysfunction and malaise. It activates the release of more pro-inflammatory mediators including IL-6 and IL-8. In human studies of sepsis TNF levels correlated highly with severity of sepsis and mortality, IL-1 levels did not. However, studies have shown that patients with who did not survive sepsis were more likely to have elevated and persistent plasma levels of IL-1β as compared to survivors.

A handful of clinical trials in the 1990s attempted to elucidate the potential utility of IL-1 receptor antagonists in sepsis. Despite evidence suggesting that inhibiting certain cytokines might improve septic outcomes, clinical trials utilizing anti-TNF and anti-IL-1 treatments have not been successful. Trials that specifically used IL-1Ra, anakinra, to prevent IL-1 signaling and thus attempt to decrease aspects of the "cytokine storm" went to phase III after some promising results in phase II. In phase III anakinra did not provide any benefit in overall 28-day survival but did show some benefit in the most severe septic patients with multiple organ dysfunction. This trial was ended however, when no statistically significant difference in mortality was found over placebo in the first analysis.

IL-6

As mentioned in earlier chapters, IL-6 is a pleiotropic cytokine which can initiate the acute phase response, act on lymphocytes, and activate coagulation. It is produced by lymphocytes, fibroblasts, and monocytes, and like IL-1 and TNF, is considered to be a pyrogen. In a clinically-relevant mouse model of sepsis, higher IL-6 levels were found 6 h after septic challenge, with higher plasma levels of >2000 pg/mL being predictive of death within 3 days. In humans, plasma IL-6 levels correlate with higher SOFA scores and mortality.

Studies of IL-6 knockout mice and mice treated with IL-6 inhibitors in sepsis support the hypothesis that IL-6 has a role in sepsis; mice lacking IL-6 have the same mortality as wild type mice but do not show the characteristic hypothermia usually seen in the first 24 h after septic

onset. Higher levels of IL-6 are also linked with decreased blood pressure and endothelial cell dysfunction. Although inhibitors have been used in septic animals with some benefit, the use of IL-6 inhibitors in human sepsis remains a difficult prospect. Not only would perspective cytokine inhibitors need to be given early on and would likely not have an effect if given too late, hindering a complex system may also prove difficult, especially since different patients appear to exhibit variable pro-inflammatory gene profiles. Additionally, IL-6 tends to be higher in Gram-positive sepsis, so the microbiological etiology would have to be known early on.

Other Cytokines Associated with Sepsis

IL-8 is a chemokine which attracts neutrophils, contributing to accumulating inflammation as well as tissue damage. It is produced by phagocytes including macrophages and neutrophils, endothelial cells, and epithelial cells in response to LPS, IL-1, and TNF, as well as cellular dysfunction. In addition to being a chemoattractant, research has suggested that IL-8 may be implicated in tissue remodeling and angiogenesis. Based on its role in inflammation and proliferation, some studies have suggested that IL-8 may be a biomarker for sepsis and subsequent mortality.

Other cytokines like IL-17 are responsible for excessive tissue damage in response to pathogens. IL-17 is produced by helper T cells and can stimulate the release of TNF-α, IL-6, IL-1β, and IL-8 as well as growth factors including G-CSF and GM-CSF. In sepsis, research has indicated that cytokines such as IL-17 are necessary for immunity against fungal infections, as well as polymicrobial sepsis.

IL-18 (formerly known as interferon-γ inducing factor) on the other hand, may play an important role in the inflammatory process initiated during sepsis; plasma IL-18 levels have been found to be elevated in septic patients and may correlate with poorer outcomes. As has been seen with other cytokines which are elevated with certain microbial etiologies, IL-18 appears to be elevated in patients with Gram-positive sepsis, thus IL-18 blockade may be an interesting therapeutic target.

HMGB-1, or high mobility group box-1 is a DNA-binding protein and is involved in gene transcription. HMGB-1 can also act as a pro-inflammatory cytokine and was found to be elevated in patients with sepsis. Work by Kevin Tracey's group was instrumental in the discovery of HMGB-1 as an inflammatory mediator, and have elucidated some of its features as a potential drug target in sepsis.

Immunosuppression and Cell Dysfunction

Failure to clear the bacterial infection as a result of immunosuppression is likely another cause of septic morbidity and mortality. This suggests that an extreme tipping of the scales exists from one extreme (the hyperinflammatory state) to the other (immunosuppressed state). As sepsis progresses, studies show a shift to compensatory anti-inflammatory response syndrome (CARS), characterized by a dominance of anti-inflammatory cytokines such as IL-10 and TGF-β, resulting in immunosuppression.

Lymphocyte Apoptosis

Research on clinically-relevant animal models of sepsis have suggested that loss of lymphocytes may contribute to immunosuppression in the later stage of sepsis, and may be due to dysregulated apoptosis of lymphocytes, leaving the host immunosuppressed and unable to fight off the microbe and lethal effects of sepsis. It is for this reason that components of the apoptotic pathways, including caspases, Bcl-2, and the Fas-FasL death receptor family have been attractive targets for therapy. Apoptosis actively eliminates cells via a specifically programmed cell-death pathway, not only during development and tissue remodeling, but also to aid in resolution of the immune response. Mediators that induce apoptosis include steroids, pro-inflammatory cytokines, oxygen free radicals, and NO. Cells that are able to induce apoptosis include NK cells and CD8 T cells expressing FasL which binds to its death receptor Fas antigen, or CD95. The apoptotic pathway may occur through three distinct paths: extrinsic, intrinsic, or the ER/stress-induced

pathway. Fas antigen is a major death receptor belonging to the TNF superfamily and represents the major mechanism by which extrinsic death signaling takes place. Fas may be expressed on thymocytes, B cells, T cells, monocytes/macrophages, and neutrophils. Non-immune cells including cells in the liver, lung, and heart may also express Fas on their surfaces. When Fas binds its ligand FasL, the downstream signaling cascade activates caspases including caspase 8, and then caspases 3, 6, or 7 which then cleave DNA in the nucleus. The intrinsic pathway can be activated by loss of growth factors such as IL-2, IL-4, or GM-CSF, or higher levels of IL-1 and IL-6. This pathway relies on mitochondria to release molecules such as cytochrome c for cellular destruction, which can activate caspase 3 and other pro-apoptotic molecules of the Bcl-2 family as well. Some Bcl-2 family members block cytochrome c and are thus anti-apoptotic, thus apoptosis can only proceed with a dominance of pro-apoptotic molecules in the cell.

Studies have shown that in sepsis, immune dysfunction and resulting immunosuppression may stem from the loss of immune cells due to dysregulated apoptosis, with lymphocytes being the most commonly affected immune cells. Animal studies of polymicrobial sepsis have shown that loss of lymphocytes correlates with a decreased survival, due to the decreased ability of the host to fight off the primary infection. While lymphocyte apoptosis may begin occurring in the thymus as early as 4 h after the onset (most likely due to glucocorticoids, NO, and C5a), apoptosis of lymphocytes is frequently seen 12+ hours after septic onset in the thymus, spleen, and GALT, and likely correlates with greater multiorgan failure and mortality. This later onset of lymphocyte apoptosis (12+ hours after onset) is thought to mainly be death receptor-driven. Since studies have suggested that lymphocyte apoptosis in sepsis may occur through both the intrinsic and extrinsic pathways, these may represent interesting targets for therapy. While caspase inhibitors have been used with positive results in septic mice, these have not been tested in humans and can be cytotoxic at too high a dose.

Why Is Sepsis So Hard to Treat?

Sepsis is caused by a complex interplay between the pro-inflammatory cytokine cascade and anti-inflammatory factors. Because sepsis is difficult to define, it is often difficult to determine when septic onset takes place in the patient. Thus, the question of when to inhibit cytokines after septic onset might be unknown in certain patients, i.e. cytokine inhibitors given too late may be actually detrimental as patients shift towards the immuno-suppressed phase of sepsis. To further complicate matters, sepsis can be caused by a wide range of microbes which may or may not be present when culture results return, which can take 1–3 days. Upon presentation, microbe status would be unknown, and any possible infections can be complicated by secondary infections. The caus-ative agent of the primary infection can result in a slightly different immune response and cyto-kine profile. Genetic variability of the pathogens and possible resistance to antibiotics can add another layer of complication when treating patients.

Current evidence-based treatment recommen-dations include initial fluid resuscitation to improve perfusion and blood pressure. Antibiotic therapies are usually given as broad-spectrum initially against likely bacterial or fungal organ-isms and then de-escalated once microbiology cultures are obtained. Vasopressors such as nor-epinephrine and epinephrine are initiated to maintain MAP. As mentioned, IV hydrocortisone may be given for septic shock when hypotension persists despite fluids and vasopressors. However, co-morbidities of the patient, as well as the stage of the acute phase response and/or coagulation may make some treatment modalities difficult.

The immune response to sepsis is a highly complex and dynamic one. With the release of pro-inflammatory mediators to eliminate patho-gens, anti-inflammatory mediators and soluble cytokine inhibitors are also released in an attempt to maintain balance and prevent excessive tissue damage. Genetic variability in hosts and their immune responses poses another barrier to an exact treatment. For this reason, a "one size fits all" approach will likely never work, and thera-pies will need to be tailored to patients and their

clinical course. Managing sepsis and therapeutic recommendations for specific patients will con-tinue to be a challenge.

Infections in Immunocompromised Patients

Tuberculosis

Throughout history, the impact of TB has been well-known as a major contributor to worldwide morbidity and mortality. Also known as "Consumption," "Pott's disease," and the "White plague," there is evidence to suggest that TB may be at least 9000 years old. In 1882, Robert Koch isolated the causative agent, a rod-shaped bacte-rium known as *Mycobacterium tuberculosis*, and showed that it can be isolated from the sputum of infected patients. It is estimated that peak infec-tions took place in the span of the nineteenth cen-tury, with approximately 450 Americans dying daily from TB in the early 1900s. Before antibi-otic advances in the late 1940s, treatment con-sisted mainly of housing the infected in sanatoriums, an idea piloted by Dr. Edward Livington Trudea, who found an improvement in his own TB infection when he escaped to his favorite Adirondack resort for rest. Therapies in sanatoriums included following a healthy diet, rest, exercise, and fresh air. Other treatments include sun therapy, removal of infected whole lung (pneumonectomy), removal of parts of the lung (lobectomy), or collapse of the lung (artifi-cial pneumothorax). With the advent of the anti-biotic streptomycin, the need for TB sanatoriums greatly diminished and many were closed by the 1960s. Today, with approximately 8–9 million new cases a year, it is estimated that roughly a third of the world's population has been exposed, and 95% of deaths occur in low and middle-income countries.

Mycobacterium tuberculosis (Mtb) is an aero-bic rod with a mycolic acid cell wall. It appears as a slender, waxy bacillus under the microscope that is either straight or curved (Fig. 9.10). Due to the lipid-rich composition, it is extremely diffi-cult to stain using Gram's stain and retains

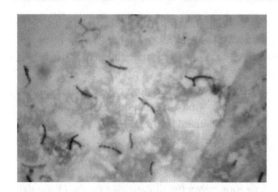

Fig. 9.10 *Mycobacterium tuberculosis* is an acid-fast bacilli which retains the initial red stain, carbol fuchsin. Magnification: 1000×. Credit: CDC/Dr. George P. Kubica

carbol-fuchsin when stained with the Ziehl-Neelsen stain despite repeated acid washes, leading to its being termed as an **'acid-fast' bacilli** or **AFB**. Due to the difficulty with staining, identification by culture is considered the gold-standard. Since it is a strict aerobe, Mtb preferentially infects the lungs. However, extrapulmonary infection with Mtb is common. Sites of extrapulmonary TB include the bone, joints, kidney, brain, pleura, lymph nodes and spine. Miliary TB occurs when bacteria enter the bloodstream. Although rare, it can be fatal and is considered a medical emergency. Children in endemic countries often present with miliary TB.

Pulmonary infection begins when Mtb bacilli are inhaled as aerosolized droplets. TLRs on macrophages and dendritic cells recognize the bacteria in the alveolar spaces, and perform phagocytosis. These APCs then present Mtb antigens on MHC II to T helper cells. Until that point, the bacilli can replicate within the phagosome of the macrophage. Once T_H1 cells are primed, they begin releasing IFN-ɣ and TNF-α to induce killing of the bacteria by macrophages. This slows replication, but does not stop it.

When first infected, macrophages mediate a robust pro-inflammatory response initiated by TLR2 signaling. TLR2 seems to preferentially recognize Mtb PAMPs, including heat shock proteins, several types of lipoproteins, glycolipids, and mannosides. It is thought, however, that continued TLR2 signaling leads to activation of regulatory T cells, IL-10 induction, and a dampened response of macrophages to IFN-ɣ. This helps Mtb evade the T_H1 immune response, and persist in its replication. The infected alveolar macrophages migrate to the lung interstitium where a granuloma is formed. The local release of TNF-α, IL-1, IL-6, IL-12, and chemokines MCP-1 and IP-10 leads to the recruitment of neutrophils, NK cells, and T and B cells, further contributing to granuloma formation.

Initially, the Mtb granuloma is composed of centralized infected macrophages encircled by extra macrophages, multi-nucleate giant cells, foamy (lipid-filled) macrophages, and granulocytes. From there, the granuloma can take several forms. The solid granuloma normally consists of a collection of infected and uninfected macrophages, as well as lymphocytes, without evidence of necrosis. This solid stage represents containment of the bacteria and latent stage of infection. The neutrophilic granuloma is characterized by more widespread granulocyte infiltration, while the caseous granuloma contains dead cells at the core (necrosis), surrounded by macrophages and neutrophils. As the granuloma progresses and hypoxia ensues which inhibits macrophage superoxide and nitric oxide formation, the intracellular killing of bacilli decreases further, and bacterial replication continues uncontrolled.

Transmission of TB occurs through the air via droplet nuclei. The bacteria can be spread when a person speaks, sings, coughs, or sneezes. Infected persons acquire the bacteria when they inhale the droplet nuclei. In most individuals, infection results in the induction of a fulminant immune response that curtails bacterial replication within granulomas. These individuals do not exhibit symptoms of TB and cannot spread the bacteria to other individuals unless reactivation occurs. They are said to have latent TB. Approximately 10% of individuals with latent TB can experience reactivation throughout their lifetime. In others, the infection results in uncontrolled replication, resulting in active TB. People with active TB are highly infectious and experience severe symptoms, including fever, weight loss, and a productive, incessant cough that lasts for several months. They can transmit the disease to other individuals. The probability of transmission depends on the infectiousness of the person, the virulence of the bacilli, the length of exposure to the infected individual and the environment in which the exposure occurred. The best way to stop transmission is to isolate the infectious person as soon as possible and initiate therapeutic regimens.

Determination of infection is usually made on the basis of cumulative results obtained from several individual tests. Latent TB is diagnosed using either a skin test, the tuberculin test, or a blood test, the interferon-gamma release assay (IGRA). The tuberculin test is also referred to as the Mantoux test based on the physician who first administered it or simply as a PPD (protein purified derivative). In the PPD test, 5 tuberculin units of PPD are dosed intracutaneously in the volar forearm. In previously-sensitized individuals, this induces a delayed-type hypersensitivity reaction resulting in the recruitment and accumulation of inflammatory cells including T_H1 cells at the injected site. This results in visible swelling which can be measured. Assessment of disease or latent TB infection (LTBI) is made based on the width of the swelling and established criteria. While the tuberculin test typically takes 48–72 h, the IGRA is a rapid read-out based on either an ELISA or ELISPOT for IFN-γ in the patient's blood.

In many countries around the world, children are given a live attenuated TB vaccine soon after birth. This vaccine is a highly attenuated strain of *M. bovis* that was developed in 1921 by the scientists Calmette and Guerin and is referred to as **Bacille Calmette-Guerin (BCG)**. Although the vaccine is not absolutely protective against pulmonary TB, it is thought to confer protection against TB meningitis in children as well as miliary TB in some cases. BCG-vaccinated individuals will often turn out to be falsely positive for infection using the PPD test. In contrast, the IGRA is much more sensitive and is recommended for BCG-vaccinated individuals.

Diagnosis of active TB is made on the basis of chest x-rays often secondary to the PPD and IGRA tests. In active pulmonary TB, damage to alveolar tissue can result in holes in the lung, referred to as pulmonary activation. These as well as granulomas can be identified on a chest X-ray. The granulomas are referred to as *Ghon's complex*. During treatment, patients are also periodically examined for the presence of bacteria in the sputum.

The risk of developing active TB is highest within the first 2 years after infection. Thus prompt treatment for LTBI is often recommended to prevent the development of active TB and stop transmission to others. Some conditions increase the probability of developing active TB with HIV infection being the highest risk factor. Other risk factors include immunosuppression due to illness or treatment with immunosuppressive drugs such as prednisone or anti-TNF-α inhibitors, substance abuse, and transplantation.

TB therapy relies on a cocktail of several antitubercular drugs including isoniazid, rifampin, pyrazinamide and ethambutol. Additionally, a number of other drugs are used depending on the patient's history and strain of the infecting bacterium. Latent TB is typically treated using monotherapy with isoniazid (INH) for 6–9 months and depending on whether the patient is HIV-infected or not. INH inhibits mycolic acid synthesis, disrupting the cell wall, and is bactericidal against both active and dormant bacteria. Although extremely effective, it comes with a black box warning for hepatitis and patients with preexisting conditions may need to be treated with alternate drugs. It can also increase the risk for concurrent peripheral neuropathy in some patients and is coadministered with pyridoxine. In some studies, treatment for 4 months with INH and rifampin has been shown to be equally efficacious for the treatment of LTBI. Rifampin inhibits RNA synthesis by binding to the beta subunit of DNA-dependent RNA polymerase. It is bactericidal against both extra- and intracellular bacilli. However, rifampin is a strong inducer of cytochrome P450 enzymes and so poses risks for several drug-drug interactions. It can also lead to an increase in hepatic enzymes.

For individuals with active TB and no other complications, a 6–9 month regimen is recommended for the treatment of drug-sensitive bacteria. This includes an initial phase consisting of treatment with INH, rifampin, pyrazinamide and ethambutol, followed by a continuous phase consisting of INH and rifampin. The mechanism of action of pyrazinamide is not well-understood and it is thought to target non-growing persistent bacteria. It is also associated with hepatotoxicity. Ethambutol inhibits arabinosyl transferase, which impairs cell wall synthesis. A common adverse effect is optic neuritis.

Second line therapy is used by experienced practitioners in the case of drug-resistant strains or patients with other complications. The emergence of drug resistance is a major confounding factor in TB therapy and a significant concern worldwide. Multi-drug resistance, poly-drug resistance as well as extensive-drug resistance (XDR) are common in some countries. Second line drugs include injectable streptomycin, fluoroquinolones, aminoglycosides, cycloserine, ethionamide and para-aminosalicylic acid.

Leprosy

Leprosy is a chronic infection caused by *Mycobacterium leprae*. Because mycobacteria tend to grow slowly, the incubation period can be between 1 and 20 years, with the average being 5 years for symptoms to become evident. *Mycobacterium leprae* can be transmitted via droplets from the nose and mouth, and through direct contact. For the most part, immunocompetent individuals (about 95%) are able to fight this infectious agent without presenting disease symptoms. However, those who do may present clinical manifestations that differ based on the type of immune response mounted against the pathogen, in particular, the type of T cell response which can be polarized to be either T_H1 or T_H2. For this reason, there are two ends of the spectrum of leprosy, tuberculoid leprosy (T-lep), and lepromatous leprosy (L-lep). In patients with T-lep, skin lesions are few, with less replicating bacilli, but tissue and nerve damage is common due to chronic inflammation. These patients are likely to have a T_H1-polarized response, dominated by T_H1 cytokines such as IL-2, lymphotoxin, and IFN-γ which helps macrophages phagocytose the bacteria. Patients with L-lep have numerous skin lesions, and persistent bacterial growth. In this case, macrophages become overwhelmed and cannot contain the multiplying bacteria. This is due to a T_H2-polarized response and the release of T_H2 cytokines including TGF-β, IL-4, IL-13, and IL-10 which can suppress macrophage activation. In L-lep skin lesions, DCs as well as costimulatory protein B7 are found in abnormally low numbers, which may be another explanation for the reduction in the T-cell mediated response. In both cases (T-lep and L-lep), the immune system is unable to clear the bacteria, and thus the condition is a chronic infection.

Toxic Shock Syndrome

Toxic shock syndrome (TSS) is an infection caused by *Staphylococcus aureus* and is commonly associated with the use of highly absorbent tampons during menstruation, particularly if the tampons are left in for longer than recommended. *S. aureus* are Gram-positive, non-motile cocci arranged in grape-like clusters and are capable of secreting toxins that can affect the host's immune system. After the exponential phase of growth, pathogenic *S. aureus* strains secrete virulence factors known as superantigens (SAgs). SAgs are non-glycosylated exoproteins of low molecular weight that are highly resistant to denaturation by acid, heat, or proteolysis. There are 23 different SAgs. One of these, namely, toxic-shock syndrome toxin (TSST-1 superantigen) is considered to be a superantigen because it can activate many different CD4 T cell clones, as well as lead to overproduction of T cell cytokines including IFN-γ, TNF-α, and IL-2. This molecule has binding sites for TCR and MHC II, and is considered to be pyrogenic because it can induce the release of IL-1β and IL-6 from antigen-presenting cells.

TSST-1 leads to barrier penetration and subsequent TSS through an "outside-in" signaling mechanism (Fig. 9.11). TSST-1 must first interact bind to vaginal epithelial cells possibly via CD40 or another unknown receptor. This stimulates the release of pro-inflammatory chemokines including IL-8 and MIP-3α which attract immune cells to the submucosa. Both innate and adaptive

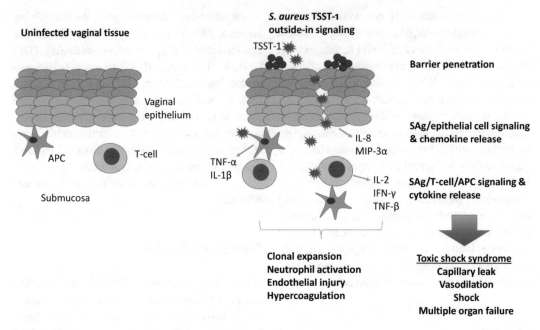

Fig. 9.11 Mechanism of toxic shock syndrome and outside-in signaling. The TSST-1 toxin binds to vaginal epithelial cells which stimulates the release of pro-inflammatory cytokines that attract immune cells to the submucosa. TSST-1 penetrates the submucosa and interacts with immune cells resulting in the effects of toxic shock syndrome

immune cells at the vaginal submucosa are now activated and contribute more inflammatory cytokines which subsequently disrupt the barrier. TSST-1 is now able to penetrate into the submucosa and interacts with macrophages and T cells which then cause the effects of TSS. During the menstrual cycle, the barrier is more susceptible to disruption, and thus TSST-1 is more easily able to cross into the submucosa to interact with immune cells. People more at risk for TSS are those who have been exposed to large quantities of TSST-1, and those who have the a receptor on vaginal mucosal epithelial receptor to which

TSST-1 can bind. Normally, vaginal epithelial cells don't interact with the SAg as well as T cells and APCs do.

As a result of TSST-1 outside-in signaling and inflammatory cytokines, there is a clonal expansion of T cells, neutrophil activation and extravasation, injury to the endothelium, and hypercoagulation. As a result of the immune response, the clinical manifestations of TSS include fever, a sunburn-like skin rash, and hypotension. Treatment strategies include antibiotics against *S. aureus*, drainage of any abscesses, and possibly IVIG.

From Bench to Bedside: Development of Vaccines

Vaccination can truly be considered one of the wonders of modern medicine, saving countless lives from deadly diseases, and eliminating pain and suffering due to disease in many parts of the world. However, although it is a routine medical procedure that is now commonly performed in any physician's office throughout the world, the history of its development has not been without challenges. The fact that some individuals are protected from disease, while others succumb to it has been observed throughout history. It has also been apparent that individuals who have previously suffered from a particular infection are far more unlikely to develop it in the future.

The modern era of vaccination began in 1796, when Dr. Edward Jenner first published his report on how inoculation with vaccinia virus from a cowpox pustule could prevent the development of smallpox in the inoculated individual. Although this was not necessarily a novel concept at the time, it was the first proof-of-principle demonstration that protection from a disease could be achieved via exposure to a similar but unrelated disease. Jenner's experiment demonstrated that this protection could safely be achieved through inoculation with agents that were not the cause of the particular disease.

In the 1700s, smallpox was one of the most feared diseases in Europe. In 1721, Lady Mary Wortley Montagu had introduced the practice of variolation, which had long been performed in many parts of Asia. This practice involved taking material from the pustules of people infected with smallpox and rubbing it onto healthy skin. Because this method of inoculation, however, utilized matter from smallpox pustules of individuals sick with smallpox, it was considered a dangerous practice it could often induce severe or fatal disease, killing 1 in 4 individuals who practiced it. Later, this method was modified slightly by Dr. Robert Sutton in Suffolk, England who took a small quantity of matter from an unripe smallpox pustule, and inject it intradermally into a healthy patient. Jenner began using this method in his native town of Berkeley and found that some patients seemed to be completely resistant to smallpox. The one thing that these individuals (who were milkmaids) had in common was that they had contracted cowpox from milking cows who had visible eruptions on their teats. This was not absolute, however, as he subsequently discovered that the cow pustules sometimes differed, and only one type of cowpox ("true cowpox" as he called it) was able to confer protection against smallpox, but only if the pustule was not too old, as was the case with Sutton's method. Based on this observation, Jenner hypothesized that cowpox (caused by vaccinia virus) might protect against contracting smallpox. It wasn't until almost 16 years later that he tested his hypothesis. On May 14, 1796, Dr. Jenner inoculated an 8-year-old boy named James Phipps with matter taken from the pustule of a milkmaid named Sarah Nelmes suffering from cowpox. Phipps did contract cowpox but recovered without incident. Nearly 2 months later on July 1, Jenner inoculated James Phipps with smallpox matter, which was unable to produce disease in the boy. While Jenner was widely mocked, he persevered and even experimented on his own 11-month old son. Nearly 2 years later, Jenner published 23 cases of cowpox inoculation successes in a book titled *An Inquiry into the Causes and Effects of the Variolae Vaccinae.* "Vaccine" was a termed coined by Jenner (*vacca* meaning cow in Latin). After the publication of his book, vaccination practices began to spread despite continued criticism and Jenner was awarded a grant by Parliament to continue his research. As a result of vaccination, smallpox deaths drastically decreased in Europe and North America, and in 1980 was announced to be eradicated by the WHO. For this important contribution to medicine, Jenner is considered by some to be the father of immunology.

The nineteenth century saw many important advancements in the field of microbiology from the germ theory of disease, to sanitation reform, to the development of anti-septic techniques. Mortality rates due to infection significantly decreased thanks to the work of many scientists including Pasteur, Koch, and Lister. Louis Pasteur, being an ardent proponent of proving that specific microbes caused specific diseases, postulated that those same diseases could be prevented by the same microbes, yet in their weakened form. After Pasteur "rescued" the French wine and vinegar industry in the mid-1800s by pointing out how to control microbial contamination, Pasteur undertook projects to not only help revolutionize industry (*i.e.* pasteurization), but also medicine, by investigating how to combat disease.

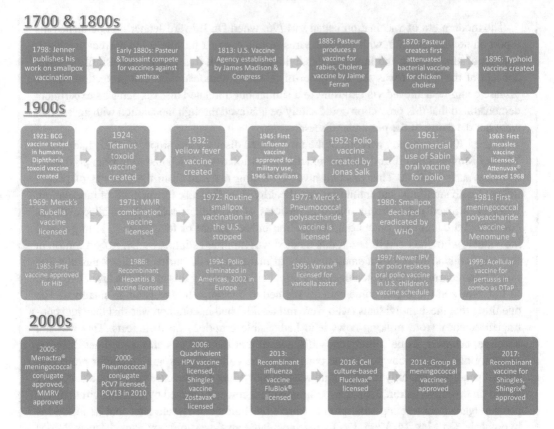

Fig. 9.12 Vaccine timeline containing the landmark vaccine discoveries since the late 1700s

Despite Edward Jenner's contributions to the field, some argue that Pasteur is the true father of immunology due to the notion that while Jenner's experiments were a proof of principle and successful, they did not describe how immunity is developed. Pasteur, however, took this idea a step further and described how this concept of vaccinating with attenuated microbes can also be applied to other infections. Pasteur postulated, keeping in mind the work of M. Toussaint on chicken cholera, that the virulence of microbes may be decreased by passing them in an alternate culture medium. In the early 1880s, he was able to apply this concept to anthrax by using weakened anthrax bacilli to develop a vaccine. By the mid1880s, Pasteur had also developed a vaccine for rabies, and in 1885 was asked to use it on a 9-year-old boy who had been attacked by a rabid dog. Pasteur injected the boy with the vaccine 13 times and the boy did not contract rabies. These early experiments laid the groundwork for future research in the field. The 1900s saw a huge increase in the amount of work being conducted on vaccination, and by the 1940s, there were vaccines available for typhoid, diphtheria, tetanus, yellow fever, and influenza (Fig. 9.12).

One of the diseases of concern and targeted for eradication was poliomyelitis, an acute paralytic disease caused by poliovirus, an enterovirus of the Picornaviridae family. One of the effects of infection with this virus is damage to the lower motor neurons, leading to asymmetric weakness and paralysis. During the U.S. epidemic of 1916, polio paralyzed roughly 27,000 people and caused 6000 deaths. Early attempts at developing a vaccine used virus particles that were taken from infected monkey spinal cords. On March 26, 1953, a researcher named

Dr. Jonas Salk announced the development of a successful vaccine for polio, which he had been researching since 1948 at the University of Pittsburgh where he was awarded a grant to study the polio virus. The findings were published in the *Journal of the American Medical Association*. Salk's injected vaccine consisted of several killed strains of the poliovirus and in 1953, he injected himself, his wife, and their three children with the experimental vaccine to demonstrate its efficacy. Subsequently, clinical trials were conducted in 1954 on almost two million American schoolchildren (one million children were used as a control population and 600,000 children injected with the vaccine). In 1955, at the end of these studies, the vaccine was deemed to be safe and effective. As a result of usage of the new vaccine, new polio cases dropped drastically and Salk was awarded several honors including the Presidential Medal of Freedom from President Jimmy Carter. In 1963 the Salk Institute for Biological Studies was opened in La Jolla, California. In the mid-1980s Salk also co-founded the Immune Response Corporation in search of an HIV vaccine. In 1961, an oral polio vaccine which was developed by Dr. Albert Sabin became commercially available and eventually phased out Salk's injected vaccine due to its superior efficacy. Due to widespread vaccination, cases of polio plummeted even further. Since there were concerns related to reversion with respect to the Sabin vaccine, and because polio was no longer endemic in the U.S., the injectable polio vaccine (IPV) was phased back in to the childhood vaccination schedule in 1997. Thanks to a consistent vaccination program, only a handful of polio cases now exist in the U.S. each year. While goals were set in 1988 by the World Health Assembly to eradicate polio worldwide by the year 2000, polio worldwide has resisted eradication, partly because of inconsistent vaccination practices in war-torn areas and in part due to the fact that polio does not always present symptoms that are easily recognizable. Thus, infected individuals may spread the disease without knowing it. Still, due to vaccination, polio was declared eliminated from the Americas in 1994 and 2002 in Europe. The rare cases that do occur yearly are brought to those continents from overseas travel. As of 2017, polio is only known to be endemic in Afghanistan, Nigeria, and Pakistan. Other African countries, as well as Ukraine, are still at risk for polio.

By the 1980s vaccines for many other diseases became available. These included the measles, rubella, pneumococcal, Hib, Hepatitis B, and typhoid vaccines. However, in the late 1980s and early 1990s, there was resurgence of measles epidemic due to lower vaccination rates. Because incidences of measles were relatively low and thus infections were considered to be under control this resulted in a lapsed sense of urgency for the vaccine and immunizations decreased. However, in the absence of effective vaccination, lower levels of disease in certain under-immunized populations served as reservoirs for the virus and measles was able to spread to more than 55,000 cases, resulting in over 120 deaths between the years 1989 and 1991. Since then, the U.S. has seen several other measles outbreaks in the last 5 years. Many of these outbreaks seem to stem from travelers acquiring the virus from overseas and infecting large numbers of unvaccinated individuals.

It can be said without a doubt that vaccination has not only protected millions of people throughout the world from developing deadly infectious diseases, but has also alleviated pain and suffering from disease in many parts of the world, and played a direct role in lifting people from poverty and allowing them to have a better quality of life. In the last century, successful vaccination campaigns have allowed the elimination or provided protection from many infectious diseases that were once feared by humans, and has significantly increased the average lifespan of humans throughout the world. While many vaccines exist today, there are still many diseases, such as AIDS, for which no vaccine is available. One reason for this failure thus far has been the ability of pathogens causing these diseases to either evade the immune system or destroy it. However, with novel discoveries in the fields of immunology, genetics, molecular biology, biochemistry, and nanotechnology, it is hoped that vaccines for these and other diseases can soon be developed. Newer technology under development including recombinant techniques will hopefully lead to more antigenically accurate vaccines which can yield better vaccine efficacy, bringing much relief to people suffering from these diseases.

Emerging Science

The Future of Influenza Vaccination

While vaccination programs have been successful in eradicating smallpox and eliminating polio in some countries, there are still several challenges with vaccination that future development techniques may be able to mitigate. Many of the vaccines used today still use either live attenuated microbes, killed microbes, or subunits that are unable to cause illness. Several factors including the immunogenicity of the antigen as well as microbial mutation may render some vaccines less effective. Newer techniques being developed include recombinant vaccines and DNA vaccines. While DNA vaccines encoding HA or NA influenza proteins have shown good results in animal models, the results have not been as promising in clinical trials. Live recombinant vaccines use either a virus or bacterial strain as a vector to deliver the antigen. Some of these types of vaccines, including FluBlok® and the Hepatitis B vaccine Recombivax-Hb® are already on the market and in circulation.

A major area of research continues to be the improvement of available flu vaccines and their ability to target many influenza strains. One particular idea is to develop a universal vaccine for influenza that may be able to replace yearly flu vaccine injections. Currently, the vaccine strains used each year are updated annually to reflect the flu strains predicted to be common in that upcoming year. These predictions, due to antigenic shift, particularly in HA, the emergence of novel surface proteins, and patterns of disease spread around the world are not often exact, rendering the vaccine only somewhat effective. Research on a universal flu vaccine has utilized double-layered nanoparticles targeting hemagglutinin to prevent viral entry of influenza into host cells. Other labs have developed artificial peptides that are able to neutralize influenza A viruses. Possible influenza targets that could serve as common epitopes for a universal vaccine include highly conserved epitopes such as the matrix M1 protein, M2 proton channel in the viral envelope, nucleoprotein (NP), and the HA2 stalk domain of hemagglutinin.

M2 plays a role in viral entry and was targeted by the influenza antivirals amantadine and rimantadine, which are no longer recommended by the CDC due to resistance. The highly conserved amino acid sequence of M2 is M2e, the extracellular domain. All influenza A virus isolates have been found to contain the N amino-terminal epitope of M2e, and in mice antibodies against M2e protect against influenza A. Due to its poor immunogenicity, M2e requires a carrier protein. Still, candidate conjugate vaccines of M2e did not produce effective antibodies. Novel approaches to using M2e include a recombinant conjugate vaccine which did elicit a good response in vaccinated mice, or a VLP vaccine of M2e. VLPs are multi-protein molecules that mimic the structure, organization, and conformation of a native virus, without containing the genetic material. Thus vaccines containing VLP are unable to replicate. Some of these recombinant vaccines based on M2e, including flagellin-adjuvanted M2 vaccines have been analyzed in clinical trials on humans. While many of them are safe and tolerable, the flagellin-adjuvanted vaccines were associated with more adverse effects. Wild-type M2 VLP vaccine used in conjunction with the inactivated influenza A vaccine improved cross-protection in mice and may be a strategy to improve the effectiveness of current vaccines.

Currently influenza vaccines utilize HA1, which is the global head domain, as the antigenic target. However, frequent mutations in this domain result in a lower efficacy of the antibodies produced from these vaccines. HA2, however, is the membrane-fusion stalk domain necessary for influenza virus entry, and appears to be more conserved among influenza A strains (sequence homology 51–80%). Many studies have been done with various combinations of HA subgroups to determine which elicits cross-reactive neutralizing antibodies.

While a live vaccine has been on the market and used, researchers are still exploring the use of a novel live vaccine based on the non-structural influenza protein NS1. NS1 is necessary for influenza viral replication as well as the inhibition of innate immune response of the host. Early clinical studies are showing that an intranasal NS1 vaccine is well tolerated and able to generate antibodies against influenza HA.

The optimal influenza vaccine must be safe, effective, elicit both cellular and humoral responses, and provide cross-strain protection, particularly against all subtypes of influenza A and B viruses. Ultimately, more studies need to be done to better understand how cross-protection mechanisms work and which adjuvants can enhance the immunogenicity of chosen antigens. In addition to the possible supplementation of existing vaccines with VLPs, future vaccines may also utilize new routes of administration, including needle-free topical skin routes, oral, sublingual, or intranasal. Recently, a microneedle flu vaccine skin patch was developed that may change how the flu vaccine is administered. The patch consists of 100 water-soluble microneedles that just penetrate into the skin and dissolve within minutes. Data showed that the antibody response elicited by the skin patch was comparable to those created by the intramuscular (IM) vaccine. This route of administration has many economic and manufacturing advantages which would reduce costs and improve usage due to the possibility that it could be self-administered and simply peeled off like a bandage. Further clinical trials will be conducted to determine the utility of the influenza vaccine skin patch as well as to investigate the possibility of using this technology with other vaccines including polio, measles, and rubella.

Summary

Active immunization relies on the principle of the adaptive immune response to create memory lymphocytes against weakened or inactivated pathogens that will allow the immune system to "see" potential pathogens as a non-harmful first exposure in order to determine how to react upon subsequent exposure(s). This exposure will allow a primary immune response to occur. Ideally, the effectiveness of the secondary response which has been built from immunization should allow clearance of the infection before symptoms develop. While earlier vaccines have used either live or killed whole microbes, newer vaccine methods are turning to recombinant DNA technology to create antigens that will stimulate an immune response. The development of vaccination in the eighteenth century followed by advances in microbiology and immunology in the next two centuries have significantly increased our ability to combat infectious diseases throughout the world. The eradication of the once feared disease smallpox in 1980 was a major medical breakthrough and may truly be considered one of the triumphs of immunology. In the last century, the discovery of many of the molecules and cells of the immune system along with discoveries of microbial structure and pathogenesis, and the DNA revolution, has further enhanced our understanding of the mechanisms by which the immune system destroys pathogens, and has enabled us to develop many drugs and other treatments for infectious diseases. Much still remains to be known, and many infectious diseases, are constantly emerging and reemerging, ensuring that our battle with infectious diseases will continue for a long time. However, as daunting as it may be, the hope is that with the scientific knowledge gained in the last few hundred years, we may be able to better prepare ourselves in the event of future epidemics or pandemics.

Practice Questions

1. Which of the following is a live, attenuated vaccine?
   - (a) Hepatitis A vaccine
   - (b) Hepatitis B vaccine
   - (c) Varicella zoster vaccine
   - (d) Meningitis vaccine

2. What is a recombinant vaccine? What does this mean? (Short answer)

3. What vaccine may contain traces of yeast, from the manufacturing process?
   - (a) Zostavax®
   - (b) Fluad
   - (c) Pneumovax®
   - (d) Recombivax-B®

4. Explain two possible mechanisms of adjuvants. (Short answer)

5. Antibiotics such as streptomycin may be found in vaccines. What is their role?
   - (a) adjuvant
   - (b) preservative
   - (c) antigen

6. Which of the following is the new recombinant vaccine for herpes zoster?
   - (a) Varivax®
   - (b) Zostavax®
   - (c) Shingrix®
   - (d) Recombivax®

7. Which flu vaccine is grown in a canine kidney cell line?
   - (a) Flucelvax®
   - (b) Fluzone®
   - (c) Afluria®
   - (d) FluBlok®

8. Which of the following would classify a patient as having AIDS?
   - (a) CD4 T cell count of 800 cells/mm^3
   - (b) CD4 T cells count <200 cells/mm^3
   - (c) Viral load of 1000 RNA copies/mL
   - (d) Viral load of 100 RNA copies/mL

9. Which of the following influenza proteins is a current target for antiviral therapies? (Select all that apply)
   - (a) Hemagglutinin
   - (b) Neuraminidase
   - (c) Reverse transcriptase
   - (d) M2 uncoating proteins
   - (e) Endonuclease

Suggested Reading

Angus DC, Linde-Zwirble WT, Lidicker J, Clermont G, Carcillo J, Pinsky MR. Epidemiology of severe sepsis in the United States: analysis of incidence, outcome, and associated costs of care. Crit Care Med. 2001;29:1303–10.

Awate S, Babiuk LA, Mutwiri G. Mechanisms of action of adjuvants. Front Immunol. 2013;4:114.

Blackwell TS, Christmas JW. Sepsis and cytokines: current status. Br J Anaesth. 1996;77:110–7.

Chaudhry H, Zhou J, Zhong Y, Ali MM, McGuire F, Nagarkatti PS, Nagarkatti M. Role of cytokines as a double-edged sword in sepsis. In Vivo. 2013;27(6):669–84.

Cooper AM. Cell mediated immune responses in tuberculosis. Annu Rev Immunol. 2009;27:393–422.

Cox MM, Hollister JR. FluBlok, a next generation influenza vaccine manufactured in insect cells. Biologicals. 2009;37(3):182–9.

Croxford S, Kitching A, Desai S, Kall M, Edelstein M, Skingsley A, et al. Mortality and causes of death in people diagnosed with HIV in the era of highly active antiretroviral therapy compared with the general population: an analysis of a national observational cohort. Lancet Public Health. 2017;2(1):e35–46.

DiazGranadose CA, Dunning AJ, Kimmel M, Kirby D, Treanor J, Collins A, et al. Efficacy of high-dose versus standard-dose influenza vaccine in older adults. N Engl J Med. 2014;371:635–45.

Eshelman E, Shahzad A, Cohrs RJ. Varicella zoster latency. Future Virol. 2001;6(3):341–55.

Gaieski DF, Edwards JM, Kallan MJ, et al. Benchmarking the incidence and mortality of severe sepsis in the United States. Crit Care Med. 2013;41:1167–74.

Gardlund B. Activated protein C (Xigris) treatment in sepsis: a drug in trouble. Acta Anaesthesiol Scand. 2006;50(8):907–10.

Grimaldi D, Turcott EWG, Taccone FS. IL-1 receptor antagonist in sepsis: new findings with old data? J Thorac Dis. 2016;8(9):2379–82.

Gul F, Arslantas MK, Cinel I, Kumar A. Changing definitions of sepsis. Turk J Anaesthesiol Reanim. 2017;45(3):129–38.

Inoue T, Tanaka Y. Hepatitis B virus and its sexually transmitted infection- an update. Microb Cell. 2016;3(9):420–37.

Iwasaki A, Pillai PS. Innate immunity to influenza virus infection. Nat Rev Immunol. 2014;14(5):315–28.

King EG, Bauzá GJ, Mella JR, Remick DG. Pathophysiologic mechanisms in septic shock. Lab Invest. 2014;94(1):4–12.

Korb VC, Chuturgoon AA, Moodley D. Mycobacterium tuberculosis:manipulator of protective immunity. Int J Mol Sci. 2016;17(3):131.

Kraft R, Herndon DN, Finnerty CC, Cox RA, Song J, Jeschke MG. Predictive value of IL-8 for sepsis and severe infections after burn injury—a clinical study. Shock. 2015;43(3):222–7.

Lambert LC, Fauci AS. Influenza vaccines for the future. N Engl J Med. 2010;363:2036–44.

Lee YT, Kim KH, Ko EJ, Lee YN, Kim MC, Kwon YM, et al. New vaccines against influenza virus. Clin Exp Vaccine Res. 2014;3(1):12–28.

Lepak A, Andes D. Fungal sepsis: optimizing antifungal therapy in the critical care setting. Crit Care Clin. 2011;27(1):123–47.

Low DE. Toxic shock syndrome: major advances in pathogenesis, but not treatment. Crit Care Clin. 2013;29(3):651–75.

Martin GS, Mannino DM, Eaton S, Moss M. The epidemiology of sepsis in the United States from 1979 through 2000. N Engl J Med. 2003;348(16):1546–54.

Modlin RL. The innate immune response in leprosy. Curr Opin Immunol. 2010;22(1):48–54.

Nascimento IP, Leite LCC. Recombinant vaccines and the development of new vaccine strategies. Braz J Med Biol Res. 2012;45(12):1102–11.

Nyamweya S, Hegedus A, Jaye A, Rowland-Jones S, Flanagan KL, Macallan DC. Comparing HIV-1 and HIV-2 infection: lessons for viral immunopathogenesis. Rev Med Virol. 2013;23(4):221–40.

Plotkin S, Gerber JS, Offit PA. Vaccines and autism: a tale of shifting hypotheses. Clin Infect Dis. 2009;48(4):456–61.

Pulendran B, Ahmed R. Immunological mechanisms of vaccination. Nat Immunol. 2011;12(6):509–17.

Rao TS, Andrade C. The MMR vaccine and autism: sensation, refutation, retraction, and fraud. Indian J Psychiatry. 2011;53(2):95.

Remick DG. Pathophysiology of Sepsis. Am J Pathol. 2007;170(5):1435–44.

Remick DG, Bolgos GR, Siddiqui J, Shin J, Nemzek JA. Six at six: interleukin-6 measured 6h after the initiation of sepsis predicts mortality over 3 days. Shock. 2002;17(6):463–7.

Rhodes A, Evans LE, Alhazzani W, Levy MM, Antonelli M, Ferrer R, et al. Surviving sepsis campaign: international guidelines for management of sepsis and septic shock: 2016. Intensive Care Med. 2017a;43(3):304–77.

Rhodes A, Evans L, Alhazzani W, et al. Surviving sepsis campaign. Crit Care Med. 2017b;45(3):486–552.658.

Rouphael NG, Paine M, Mosley R, Henry S, McAllister DV, Kalluri H, et al. The safety, immunogenicity, and acceptability of inactivated influenza vaccine delivered by microneedle path (TIV-MNP 2015): a randomised, partly blinded, placebo-controlled phase I trial. Lancet. 2017;390(10095):649–58.

Singer M, Deutschman CS, Seymour CW, Shankar-Hari M, Annane D, Bauer M, et al. The third international consensus definitions for sepsis and septic shock (Sepsis-3). J Am Med Assoc. 2016;315(8):801–10.

Smith KA. Louis Pasteur, the father of immunology? Front Immunol. 2012;3(68):1–10.

Srisangthong P, Wongsa A, Kittiworawitkul P, Wattanathum A. Early IL-6 response is correlated with mortality and severity score. Crit Care. 2013;17(Suppl 2):P34.

Stach CS, Herrera A, Schlievert PM. Staphylococcal superantigens interact with multiple host receptors to cause serious diseases. Immunol Res. 2014;59(1–3):177–81.

Suarez De La Rica A, Gilsanz F, Maseda E. Epidemiologic trends of sepsis in western countries. Ann Transl Med. 2016;4(17):325.

Wesche-Soldato DE, Lomas-Neira JL, Perl M, Jones L, Chung CS, Ayala A. The role and regulation of apoptosis in sepsis. J Endotoxin Res. 2005;11(6):375–82.

Wesche-Soldato DE, Swan RZ, Chung CS, Ayala A. The apoptotic pathway as a therapeutic target in sepsis. Curr Drug Targets. 2007a;8(4):493–500.

Wesche-Soldato DE, Chung CS, Gregory SH, Salazar-Mather TP, Ayala CA, Ayala A. CD8+ T cells promote inflammation and apoptosis in the liver after sepsis: role of Fas-FasL. Am J Pathol. 2007b;171(1):87–96.

Wilcox MH, Gerding DN, Poxton IR, Kelly C, Nathan R, Birch T, Cornely OA, et al. Bezlotoxumab for prevention of recurrent Clostridium difficile infection. N Engl J Med. 2017;376:305–17.

Cancer Immunotherapy

10

Doreen E. Szollosi, Shannon R. M. Kinney,
A. R. M. Ruhul Amin, and Ngumbah Chumbow

Learning Objectives

1. Identify common features that distinguish cancer cells from normal cells.
2. Identify the pathological stages of cancer from benign/precancerous *in situ*, to invasive vascularized cancer, and finally metastatic disease.
3. Identify the role of MHC class I in the killing of tumor cells by cytotoxic T-cells.
4. Identify tumor-associated antigens, tumor-specific antigens, and the mechanisms by which successful tumors evade the immune system.
5. Discuss the pharmacology of cancer immunotherapies including their mechanism of action, functional responses, clinical uses, and adverse effects.

Drugs discussed in this chapter

Drug	Classification
Aldesleukin (Proleukin®)	Recombinant human IL-2
Atezolizumab (Tecentriq®)	Anti-PD-L1 monoclonal antibody
Avelumab (Bavencio®)	Anti-PD-L1 monoclonal antibody
Axicabtagene ciloleucel (Yescarta®)	CAR-T cell therapy
Bevacizumab (Avastin®)	Anti-VEGF-A monoclonal antibody
Blinatumomab (Blincyto®)	Anti-CD19/CD3 monoclonal antibody, bi-specific T-cell engager (BiTE)
Brentuximab vedotin (Adcetris®)	Anti-CD30 monoclonal antibody conjugated to an antineoplastic agent, Monomethyl auristatin E (MMAE)
Cetuximab (Erbitux®)	Anti-EGFR monoclonal antibody
Daratumumab (Darzalex®)	Anti-CD38 monoclonal antibody
Darbepoetin (Aranesp®)	Erythropoietin
Denosumab (Xgeva®, Prolia®)	Anti-RANKL monoclonal antibody
Durvalumab (Imfinzi®)	Anti-PD-L1 monoclonal antibody
Elotuzumab (Empliciti™)	SLAMF7-directed immunostimulatory antibody
Eltrombopag (Promacta®)	Thrombopoietin receptor agonist
Epoetin (Epogen®, Procrit®)	Erythropoietin
Filgrastim (Neupogen®)	G-CSF

D. E. Szollosi (✉)
Department of Pharmaceutical Sciences,
School of Pharmacy and Physician Assistant Studies,
University of Saint Joseph, Hartford, CT, USA
e-mail: dszollosi@usj.edu

N. Chumbow
School of Pharmacy and Physician Assistant Studies,
University of Saint Joseph, Hartford, CT, USA

S. R. M. Kinney
College of Pharmacy and Health Sciences, Western
New England University, Springfield, MA, USA

A. R. M. Ruhul Amin
Marshall University School of Pharmacy, Huntington,
WV, USA

© Springer Nature Switzerland AG 2020
C. B. Mathias et al., *Pharmacology of Immunotherapeutic Drugs*,
https://doi.org/10.1007/978-3-030-19922-7_10

Drug	Classification
Ibritumomab tiuxetan (Zevalin®)	Anti-CD20 Radioimmunotherapy
Imiquimod (Aldara®, Zyclara®)	TLR7 agonist
Interferon alfa-2b (Intron A®)	Interferon
Ipilimumab (Yervoy®)	Anti-CTLA4 monoclonal antibody
Lenalidomide (Revlimid®)	IMiD
Methoxy polyethylene glycol-epoetin beta (Mircera®)	Erythropoietin
Moxetumomab pasudotox (Lumoxiti®)	Anti-CD22 monoclonal antibody
Necitumumab (Portrazza®)	Anti-EGFR monoclonal antibody
Nivolumab (Opdivo®)	Anti-PD1 monoclonal antibody
Obinutuzumab (Gazyva®)	Anti-CD20 monoclonal antibody
Ofatumumab (Arzerra®)	Anti-CD20 monoclonal antibody
Oprelvekin (Neumega®)	Recombinant IL-11
Panitumumab (Vectibix®)	Anti-EGFR monoclonal antibody
Pegfilgrastim (Neulasta®)	Pegylated G-CSF
Peginterferon alfa-2b (Sylatron®)	Pegylated interferon
Pembrolizumab (Keytruda®)	Anti-PD1 monoclonal antibody
Pertuzumab (Perjeta®)	Anti-HER2 monoclonal antibody
Pomalidomide (Pomalyst®)	IMiD
Ramucirumab (Cyramza®)	Anti-VEGFR2 monoclonal antibody
Rituximab (Rituxan®)	Anti-CD20 monoclonal antibody
Romiplostim (Nplate®)	Thrombopoietin analog
Sargramostim (Leukine®)	GM-CSF
Sipuleucel-T (Provenge®)	Dendritic cell-based prostate cancer vaccine
Talimogene laherparepvec (Imlygic®)	Modified HSV1 therapy
Thalidomide (Thalomid®)	IMiD
Tisagenlecleucel (Kymriah™)	CAR-T cell therapy
Trastuzumab (Herceptin®)	Anti-HER2 monoclonal antibody

Introduction

Cancer is a class of diseases characterized by uncontrolled cell growth. There are at least 100 different types of cancer arising at different sites in the body. These diverse types of cancer together lead to approximately a quarter of all deaths in the United States, making cancer second to only cardiovascular disease as a cause of death. Cancer development is a multifactorial and multistep process, involving a complex interplay between the environment (broadly defined) and inherited, as well as *de novo*, genetic mutations. As a result of these processes, cancer cells take on abnormal features that may resemble virus-infected cells. It is well known that the immune system can identify, control, and eliminate cancer cells the same way it would a virus-infected cell via recognition of MHC I. This mechanism provides an explanation for anecdotal cases where patients' tumors have spontaneously regressed without treatment. However, some cancer cells can avoid immune system recognition and removal, which is one of several crucial steps in the development of progressive disease. As a result of this multistep process, cancer cells acquire various characteristics that set them apart from normal cells. These characteristics were described in two seminal papers authored by Douglas Hanahan and Robert Weinberg entitled The hallmarks of cancer and Hallmarks of cancer: the next generation, in 2000 and 2011, respectively.

Pathophysiology of Cancer

Hallmarks of Cancer

Tumor cells can be derived from various normal cells in the body, such as epithelial cells, connective tissue cells, and hematopoietic cells, resulting in what are referred to as **carcinomas**, **sarcomas**, and **myelomas**, **leukemias**, and **lymphomas**, respectively. These cells must acquire the hallmark characteristics described in the Hanahan and Weinberg articles mentioned above, including:

1. Self-sufficiency in growth signals
2. Insensitivity to anti-growth signals
3. Evading apoptosis
4. Tissue invasion and metastasis
5. Limitless replicative potential

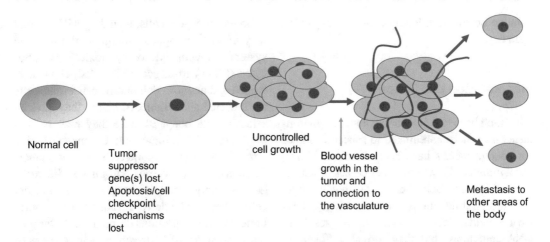

Fig. 10.1 The steps leading to carcinogenesis often begin with loss of tumor suppressor ability in the cell cycle due to genetic mutations. Thus, cellular damage which would normally lead to apoptosis during the cell cycle are essentially ignored, allowing cells with mutations to continue replicating. Because of this, cells may acquire limitless replicative potential and other oncogenic characteristics. Once a developing tumor has outgrown its normal blood supply, it may promote growth of new blood vessels, which allow the tumor to continue growing. Cancer cells lose their normal cellular structure, taking on a migratory phenotype and reducing connections with neighboring cells, increasing their ability to invade nearby normal tissues and metastasize through the lymphatic and vascular systems to distant locations in the body

6. Sustained angiogenesis
7. Deregulating cellular energetics
8. Tumor promoting inflammation
9. Avoiding immune destruction
10. Genome instability and mutation

As cancer cells within a tumor undergo these changes, they can invade beyond the basement membrane or normal boundaries of the organ or tissue in which they originate, differentiating cancerous tumors from benign disease (Fig. 10.1). Tumors that continue to grow have an increased requirement for oxygen and nutrients, as well as increased production of waste. Larger tumors begin to produce pro-angiogenic factors that stimulate growth of blood vessels to supply the tumor with what it requires. These new vessels, as well as lymphatic vessels, often serve as a conduit for tumor cells, that have detached from the primary tumor and taken on phenotypes that allow for migration, to spread to other locations in the body. This process of metastasis is complex, and many cancer cells will not survive the many steps involved. Those that do often colonize crucial organs, such as the brain, liver, and lungs, resulting in the death of the patient.

The hallmarks of cancer are acquired through a stepwise process that often begins with a sporadic mutation in a gene, such as a tumor suppressor gene or proto-oncogene that is involved in cellular growth, apoptosis, DNA damage repair, or another relevant pathway. As a result, tumor cell DNA becomes unstable and mutations occur at a much higher rate than normal. This allows for heterogeneity within the tumor and development of resistance mechanisms to therapies, including increased efflux of drugs from cancer cells, increased inactivation of drugs via metabolism, and altered structure and levels of drug targets. Resistance is a major concern when treating cancer patients as many will either not be sensitive to certain drugs to begin with or develop refractory disease after being treated with a particular agent. While mutations are often selected for within the tumor that allow for cancer development and progression, the one benefit is that the resulting products may also provide therapeutic targets that can be taken advantage of to treat the disease.

There are two hallmarks of cancer that directly relate to the immune system (1) tumor promoting inflammation and (2) avoiding immune destruction. Each of these is expanded upon here.

Inflammation and Cancer

It has long been understood that both the environment and genetics are linked to cancer. Some of the genetic factors have been described above, and a number of environmental causes of cancer are well known, such as cigarette smoking, obesity, and viral infections. Not surprisingly, these environmental factors often directly result in DNA mutations, but they are also linked to chronic inflammation. Chronic inflammation can cause DNA damage through production of reactive oxygen species and this serves as part of the mechanism whereby inflammation promotes tumors.

In addition to this and other possible mechanisms, the balance of various innate and adaptive immune cells, as well as the cytokines and chemokines they produce may change such that the tumor microenvironment can switch from tumor-preventing (IL-12, TRAIL, IFN-γ) to tumor-promoting (IL-6, IL-17, IL-23). Inflammatory cells can also produce proteases and angiogenic factors that would be beneficial for the tumor as it grows and becomes invasive. It remains unclear why only some inflammatory syndromes, such as irritable bowel disease, are tumor promoting and others are not.

Cancer Immunosurveillance

The role of the immune system is important in the constant monitoring for and removal of abnormal cells in the body. This is evident among patients who are on immunosuppressive therapies, have immunosuppressive diseases (HIV), or who have genetic immunodeficiencies, all of who are at an increased risk of developing cancer. Normally, immune cells including NK cells and T cells "survey" the body for cancer; killing those cells before they cause clinically relevant disease. Oftentimes, malignant transformation alters protein expression or

structure in cancer cells, including MHC I, that may make them appear foreign to the immune system, allowing NK or cytotoxic T lymphocytes (CTLs) to target these cells. Thus, it is believed that most potentially cancerous cells are detected and eliminated before they have an effect on the body. Because they may be displayed on MHC I, tumor antigens may also play a role in whether immune cells can (or cannot) detect a cell as cancerous. **Tumor-specific antigens** are only found on tumor cells, not normal cells. They can be derived from oncogenic viral proteins, altered portions of mutant cellular proteins, such as p53, or amino-acid sequences spanning tumor-specific recombination sites between genes, such as Bcr/Abl. They can be presented on MHC I or II to CD8 and CD4 T cells. **Tumor-associated antigens** are expressed in tumor cells in greater amounts than on their normal counterparts or may only normally be expressed in certain cells at particular stages of development. The expression of these genes is often regulated through epigenetic mechanisms. For example, the type I members of the melanoma antigen gene (MAGE) family are normally only expressed in testis or placenta but are transcriptionally silenced via DNA methylation in other normal adult tissues. In cancer cells, these genes' promoters can become demethylated and activated resulting in antigen production.

Successful Tumors Evade the Immune Response

It is important to understand how cancer cells circumvent immune attack. Because the mechanisms seem to be quite complex, much is still being elucidated to determine how various cancers accomplish this. As more mutations are acquired during the development of a cancer, there is more selective pressure for cells that successfully evade immune system surveillance. These cells may display a reduced expression of tumor antigens or mutant epitopes, which will allow the cell to not be as easily recognized by the immune system. Additionally, cancer cells

Tumor oncogenes and antigens

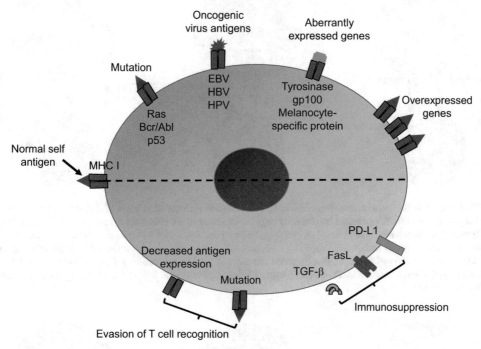

Fig. 10.2 Tumor-associated antigens, tumor-specific antigens, and tumor immune escape. Tumor-associated antigens are normal self-antigens that can be overexpressed on tumor cells. Tumor-specific antigens are abnormal antigens that are expressed on tumor cells due to mutations that cause novel protein sequences or expression of proteins derived from oncogenic viruses. Tumor cells can avoid the immune response in various ways, including decreased MHC I/antigen expression, as well as expression of immunosuppressive molecules that are anti-inflammatory or suppress activation of T cells that are involved in tumor cell killing (figure contributed by Jeremy P. McAleer)

may stop expressing MHC class I molecules that would be recognized by T cells, or even secrete anti-inflammatory cytokines such as TGF-β (Fig. 10.2).

Early on in carcinogenesis, tumor cells are often vulnerable to the anti-tumor immune response, mediated for the most part by tumor infiltrating cells—CD8 T cells and NK cells (Figs. 10.3 and 10.4), which recognize them as abnormal and kill them, thus impeding their growth. However, an altered tumor microenvironment can allow for genetic changes and malignant cells that acquire the ability to avoid being killed by tumor-infiltrating cells. MHC I on the surface of self cells displays the cell's internal proteins and signals to T cells that it is normal. Abnormal MHC I display can signal

that a cell is either infected with an internal pathogen or its normal cellular mechanisms have been altered genetically. CD8 T cells recognize foreign and abnormal antigen display on MHC I. In many cases, however, tumors downregulate their MHC I expression to avoid CTL killing. NK cells can still kill tumor cells that lack MHC I, considering that they do not have antigen-specific cell surface receptors and do not require any prior antigen exposure. In normal instances, MHC class I is recognized by inhibitory receptors on NK cells which prevents them from becoming activated. Cells that have downregulated or have stopped expressing MHC I recognized by inhibitory receptors results in the activation of NK cells. This activation includes the release of cytotoxic granules or

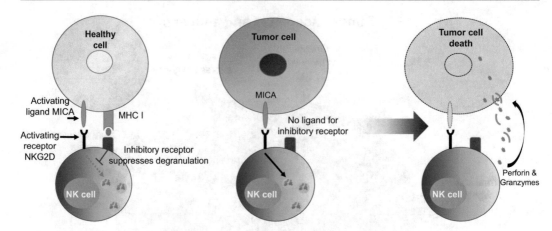

Fig. 10.3 Tumor immunosurveillance and killing by NK cells involves the integration of signals from activating and inhibitory receptors. MICA expressed on potential target cells serves as an activating ligand for NKG2D on NK cells. This interaction can potentially stimulate NK cell degranulation and death of the target cell. MHC class I expressed on healthy cells interacts with an NK cell inhibitory receptor (red), suppressing the activation of NKG2D and degranulation. The downregulation of MHC class I by some tumors will prevent this inhibitory signal from being delivered, resulting in activation of the NKG2D signaling pathway, degranulation, and tumor cell death (figure contributed by Jeremy P. McAleer)

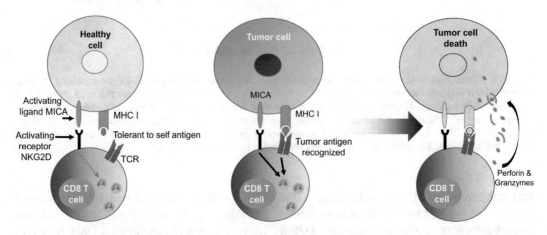

Fig. 10.4 Tumor immunosurveillance and killing by CD8 T cells involves the integration of multiple signals. MICA expressed on potential target cells serves as an activating ligand for NKG2D on CD8 T cells. This interaction is not sufficient to stimulate CD8 T cell degranulation and death of the target cell. On healthy cells, tumor peptide/MHC I complexes are generally not recognized by TCRs due to self-tolerance. Tumor-associated or tumor-specific antigens can be targeted by effector CD8 T cells. In this case, signaling through the TCR synergizes with NKG2D activation, leading to CD8 T cell degranulation and tumor cell death (figure contributed by Jeremy P. McAleer)

induction of cell death of the target cell. Certain MHC class I chain related molecules including MICA, MICB and UL-16 binding proteins are also recognized by activating receptors on NK and CD8 T cells, leading to killing of abnormal cells (Figs. 10.3 and 10.4). Tumor cells that successfully evade the effects of these cytotoxic cells may also down-regulate expression of MHC class I chain related molecules such as MIC or cleave them off all together to avoid ligation of activating receptors that could result in their death.

As discussed in Chap. 3, cancer cells can also side step T cell cytolysis by expressing a molecule known as PD-L1. PD-1 and PD-L1 and their mechanism are described in further detail below.

This mechanism has been exploited as a target for allowing for T cells to be activated to kill tumor cells. The drugs that target this mechanism are known as the checkpoint inhibitors.

Macrophages are also integral in destroying and phagocytosing aberrant cells. Some cancer cells, aggressive forms in particular, express a protein that can signify to macrophages that they should not be consumed (i.e. a "don't eat me" signal). This protein signal is CD47 which binds to a protein known as SIRPalpha on the surface of macrophages. The ligation of these two proteins sends an inhibitory signal that decreases their ability to consume cancer cells. Animals treated with anti-CD47 antibodies show normal macrophage phagocytosis and clearance of cancer cells due to inhibition of CD47 and SIRPalpha binding. On the other hand, macrophages can be recruited to the tumor and become polarized to promote tumor growth and angiogenesis. These are referred to as **tumor-associated macrophages (TAMs).** Tumors that reveal infiltration of TAMs are often associated with poor prognosis. These macrophages derive from peripheral blood monocytes and are recruited to the tumor by chemokines. Depending on signals within the tumor microenvironment, they may be polarized to promote blood vessel growth within the tumor as well as suppress adaptive immune responses which allow for tumor metastasis.

In addition to immune ligands such as PD-L1 and CD47, tumor cells are capable of expressing various antigens that promote their avoidance of immune recognition and clearance. Some of these molecules are summarized in Table 10.1.

Immunosuppressive Effects of Cytotoxic Chemotherapy

Prior to the middle of the twentieth century, the main treatments for cancer were surgery and radiation therapy. It eventually became evident that these treatment modalities were only effective in a small percentage of cancer cases due to the presence of metastases with more advanced disease. In the early 1900s scientists began developing murine models to test chemical agents for their activity against cancer. The first cytotoxic chemo-

Table 10.1 Examples of molecules that are associated with tumor cell immune response evasion

Molecule expressed	Role in immune evasion
PD-L1	Binds to PD-1, inhibiting activation of T cells
CD47	Inhibits phagocytosis by macrophages
CD73	Aids in generation of adenosine which may inhibit anti-tumor actions of NK cells, macrophages, and T cells
CD14	May recruit monocytes and macrophages that are polarized to become immunosuppressive
CD68	Expressed on tumor-associated macrophages (TAMs) which appear to aid in promoting tumor growth and angiogenesis
MAC387	Expressed on TAMs
CD163	A scavenger receptor on M2 macrophages, particularly TAMs
DAP12	Reduced levels in NK cells surrounding the tumor have a reduced ability to kill tumor cells

therapy agents to be studied became of interest after an accidental spill of sulfur mustards used in World War II caused marked suppression of bone marrow and lymph nodes in the men who were exposed. This eventually led to the introduction of these chemicals to Alfred Gilman and Louis Goodman and the discovery that nitrogen mustards were very effective in treating non-Hodgkin's lymphoma in the 1940s. This caused a flurry of research that lead to the development of several anticancer agents, including methotrexate and the anticancer antibiotic actinomycin D. Nitrogen mustards, methotrexate, and antitumor antibiotics are all used to this day to treat lymphomas and leukemias because of their DNA damaging and antimetabolite activities, which are especially effective against the fast-growing cells of these cancers. In addition to the drugs already mentioned, several other cytotoxic chemotherapies have been developed since the middle of the twentieth century. These agents can be effective against both hematopoietic and solid tumors and are still commonly used despite major efforts towards the creation of molecular targeted therapies. The mechanism of action of these traditional drugs acts as a double-edged sword however, as in addition to a number of other toxicities, their use severely represses normal hematopoiesis, allowing for the development of deadly infections. Therefore, it is crucial to monitor the white cell counts of any patient that is administered cytotoxic chemotherapeutic agents.

Immune Cell Cancers

There are several terms used for various immune cell cancers. There are many different cancers of the immune system, and it is important to know that immune cells at various stages of development can become cancerous.

Leukemia is a broad term describing cancer of circulating cells, particularly white blood cells, but can also affect red blood cells, and platelets. Leukemia is the most common type of cancer in children under 15. It also occurs in adults who are generally over the age of 55.

Acute lymphoblastic leukemia (ALL) is a type of leukemia seen in both adults and children. ALL is characterized by an abnormally high amount of stem cells in the bone marrow differentiating to become B or T cells that do not function normally. The increase in abnormal lymphocytes which are not capable of fighting infection leads to decreased space for functional circulating platelets, and white and red cells. This results in anemia, as well as the patient being at an increased risk for infection or bleeding. Common symptoms of ALL include fever, bone and joint pain, petechiae, painless lumps in lymph nodes in the neck, inguinal and axillary regions, as well as weakness, fatigue, and decreased appetite. Cytogenetic analysis of chromosomes in the cancerous lymphocytes may reveal a Philadelphia chromosome, which results from a reciprocal translocation or when a portion of one chromosome is switched with a portion of another chromosome. The Philadelphia chromosome, in particular, occurs between chromosomes 22 and 9. The resultant cancer-causing chromosome contains a fusion gene, BCR-ABL. This gene encodes for a fusion protein, which is a constitutively active tyrosine kinase signaling factor that causes the cell to divide uncontrollably. The Philadelphia chromosome is found in approximately 25–30% of cases of adult ALL and up to 10% of cases of pediatric

ALL. **Chronic lymphocytic leukemia (CLL)** indicates a leukemia of the same lymphoid cell types. However, the term "chronic" refers to the fact that it progresses at a much slower rate than ALL. Additionally, CLL most commonly affects older adults.

Acute myeloid, (or myelogenous) leukemia (AML) is another type of leukemia that can occur in both children and adults. As opposed to ALL which generally affects lymphocytes, AML affects myeloid stem cells which can become red blood cells, platelets, or granulocytes. These cancerous myeloid cells can build up in the bone marrow and blood and take away space from healthy circulating cells. As in ALL, patients with AML are also prone to infection, anemia, and bleeding. These cells may also end up in the CNS, skin, or gums, or may even form a solid tumor known as a chloroma or granulocytic sarcoma. As with CLL, **chronic myelogenous leukemia (CML)** refers to a type of leukemia that affects the same myeloid cells as AML but progresses much more slowly. While it can occur at any age, it is much more common in older adults and less common in children. The BCR-ABL gene (Philadelphia chromosome) is present in almost all cases of CML.

Hairy cell leukemia is a slowly progressing cancer of B lymphocytes. Under the microscope these abnormal B cells appear "hairy", hence the name. With the aberrant growth of abnormal B cells, fewer healthy leukocytes are produced leaving the patients more vulnerable to infection. Hairy cell leukemia seems to affect men more commonly than women, and in middle-aged to older adults. This type of leukemia is sometimes not diagnosed immediately, as patients may not experience signs and symptoms, or may experience signs that are common to other conditions such as fatigue, recurrent infections, bruising, weakness, weight loss, or fullness in the abdomen. A blood test can reveal the abnormally appearing "hairy" B lymphocytes.

The term **lymphoma** refers to a solid lymphoid tumor that often originates in the lymph nodes or other lymphoid tissues. Cancerous lymphocytes have the ability to travel through the blood and lymphatic systems like their normal

Fig. 10.5 37-year old male patient with enlarged cervical lymph nodes due to Hodgkin lymphoma. Credit: CDC/Robert E. Sumpter

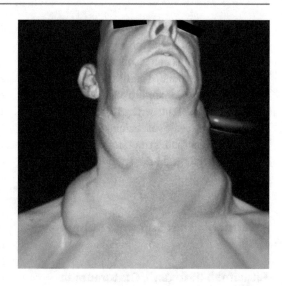

counterparts and thus can easily metastasize to other parts of the body. Lymphomas may differ based on which type of lymphocyte they affect (T or B) and how fast or slow they are growing. Indolent lymphocytes are generally slow-growing and are not always treated immediately. Aggressive lymphomas, on the other hand, grow and metastasize at a much quicker rate and require immediate treatment. In the U.S. the most common form of aggressive lymphoma is **diffuse large B cell lymphoma (DLBCL)**.

Hodgkin lymphoma is an uncommon type of lymphoma (approximately 9000 new cases in the U.S. each year) of which there are five different classifications. Hodgkin lymphoma is character-ized by the presence of Reed-Sternberg cells. Reed-Sternberg cells (RSCs) are usually B cell in origin and are large in appearance under a light microscope. A type of RSC is the lacunar histio-cyte which looks like cells that are lying within empty spaces, due to the retraction of their cyto-plasm after formalin fixation. Other types of RSCs include popcorn cells which are small cells with lobulated nuclei and small nucleoli as well as mummified RSCs that have a compact nucleus and no nucleolus. From these characteristics, his-topathology can determine the type of Hodgkin lymphoma. Unlike normal lymphocytes, RSCs appear to express high levels of the lipoxygenase ALOX15 which results in a variety of arachi-donic acid metabolites that may contribute to

their abnormal morphology. Some of the symp-toms include enlarged lymph nodes (Fig. 10.5), weight loss, fatigue, fever, or night sweats.

Non-Hodgkin lymphoma (NHL) is a cancer of lymphocytes that most often originates in the lymph nodes or other lymphoid tissues such as the spleen, bone marrow, thymus, adenoids/tonsils, or digestive tract. There are more than 90 types of NHL, all of which do not involve Reed-Sternberg cells. To determine the best treatment strategy, it is important to deter-mine if the lymphoma is affecting B or T cells.

AIDS-related lymphoma occurs in HIV patients whose disease has progressed to AIDS. The lymphoid cancer cells form in the lymphatic system and result in weight loss, night sweats, and fever. One type of lymphoma that AIDS patients could be at risk for is **Primary CNS lymphoma** which is characterized by the forma-tion of malignant cells in the lymphoid tissues of the brain and/or spinal cord. Other patients who are immunocompromised may also be at increased risk of developing this type of lymphoma.

Multiple Myeloma (MM) is another cancer that begins in the bone marrow and is character-ized by abnormal plasma cells. Because of the overgrowth of these abnormal plasma cells, they may crowd out the normal formed elements of the blood, leading to anemia, leukopenia, and thrombocytopenia. These abnormal plasma cells produce abnormal antibodies called M proteins that can build up in the kidney and cause kidney damage. MM cells can also stimulate osteoclasts to break down bone, resulting in weak, brittle bones. When bones are broken down, calcium is released, thus patients with MM may have higher than normal levels of calcium in the blood. Common signs and symptoms of MM include frequent infections, kidney problems, bone problems, and fatigue.

Treatments That Suppress Immune Cells

Rituximab (Rituxan®), Ofatumumab (Arzerra®), and Obinutuzumab (Gazyva®)

As mentioned in Chap. 7, rituximab is a B cell inhibitor which can be used to treat Rheumatoid arthritis as well as certain types of cancers. Rituximab is a chimeric antibody which binds to

CD20 found on the surface of B cells, resulting in complement-dependent cytotoxicity and antibody-dependent cellular cytotoxicity (ADCC) and thus death of targeted tumor cells (Fig. 10.6). Ofatumumab is a fully human anti-CD20 monoclonal antibody while obinutuzumab is humanized. CD20 is necessary for B cell cycle initiation and may also function as a calcium channel. Its expression may be increased on certain B cell tumors. It is important to note that CD20 is not expressed on plasma cells, thus, patients will not lose antibodies that they have already produced. These drugs are approved for certain lymphomas as well as chronic lymphocytic leukemia (CLL). Rituximab is given as an IV infusion and because it is a chimeric antibody (34% mouse) it can potentially cause a serious infusion reaction which can be fatal. For this reason, patients should be monitored closely, especially during the first infusion. Infusion reactions may be prevented with a gradual increase in dosing. Pre-medicating with antihistamines and

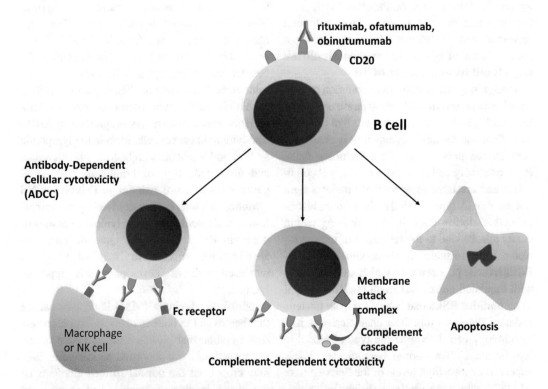

Fig. 10.6 Rituximab, ofatumumb, and obinutuzumab are monoclonal antibodies which bind to CD20, resulting in antibody-dependent cytotoxicity, complement-dependent cytotoxicity, or apoptosis of B cells

acetaminophen may reduce severity. Rituximab should also not be administered as an IV push or bolus. Ofatumumab and obinutuzumab should also not be administered via IV push or bolus. Obinutuzumab should be administered through a dedicated IV line and should not be mixed or infused with other medications. HBV reactivation can occur in some patients; therefore, it is important to test patients for HBV before beginning therapy. Other adverse effects seen with rituximab include cardiovascular events such as peripheral edema, cardiac arrhythmias, as well as kidney failure caused by a condition called **tumor lysis syndrome (TLS)** which results from the quick breakdown of cancer cells. TLS can happen within 12–24 h after a rituximab infusion. The symptoms of TLS include nausea, vomiting, diarrhea, or lack of energy. Patients receiving rituximab can also experience painful sores or ulcers on the skin, mouth, or lips. Rituximab does cross the placenta and may be excreted into breast milk which can possibly lead to B-cell lymphocytopenia in the infant, thus it is contraindicated in pregnancy and lactation. Because of the immunosuppressive nature of these treatments, patients with chronic lymphocytic leukemia (CLL), *Pneumocystis jirovecii* pneumonia (PCP) and antiherpetic viral prophylaxis is recommended during treatment (and for up to 12 months following treatment). Lastly, **progressive multiforme leukencephalopathy (PML)**, a rare but serious infection of the brain is also a risk.

Ibritumomab tiuxetan (Zevalin®) is an anti-CD20 monoclonal antibody conjugated to a chelator (tiuxetan) to which a radioisotope is added (Yttrium-90, Y-90). This drug is approved for non-Hodgkin's lymphoma and is used in conjunction with rituximab.

Blinatumomab (Blincyto®)

Blinatumomab is a bispecific T-cell engager (BiTE) diabody. It has two binding sites that simultaneously engage and activate the CD3 receptor on T cells which targets the activated T cell to the tumor cell by binding to CD19 surface antigen. This results in the cytotoxic destruction of the CD19 B cell (Fig. 10.7). Blinatumomab is made up of a heterodimer composed of the CD3 light or heavy chain linked to the CD19 heavy or light chain peptides. Each polypeptide contains one light and one heavy chain from each binding target, allowing it to have two binding sites. Blincyto® is approved for relapsed/refractory Philadelphia chromosome-negative B-cell ALL. In clinical trials, patients taking Blincyto® had a median survival of nearly 8 months compared to 4 months for the patients taking standard chemotherapy regimens. Adverse reactions can include symptoms of cytokine release syndrome and infusion reaction, such as fever, fatigue, weakness, dizziness, headache, nausea, vomiting, or chills. Blincyto® may also induce neurologic symptoms such as seizures, slurred speech, confusion, and disorientation. This therapy is given as a continuous IV infusion for 28 days per cycle. Patients typically spend the first 9 days in the hospital receiving treatment in order to be monitored for adverse effects. Blincyto® can continue to be administered at home via a small portable pump. After the first 1-month cycle, the patient has 2 weeks off before beginning a second cycle. This treatment is approved for both pediatric and adult patients with relapsed ALL.

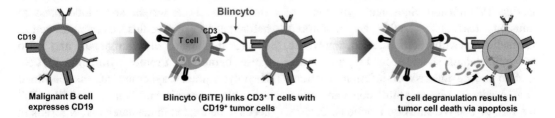

Fig. 10.7 Mechanism of action of blinatumomab (BiTE). Blinatumomab is a diabody that binds to both CD19 on tumor cells and CD3 on T cells that are capable of inducing apoptosis. Linking these two cells together increases the chances of T cell induction of tumor cell apoptosis (figure contributed by Jeremy P. McAleer)

Brentuximab Vedotin (Adcetris®)

Brentuximab is a monoclonal antibody targeting CD30 antigen conjugated to **MMAE (monomethyl auristatin E**, a cytotoxic synthetic microtubule polymerization disruptor) and is approved for several refractory types of lymphoma. Certain cells express the CD30 transmembrane glycoprotein, including subtypes of NHL and Reed-Sternberg cells. This drug is unique because when the antigen/antibody complex is endocytosed, the cytotoxic drug is brought into cell where it is cleaved off the antibody in the lysosome. The cleaved drug can then also escape the cell and kill nearby cancer cells, which is known as bystander cell killing.

Daratumumab (Darzalex®)

Daratumumab is a human monoclonal antibody which binds to and blocks CD38, a marker which is highly expressed on MM cells and is approved for refractory MM. By blocking CD38, daratumumab acts through apoptosis and multiple immune-mediated mechanisms including complement-dependent cytotoxicity, antibody-dependent cellular phagocytosis, and antibody-dependent cellular cytotoxicity. In many cases, daratumumab is used in combination with an immunomodulatory agent (IMiD) and/or a proteasome inhibitor or glucocorticoid. It may also be used alone for patients who did not respond to at least three prior treatments. Adverse effects include anemia, thrombocytopenia, infusion reactions, joint pain, muscular chest pain, hypertension, and fatigue. Complete blood cell counts should be done periodically. Infusion-related reactions with daratumumab often manifest as nasal congestion, cough, throat irritation, nausea, vomiting, and chills. During IV infusion signs and symptoms of infusion reactions should be monitored. Premedication with a corticosteroid, antipyretic, and antihistamine should occur 1 h prior to infusion to reduce the risk of infusion reactions. Oral corticosteroids post-infusion can reduce the risk of delayed infusion reactions. Patients should have their blood type tested prior to initiating therapy due to the fact that it can give false positive results for the Coombs test to detect irregular blood group antibodies. Thus, all providers, blood banks, and pathology labs should be aware that the patient is receiving daratumumab. Because patients with MM are at a great risk of viral infection such as herpes zoster, antiviral prophylaxis for herpes zoster within 1 week is recommended to prevent reactivation of the virus. This should be continued for 3 months following completion of treatment.

Moxetumomab Pasudotox (Lumoxiti®)

In 2018 the FDA approved a new biologic for treatment of patients with Hairy Cell Leukemia who have already undergone two standard lines of treatment. Moxetumomab is a novel treatment in that it is composed of the immunoglobulin heavy and light variable domains (Fv fragment) of an anti-CD22 monoclonal antibody fused to Pseudomonas exotoxin A, known as PE38. When the drug binds to CD22 on the surface of cancerous B cells in Hairy Cell Leukemia patients, the complex is internalized and processed in the endosome, where the toxin is then released. PE38 is then processed through the endoplasmic reticulum and subsequently inhibits protein synthesis leading to death of the cell. In clinical trials, approximately 30% of patients had a complete response, with 75% of total patients having a complete or total response. Adverse effects related to moxetumomab treatment include **capillary leak syndrome (CLS)**. CLS is a condition caused by leak of fluid from blood vessels to body tissues, resulting in swelling and weight gain, decrease in blood pressure, weakness, dizziness, and difficulty breathing; thus, it needs to be treated immediately. For this reason, healthcare providers should check weight and blood pressure before patients receive this treatment as well as during treatment. Moxetumomab may also cause **hemolytic uremic syndrome (HUS)**. Hemolytic uremic syndrome affects the blood cells, blood vessels, and kidneys and like CLS needs to be treated immediately. HUS results in destruction of platelets, anemia, and kidney failure. Symptoms of HUS include dark urine, stomach pain, unusual skin bruising, rapid heartbeat, seizures, shortness of breath, confusion, and fever. In addition to their serious conditions, common side effects include nausea, diarrhea, fatigue, fever, headache, constipation, and edema of the face, arms, or legs.

Elotuzumab (Empliciti®)

Elotuzumab is a humanized monoclonal antibody which binds to **SLAMF7 (Signaling Lymphocyte Activation Molecule F7)** which is found to be highly expressed on MM cells. While SLAM receptors are often expressed on cells of leukocytes, they are generally not expressed on nonhematopoietic cells. Uniquely, the SLAM receptors can act as "self-ligands" and in essence recognize the receptor on another cell as a ligand to which it can bind. SLAMF7 in particular seems to play a role in the adhesion of MM cells to bone marrow stromal cells (BMSCs). Elotuzumab, the first monoclonal antibody therapy that was approved for MM, acts through NK-mediated cell death by tagging MM cells, and thus stimulates NK cells to kill by ADCC, releasing perforin and granzyme B that results in MM cell lysis. Binding to SLAMF7 by elotuzumab also blocks adhesion of MM cells to BMSCs. Adverse effects include neutropenia, thrombocytopenia, hyperglycemia, changes in blood pressure, elevated liver enzymes, fatigue, diarrhea, constipation, peripheral neuropathy, and infusion reactions. Patients undergoing IV infusion should be monitored for signs and symptoms of infusion reactions (including pyrexia, chills, and hypertension). Premedication with dexamethasone, antihistamines, and acetaminophen 45–90 min prior to infusion is recommended. Because of the potential effect on the liver, liver function tests should be monitored periodically as well as risk of infection and secondary primary malignancies. There may be a small risk of developing a solid tumor or skin cancer years after finishing treatment with elotuzumab.

CAR-T Cell Therapy

In 2017, the FDA approved two **chimeric antigen receptor (CAR-T) therapies- tisagenlecleucel (Kymriah™)** an **axicabtagene ciloleucel (Yescarta®)** for the treatment of specific types of leukemia and lymphoma. This type of treatment could revolutionize approaches to cancer treatments. CAR-T cell therapy uses the patient's own T cells to initiate an immune response against the cancer. To do this, the patient's blood is drawn for harvesting of T cells (Fig. 10.8). The T-cells are then genetically engineered using an attenuated (disarmed) virus to produce surface antigen receptors referred to as chimeric antigen receptors (CARs) (Fig. 10.9). These engineered CARs are synthetic receptors because they are not naturally occurring receptors found in the body. These receptors provide specificity to the T-cells by allowing them to attach to specific proteins or antigens on cancer cells. Once the T-cells have been successfully engineered to express the CARs, they are further cloned to produce millions of copies in the lab. The T-cells can then be infused back into the patient once the patient has undergone a lymphodepleting chemotherapy regimen. Once in the body, the engineered T-cells further multiply and can detect and kill tumor cells that have the surface antigen with guidance from the expressed receptors. Because CAR-T cell therapies have pseudo-living components associated with them, they are sometimes referred to as "living drugs." Since the patients T-cells are genetically engineered to contain the unique receptor, they are also considered to be the first FDA-approved gene therapies. The two approved therapies both contain an extracellular component of the CAR that has anti-CD19 properties to target B cells. Studies of B-cell lymphopoiesis have found that there is a common lymphoid progenitor (CLP) cell that forms in the bone marrow. Some of these have been found to have thymus-seeding properties and are likely to be early T cell progenitors. Some CLPs stay in the bone marrow and are likely to become B cells or NK cells. Pre-pro B cells that are destined to become B cells from these CLPs express B220. Once these cells are committed to the B cell lineage, they are considered to be pro-B cells and express CD19. From this point of B cell development on, B cells (including mature and memory) express CD19. Thus, the patient's engineered T cells will bind to hematopoietic cancer cells that often overexpress CD19, allowing for some specificity to the cancer

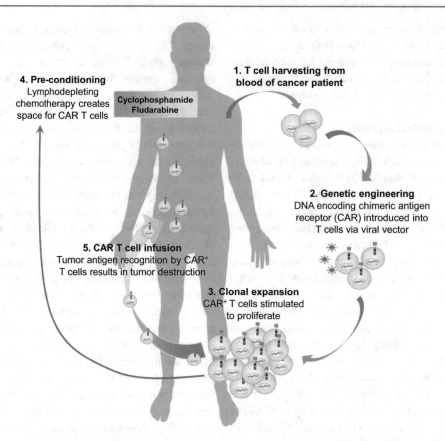

Fig. 10.8 Process of harvesting patient's T cells for reprogramming with CAR. T cells from patients receiving chimeric antigen receptor (CAR) therapy are infected with a virus encoding the CAR. This receptor is engineered to recognize a tumor-associated antigen and to stimulate T cell activation upon antigen recognition. The genetically modified T cells are then stimulated to proliferate in vitro in order to generate high numbers of activated, tumor-specific T cells. Prior to T cell infusion, patients are pre-conditioning with a Lymphodepleting regimen (cyclophosphamide, fludarabine) in order to create space for the genetically-modified T cells. Following injection, CAR T cells recognize and destroy the tumor (figure contributed by Jeremy P. McAleer)

cells. Binding to CD19 activates the intramembrane component of the CAR, which contains several T-cell activation domains (e.g. CD28, CD137, and CD3), as well as a co-stimulatory domain, ensuring that the T-cell response will be effective.

For patients with relapsed/refractory (r/r) acute lymphoblastic leukemia (ALL) the prognosis is poor. Many often undergo several rounds of chemotherapy, radiation, or bone marrow transplants with the result still being only 10% of patients surviving 5 years after diagnosis. Tisagenlecleucel (Kymriah™) was approved by the FDA in 2017 for the treatment of ALL in patients up to 25 years of age. For patients in this age category with r/r ALL and few treatment

options, Kymriah demonstrated a 83% remission rate 3 months after infusion. While not all patients experience adverse effects from Kymriah, one of the most common is **cytokine release syndrome (CRS)** likely due to the activation of the newly introduced engineered T cells. CRS was managed in these patients via the CRS treatment algorithm. Other adverse effects include headache, delirium, increased risk of infection, decrease in appetite, hypotension, and acute kidney injury. To manage these as well as inform patients of the possible risk of treatment with Kymriah, the FDA has approved a REMS program for this treatment.

Axicabtagene ciloleucel (Yescarta®) was also approved in 2017 for treatment of non-Hodgkin's

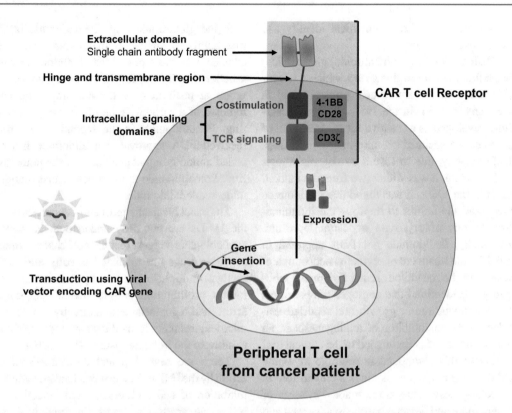

Fig. 10.9 Expression of CAR-T cell receptor on the cancer patient's own T cells. Peripheral T cells from a patient receiving CAR-T cell therapy are infected (transduced) with a virus encoding a gene for the chimeric antigen receptor (CAR). The gene is inserted into chromosomal DNA and expressed using the host cell machinery. The structure of a CAR includes an extracellular domain recognizing the tumor-associated antigen, flexible transmembrane region, and intracellular signaling domains derived from costimulatory molecules and the TCR (figure contributed by Jeremy P. McAleer)

lymphoma (CD19+ diffuse large B cell lymphoma [DLBCL]). In a clinical trial of 101 DLBCL patients who had failed other treatments, 51% achieved complete remission and another 21% achieve partial remission. Fifteen months later, 40% of patients still had a complete response. Responses occurred within a month of receiving treatment. While this therapy also comes with risk of CRS, other adverse effects experienced include fever, leukopenia, anemia, hypotension, rapid heartbeat, confusion, fatigue, and GI side effects.

Because of the specificity of both treatments and the possible adverse effects and monitoring required, the FDA specified that healthcare institutions must be certified to carry out these treatments.

Immunomodulatory Imide Drugs (IMiDs)

Research over the last decade has identified "avoiding immune destruction" as an emerging hallmark in the pathogenesis of cancer. At the same time, efforts have been made to reactivate or boost the immune system to attack and destroy premalignant and or malignant cells. Multiple approaches to reactivate or boost the immune system to attack premalignant or malignant cells have been successful and thus have gotten regulatory approval. **Thalidomide (Thalomid®), lenalidomide (Revlimid®)** and **pomalidomide (Pomalyst®)** constitute a group of orally active compounds that modulate the patient's immune system to destroy cancer cells as their major mechanism of action. These drugs are collectively known as immunomodulatory imide drug

(IMiD) because of their chemical identity and mechanism of action.

Thalidomide (α-(N-phthalimido) glutaramide) is the first member of this group, which was synthesized from the amino acid glutamic acid in Germany in 1954. In the 1950s, it was successfully developed as a sedative for the treatment of pregnancy-associated morning sickness. Unfortunately, due to severe teratogenic effects and dysmelia, it was withdrawn from the market. Later in the 1960s, it was found that thalidomide possessed the ability to improve the inflammatory lesions of erythema nodosum leprosum. Eventually, thalidomide got FDA approval in 1998 for the treatment of erythema nodosum leprosum. In the meantime, Judah Folkman's laboratory had identified that angiogenesis is critical for continuous tumor growth and reported thalidomide as an inhibitor of angiogenesis in an animal model. This finding led to the clinical trial testing of this compound in multiple myeloma (MM) since angiogenesis plays a crucial role in its pathogenesis. Due to the marked synergy of thalidomide and dexamethasone in advanced and refractory MM patients, the FDA approved this combination as first-line therapy for patients with newly diagnosed MM in 2006. Efforts were also continued to synthesize and develop analogues that were more potent and safer with the goal of eliminating adverse side effects. These efforts led to the development of lenalidomide (second generation) and pomalidomide (third generation IMiD). Lenalidomide was approved by the FDA for the treatment of red blood cell transfusion-dependent anemia due to myelodysplastic syndrome in 2005 and for the treatment of patients with refractory/relapsed MM in the United States and the European Union, in combination with dexamethasone in 2006. The third generation analogue pomalidomide (Pomalyst®) was approved, in combination with dexamethasone, for patients with MM in 2013.

Chemically, thalidomide and related drugs are imide, a functional group consisting of two acyl groups bound to nitrogen. The first member thalidomide was synthesized from amino acid glutamic acid and named α-(N-phthalimido) glutaramide. IMiDs contain a phthalimide ring fused with the glutarimide ring. Lenalidomide is the first approved analog of thalidomide which is considerably more potent than thalidomide with a better toxicity profile. It has an added amino group at position 4 of the phthaloyl ring and removal of a carbonyl group from the phthaloyl ring. Pomalidomide is the second analog that received FDA approval. Pomalidomide has an added amino group at position 4 of the phthaloyl ring. Pomalidomide is more potent that thalidomide and lenalidomide.

The exact mechanisms of anti-cancer action of the IMiDs are not fully understood. However, available data suggest that the anti-cancer effects of these drugs are mediated directly and indirectly at multiple levels: directly on tumor cells to inhibit proliferation and to induce cell cycle arrest and apoptosis and indirectly on tumor microenvironment to modulate angiogenesis and to activate the immune system (Fig. 10.10).

There are several potential mechanisms of action by the IMiDs. The first mechanism includes inhibition of cell proliferation and induction of cell cycle arrest and apoptosis through direct effect on cancer cells: These effects of IMiDs are mediated by inactivation of nuclear factor-κB (NF-κB), down-regulation of C/EBPβ and activation of caspase 8. The IMiDs are also thought to have anti-angiogenic and anti-proliferative and anti-inflammatory effects: IMiDs alter the interaction between cancer cells and non-cancerous cells in the bone marrow (BM) microenvironment including BM stromal cells (BMSCs), osteoclasts (OCs) and immune cells. The interaction of MM cells with the BM microenvironment enhances MM cell growth, survival, migration and drug resistance. IMiDs block this interaction of MM cells and BMSCs through inhibition of the expression of surface adhesion molecules on both MM cells and BMSCs, such as selectins and VCAM. As a result, the production of interleukin-6 (IL-6), insulin-like growth factor 1 (IGF-1), TNF-α, vascular endothelial growth factor (VEGF), basic fibroblast growth factor (bFGF) are inhibited. IL-6 and TNF-α are important for inflammation and VEGF and bFGF mediates angiogenesis. Lastly, the IMiDs may activate cell-mediated cytotoxicity. IMiDs increase the activation and

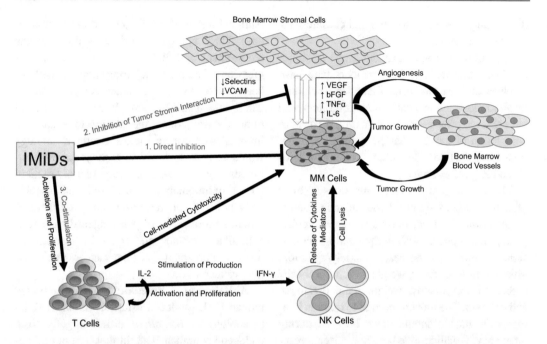

Fig. 10.10 Schematic overview of proposed mechanisms of anti-cancer activity of thalidomide and its derivatives. (1) Direct anti-proliferative, growth arrest and apoptotic effects on tumor cells. This effect is attributed to the inhibition of NF-κB and CEBP and activation of caspase 8. (2) Inhibition of tumor-stroma interactions leading to anti-angiogenesis and anti-proliferative effects. IMiDs inhibit tumor cell adhesion to stromal cells, which decreases production and secretion of cytokines and growth factors (VEGF, bFGF, TNF-α, IL-6) important for angiogenesis and proliferation. (3) Enhanced immune-mediated cytotoxicity. IMiDs increase T-cell production of IL-2 and INF-γ, that increase the number and cytotoxic functionality of NK cells (figure contributed by A.R.M. Ruhul Amin)

proliferation of T-cells by serving as co-stimulators. Activated T cells secrete IL-2 and IFN-γ, which subsequently activate NK cells and more T-cells, thus enhancing both innate and adaptive cellular immunity.

Thalidomide has been approved by the FDA for the treatment of erythema nodosum leprosum. In combination with dexamethasone, thalidomide has been approved by the FDA for the treatment of newly diagnosed MM as first line therapy. The European Medicines Agency has also approved thalidomide in combination with prednisone and/or melphalan for the treatment of newly diagnosed MM. Orphan indications for thalidomide by the FDA include graft-versus-host disease, mycobacterial infection, recurrent aphthous ulcers, severe recurrent aphthous stomatitis, primary brain malignancies, AIDS-associated wasting syndrome, Crohn's disease,

Kaposi's sarcoma, myelodysplastic syndrome and hematopoietic stem cell transplantation.

Lenalidomide, on the other hand, is approved by the FDA for the treatment of red blood cell transfusion-dependent anemia due to myelodysplastic syndrome. In combination with dexamethasone, it is also approved for the treatment of patients with refractory/relapsed MM. Lenalidomide is approved in nearly 70 countries, in combination with dexamethasone for the treatment of patients with MM who have received at least one prior therapy, or who are not eligible for autologous stem cell transplant. It is also approved as maintenance therapy for patients with MM following autologous stem cell transplant, and Mantle cell lymphoma (MCL) whose disease has relapsed or progressed after two prior therapies, one of which included bortezomib. Orphan indications for lenalidomide include diffuse large B-cell lymphoma and chronic lymphocytic leukemia.

In combination with dexamethasone, pomalidomide is indicated for MM patients who have received at least two prior therapies (including lenalidomide and a proteasome inhibitor) and have disease progression on or within 60 days of completion of the last therapy. Orphan designations for pomalidomide include Systemic sclerosis and Kaposi sarcoma.

The most common adverse reactions ($\geq$20%) of thalidomide are fatigue, hypocalcemia, edema, constipation, dyspnea. muscle weakness, leukopenia, neutropenia, rash/desquamation, confusion, anorexia, nausea, anxiety/agitation, asthenia, tremor, fever, weight loss, thrombosis/embolism, neuropathy, weight gain, dizziness, and dry skin. The most important toxicity is teratogenesis, thus it should never be used during pregnancy. Lenalidomide common adverse reactions ($\geq$20%) include teratogenicity (much less than thalidomide), low blood counts (neutropenia, thrombocytopenia, anemia), diarrhea, constipation, muscle cramp, pyrexia, peripheral edema, nausea, back pain, upper respiratory tract infection, dyspnea, dizziness, tremor and rash. A rare, but serious side effect of Lenalidomide is blood clots, including **deep vein thrombosis (DVT) and pulmonary embolus (PE)**. The most common (>20%) adverse reactions of pomalidomide are severe life-threatening human birth defects if taken during pregnancy, fatigue, weakness, low white blood cell count, anemia, constipation, nausea, diarrhea, shortness of breath, upper respiratory infections, back pain and fever. Less common effects include neuropathy (numbness and tingling), dizziness, and confusion. A serious but rare side effect of pomalidomide is blood clots forming in the legs or lung.

Non-immune Cell Cancers

Treatments for Cancer That Stimulate Immune Cells to Kill

Historically, cancer treatment has consisted of a combination of "Slash, Burn, and/or Poison" (surgical resection, radiation, and/or chemotherapy). These approaches primarily focus on the requirement of cellular growth for cancer progression. More recently, various approaches have been developed that take other cancer characteristics into consideration. Because successful tumors have gained the ability to evade the immune response, a logical treatment strategy would also be to boost immunity against non-immune system cancers. Drugs like aldesleukin (IL-2), ipilimumab, and pembrolizumab specifically boost T cell responses, allowing them to mount a more active response against cancerous cells like metastatic melanoma, bladder cancer, prostate, non-small cell lung cancer, renal, and liver cancers.

Aldesleukin (Proleukin®) is recombinant human IL-2, produced using recombinant DNA technology in *E. coli*. It differs slightly from endogenous human IL-2, in that it is not glycosylated, nor does it have an N-terminal alanine. As mentioned in Chap. 3, IL-2 activates and promotes proliferation of T cells. Similarly, aldesleukin binds to the IL-2 receptor leading to dimerization of IL-2R β and γ chain cytoplasmic regions. This activated receptor complex leads to recruitment of cytoplasmic signaling molecules resulting in growth and differentiation of T cells, and their enhanced cytotoxicity. It is also thought that it may interfere with tumor blood supply. While it is given intravenously and used in renal cell carcinoma and metastatic melanoma, its adverse effects are many. These include fever, chills, dry skin, mouth sores, and severe nausea and vomiting. Because of the severity of high-dose IL-2 side effects, patients are often hospitalized to help mitigate these effects. Low-dose IL-2 may be used in some regimens and can be given outpatient subcutaneously.

Ipilimumab (Yervoy®) was approved by the FDA in 2011 and is a fully human monoclonal antibody against CTLA4. Normally, CTLA4 is inhibitory for CD8 T cells. Shutting off this inhibitory signal allow CTLs to maintain their cytotoxicity and kill cancer cells (Fig. 10.11). Ipilimumab is given intravenously and is approved for treatment of unresectable or metastatic melanoma, and renal cell carcinoma. Its

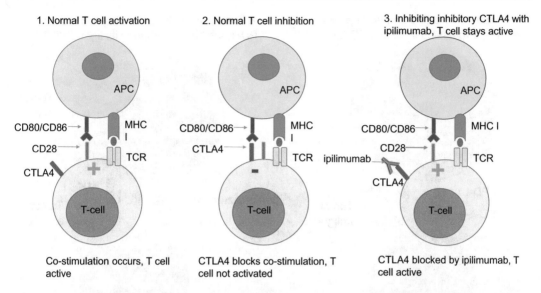

Fig. 10.11 Mechanism of action of ipilimumab. Under normal conditions, CD28 is a ligand for CD80/86 on the APC. This binding is necessary for the costimulatory signal that allows the T cell to become active. CTLA4 is a competitive inhibitor of CD28 on the CD80/86 binding site; this binding blocks costimulation. Ipilimumab binds to CTLA4 to prevent it from inhibiting costimulation, and allows the T cell to receive the costimulation signal from the APC to become active

adverse effects include stomach pain, nausea, vomiting, pruritis, fatigue, bloating, fever, and breathing problems (for which risk versus benefit must be weighed). Some of these can occur weeks or even months after discontinuation. Other severe immune-mediated adverse events (Black box warnings) which may occur due to T-cell activation include inflammation of the intestines and intestinal tears, hepatitis, dermatitis (including toxic epidermal necrolysis), endocrinopathy, as well as inflammation of the skin or eyes. Patients should be monitored for adrenal insufficiency, thyroid disorders, and hypophysitis (inflammation of the pituitary gland). Patients should also receive liver functions tests and adrenocorticotropic hormone should be measured at baseline and prior to each dose.

Checkpoint Inhibitors

As discussed in Chap. 3, PD-1, or programmed cell death protein 1, is an inhibitory co-stimulatory molecule on the T cell surface and is a member of the CD28/CTLA4 family of T cell regulatory proteins. It can be expressed on activated T cells, B cells, and macrophages. This suggests that PD-1 regulates immune responses more broadly than CTLA-4. While PD-1 can suppress autoreactive T cell activity and autoimmunity, expression of PD-1 is upregulated on some tumors. As mentioned earlier in this chapter, expressing an immunosuppressive molecule on the cell surface allows some tumors to escape immune surveillance, thus, blocking PD-1/PD-L1 interactions with monoclonal antibodies such as atezolizumab, pembrolizumab, and nivolumab is a novel therapeutic target in cancer. These therapies are referred to as checkpoint inhibitors.

Pembrolizumab (Keytruda®) is used for metastatic melanoma as well as non-small cell lung cancer. It is a humanized monoclonal antibody which blocks the inhibitor ligand of PD-1 (programmed cell death receptor 1) located on lymphocytes (Fig. 10.12). This essentially blocks the inhibition of lymphocytes, allowing the immune system to kill these abnormal cells. **Nivolumab (Opdivo®)** is another possible treatment for metastatic melanomas that do not have a mutation in BRAF and is sometimes used in combination with

1. Cancer cell evading immune system
killing by expressing inhibitory PD-L1

2. Treatment with pembrolizumab blocks
PD-1, inhibiting binding to its ligand PD-L1

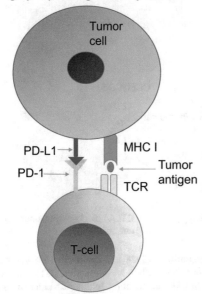

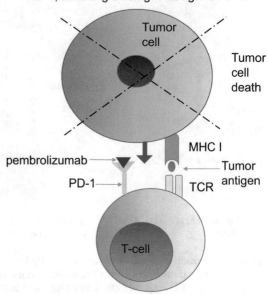

Fig. 10.12 Mechanism of action of the checkpoint inhibitors. To avoid the immune response, tumor cells may express higher than normal levels of PD-L1 in order to bind to T cells and inhibit their activation. These monoclonal antibodies can be used to bind to PD-1 or PD-L1 to block their interaction, allowing the T cell to become active

ipilimumab. Nivolumab is a fully human monoclonal antibody against PD-1. **Atezolizumab (Tecentriq®)** is a humanized monoclonal antibody which binds to PD-L1, which is the ligand for PD-1. Thus, the mechanism of action of atezolizumab is similar to the action of pembrolizumab and nivolumab because it still blocks the inhibitory activity of the PD-1/PD-L1 binding, allowing lymphocytes to kill tumor cells. **Avelumab (Bavencio®)** and **durvalumab (Imfinzi®)** are also PD-L1 inhibitors. FDA-approved indications for the checkpoint inhibitors is outlined in Table 10.2.

In general, the checkpoint inhibitors may induce severe inflammation due to their mechanism of action. This inflammation may occur in the lungs, colon, liver, kidneys, intestines, and thyroid. More common adverse effects of these drugs may include skin rash, pruritis, fatigue, cough, nausea, or loss of appetite. Rare but severe side effects include immune-mediated pneumonitis, immune-mediated colitis, immune-mediated hepatitis, immune-mediated nephritis and renal dysfunction, as well as immune-mediated hypothyroidism and hyperthyroidism.

Interferons (IFN)

Interferon therapy, IFN-alfa in particular, can activate NK cells, T cells, DCs, and innate lymphoid cells to respond to cancer cells. IFN-alfa may also affect cancerous cells by inhibiting their proliferation and differentiation as well as promoting apoptosis. While IFN seems to have a marginal role in cancer therapy, it may still be used in melanoma, in addition to Kaposi sarcoma, CML, NHL, MM, and even renal cancer as an adjuvant therapy. **Interferon alfa-2b (Intron A®)** and **peginterferon alfa-2b (Sylatron®)** are two products which may be used in addition to other cancer therapies. Adverse effects, as with any IFN therapy tend to be fatigue, flu-like symptoms, and injection site reactions.

Table 10.2 FDA indications for the checkpoint inhibitors

Checkpoint inhibitor	Target	FDA-approved indications
Pembrolizumab	PD-1	NSCLC[a], metastatic melanoma, head and neck squamous cell carcinoma, classical Hodgkin lymphoma, urothelial bladder carcinoma, cervical cancer, gastric cancer, hepatocellular carcinoma, microsatellite instability high cancer, Merkel cell carcinoma, primary mediastinal B cell lymphoma
Nivolumab	PD-1	NSCLC, SCLC[a], metastatic melanoma, head and neck squamous cell carcinoma, classical Hodgkin lymphoma, urothelial bladder carcinoma, hepatocellular carcinoma, metastatic colorectal carcinoma, renal carcinoma
Atezolizumab	PD-L1	NSCLC, urothelial bladder carcinoma
Avelumab	PD-L1	Merkel cell carcinoma
Durvalumab	PD-L1	NSCLC

[a]NSCLC non small cell lung cancer, SCLC small cell lung cancer

Imiquimod (Aldara®)

Imiquimod is a prescription cream used to treat superficial basal cell carcinoma, genital warts, and actinic keratosis. Imiquimod activates Toll-like receptor 7 (TLR7) to induce an immune response. Cytokines released by activated cells, likely DCs, include IL-12, IL-8, IFN-α, IFN-γ, TNF-α. This results in recruitment of NK cells and CD8 T cells which aid in killing of cancerous cells. Studies have shown that imiquimod upregulates MHC Class I on tumor cells and mobilizes Langerhans cells and inflammatory DCs. While keratinocytes generally don't express TLR7, imiquimod is also thought to have an effect on this cell type independent of TLR signaling, since it has been shown to increase keratinocyte release of IL-8 and TNF-α through activation of NF-κB. In the treatment of basal cell carcinoma, it is generally applied to the affected skin 5 times a week for 6 weeks. Because the cream induces inflammation in an effort to remove cancerous skin cells, the treatment area may become red and irritated, with a flaky/crusty scab that eventually heals after discontinuing the cream. Other adverse effects may include headache, nausea, and flu-like symptoms.

Bacille Calmette-Guerin (BCG)

Bacillus of Calmette-Guerin (BCG), also known as *Mycobacterium bovis*, is a bacterium first described by two French scientists, Albert Calmette and Camille Guerin who developed it as a vaccine for M*ycobacterium tuberculosis* during the twentieth century. In cancer treatment, BCG has been approved as an intravesical therapy for bladder cancer, meaning that it is introduced directly into the bladder through a catheter. This method of administration activates lymphocytes and potentiates T-helper type 1 immune responses to eliminate tumor cells in the bladder. Traditionally, one dose is instilled in the bladder of the patient once weekly for 6 weeks beginning 7–14 days after biopsy or transurethral resection of the bladder tumor (TURBT). This treatment is used for early-stage bladder cancer, including carcinoma *in situ* (CIS) and minimally invasive papillary tumors, as the lymphocytes attracted to the bladder will generally only affect the innermost cells lining the bladder and will not reach cells that have grown deeper into the bladder wall. More common side effects include painful or difficult urination, urinary urgency or frequency, hematuria, and flu-like symptoms. Because this treatment uses live attenuated mycobacteria, it could lead to a systemic infection and sepsis. Therefore, patients should be monitored for fever (especially ≥103 °F lasting longer than 24 h) and other signs of infection.

Sipuleucel-T (Provenge®)

Sipuleucel-T cell therapy was approved in 2010 for asymptomatic (minimal) metastatic hormone-refractory prostate cancer (HRPC). It is an autologous cellular immunotherapy in which the patient's dendritic cells are extracted via leukapheresis and activated with a fusion protein consisting of prostate cancer specific antigen (Prostatic Acid Phosphatase—PAP), which is present in 95% of prostate cancers and GM-CSF to mature the dendritic cells. Data has shown that men who received Provenge® therapy had a median survival time of 4.4 months longer than men who did not receive the therapy. While the therapy is generally well-tolerated, an acute infusion reaction can occur, including chills, fatigue, fever, headache, joint ache, nausea and back pain. Most of these effects seem to last for only 1 or 2 days.

Talimogene Laherparepvec, T-VEC (Imlygic®)

Talimogene laherparepvec, or T-VEC, is the first of its kind to be approved for cancer treatment and was approved for the treatment of metastatic melanoma in 2015. Its novel mechanism of action includes the injection of a genetically modified herpes simplex type 1 virus directly into the tumor, which selectively replicates in the tumor to destroy tumor cells and produces GM-CSF to produce systemic antitumor immune responses.

Patients who experience side effects usually report mild to moderate fever, nausea, flu-like symptoms, and pain at the injection site. Because this treatment includes the injection of a virus, patients who are pregnant or are immunocompromised with an immune deficiency, on steroid treatments, or have HIV should not use T-VEC.

Treatment of Solid Cancers That Target Tumor-Associated Signaling Pathways

Several other unique cancer characteristics are also targeted by immunological therapies for the treatment of solid tumors. As described above, cancer is a disease caused by uncontrolled growth of cells. The mitogenic signaling pathways that normally regulate cell growth are disrupted through mutations resulting in loss of tumor suppressor gene function and gain of

oncogene function. Once this occurs, cancer cells become dependent on this growth promoting signaling, which has been described as oncogene addiction. Cancer also requires growth of tumor vasculature for oxygen and nutrients, as well as a potential outlet for metastasis to occur. Several pharmacological therapies, including biologics, have been developed that inhibit the ligands or downstream signaling pathways regulating these mechanisms.

Trastuzumab (Herceptin®) and Pertuzumab (Perjeta®)

Trastuzumab was the first therapy of its kind approved for solid tumors, specifically breast cancer, in 1998, only 1 year after the FDA approval of rituximab. Trastuzumab and the more recently developed **pertuzumab**, are monoclonal antibodies that bind to and inhibit the transmembrane HER2 receptor tyrosine kinase. **HER2** is a member of the epidermal growth factor receptor family and becomes mutated, overexpressed, and constitutively activated in cancer cells. While this particular mutation occurs primarily in breast cancer, these drugs are also approved to treat HER2 positive **gastrointestinal stromal tumors (GIST)** and HER2 mutations have been detected in almost all types of solid cancer. Because the cancer cells that contain this mutation are dependent on the HER2 signaling pathway for growth and survival, blockade of HER2 is a very effective anticancer treatment. Since trastuzumab and pertuzumab bind to different domains of the extracellular portions of HER2, they inhibit ligand independent and dependent HER2 signaling, respectively, and can be used in combination. In addition, because these are monoclonal antibodies, as opposed to small molecule inhibitors like some other growth factor targeting therapies, they are believed to activate antibody dependent cellular cytotoxicity of the HER2 overexpressing cancer cells that the antibody has bound to. The major concerns for a patient being administered these therapies are infusion reactions and pulmonary toxicity, neutropenia, cardiomyopathy, and teratogenicity. These effects are likely due to target or off-target binding in other tissues and are generally reversible. Patients should be monitored for vital signs during infusions and may be premedicated with antihistamines and/or corticosteroids. Cardiac function should also be assessed regularly in patients that are on this medication.

Cetuximab (Erbitux°), Panitumumab (Vectibix°), and Necitumumab (Portrazza°)

Epidermal Growth Factor Receptor (EGFR) is overexpressed or mutated in a number of cancer types and has proved to be an effective target in colorectal cancer, head and neck cancer, and lung cancer. EGFR signaling is important for cellular growth, but also has roles in differentiation and survival. The monoclonal antibodies that have been developed to target EGFR either bind to the extracellular domain of the receptor (**cetuximab** and **necitumumab**) preventing activation by its ligands epidermal growth factor (EGF) and transforming growth factor alpha (TGF-α) or binding to the EGF ligand itself (**panitumumab**) to disrupt its ability to bind to the receptor. Similar to the therapies that target HER2, these drugs inhibit EGFR signaling that the cancer cells have become dependent on for their growth and survival. However, it has been found that patients whose tumors carry a Ras mutation are unlikely to respond to these therapies, as Ras is downstream of EGFR signaling. Thus, it is required that patients be genetically tested, not only for EGFR mutations, but also Ras mutations prior to the start of therapy. It is likely that anti-EGFR antibodies also activate immune-mediated death of the cancer cells as a component of their mechanism of action. The warnings for these medications include risk of infusion reactions, cardiopulmonary arrest, pulmonary toxicity, dermatologic toxicity, hypomagnesemia, and teratogenicity. Patients should be monitored for vital signs during infusions and regularly assessed for electrolyte abnormalities. Another less severe, but more common side effect is an acne-like rash caused by inhibition of EGFR in the skin. This acneiform rash and other dermatologic toxicities may be a sign that complications are more likely to occur and should be considered when monitoring a patient.

Bevacizumab (Avastin°) and Ramucirumab (Cyramza°)

Angiogenesis is the process by which new vasculature is formed, which normally occurs during embryonic and fetal development, as well as wound healing. As tumors develop, they outgrow the blood supply in the vicinity and an "angiogenic switch" occurs whereby **vascular endothelial growth factor (VEGF)** signaling is dramatically increased causing growth of substantial, yet abnormal, tumor vasculature. As mentioned earlier, it was proposed by Judah Folkman in the early 1970s that an effective anticancer therapy would be to target this angiogenic process. This approach has resulted in a number of FDA approved treatment options for solid tumors, ranging from small molecule inhibitors to biologics. Two monoclonal antibodies that target VEGF signaling are used for the treatment of metastatic solid tumors, including ovarian, cervical, renal, and colorectal cancers. **Bevacizumab** binds to the VEGF-A ligand and ramucirumab binds to the extracellular domain of the VEGF receptor (VEGFR2) on endothelial cells, preventing the activation of downstream signaling and growth. Because VEGF signaling is not unique to the tumor vasculature, normal blood vessels and VEGF signaling in the kidney may be affected. As a result, these medications carry the black box warnings of gastrointestinal perforations, surgery and wound healing complications, and hemorrhage. Some other more common adverse effects are hypertension, arterial thromboembolic events, proteinuria, non-gastrointestinal fistula formation, reversible posterior leukoencephalopathy syndrome, and infusion reactions. Antiangiogenic therapies are somewhat unique in that they do not directly cause death of tumor cells, rather they prevent the tumor from growing and spreading. Thus, these therapies are generally administered chronically, until patients show signs of resistance and disease progression.

Denosumab (Xgeva°)

Different types of cancer tend to metastasize to certain other regions or organs in the body. There are several mechanisms for how this occurs, including ease of disbursement through blood or lymph and local signaling that is advantageous to the tumor cells. Prostate cancer, for example, often metastasizes to the bone, forming osteolytic lesions. These lesions can be painful and weaken the bones of these patients. Furthermore, hormonal therapies for prostate and breast cancers lead to reduced sex hormone signaling and osteoporosis. The **Receptor activator of nuclear factor kappa-B (RANK)** is involved in the mechanism of bone resorption. **Denosumab** binds to its ligand, **RANKL**, and inhibits this signaling pathway suppressing osteoclast function. This reverses the breakdown of bone caused by the tumor and/or treatments. One concern of treating patients with denosumab is the increased risk of infections, which has been linked to the expression and activity of RANK signaling in various immune cells, such as T cells and dendritic cells.

Cancer Prevention by Viral Vaccines

It was discovered in the early 1900s, by Peyton Rous, that viruses can cause cancer. In the century since, scientists have learned which human cancers are caused by viruses and the potential mechanisms of this process. One such mechanism is through integration of the viral DNA into the host genome. This integration can cause a genetic mutation and depending on where in the genome this occurs (e.g. in a tumor suppressor gene or proto-oncogene) may be sufficient to initiate cancer development. A second mechanism by which viruses may play a role in cancer is through expression of oncogenic viral proteins. For example, the **human papillomavirus (HPV)** early gene products, E6 and E7, repress both p53 and Retinoblastoma (Rb) tumor suppressor activity. In addition, a number of studies suggest various mechanisms whereby viruses alter immune system function resulting in tumor promoting inflammation and/or lack of immune surveillance, which also likely affect cancer development and progression as described above.

Although a number of malignancies are associated with viruses, the two most common cancers in humans that are linked to viral causes are liver and cervical cancers. The risk of developing hepatocellular carcinoma (HCC) is increased 100-fold in those that have chronic hepatitis infections and it is estimated that 80% of HCC cases are caused by viral hepatitis. Prevention of acute and chronic hepatitis, as well as HCC, has been shown to be highly effective with the hepatitis B virus (HBV) vaccine.

Over 99% of cervical cancers are associated with human papillomavirus (HPV), 70% of which are specifically caused by HPV types 16 and 18. More recently, HPV has also been linked to certain head and neck cancers and various anogenital cancers. Thus, it is recommended by the Centers for Disease Control (CDC) that both male and female children aged 11–12 years be vaccinated to prevent genital warts and these types of cancer.

Managing Chemotherapy-Induced Myelosuppression

Hematopoietic Agents

The three cellular components of blood perform three major functions for our body: (1) RBCs transport oxygen to various parts of the body; (2) WBCs protect our body from infections and cancers and (3) platelets prevent excessive blood loss. Interestingly, all of the blood cells arise from the same type of stem cell, the hematopoietic stem cell or hemocytoblast (Fig. 10.13). Differentiation to a specific cell type requires specific growth factors/cytokines and cofactors. Like cancer cells, blood cells are fast growing/dividing cells (adults produce 400 billion platelets, 200 billion RBCs, and 10 billion WBCs every day) and are affected by chemotherapeutic drugs more than other cell types in the body with a slower turnover rate. As introduced earlier in the chapter, **myelosuppression** is a common and serious adverse effect of most chemotherapy and some molecularly targeted anticancer drugs resulting in a decrease in the number of all blood cells. Chemotherapy drugs are administered in cycles and blood cells must return to a "safe" level prior to each treatment cycle. Based on the blood counts, drugs are prescribed to stimulate the production of the required type of blood cells. Collectively, these drugs are called hematopoietic drugs (Table 10.3).

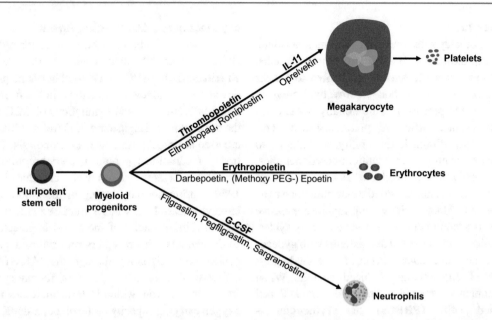

Fig. 10.13 Hematopoietic agents that stimulate myelopoiesis mimic the action of endogenous growth factors. Myeloid progenitor cells can differentiate into platelet-producing megakaryocytes, erythrocytes or neutrophils in response to growth factors, as shown. Medications that mimic the function of these growth factors can be used to increase the production of certain myeloid-derived lineages in the bone marrow of patients (figure contributed by Jeremy P. McAleer)

Table 10.3 Overview of hematopoietic agents

Hematopoietic agent	Indication	Mechanism of action
Epoetin	Anemia	Binds to EPO receptor on RBCs, activates JAK/STAT pathway to stimulate proliferation of RBCs
Darbepoetin	Anemia	Binds to EPO receptor on RBCs, activates JAK/STAT pathway to stimulate proliferation of RBCs
Methyl PEG epoetin beta	Anemia	Binds to EPO receptor on RBCs, activates JAK/STAT pathway to stimulate proliferation of RBCs
Filgrastim	Neutropenia	G-CSF (granulocyte colony stimulating factor) binds to receptor on granulocyte precursor cells in bone marrow to activate JAK/STAT pathway which stimulates proliferation of granulocytes, mainly neutrophils
Pegfilgrastim	Neutropenia	G-CSF (granulocyte colony stimulating factor) binds to receptor on granulocyte precursor cells in bone marrow to activate JAK/STAT pathway which stimulates proliferation of granulocytes, mainly neutrophils
Sargramostim	Neutropenia	GM-CSF (granulocyte macrophage colony stimulating factor) binds to receptor on precursor cells in the bone marrow to activate JAK/STAT pathways which stimulates proliferation of granulocytes as well as monocytes
Romiplostim	Thrombocytopenia	TPO mimetic which binds to TPO receptor to activate JAK/STAT and MAPK pathways for proliferation of megakaryocytes
Eltrombopag	Thrombocytopenia	TPO receptor agonist which activates JAK/STAT and MAPK pathways for proliferation of megakaryocytes
Oprelvekin	Thrombocytopenia	IL-11, binds to IL-11 receptor to activate JAK/STAT pathways for proliferation and maturation of megakaryocytes

Anemia

Chemotherapy- or cancer-induced anemia is seen in approximately 30–90% of cancer patients. Chemotherapeutic agents are known to impair hematopoiesis in the bone marrow by decreasing erythrocyte precursors. Additionally, some cytotoxic agents, particularly platinum-based therapies, may diminish the ability of kidneys to release erythropoietin. Platinum-based therapies, commonly used in head and neck cancers, lung, and ovarian cancers tend to cause both bone marrow and kidney toxicity, with myelosuppressive effects accumulating over several therapy cycles. Studies have suggested that patients with gynecologic and lung cancers seem to have the highest risk of chemotherapy-induced anemia. When treatment of anemia is warranted, **packed red blood cells (PRBCs)** or **erythropoiesis-stimulating agents (ESAs)** are used, however both come with drawbacks. PRBCs generally come from whole blood donations or are collected through apheresis. Some may undergo leukoreduction, irradiation, and testing for pathogens. Before transfusion, donor blood and the patient receiving the transfusion are cross-matched for ABO compatibility. The main benefit of PRBC transfusion is that it provides a quick increase in hemoglobin and hematocrit levels, and for this reason it is the preferred method to remedy anemia. For myelosuppressed chemotherapy patients who need immediate action to correct anemia, it is the only possible method. One of the biggest risks of PRBCs is transfusion-related reaction, however leukoreduction of the blood beforehand reduces the risk of this, and usually is done if the patient will require several transfusions. Other potential risks include congestive heart failure, bacterial contamination, viral infection, thromboembolism, or iron overload, which is generally only seen in patients who are receiving frequent transfusions over several years. Iron overload generally does not occur (or is less likely to occur) in patients who receive transfusions during chemotherapy treatment (over a period of less than 1 year). Due to the limited supply of blood in the United States, not every patient with chemotherapy-induced anemia will receive PRBCs, hence the reliance on ESAs.

Erythropoiesis-Stimulating Agents

Erythropoiesis is the production of erythrocytes (RBC) from hematopoietic stem cells. **Erythropoietin (EPO)** is a natural hormone produced by the kidney that is critical in the formation (differentiation and maturation) of RBC by the bone marrow. Engineered EPO (recombinant) are used as drugs to stimulate erythropoiesis. The first recombinant human erythropoiesis-stimulating agents (ESAs) were introduced in 1989. During normal filtering of the blood, the kidneys release EPO when a decrease in the oxygen carrying capacity of the blood is detected. EPO interacts with receptors on erythroid progenitor cells, signaling through the JAK/STAT pathway. This induces release of reticulocytes from bone marrow which in turn, increases the oxygen carrying capacity of the blood, a signal to the kidneys to stop releasing EPO. This feedback loop maintains red blood cell levels. Certain conditions, including chronic kidney disease (CKD) or toxicity to the bone marrow or kidney by chemotherapy agents can disrupt this feedback loop. Thus, the levels of erythropoietin released are inversely related to hemoglobin or hematocrit levels. Unlike PRBC transfusion, it can take weeks to detect an increase in hemoglobin with ESA therapy.

Due to some risks associated with ESAs, the FDA mandated black box warnings as well as a Risk Evaluation and Mitigation Strategies (REMS) program. While there is conflicting study data regarding worsening health outcomes and increased mortality, other possible increased risks include risk of venous thromboembolism in patients with cancer, and increased hypertension and seizures in patients with chronic renal failure. Patients on ESAs should have their hemoglobin levels monitored. Additionally, patients who have a sudden loss of response should be checked for erythropoietin antibodies. A rare condition known as pure red cell aplasia (PRCA) is characterized by low levels of reticulocytes, loss of erythroblasts in the bone marrow, as well as neutralizing antibodies against EPO. While a rise in cases of PRCA occurred from 1998 to 2004, the vast majority of these cases were associated with a formulation used outside of the United States.

Epoetin alfa (Procrit®, Epogen®) is a human recombinant EPO, is 34–39 kDa glycoprotein hormone manufactured by recombinant DNA technology and is measured in IU. EPO binds with the EPO receptor on the surface of RBCs. This interaction activates several signal transduction pathways including the JAK-STAT pathways. STATs are transcription factors that transcribes genes which stimulate proliferation and terminal differentiation of erythroid precursor cells and providing protection from RBC precursor apoptosis. Epoetin is generally given once to three times weekly until the completion of chemotherapy. Other common adverse effects include hypertension due to a quick rise of hemoglobin, fever, pruritis, rash, GI effects, and arthralgia. Chronic kidney disease (CKD) patients may experience seizures. Its therapeutic uses include anemia of chronic renal failure patients, anemia in zidovudine-treated HIV-infected patients, anemia in cancer patients with chemotherapy, and reduction of allogenic blood transfusion in surgery patients.

Darbepoietin alfa (Aranesp®) is a 37 kDA heavily glycosylated form of epoetin. It contains two additional N-linked carbohydrate chains at positions 30 and 88, as a result of five amino acid substitutions (Ala30Asn, His32Thr, Pro87Val, Trp88Asn, Pro90Thr). This glycosylation improves pharmacokinetic properties. Compared with epoetin, not only does darbepoetin have a threefold longer serum half-life (25.3 h), but it also has a lower receptor-binding affinity and enhanced *in vivo* bioactivity. Because of its longer half-life, darbepoetin can be dosed once weekly or even every 2–3 weeks until the completion of chemotherapy. Adverse effects include hypertension, peripheral edema, dyspnea, cough, and seizures in CKD patients. Perisurgical patients should receive DVT prophylaxis. Darbepoetin can be used to treat anemia due to CKD in patients on dialysis and patients not on dialysis. It can also be used for minimizing the effects of concomitant myelosuppressive chemotherapy, if there is a minimum of two additional months of planned chemotherapy upon initiation.

Methoxy polyethylene glycol-epoetin beta (Mircera®) was approved in June 2018 for the treatment of pediatric patients aged 5–17 years who are on hemodialysis from CKD and are converting from another ESA after stabilization of hemoglobin levels with an ESA.

Neutropenia

Neutropenia is a condition characterized by decreased neutrophil counts and is a disorder common with many traditional chemotherapies. As mentioned earlier, all blood cells are derived from same stem cell precursors. Granulocyte colony stimulating factor (G-CSF) or granulocyte macrophage colony stimulating factor (GM-CSF) are glycoproteins that stimulate the bone marrow to produce granulocytes and release them into the bloodstream. G-CSF is relatively specific and promotes neutrophil proliferation and maturation. On the other hand, GM-CSF is non-specific and promotes macrophages, eosinophils, and neutrophil proliferation and maturation. Bone marrow suppression and hematopoiesis is an inevitable result of cytotoxic chemotherapy. Decreases in neutrophil counts leaves the patient at great risk of infection. Since neutropenia can mask the signs and symptoms of infection, fever may be the only sign of infection. For patients with febrile neutropenia (neutropenia with fever), treatment with IV antibiotics must be initiated immediately to reduce the risk of spreading severe infection. The mortality rate from this complication is over 50%.

Colony Stimulating Factors

Filgrastim (Neupogen®) is recombinant human granulocyte-colony stimulating factor (rHuG-CSF). It is a non-glycosylated 18 kDA peptide of 175 amino acids with an amino acid sequence that is identical to the natural sequence predicted from human DNA sequence analysis, except for the addition of an N-terminal methionine necessary for expression in *E coli*. Filgrastim was introduced in 1991 for chemotherapy-induced neutropenia and interacts with a receptor on precursor cells in the bone marrow and stimulates proliferation and differentiation into mature granulocytes (the neutrophil lineage) through JAK/STAT signaling. Filgrastim more specifically stimulates and regulates neutrophils within the bone marrow. It is a hematopoietic growth factor, which regulates the production and function of neutrophils by controlling the proliferation of committed progenitor cells and influences their maturation into mature neutrophils. Filgrastim also stimulates the release of neutrophils from bone marrow storage pools and reduces their maturation time. Filgrastim binds with the receptor at the cell surface and activates the JAK-STATs pathways. STATs are transcription factors which upon activation, transcribes genes critical for cell including WBC differentiation and maturation. Filgrastim promotes survival, proliferation, and differentiation of neutrophil precursors and mature neutrophils, as well as mobilizes hematopoietic stem cells to the peripheral blood. Filgrastim can be given IV or subcutaneously daily for up to 2 weeks and should not be used 24 h before or after administration of cytotoxic chemotherapy; it may potentially act as a growth factor for tumors of myeloid origin. Adverse effects include fever, petechiae, rash, elevated LDH/uric acid levels, diarrhea, splenomegaly—severe chronic neutropenia, bone/skeletal pain in the lower back/posterior iliac crest or sternum, epistaxis, temporary increase in alkaline phosphatase. Common uses of filgrastim include treatment of cancer patients receiving myelosuppressive chemotherapy, patients with acute myeloid leukemia receiving induction or consolidation chemotherapy, as well cancer patients with cancer bone marrow transplantation (BMT) or hematopoietic stem cell transplantation (HSCT). Other possible uses include autologous peripheral blood progenitor cell collection and therapy, severe chronic neutropenia, and exposure to myelosuppressive doses of radiation (Hematopoietic Syndrome of Acute Radiation Syndrome). It should be noted that there are other products on the market similar to filgrastim. **Tbo-filgrastim (Granix®)** was approved in 2014 for self-administration to treat severe neutropenia in patients with non-myeloid malignancies. It is recombinant G-CSF and is not considered a biosimilar. There are two biosimi-

lars of filgrastim on the U.S. market, however, **filgrastim-sndz (Zarxio®)**, the first biosimilar ever approved by the FDA (in March 2015) and **filgrastim-aafi (Nivestym®)**.

Pegfilgrastim (Neulasta®) is the pegylated form of G-CSF, and thus has a longer half-life which allows for less frequent dosing. Pegfilgrastim should not be used 14 days before or 24 h after administration of cytotoxic chemotherapy; it may potentially act as a growth factor for tumors of myeloid origin. Adverse effects include peripheral edema, headache, GI side effects, bone pain, myalgias, and arthralgias. Neulasta® Onpro® is an on-body-injector applied by the healthcare provider after a strong chemotherapy treatment and automatically delivers the patient's dose of pegfilgrastim the following day (27 h following treatment). The injector delivers the dose over a period of 45 min. This prevents the patient from having to travel back to the hospital the day after chemotherapy. Common uses of pegfilgrastim include treatment of cancer patients receiving myelosuppressive chemotherapy, as well as patients exposed to myelosuppressive doses of radiation. There are currently two pegfilgrastim biosimilars on the market, **pegfilgrastim-jmdb   (Fulphila®)   and pegfilgrastim-cbqv (Udenyca®)**.

Sargramostim (Leukine®) is known as granulocyte-macrophage colony stimulating factor (GM-CSF). It is a recombinant human GM-CSF produced in a yeast expression system and is a partially glycosylated peptide of 127 amino acids available in 3 molecular species. It is relatively non-specific and promotes macrophages, eosinophils, and neutrophil survival, proliferation, differentiation, and maturation and to some extent RBC and platelets. It binds to the GM-CSF receptor (GM-CSF-R-alpha or CSF2R). This receptor activation stimulates JAK2-STAT and other signal transduction pathways including PI3K and MAPK. Thus, sargramostim stimulates proliferation and differentiation of granulocytes (neutrophils, basophils, eosinophils) and monocytes, as well as stimulates function of mature neutrophils. Adverse effects can include fever, arthralgia, myalgia, and capillary leak syndrome. It is used for various treatments including acute myeloid leukemia following induction chemotherapy, autologous peripheral blood progenitor cell mobilization and collection, autologous peripheral blood progenitor cell and bone marrow transplantation, allogeneic bone marrow transplantation, as well as allogeneic or autologous bone marrow transplantation: treatment of delayed neutrophil recovery or graft failure.

Thrombopoiesis-Stimulating Agents

Platelets, also known as thrombocytes, are fragments of larger precursor cells called megakaryocytes. The main function of platelets or thrombocytes is to stop excessive bleeding during accidents or injuries. Platelets are derived from the myeloid stem cells. **Thrombopoietin (TPO)** and **interleukin-11 (IL-11)** are two hematopoietic growth factors and cytokines that are responsible for the proliferation and differentiation of myeloid stem cells to platelets. TPO is a 332 amino acid glycoprotein produced primarily in the liver and kidney that stimulates the formation of megakaryocytes from CFU-Meg (colony forming unit, megakaryocyte). On the other hand, interleukin 11 is a 19 kD protein consisting of 199 amino acids and a member of a family of human growth factors which include human growth hormone, G-CSF etc. IL-11 stimulates megakaryopoiesis (differentiation and maturation of megakaryocytes). Megakaryocytes are cells from which platelets derive. Thrombocytopenia is a pathophysiologic condition with reduced platelet counts (circulating platelets <50,000/L) and presents bleeding risks. The causes of thrombocytopenia include spontaneous bleeding from small blood vessels all over the body, deficiency of clotting factors due to impaired liver function, hemophilia (hereditary bleeding disorders due to deficiency of clotting factors) and chemotherapy and immune-mediated destruction of platelets. Because platelets are essential to blood clotting, thrombocytopenia, or a decrease in blood platelets results in an increased bleeding risk. When platelet counts fall to below 10,000/μL, the risk of spontaneous bleeding increases. This is a major problem for cancer patients undergoing chemotherapy. Several drugs have been approved to stimulate megakaryopoiesis in thrombocytopenia. There are several mechanisms by which chemo-

therapeutic agents aid in decreased platelet numbers. Some treatments promote platelet apoptosis, while others, such as alkylating agents, affect hematopoietic stem cells in the bone marrow. Some treatments affect megakaryocytes directly and prevent platelets from being released from them. Unsurprisingly, a dose reduction in chemotherapy due to thrombocytopenia can impact a patient's survival. Transfusion with donor platelets is a common practice, however it can create infusion complications. Thrombopoietic agents were first introduced in 1994 and work to differentiate hematopoietic progenitor cells to become megakaryocytes, either through agonistic activity of the TPO receptor on the megakaryocyte surface or through growth factors. It takes approximately 10–14 days to increase platelet count after beginning a thrombopoietic agent.

Romiplostim (Nplate®) is a recombinant Fc-peptide fusion protein produced in *Escherichia coli* containing two side-chain subunits that each of a region of two TPO receptor-binding domains. Thus, it is considered to be a TPO mimetic and thus a TPO receptor agonist. It does not, however, have any amino acid sequence homology to TPO. It directly binds to the TPO receptor (TpoR, Mpl, or CD110 antigen), a cytokine receptor belonging to the hematopoietin receptor superfamily and activates the receptor. Activation of TpoR activates the JAK-STAT and Ras-MAPK pathways and transcribes genes that stimulates the proliferation and differentiation of megakaryocytes, resulting in an increase in the production of blood platelets. It works similarly to endogenous TPO. Romiplostim is given subcutaneously once weekly and should only be used when the degree of thrombocytopenia and clinical condition increase the risk for bleeding. Inadequate platelet response may be due to neutralizing antibodies to the drug or bone marrow fibrosis. The lowest dose should be used to maintain platelet counts of ≥50,000/μL. Adverse effects include headache, dizziness, insomnia, abdominal pain, fatigue, arthralgia, and myalgia. Romiplostim is indicated for the treatment of thrombocytopenia in patients with chronic immune thrombocytopenia (ITP) who have had an insufficient response to corticosteroids, immunoglobulins, or splenectomy.

Eltrombopag (Promacta®) is a small molecule drug which acts as an agonist of the thrombopoietin receptor (TpoR). Eltrombopag is taken once daily and is approved for the treatment of patients with immune (idiopathic) thrombocytopenia purpura (ITP) who have not responded to treatment with corticosteroids, splenectomy, or immunoglobulin therapy and should only be used when the degree of thrombocytopenia and clinical condition increase the risk for bleeding. An inadequate platelet response may be due to neutralizing antibodies or bone marrow fibrosis. Possible adverse effects include cataract formation, thromboembolism, GI upset, fatigue, headache, and jaundice. Eltrombopag does come with a black box warning for hepatotoxicity which is detected by increased liver enzymes and bilirubin. Additionally, as a counseling point it should be separated from antacids, foods high in calcium, or minerals such as iron, calcium, aluminum, magnesium, and zinc by at least four (4) hours.

Oprelvekin (Neumega®) is a recombinant IL-11 produced in E. coli. It is a 177 amino acid polypeptide with a molecular mass of approximately 19,000 g/mol and is non-glycosylated. Natural IL-11 has 178 amino acids. Oprelvekin binds to IL-11 receptor (IL-11R) and forms a high-affinity hexameric complex comprising IL-11 itself, IL-11R, and gp130. This leads to the activation of the JAK/STAT pathway, which transcribes genes important for proliferation of hematopoietic stem cells and megakaryocyte progenitor cells and for maturation of megakaryocytes. The end result is an increased platelet production. Oprelvekin is given subcutaneously once daily 6–24 h after chemotherapy treatment. Possible adverse effects include hypersensitivity, bone pain which typically occurs in the thighs, hips, or upper arms, flu-like symptoms, arrhythmias, fluid retention, or anemia. Rarely, administration of IL-11 can cause eye problems including swelling of the optic nerve, blurry vision, or vision loss. Oprelvekin is indicated for the prevention of severe thrombocytopenia and the reduction of the need for platelet transfusions following myelosuppressive chemotherapy in adult patients with non-myeloid malignancies who are at high risk of severe thrombocytopenia.

From Bench to Bedside: Development of Rituximab

Commentary by Kaitlin Armstrong

Rituximab is a chimeric monoclonal antibody that was originally developed to treat Non-Hodgkin's Lymphoma (NHL) and now is additionally FDA indicated for several other B cell-related cancers and autoimmune disorders, specifically rheumatoid arthritis and pemphigus vulgaris. Rituximab's approval in 1997 revolutionized lymphoma treatment. It targets the CD20 antigen, which is expressed on mature B cells, in order to initiate cell death through complement-mediated cytotoxicity and antibody-dependent cellular toxicity.

The first step towards the development of rituximab was the discovery and identification of NHL. Cancer of the lymphatic system was first characterized by a British physician named Thomas Hodgkin in 1832. Hodgkin described a disease of the lymph nodes and spleen which caused inflammation seemingly independent of an infection. His work was brought to light in 1865 by Samuel Wilk who found Hodgkin's observations from 1832 strikingly similar to his own and subsequently referred to the disease as "Hodgkin's lymphoma" (HL) in his paper. In the century that followed, work from dozens of different scientists went into the task of classifying and characterizing the numerous types of lymphomas based on organization and cell size, cell type, site of origin, tumor grading, clinical features, morphology, immunology, genetics, and cell lineages. The classification of HL based on cytology is attributed to the work of Sternberg et al.

in 1898 and Dorothy Reed in 1902 in the discovery of large, abnormal, multinucleated B cells which would later be called Reed-Sternberg cells. The presence of these Reed-Sternberg cells in a tumor biopsy is one of the differentiating factors between HL and NHL.

At the same time as the frenzy of research defining and classifying the types of lymphomas, work was being done in the realm of immunology which moved the scientific world closer to the discovery of rituximab through elucidating the types of lymphocytes and their respective receptors and signaling pathways involved in the pathogenesis of lymphomas. While thymectomy was found to prevent lymphocytic leukemia in the late 1950s, a landmark paper in 1961 from Jacques Miller identified the thymus as also playing a major role in immunity. Further studies supported this by demonstrating that a certain class of white blood cells, later termed T-lymphocytes, developed in the thymus. The distinction between B and T lymphocytes specifically was made 3 years later in 1965 by Cooper et al. who demonstrated that the cells producing antibodies originated in the chicken-equivalent of bone marrow and the cells that were responsible for hypersensitivity responses originated in the thymus. The CD20 antigen, at the time called B1, was the first surface protein identified on the B cell and was characterized using a monoclonal antibody in 1980.

As recombinant DNA techniques and tools became more widespread and monoclonal antibody technology improved, IDEC pharmaceuticals developed a chimeric monoclonal antibody specific for the CD20 receptor in 1991, which would become rituximab. Targeting CD20 induced mature B cell apoptosis, which was successful in combating the lymphoma and in the following clinical trials 40% of patients with NHL responded to rituximab alone with no dose limiting toxicity. In phase III of the clinical trials, rituximab was shown to significantly prolong time to treatment failure, duration of remission, and overall survival rates when combined with cyclophosphamide, hydroxydaunorubicin, oncovin, and prednisone (CHOP), which was the gold standard of treatment, compared to CHOP alone. Rituximab was approved in 1997 for NHL and become an essential component of RCHOP, which is the paradigm of treatment for NHL.

In 2006, rituximab was approved by the FDA for moderate-to-severe rheumatoid arthritis when used with methotrexate for individuals who had not seen a response to tumor necrosis factor antagonist therapies. Over half of the phase III clinical trial participants saw a 20% reduction in swollen and tender joints, demonstrating clinical effectiveness in treating B cell mediated autoimmune disorders through targeting CD20. In 2018, another indication for rituximab was approved by the FDA, allowing treatment of pemphigus vulgaris (PV) with this drug. In the Ritux-3 clinical trial, participants demonstrated remission of PV at the end of 24 months when treated with rituximab and a tapered corticosteroid compared 28% when treated with a corticosteroid alone. Rituximab was the first new drug for PV in over 60 years and has been a landmark therapy in both cancer and autoimmunity.

Summary

Cancer involves a complex interplay between the environment and inherited and acquired genetic mutations. Cancers that occur in immune cells are generally classified as leukemias or lymphomas, and many of the treatments are immunosuppressive in nature to promote the cell death of cancerous leukocytes. Many of these treatments are monoclonal antibody therapies targeting markers such as CD20, CD30, CD38, CD22, and SLAMF7. These may be expressed in greater amounts on immune cell cancers such as multiple myeloma, Hodgkin and Non-Hodgkin lymphoma, or Hairy cell leukemia. Other immunosuppressive-type therapies, including the Bi-specific T-cell engager therapy and CAR-T cell therapy utilize novel mechanisms of alerting and stimulating T-cells to target cancerous CD19 B cells in ALL. In contrast, the thalidomide drugs are small molecules which are immunomodulatory and may act directly on tumor cells to inhibit proliferation and to induce cell cycle arrest and apoptosis. They may also act indirectly on the tumor microenvironment to modulate angiogenesis and to activate the immune system.

Immunotherapies for both immune and non-immune cell cancers are aimed at stimulating the immune system in an effort to remove cancerous cells. The mechanisms by which many of these treatments work boost the immune response by inducing acute inflammation, promoting T cell growth and differentiation, or blocking inhibition of T cell activation, allowing them to remain functional. A novel treatment for prostate cancer, sipuleucel-T, acts as a cancer vaccine by activating and loading patient-derived DCs with an antigen from prostatic acid phosphatase, which is overexpressed on prostate cancer to promote cancer-targeted T cell activation. Other treatments utilize monoclonal antibodies to tumor-associated signaling pathways, including growth factor signaling through EGFR and angiogenic signaling through VEGF.

Because many cancer therapies can cause anemia, neutropenia, and/or thrombocytopenia, cancer patients may need to be prescribed a hematopoiesis-stimulating agent. Many of these medications mimic the functions of growth factors that increase the production of certain myeloid-derived lineages (red blood cells, leukocytes, or platelets) in the bone marrow of patients.

From discovery of the cells constituting various immune derived cancers to the many immunomodulating and antibody-based targeted therapies, as well as agents that reduce the deadly toxicity of bone marrow suppression to allow for treatment with cytotoxic chemotherapies, the field of immunology has been at the forefront of cancer pharmacology and revolutionized the way cancer is treated.

Case Study: Leukemia

Sarah Woods is a 62-year-old Caucasian female who is seeing her primary care physician. Her major complaint is that she has been fighting off a cold and feeling very fatigued over the last couple of weeks, but she thought it might just be because she is getting older. Her physical exam reveals bilateral lymph node enlargement. Her blood cell counts indicate that she is thrombocytopenic and has elevated leukocytes.

Sarah is referred to a local oncologist and undergoes a bone marrow biopsy, which reveals a diagnosis of acute lymphocytic leukemia (ALL) with 85% bone marrow involvement, primarily consisting of immature blasts carrying the following immunophenotype: HLA-DR+, CD19+, CD79a+, and CD22+. Further cytogenetic analysis reveals that Sarah's ALL is Philadelphia chromosome negative.

Sarah's oncologist decides to begin treatment immediately with a combination chemotherapy regimen Hyper-CVAD, which contains doxorubicin, vincristine, cyclophosphamide, methotrexate, cytarabine, mesna, and dexamethasone, while awaiting a bone marrow transplant. Sarah initially develops symptoms of nausea and vomiting from the treatment, but antiemetic medications provide relief and she continues with the cycle. After 2 weeks on the regimen, Sarah develops a fever and is admitted to the intensive care unit with a neutrophil count of 530/mm^3.

Sarah recovers from her infection, and after taking an extended break to allow for recovery of her immune cells, continues the rest of the cycles of chemotherapy and eventually undergoes a bone marrow transplant (BMT). Sarah's ALL is in remission for 3 years, when blood cell count monitoring reveals that her disease has relapsed. Her oncologist makes the recommendation that Sarah be treated with blinatumomab. Shortly after Sarah's infusion begins, her blood pressure drops and she has difficulty breathing. Her infusion is stopped and she is treated for her infusion reaction. A week later she is re-challenged and this second time does not have a reaction to the treatment. Treatment with blinatumomab is a long and difficult process, but Sarah eventually completes her course of treatment and her ALL again goes into remission.

1. What symptoms does Sarah have that are indicative of leukemia? Why?
2. Based on your knowledge of hematopoietic cell lineages and differentiation, why was Sarah diagnosed with ALL versus other types of leukemia or lymphoma?
3. Why does Sarah become neutropenic with the Hyper-CVAD therapy?
4. Sarah develops an infusion reaction in response to blinatumomab. Why is this a common concern with antibody-based therapies? What other toxicities could arise with blinatumomab and other immunotherapies having a similar mechanism of action?

Practice Questions

1. Which of the following is NOT a Hallmark of cancer?
   (a) Self-sufficiency in growth signals
   (b) Enhancing apoptosis
   (c) Sustained angiogenesis
   (d) Genome instability and mutation
2. All of the following describe ways in which tumor cells evade the immune response EXCEPT which?
   (a) Down-regulation of MHC I
   (b) Cleaving off MICA
   (c) Promotion of proinflammatory cytokines such as IL-6
   (d) Expression of PD-L1
3. Cancers derived from epithelial cells are considered
   (a) Leukemias
   (b) Sarcomas
   (c) Carcinomas
   (d) Blastomas
4. What differentiates a benign versus malignant tumor?
   (a) A tumor is considered malignant when it is larger than 10 cm
   (b) Benign tumors only develop in adipose tissue
   (c) A tumor is considered benign if it responds to therapy
   (d) A tumor is considered malignant once it had invaded beyond the basement membrane of the organ in which it is derived
5. Which of the following recombinant drugs is a cytokine that stimulates T cells?
   (a) oprelvekin
   (b) aldesleukin
   (c) ipilimumab
   (d) darbepoietin
6. Which of the following drugs binds to PD-1?
   (a) pembrolizumab
   (b) rituximab
   (c) atezolizumab
   (d) bevacizumab
7. Patient DF is on chemotherapy and has a neutrophil count of 1000/mm³ putting him at risk of infection. Which of the following drugs may be useful for patient DF?
   (a) romiplostim
   (b) epoietin
   (c) eltrombopag
   (d) filgrastim
8. All of the following drugs utilize and reprogram the patient's own immune cells EXCEPT which?
   (a) Kymriah™
   (b) Opdivo®
   (c) Provenge®
   (d) Yescarta®

9. Which of the following drugs is a thrombo-poietin receptor agonist?
   (a) oprelvekin
   (b) eltrombopag
   (c) filgrastim
   (d) brentuximab
10. Which of the following statements best describes multiple myeloma?
    (a) A cancer of pigmented skin cells.
    (b) A cancer of plasma cells
    (c) A cancer of T lymphocytes
    (d) A solid tumor of lymphoid cells
11. Is ipilimumab considered an immunosuppressant or immune stimulant? Explain.
12. Which statement best describes the mechanism of blinatumomab?
    (a) Binds to CD20 to induce apoptosis of B cells.
    (b) Binds to CTLA4 to inhibit suppression of T cell action.
    (c) Binds to CD30 and contains a cytotoxic microtubule disruptor which kills cancer cells.
    (d) Binds to CD3 on T cells and links them with CD19-expressing B cells to promote killing of cancerous B cells.
13. Which of the following drugs targets an EGFR family receptor? (Select all that apply)
    (a) Cetuximab (Erbitux®)
    (b) Denosumab (Xgeva®)
    (c) Trastuzumab (Herceptin®)
    (d) Necitumumab (Portrazza®)
14. What is the brand name of Bevacizumab
    (a) Avastin®
    (b) Darzalex®
    (c) Promacta®
    (d) Keytruda®
15. Which virus is considered the cause of over 99% of cervical cancers?
    (a) EBV
    (b) HIV
    (c) HPV
    (d) HBV
16. Which of the following is a major adverse effect that can be caused by necitimumab treatment?
    (a) cardiopulmonary arrest
    (b) hypertension

(c) neutropenia
(d) hyperthyroidism

17. Which of the following cancer types is trastuzumab approved by the FDA to treat? Select all that apply.
    (a) Breast cancer
    (b) Lung cancer
    (c) GIST
    (d) Colorectal cancer
18. Which of the following should be monitored in patients receiving BCG treatment?
    (a) neutropenia
    (b) high fever lasting longer than a day
    (c) creatinine clearance
    (d) cardiac function
19. How is treatment with denosumab beneficial for cancer patients?
    (a) It is a very effective anticancer agent
    (b) It reduces symptoms associated with bone loss caused by osteolytic lesions
    (c) It reduces bone marrow suppression caused by cytotoxic chemotherapy
    (d) It is an antidote for infusion reactions
20. What mutation is most common in chronic myeloid leukemia?
    (a) CTLA4
    (b) BCR-ABL
    (c) BRAF
    (d) EML4-ALK

Suggested Reading

Barkal AA, Weiskopf K, Kao KS, Gordon SR, Rosental B, Yiu YY, et al. Engagement of MHC class I by the inhibitory receptor LILRB1 suppresses macrophages and is a target of cancer immunotherapy. Nat Immunol. 2018;19:76–84.

Connell CM, Doherty GJ. Activating HER2 mutations as emerging targets in multiple solid cancers. ESMO Open. 2017;2(5):e000279.

Cooper MD, Peterson RD, Good RA. Delineation of the thymic and bursal lymphoid systems in the chicken. Nature. 1965;205:143–6.

Crawford J, Dale DC, Lyman GH. Chemotherapy-induced neutropenia: risks, consequences, and new directions for its management. Cancer. 2004;100(2):228–37.

D'Amato RJ, Loughnan MS, Flynn E, Folkman J. Thalidomide is an inhibitor of angiogenesis. Proc Natl Acad Sci U S A. 1994;91:4082–5.

DeVita VT, Chu E. A history of cancer chemotherapy. Cancer Res. 2008;68(21):8643–53.

Du FH, Mills EA, Mao-Draayer Y. Next-generation anti-CD20 monoclonal antibodies in autoimmune disease treatment. Auto Immun Highlights. 2017;8(1):12.

Ferreira JN, Correia LRBR, Oliveira RM, Watanabe SN, Possari JF, Lima AFC. Managing febrile neutropenia in adult cancer patients: an integrative review of the literature. Rev Bras Enferm. 2017;70(6):1301–8.

Franks ME, Macpherson GR, Figg WD. Thalidomide. Lancet. 2004;363:1802–11.

Gajria D, Chandarlapaty S. HER2-amplified breast cancer: mechanisms of trastuzumab resistance and novel targeted therapies. Expert Rev Anticancer Ther. 2011;11(2):263–75.

Gao Z-W, Ke Dong K, Zhang H-Z. The roles of CD73 in cancer. Biomed Res Int. 2014;2014:460654.

Grivennikov SI, Greten FR, Karin M. Immunity, inflammation, and cancer. Cell. 2010;140:883–99.

Hanahan D, Weinberg RA. The hallmarks of cancer. Cell. 2000;100(1):57–70.

Hanahan D, Weinberg RA. Hallmarks of cancer: the next generation. Cell. 2011;144(5):646–74.

Hassan MN, Waller EK. Treating chemotherapy-induced thrombocytopenia: is it time for oncologists to use thrombopoietin agonists? Oncology. 2015;29(4):295–6.

Javier RT, Butel JS. The history of tumor virology. Cancer Res. 2008;68(19):7693–706.

King T, Jagger J, Wood J, Woodrow C, Snowden A, Haines S, Crosbie C, Houdyk K. Best practice for the administration of daratumumab in multiple myeloma: Australian myeloma nurse expert opinion. Asia Pac J Oncol Nurs. 2018;5(3):270–84.

Kourlaba G, Dimopoulos MA, Pectasides D, Skarlos DV, Gogas H, Pentheroudakis G, et al. Comparison of filgrastim and pegfilgrastim to prevent neutropenia and maintain dose intensity of adjuvant chemotherapy in patients with breast cancer. Support Care Cancer. 2015;23(7):2045–51.

Kuter DJ. Managing thrombocytopenia associated with cancer chemotherapy. Oncology. 2015;29(4):282–94.

Leibbrandt A, Penninger JM. Novel functions of RANK(L) signaling in the immune system. Adv Exp Med Biol. 2010;658:77–94.

Li S, Pal R, Monaghan SA, Schafer P, Ouyang H, Mapara M, Galson DL, Lentzsch S. IMiD immunomodulatory compounds block C/EBP{beta} translation through eIF4E down-regulation resulting in inhibition of MM. Blood. 2011;117:5157–65.

Lian Y, Meng L, Ding P, Sang M. Epigenetic regulation of MAGE family in human cancer progression-DNA methylation, histone modification, and non-coding RNAs. Clin Epigenetics. 2018;10:115.

Magen H, Muchtar E. Elotuzumab: the first approved monoclonal antibody for multiple myeloma treatment. Ther Adv Hematol. 2016;7(4):187–95.

Miller JF. Immunological function of the thymus. Lancet. 1961;2(7205):748–9.

Millrine D, Kishimoto T. A brighter side to thalidomide: its potential use in immunological disorders. Trends Mol Med. 2017;23:348–61.

Mitsiades N, Mitsiades CS, Poulaki V, Chauhan D, Richardson PG, Hideshima T, et al. Apoptotic signaling induced by immunomodulatory thalidomide analogs in human multiple myeloma cells: therapeutic implications. Blood. 2002a;99:4525–30.

Mitsiades N, Mitsiades CS, Poulaki V, Chauhan D, Richardson PG, Hideshima T, et al. Biologic sequelae of nuclear factor-kappaB blockade in multiple myeloma: therapeutic applications. Blood. 2002b;99:4079–86.

Neelapu SS, Locke FL, Bartlett NL, Lekakis LJ, Miklos DV, Jacobson CA, et al. Axicabtagene ciloleucel CAR T-cell therapy in refractory large B-cell lymphoma. N Engl J Med. 2017;377:2531–44.

Nutt SL, Kee BL. The transcriptional regulation of B cell lineage commitment. Immunity. 2007;26(6):715–25.

Parcesepe P, Giordano G, Laudanna C, Febbraro A, Massimo Pancione M. Cancer-associated immune resistance and evasion of immune surveillance in colorectal cancer. Gastroenterol Res Pract. 2016;2016:6261721.

Ronson A, Tvito A, Rowe JM. Treatment of relapsed/refractory acute lymphoblastic leukemia in adults. Curr Oncol Rep. 2016;18(6):39.

Scott AM, Wolchok JD, Old LJ. Antibody therapy of cancer. Nat Rev Cancer. 2012;12(4):278–87.

Sharma P. Kumar P,2 and Sharma R. Natural killer cells—their role in tumour immunosurveillance. J Clin Diagn Res. 2017;11(8):BE01–5.

Sheskin J. Thalidomide in the treatment of Lepra reactions. Clin Pharmacol Ther. 1965;6:303–6.

Weiner GJ. Building better monoclonal antibody-based therapeutics. Nat Rev Cancer. 2015;15(6):361–70.

Answer Key

Chapter 1

1. The following are three examples of innate immune cells: (1) Macrophages are sentinel cells that are present at sites of pathogen entry such as the skin. In response to infection, macrophages produce a number of cytokines and chemokines such as TNFα and CXCL8 that enhance inflammation and promote the recruitment of leukocytes such as neutrophils to infected tissues. (2) Natural Killer (NK) cells are innate lymphocytes that are involved in immune responses to viral infections. When activated, NK cells produce potent cytokines such as IFN-γ, which induces viral elimination and promotes macrophage activity. (3) Dendritic cells are phagocytic cells that capture pathogens and present pathogenic peptides to naïve T cells to induce their activation. They are critical for the initiation of T cell responses during immunity.

   The following are three examples of adaptive immune cells: (1) CD4 T cells, also called helper T cells, are instrumental in the development of adaptive immune responses to specific antigens. They are required for the activation of CD8 T cells to some types of antigens and 'help' B cells in their production of antibodies. Distinct helper T cell subsets coordinate responses to different types of antigens. Examples include T_H1 cells, which mediate responses to intracellular bacteria and T_H2 cells, which mediate responses to parasites. (2) CD8 T cells, also called cytotoxic T cells, are important for the killing of virally-infected cells and mediate immune responses to tumor antigens. (3) B cells are adaptive immune cells that produce antibodies in response to foreign or cellular antigens.

2. The microbial composition of the gastrointestinal tract plays a pivotal role in the development of immune responses. Mice bred in a germ-free environment tend to have smaller secondary lymphoid organs, have lower levels of serum immunoglobulin, and generate weaker immune responses to foreign antigens. A number of studies suggest an important role for the microbiota in the development or prevention of inflammation in a wide variety of diseases, including inflammatory bowel disease, food allergy, and other diseases. The composition of the microflora is dynamic and can change as a consequence of environmental modulation such as treatment with antibiotics. Bacterial death after antibiotic treatment results in the recolonization of the GI tract with new species of bacteria that have the potential to further shape the immune system.

3. The four cardinal characteristics of inflammation are *rubor* (redness), *calor* (heat), *tumor* (swelling), and *dolor* (pain). Infection or injury to the host induces the production of cytokines by epithelial cells, macrophages, and mast cells that promote the recruitment of leukocytes to the infected or injured tissue. TNF-α and histamine promote

© Springer Nature Switzerland AG 2020
C. B. Mathias et al., *Pharmacology of Immunotherapeutic Drugs*,
https://doi.org/10.1007/978-3-030-19922-7

vasodilation and enhance vascular permeability, making blood vessels leaky, and facilitating the migration of leukocytes. This is responsible for the redness and heat associated with inflammation. The infiltration of cells such as neutrophils and leakage of fluid from blood vessels causes the swelling, and the pinching of the nerves associated with the blood vessels causes pain.

4. (a)

5. (a)

6. (b), (c)

7. (b)

8. (a), (d)

9. When cells such as epithelial cells are infected by viruses, they rapidly produce a number of molecules including various cytokines and chemokines. Of these, the type I interferons, IFN-α and IFN-β play a critical role in the induction of anti-viral responses. They increase the innate resistance of the cell to viral infection by turning on a number of genes that are involved in antiviral immunity. They also increase the expression of cell surface ligands for activating receptors on NK cells, and increase the activation and recruitment of NK cells.

10. NK cells express a number of receptors on their surface, the balance of which controls the activation of NK cells and the NK cell-mediated killing of virally infected cells. Inhibitory receptors on NK cells recognize MHC I molecules on host cells and prevent their activation-induced cytotoxic function. In contrast, activating receptors such as NKG2D recognize stress proteins on the surface of infected cells. During infection, the expression of HLA-E on cells is downregulated, while the expression of stress ligands is increased by type I interferons and other cytokines. This shifts the balance of receptor engagement on NK cells towards activation, resulting in activation-induced signals that initiate cytotoxic activity.

11. The process of activation of naïve T cells begins with the capture of antigens by APCs such as dendritic cells at sites of antigen entry. Pathogen-laden dendritic cells travel to secondary lymphoid organs such as the lymph node, expressing various costimulatory molecules such as B7.1 and B7.2 during the course of migration. They also upregulate the expression of MHC II in preparation to engage naïve helper T cells. In the lymph node, APCs make contact with naïve T cells, and present processed antigenic peptides on the surface of MHC molecules to T cell receptors on CD4 and CD8 T cells. This is then followed by the simultaneous engagement of costimulatory molecules on APCs to their receptors (such as CD28) on T cells. A number of other adhesive interactions occur strengthening the immunological synapse. The TCR-mediated activation of T cells induces a signaling cascade involving various tyrosine kinases and transcription factors, resulting in the activation of the gene for IL-2. IL-2-driven T cells further differentiate under the control of transcription factors in response to cytokine stimuli such as IL-12 or IL-4. Subsets of effector T cells and memory T cells are generated during the course of the response.

12. (a)

13. (c)

14. Several subsets of helper T cells have been characterized, based on the type of transcription factor they express, the cytokines responsible for their differentiation, and their immunological function. T_H1 cells produce cytokines such as IFN-γ and coordinate responses to intracellular bacteria. T_H2 cells produce IL-4 and IL-5 in response to parasitic antigens. T_H17 cells respond to extracellular bacteria and fungi by producing IL-17 and IL-22. T_H9 cells produce IL-9 and are involved in the generation of mast cell-specific responses. T_{FH} cells produce IL-4, IL-5, and IL-6 and promote the activation and maturation of B cells. T_{reg} cells produce IL-10 and TGF-β and suppress T cell-mediated inflammatory responses.

15. Antibodies employ a number of different mechanisms during protection against infectious organisms. These include neutralization,

opsonization, and antibody-dependent cellular cytotoxicity (ADCC). Neutralization involves the binding of antibodies to free pathogens or other pathogenic components and the prevention of their molecular or cellular activity. For example, the binding of hemagglutinin by dimeric IgA antibodies prevents the attachment of influenza virus to epithelial cells. Similarly IgG antibodies neutralize bacterial toxins by preventing the engagement of their receptors on cell surfaces. Opsonization involves the Fc receptor or complement receptor-mediated phagocytosis of pathogens or their components. The Fc portion of pathogen-bound antibodies such as IgG binds its corresponding Fc receptor on cells such as macrophages. This results in the phagocytosis or endocytosis of the pathogen and its degradation in vesicular compartments. ADCC involves the binding of IgG molecules to specific Fc receptors on NK cells. This antibody-mediated activation of NK cells induces their cytotoxic activity and promotes the killing of target cells expressing the specific antigen.

16. (b)
17. Somatic hypermutation is the process by which numerous mutations are induced in the complementarity determining regions of the variable portions of antibody molecules. The process is driven by the enzyme activation-induced cytidine deaminase (AID) and enhances the specificity and the affinity of the antibody molecule for the specific antigen. Successive mutations enhance the quality of the type of antibody produced, leading to the generation of a potent B cell repertoire containing highly effective neutralizing antibodies.
18. (b)
19. (b)
20. (a)
21. (a)
22. (a)
23. (a), (b), (c)
24. (b)
25. (a)
26. (c)

Chapter 2

Practice Questions

1a, 2b, 3c, 4a, 5b, 6b, 7d, 8d, 9d, 10b, 11ab, 12d

Chapter 3

Case Study: RhoGAM®

Questions:
1. It is an anti-D polyclonal antibody.
2. Anti-D antibodies bind to Rh+ erythrocytes that may cross the placenta during the pregnancy, and thus prevent naive B cells from binding to the erythrocytes and becoming active. Thus, memory B cells are not formed which would produce higher-affinity IgG bind to Rh+ erythrocytes in subsequent pregnancies.
3. Hemolytic disease of the newborn is a disease in which maternal antibodies against D-polypeptide cross the placenta and destroy fetal red blood cells.
4. Because it is IgG, RhoGAM® can cross the placenta, but it is not enough to cause hemolytic disease of the newborn on its own.
5. Yes, Carrie should receive injections of RhoGAM with each pregnancy to protect possible future pregnancies.
6. An Rh− mother would not need RhoGAM if the fetus was also Rh−

Practice Questions
1b, 2cd, 3b, 4c, 5d, 6b, 7c, 8c, 9d, 10c, 11cd

Chapter 4

1. The development of acute episodes of asthma is driven by mast cells which are activated by IgE and allergen exposure. Binding of allergen to IgE antibodies on mast cells induces signaling events via FcεRI, resulting in mast cell degranulation and the release of preformed mediators such as histamine which can induce smooth muscle contraction and

difficulty breathing. Subsequently, the release of lipid mediators such as leukotrienes and *de novo* synthesized cytokines also contribute to the development of inflammation and bronchoconstriction.

2. (d)
3. (e)
4. (a), (b)
5. (c)
6. (c)
7. (c)
8. (b)
9. (c)
10. (c)
11. (b)
12. (a), (c)
13. (a), (b)
14. (c), (d)
15. (c)
16. (a)
17. (b)
18. (d)
19. (b), (c)
20. (c)

Chapter 5

Case Study 1: Atopic Dermatitis

1. The development of atopic dermatitis involves the participation of a wide variety of immune cells and molecules that contribute to the pathogenesis of the disease. This includes T_H2 cells and cytokines produced by them such as IL-4 and IL-5, mast cells, eosinophils, and B cells. Topical corticosteroids suppress immune cell function and activity by inhibiting their activation, differentiation and migration. They also suppress the production of cytokines, chemokines, and lipid mediators from immune cells. Suppression of inflammation resolves the symptoms of atopic dermatitis and induces the processes of healing and tissue repair.

2. The atopic march refers to the tendency to develop a number of inter-related atopic conditions that progress throughout life, beginning during infancy or childhood and continuing into adult life. The diseases that comprise the atopic march include atopic dermatitis, food allergies, allergic rhinitis, and asthma. The progression of the atopic or allergic march is thought to typically begin with atopic dermatitis which transitions or is followed later on by other atopic conditions. This is why the doctor asked Janet's mother about her previous medical history.

3. Classical allergic eczema is thought to be mediated by T_H2 cells which produce elevated levels of T_H2 cytokines such as IL-4, IL-5, and IL-13. Increased IL-5 production has a potent effect on the generation, activation, and function of eosinophils, which contribute to tissue damage in the skin. Patients with atopic dermatitis therefore have elevated eosinophil counts.

4. Mechanical injury to the skin results in the introduction of allergens that penetrate the epithelial barrier and induce the activation of cells such as Langerhans cells and keratinocytes. Keratinocytes produce a number of cytokines and chemokines including TSLP, IL-33, and IL-25, which can stimulate type 2 immune responses. TSLP in particular modulates dendritic cell function, biasing them toward a phenotype that favors the activation of T_H2 cells.

5. (c)
6. (c)
7. Skin lesions in the dermis of patients with atopic dermatitis have been found to contain activated memory T_H2 cells and macrophages. T_H2 cells produce a number of cytokines that have potent effects on the allergic response. IL-4 and IL-13 cause keratinocytes and fibroblasts to release chemokines for T cells and eosinophils(including eotaxin), and increase the levels of IgE antibodies by promoting B cell class switching. IL-5 increases the differentiation and survival of eosinophils. IL-3 induces the generation of granu-

locytes and macrophages, and IL-3, IL9, and IL-10 stimulate mast cells and induce their activation. IL-31 causes the development of pruritis. Fas ligand and TNF-α expressed by activated T_H2 cells induce keratinocyte damage. T_H2 cytokines also downregulate the expression of antimicrobial peptides such as defensins increasing susceptibility to cutaneous infections with *S. aureus* and Herpes Simplex Virus-1.

8. Inflammation induced by T_H2 cells in the skin causes the downregulation of various antimicrobial peptides and other factors produced by keratinocytes in response to bacterial exposure. This facilitates infection of the skin by opportunistic skin bacteria such as *Staphylococcus*. The induction of immune responses against invading bacteria by T_H1 and T_H17 cells further increases skin inflammation and exacerbates the rash associated with eczema. This is the reason the doctor checked Janet for the presence of infection with *S. aureus*.

9. Dupixent® or dupilumab is an FDA-approved drug that inhibits signaling mediated via the IL-4Ra. This subunit is a component of both the type I IL-4 receptor on hematopoietic cells which binds IL-4, and the type II IL-4 receptor on non-hematopoietic cells, which can bind both IL-4 and IL-13. Dupilumab inhibits both the IL-4 and IL-13-mediated effects of allergic inflammation. It suppresses T_H2, T_H17, and T_H22 responses, and decreases the S100A anti-inflammatory proteins. It has been found to be extremely effective in eczema and thus may significantly improve Janet's condition.

10. (b)

Case Study 2: Plaque Psoriasis

11. Sarah's symptoms are indicative of moderate-to-severe plaque psoriasis. She also has psoriatic arthritis.

12. Since Sarah has plaque psoriasis with greater than 40% of body surface area involved, she is a candidate for systemic therapy. The first line drugs for systemic treatment include calcineurin inhibitors such as cyclosporine, methotrexate, and biologics. The physician decides to use short-course cyclosporine therapy which has been found to be very effective, along with anti-TNF inhibitors. Methotrexate is not recommended due to the potential for pregnancy, since it is known to be a teratogen. Adalimumab has been found to be very effective against psoriatic arthritis, reducing axial and distal joint swelling, and decreasing patient pain scores.

13. Since adalimumab is a TNF antagonist, care must be taken to prevent the onset of infections. Reactivation of latent tuberculosis is of particular concern since it is typically controlled *via* TNF-α-secreting activated macrophages.

14. The effects of adalimumab during pregnancy have not been well studied. It is a category B pregnancy agent that must be used with caution and where the benefits outweigh the risk for the patient. Adverse effects associated with adalimumab include the increased risk of development of infections during pregnancy. There is also the potential for increased placental transfer of the drug during the final trimester of pregnancy, with the possibility of affecting the fetus. Lastly, studies suggest that for dermatologic conditions, adalimumab during pregnancy is only advisable in the case of severe, recalcitrant disease. In Sarah's case, the physician prefers that she not be taking any oral medications during pregnancy.

15. Cyclosporine is a calcineurin inhibitor. It binds cyclophilin A within cells and forms a complex with calcineurin, preventing its ability to activate NFAT and induce the proliferation of T cells *via* IL-2 production.

16. Secukinumab is a human IgG1 monoclonal antibody against IL-17A. By blocking IL-17-mediated effects, it inhibits the activity of T_H17 cells, which are known to be major culprits in the development of psoriasis and psoriatic arthritis.

17. (b), (c)

18. (a)

Chapter 6

1. The type of IBD that most matches Ethan's prior history and current symptoms is Crohn's Disease (CD). Ethan has been experiencing weight loss and several bouts of unbloody diarrhea. He has had a history of chronic smoking which is a risk factor for CD.
2. Ibuprofen (Advil®) is associated with IBD flare-ups and can cause the disease to progress.
3. The colonoscopy is indicative of Crohn's Disease which is characterized by inflammation in the GI tract interspersed by normal bowel or "skip" areas.
4. (c)
5. (b), (c), (d)
6. Based on the information provided in the case, it is not possible to determine whether Brenda's symptoms may be due to IBD or other conditions such as irritable bowel syndrome.
7. Inflammation within the colon and rectum areas indicate that the type of IBD may likely be ulcerative colitis (UC). However, Crohn's Disease of the colon can present similarly. UC may also be indicated by the presence of blood within the stool. Further clarification will be dependent on the results from pathology.
8. Crypt abscesses may be found in both UC and CD. In CD however, they often progress to become aphthoid ulcers which may be accompanied in the future by non-caseating granulomas. It is therefore not possible to determine whether Brenda has UC or CD based on the presence of crypt abscesses.
9. A depletion of goblet cells and the absence of mesenteric lymph node involvement or non-caseating granulomas strongly suggest that the type of IBD is UC.
10. Aphthous ulcers are an extra-intestinal manifestation (EIM). They are linked to the inflammation from UC due to the release of cytokines such as TNF-α and IL-6 from immune cells.
11. Aminosalicylates (ASAs) are the most commonly used drug type to treat UC.
12. Corticosteroids are often used along with aminosalicylates to induce remission in patients with UC.
13. Immunomodulatory drugs such as TNF inhibitors are the next best option for the treatment of UC. Calcineurin inhibitors and antiproliferative drugs such as azathioprine may also be considered.
14. The integrin inhibitors natalizumab and vedolizumab have been linked to a significant increase in the risk of development of progressive multifocal encephalopathy in patients who have been infected with JC virus. Patients on these drugs must be monitored for infection with JC virus.

Chapter 7

Case Study 1

1. This patient is exhibiting signs and symptoms of MG deterioration, such as exhaustion, shortness of breath, difficulty walking and muscle cramping. If left untreated she may develop MG crisis where she will develop difficulty in breathing and require mechanical ventilation. She should be admitted as an inpatient.
2. For patients who have respiratory symptoms, bulbar symptoms, who are deteriorating, treatment should include either plasma exchange or IVIG. When choosing one treatment or the other, patient factors should be taken into consideration. For example plasma exchange is not recommended if she has sepsis, and IVIG is not recommended if she has deteriorating renal function, risks for thrombosis or previous reactions to IVIG such as anaphylaxis. Advantages of IVIG over plasma exchange is ease of administration and it requires less time. Advantages of plasma exchange is it has greater effectiveness and works quickly.
3. Immune globulin is a blood product (pooled plasma from blood donors) that contains IgG antibodies. Its mechanism of action in the

treatment of MG is not fully known but may be due to its effects of the body's production of antibodies. The dose for IVIG for MG is 1–2 g/kg total dose given over 2–5 days. If the patient has anti IgA antibodies and a history of IVIG reactions a very low IgA immune globulin should be chosen such as Gammagard S/D®. Initial infusion rates for IVIG are slow and then titrated up to a maintenance goal if tolerated by the patient. Starting infusions slowly help minimize infusion reactions.

4. IgA levels, CBC, baseline kidney function tests and electrolytes should be obtained. This patient should be monitored for infusion reactions.

5. Side effects of IVIG include increased temperature, body aches, urticaria, pruritis, infusion reactions and hypersensitivity reactions including anaphylaxis. Reactions can occur while IVIG is infusing and after the infusion is complete. Pre-medications are advisable 30–60 min prior to starting IVIG and should be tailored to each individual patient. Premedications include acetaminophen, diphenhydramine, an H2 blocker, and an IV steroid. Decreasing the IVIG infusion rate can also help treat mild reactions.

6. IVIG can be used for MG deterioration and MG crisis. It can be used in patients for chronic treatment who cannot tolerate immunosuppressants. This patient has an allergy to mycophenolate, corticosteroids, pyridostigmine. A thorough medication allergy history should be obtained because there are other medication options such as azathioprine, cyclosporine, tacrolimus and rituximab. For Samantha, she has been receiving IVIG with a good response. Due to her history of multiple medication allergies (with the assumption that she is not a candidate for other medication treatment options) it would be appropriate for her to continue her IVIG for chronic treatment of MG as an outpatient.

7. Currently subcutaneous infusions of immune globulin are being studied for the treatment of MG, for maintenance therapy and exacerbations. This route allows the patient to self-administer the medication via an infusion pump at home, instead of receiving IVIG as an outpatient through an infusion center.

8. Her serum AchR antibody status, and thyroid function tests would be helpful in evaluating her condition.

Case Study 2

1. Patients that have positive anti-cyclic citrullinated peptide (CCP) antibodies and rheumatoid factor, tend to develop worse disease. This patient has an established RA because she has had symptoms for ≥6 months.

2. Methotrexate is a folic acid antagonist and can cause folic acid deficiency. The recommended dose of folic acid is 1–4 mg daily. Folic acid supplementation can also help reduce methotrexate's adverse effects.

3. Yes, despite being on two DMARD medications it is appropriate to add a TNF-α inhibitor such as golimumab. For this patient who has moderate to severe rheumatoid arthritis adding another DMARD such as hydroxychloroquine can be tried, or a non-TNF biologic medication can be initiated or adding a TNF-α inhibitor to her drug regimen is another option. TNF-α inhibitors are monoclonal antibodies that reduce pro-inflammatory cytokines that are found in the synovium and decreases the pain and swelling in the joints. An advantage TNF-α inhibitors have is that they work faster than DMARD medications when they are used alone. Patients may respond even after one dose. Also when they are combined with DMARD medications they have an increased effectiveness. There are several TNF-α inhibitors on the market. Choosing which TNF-α inhibitor depends on the provider's experience and preference, patient response, dosing (weekly administration vs monthly) and insurance coverage (drug formularies). If a patient does not respond to one TNF-α inhibitor another TNF-α inhibitor can be tried.

4. This patient should have a complete blood counts, liver transaminase levels and serum creatinine levels monitored while on DMARD medications. TNF-α inhibitors can increase the risk for developing infections. Baseline

TB testing should be performed prior to initiating a TNF-α inhibitor. While receiving TNF-α inhibitors complete blood counts, liver transaminase levels should also periodically be monitored.

5. Yes, clarification should be obtained to indicate if her "sulfa" allergy is a sulfonamide allergy. If the patient is receiving sulfasalazine which contains an arylamine structure, there can be a cross reaction to sulfonamides.

6. This patient increased her prednisone to 20 mg to treat her RA symptoms despite receiving 2 DMARD medications and a TNF-α inhibitor. Golimumab can be discontinued and another TNF-α inhibitor can be initiated. A non TNF biologic can also be trialed.

7. Tocilizumab is a anti-IL-6 biologic agent and a monoclonal antibody that inhibits the pro-inflammatory cytokine Interleukin-6 from binding to its receptors. It can be given as an IV infusion over 60 min every 4 weeks or subcutaneously every week to every other week.

8. Side effects of tocilizumab include hypersensitivity reactions, headache and injections site reactions. Premedication prior to starting tocilizumab infusions is not required unless she experienced reactions in the past.

This patient should have complete blood counts, liver transaminase levels, and a lipid panel monitored while on tocilizumab. Tocilizumab can increase the risk for developing infections. Baseline TB testing should be performed prior to initiating tocilizumab and during tocilizumab treatment.

Practice Questions
1a, 2b, 3c, 4c, 5a, 6a, 7d, 8a, 9c, 10acde, 11d, 12c, 13b, 14d, 15ab

---

Chapter 8

Case Study

1. Antithymocyte globulin is reactive against T cells, B cells, NK cells, DCs, and macrophages among other cells, effectively depleting cells expressing CD2, CD3, CD4, CD8, CD11a, or CD18, through opsonization/phagocytosis, complement-mediated lysis, or ADCC. In addition to depletion, this treatment can suppress antigen-dependent T cell proliferation.

2. Tacrolimus is a calcineurin inhibitor which inhibits the activation of the transcription factor NFAT. This prevents the production of IL-2 and suppresses the expansion of alloreactive T cells.

3. Omeprazole interacts with the Cytochrome P450 (CYPE 3A4) enzyme system, increasing the levels of cyclosporine.

4. Rituximab is a humanized antibody targeting the CD20 antigen on mature B cells. In this way, rituximab labels B cells for complement-mediated lysis, macrophage-mediated phagocytosis, and NK cell-dependent lysis (ADCC).

Practice Questions

1. An autograft is a graft that is transferred from one part of a body to another. An example of an autograft is transfer of skin from one part of the body to another site.

   An isograft involves the transfer of grafts between genetically identical individuals, such as the transfer of a kidney to a genetically identical twin.

   An allograft is a transfer of organs between members of the same species such as the transfer of a liver between two HLA-compatible individuals.

   A xenograft involves the transfer of organs between members of different species, such as the transfer of a heart from a pig to a human.

2. Hyperacute rejection can occur within minutes to hours of the transfer of a graft. It is mediated by pre-existing antibodies against blood group antigens on the donor graft or against donor HLA molecules. Pre-existing antibodies against donor HLA may have been generated as a result of previous pregnancies, blood transfusions, or transplantation procedures.

3. Blood cells express the polymorphic antigens O, A, and B on their surface. The A and B

antigens are glycosylated modifications of the O antigen. In addition, blood cells also express a number of other antigens including the Rh factor. Different individuals within the population express distinct combinations of these blood antigens and in general may be classified to be either positive for O, A, or B, negative for O, A, or B, and positive or negative for A and B. Some commensal bacteria share epitopes that are similar to those expressed on the A and B antigens, resulting in the production of antibodies against these antigens. When individuals of a particular blood group such as O$^+$ are transfused with blood from a different group such as A$^+$, these cross-reactive antibodies initiate type II hypersensitivity reactions that induce destruction of the blood cells accompanied by fever, chills, and other symptoms. Therefore, successful blood transfusions involve the assessment of a cross-match test which determines the compatibility of blood group antigens between the donor and the recipient.

4. (c)
5. (b)
6. Acute rejection occurs when dendritic cells from the donor graft travel to secondary lymphoid organs in the recipient and activate recipient T cells against the graft. This is referred to as the direct pathway of allorecognition. In contrast, chronic rejection occurs much later, when recipient dendritic cells present HLA molecules from donor cells to recipient T cells. This results in the activation of recipient helper T cells, which then activate B cells to produce antibodies. Activated antibodies attack the vasculature of the graft, causing fibrosis, tissue damage, and graft rejection. This process is termed as the indirect pathway of allorecognition.
7. A number of drugs may be used to suppress acute rejection after solid organ transplantation. Calcineurin inhibitors such as cyclosporine prevent the activation of NFAT in T cells and suppress their proliferation by inhibiting IL-2 production. Some adverse effects associated with these drugs include nephrotoxicity, hepatotoxicity, and hypertension.

Prednisone is a glucocorticoid that may be used to suppress acute rejection. It has a variety of effects on leukocyte gene transcription, activation, cytokine production, phospholipase production, and migration. Long-term treatment with corticosteroids is associated with a number of symptoms including weight gain, diabetes, and Cushing syndrome among others. Basiliximab is a monoclonal antibody against CD25, which is expressed on T cells. It prevents the binding of IL-2 to its receptor and inhibits T cell proliferation. In general, basiliximab is not associated with serious adverse effects. However, precautions must be taken, when administered along with other immunomodulatory drugs.

8. (b)
9. (b)
10. (a)
11. (a)
12. (b)
13. (a), (c)
14. (c)
15. (c)
16. Alemtuzumab is an example of a depleting antibody used in induction regimens for transplantation. It depletes leukocytes by binding CD52 on NK cells, T cells, B cells, and other leukocytes. Daclizumab is an example of a non-depleting antibody used in transplantation. It binds the IL-2Rα chain (CD25) on T cells and prevents their expansion without causing cellular lysis. It may be used as a prophylactic agent or to prevent acute rejection.
17. (a), (d)
18. (a), (b), (d)
19. (b)
20. (c)

Chapter 9

Case Study

Questions:

1. Gerald should receive an influenza vaccine, herpes zoster vaccine, and pneumococcal

vaccine. Gerald may also be a candidate for the Hepatitis B vaccine due to the risk associated with blood borne infection.*

2. Since Gerald is older than 65, he should receive a PCV13 vaccine, followed by PPSV23 1 year later. Had he been in the 19–64 age group, he would have received PPSV23 first due to his type II diabetes.*

3. Adults 65 and older with no history of prior pneumococcal vaccination should receive one dose of PCV13. They should then receive PPSV23 at least one year after the dose of PCV13.*

4. PCV13 is a conjugate vaccine which protects against 13 strains of pneumococcus, while PPSV23 is a polysaccharide vaccine which protects against 23 strains of pneumococcus.

5. Gerald does not appear to have any contraindications to being immunized at this time.

6. Based on his age, Gerald could receive the standard IIV3 or IIV4 vaccine, the adjuvanted Fluad™ vaccine, or the high dose Fluzone®. *

*Immunization guidelines may be periodically re-evaluated and updated based on a number of factors. Please refer to current immunization guidelines before making clinical decisions.

Practice Questions

1c

2. A recombinant vaccine utilizes DNA technology to create an antigen that will be utilized in the vaccine. The gene for this antigen is inserted into a vector and is then grown in a cell line which subsequently begins producing the protein of interest. This protein can then be isolated, purified, and used in the vaccine.

3d

4. Adjuvants are substances that enhance immune response by inducing inflammation and uptake of an antigen (which is usually stand-alone or part of an inactivated vaccine) by an APC, such as a dendritic cell.

5b, 6c, 7a, 8b, 9be

Chapter 10

Case Study

1. Sarah is fatigued and it has taken her several weeks to fight a cold virus. This is because abnormal leukocytes are being produced and crowding out stem cells in the bone marrow that would become normal functioning red and white blood cells. This can then result in anemia which may contribute to Sarah's fatigue, as well as her decreased ability to fight infection.

2. Sarah's bone marrow biopsy revealed mainly immature blasts that are HLA-DR+, CD19+, CD79a+, and CD22+. Because these surface molecules are associated with B cells, it suggests that this cancer is lymphocytic in nature. This differs from AML or CML, which affect myeloid stem cells which become red blood cells, platelets, or granulocytes. It is also likely that Sarah has acute leukemia, as opposed to chronic leukemia, as a majority of the cancer cells are immature. Additionally, because her bone marrow biopsy revealed abnormal cells, it probably originated there and not in the lymph nodes or other lymph tissues, as a lymphoma would.

3. There are several cytotoxic chemotherapies in the Hyper-CVAD regimen, including Doxorubicin, Vincristine, Cyclophosphamide, Methotrexate, and Cytarabine, which can cause myelosuppression resulting in neutropenia. Filgrastim, or pegfilgrastim, is often given after chemotherapy to patients who become neutropenic.

4. Blinatumomab is derived from mouse monoclonal antibodies. Non-human portions of antibodies tend to induce an immune response during infusion, including cytokine release syndrome

(fever, fatigue, rapid heartbeat, low blood pressure, trouble breathing, weakness, dizziness, headache, nausea, vomiting, or chills), which ranges from mild to life threatening. This results from a flood of cytokines into the bloodstream from the immune cells activated by the therapy.

Practice Questions

1b, 2c, 3c, 4d, 5b, 6a, 7d, 8b, 9b, 10b

11. It is an immune stimulant given that it inhibits an inhibitory mechanism (CTLA4), allowing T cells to stay active.

12d, 13ad, 14a, 15c, 16a, 17ac, 18b, 19b, 20b

Glossary

5-aminosalicylic acid (5-ASA) Aminosalicylic acid, a salicylate that is used for its local anti-inflammatory properties in the treatment of inflammatory bowel disease.

5-lipoxygenase Enzyme involved in the synthesis of cysteinyl leukotrienes from arachidonic acid in cells; it is targeted by the drug *Zileuton*.

6-mercaptopurine (6-MP) The active form of azathioprine in the body.

$\alpha_4\beta_7$ Integrin expressed on lymphocytes that preferentially migrate to the GI tract. Interacts with MAdCAM-1 on intestinal vascular endothelium.

AchR Acetylcholine receptor, nicotinic receptors bind to acetylcholine at the neuromuscular junction resulting in innervation of the muscle.

Acid fast bacilli (AFB) General nomenclature used to refer to certain species of bacteria, including mycobacteria, which resist decolorization during staining procedures despite multiple acid washes. Mycobacteria such as *Mycobacterium tuberculosis* appear bright red when stained with an acid-fast stain such as Ziehl Neelson's stain. The resistance to decolorization with acids occurs due to the presence of a large number of lipids in the bacterial cell wall, known as mycolic acids.

Acquired immunodeficiency syndrome (AIDS) Disease caused as a result of infection with the Human Immunodeficiency Virus. AIDS occurs during the final stage of HIV infection, concurrent with a dramatic reduction in CD4 helper T lymphocytes. This results in immune compromise and susceptibility to the development of a number of opportunistic infections.

Activation Induced Cytidine Deaminase (AID) Enzyme expressed in B cells following CD40 ligation and required for antibody somatic hypermutation and isotype switching. It deaminates DNA at cytosine residues, converting them to uracil. The repair of damaged DNA contributes to somatic hypermutation and isotype switching.

Active immunization Resistance acquired after the production of antibodies by the immune system after exposure to a foreign antigen.

Acute lymphoblastic leukemia (ALL) A cancer of the bone marrow resulting in abnormal immature white blood cells.

Acute Myeloid Leukemia (AML) A cancer originating in the bone marrow that affects myeloid stem cells which can become red blood cells, platelets, or granulocytes.

Acute phase proteins Proteins released by the liver as a result of an acute phase reaction in response to inflammation. Positive acute phase proteins act to inhibit the growth of microbes.

Acute phase response Innate immune response that occurs soon after infection. It involves the production of acute-phase proteins by the liver and their secretion into blood, changing the profile of proteins that can be enumerated in the serum.

Acute rejection Rejection of a transplanted organ from a genetically incompatible donor due to T cell responses against HLA differences between the donor and the recipient. Acute rejection can occur within a week to three months after the transplant.

Acute rheumatic fever (ARF) Occurs secondary to a Group A streptococcal infection and

© Springer Nature Switzerland AG 2020
C. B. Mathias et al., *Pharmacology of Immunotherapeutic Drugs*,
https://doi.org/10.1007/978-3-030-19922-7

can manifest as carditis, arthritis, involuntary movements (chorea), red pink rings on the skin known as erythema marginatum, or subcutaneous nodules.

ADAM 33 A glycoprotein belonging to the "*a disintegrin and metalloproteinase*" gene family that is involved in cellular proteolysis, cleavage, cell adhesion and cell signaling during many cellular processes including fertilization, myogenesis, neurogenesis, the inflammatory response and apoptosis. It has been linked to various features of asthma including bronchial hyperresponsiveness and airway remodeling.

Adaptation Organ transplant recipient becoming tolerant to alloantigens over time due to immunosuppressive therapy.

Adaptive immunity Pathogen specific immunity in which T and B lymphocytes mount a response to an antigen, creating immunological memory, resulting in a faster and more enhanced response upon a second exposure.

Agammaglobulinemia The inability to make antibodies, which can occur due to a primary immunodeficiency such as a hereditary defect in immune function, or due to secondary effects such as leukemias, poor nutrition, or certain types of drugs. It is reflected by abnormal or low amounts of antibodies in serum.

Antibody dependent cellular cytotoxicity or ADCC The process by which IgG antibodies coat surface antigens on target cells and induce the activation of FcγRIII (CD16)-bearing NK cells which destroy the target via NK cell mediated cytotoxicity.

Adjuvant Substances found in a vaccine that enhance immune response by inducing inflammation and uptake of the antigen by an APC, such as a dendritic cell.

Affinity maturation Process coupled with somatic hypermutation in which B cells with antibodies that acquire mutations that increase binding affinity to antigens are selected to survive.

AIRE Autoimmune regulator, a transcription factor expressed in the thymus that is involved in the elimination of self-reactive T cells.

Airway hyperresponsiveness (AHR) AHR or bronchial hyperresponsiveness (BHR) is the increased sensitivity of the airways to inhaled stimuli or constricting agonists. It is caused as a result of bronchoconstriction or bronchospasm due to constricting bronchioles and is a defining characteristic of asthma.

Airway remodeling Structural changes that occur in the small and large airways during inflammatory diseases. These changes can occur due to subepithelial fibrosis, increase in smooth muscle mass, epithelial changes, gland enlargement, and vascularization of tissues.

Allergen Antigenic substance that induces the development of allergy in susceptible individuals. Types of allergens include low molecular weight proteins, certain types of drugs, occupational chemical antigens, food-derived substances, pollutants, and other antigens derived from plants or animals.

Allergy A condition that is caused by the development of an immune response to non-cellular antigens that do not pose a threat to the well-being or survival of a host. Various types of hypersensitivity reactions may be involved during an allergic response.

Alloantibodies Antibodies recognizing antigens from non-self HLA alleles or erythrocyte AB antigens. They may play a role in organ transplant rejection.

Alloantigen Antigens derived from non-self HLA alleles that are recognized by recipient- or donor-derived lymphocytes following transplantation.

Allogeneic transplantation Transplantation procedure in which a patient receives an organ, tissue, or cells from another individual.

Allograft Tissue transplanted from a donor of the same species as the recipient.

Alopecia Areas of hair loss. May be an adverse effect of certain drugs.

Alveolar macrophage (AM) A type of macrophage found in the lung that is involved in pulmonary defense. It is generally immunosuppressive but can be stimulated during inflammation.

Alveolus (alveoli) Lung alveoli are the basic unit of ventilation and are the terminally differentiated components of the respiratory tree. Their primary function is the exchange of the gases, oxygen and carbon dioxide. They participate in ventilation, diffusion, and perfusion of lung tissue.

Anaphylaxis Severe, potentially life-threatening, systemic allergic reaction involving one or more organ systems that typically occurs within seconds to minutes. It occurs as a result of systemic IgE-mediated mast cell and basophil activation upon IgE cross-linking of an allergen.

ANCA Anti-neutrophil cytoplasmic antibodies, autoantibodies produced that can target and attack neutrophils.

Anemia A condition resulting from low levels of healthy red blood cells or hemoglobin.

Anergy Non-responsiveness of a T cell or B cell following exposure to its cognate antigen.

Angiogenesis The process by which new vasculature is formed.

Ankylosing spondylitis Inflammation primarily of the axial skeleton but peripheral joints and extraarticular structures may be involved. The hallmark sign is involvement of the sacroilliac joints.

Anti-CCP antibodies Anti-cyclic citrullinated protein antibody. Diagnostic antibodies against citrullinated proteins that are a diagnostic marker of Rheumatoid arthritis.

Anti-GBM antibodies Antibodies against glomerular basement membrane maybe seen in autoimmune disorders that affect the kidney, such as Goodpasture's disease.

Anti-nuclear antibodies (ANA) A common autoantibody found in lupus.

Anti-Smith antibodies Antibodies that target seven proteins that constitute the common core of small nuclear ribonuclear protein particles, often found in lupus.

Antibody Secreted immunoglobulin molecules produced by plasma cells (differentiated form of B cells) that protect the host during infection and evolved to destroy pathogens and other causes of host damage.

Antigen Macromolecules (proteins, polysaccharides, glycoproteins, glycolipids, nucleic acids) or peptides recognized by antigen receptors on T cells and B cells.

Antigen presentation The process by which antigens are processed into short peptide fragments that are displayed on MHC molecules to induce the activation of naive T cells.

Antigen presenting cell (APC) Cells that present antigen on their surface via major histocompatibility complex class I (MHC I) and MHC class II to naive and activated T cells. They include dendritic cells, macrophages and B cells.

Antigen receptor repertoire The total variety of antigen receptors present in an individual.

Antigenic drift Small changes or point mutations in influenza genes that happen over time as the virus continues to replicate. Antigenic drift is responsible for seasonal changes in the strains of influenza virus.

Antigenic shift A major change in genetic makeup of influenza virus. Antigenic shift typically occurs when genetic material from two different influenza viruses is recombined in a foreign species. Viruses arising from antigenic shifts are the usual causes of influenza pandemics.

Antimicrobial peptides (AMPs) Innate immune proteins that can help kill both Gram-positive and Gram-negative bacteria, as well as fungi and enveloped viruses.

AP-1 Transcription factor complex involved in lymphocyte activation.

Apoptosis Programmed cell death occurring as a normal part of growth and development.

ART/HAART Antiretroviral therapy/Highly active antiretroviral therapy used to manage HIV infection. In HAART, a cocktail of anti-retroviral drugs is used to decrease the viral load and prevent the development of resistance to anti-retroviral therapy.

Arthralgia Pain in a joint, including stiffness, and reduced mobility.

Arthritis Joint pain as a result of inflammation resulting in swelling and loss of cartilage and bone leading to reduced mobility.

Asthma Respiratory disease of the airways that is characterized by wheezing, chest tightness, and shortness of breath. The pathophysiological features of the disease include chronic bronchial inflammation predominantly involving eosinophils, bronchoconstriction, mucus hyperplasia, and airway remodeling. The disease is driven by subsets of helper T cells (TH2), mast cells, eosinophils, IgE antibodies, and other immune mediators.

Ataxia Lack of coordination of voluntary muscle movements. Can be caused be genetic factors, certain drugs, stroke, alcohol abuse, cerebral palsy, brain degeneration, or multiple sclerosis.

Atopic dermatitis (AD) Allergic inflammatory disease of the skin characterized by a red, scaly, itchy rash. It is an IgE-mediated disease driven by T_H2 cells, eosinophils, mast cells, and other immune mediators.

Atopy The genetic predisposition to develop allergies to common innocuous environmental allergens. It is associated with heightened sensitivity to allergens and the production of elevated levels of IgE antibodies.

Attenuated vaccine A vaccine that contains live pathogen with reduced virulence.

Autoantibodies Antibodies which target autoantigens, or self-antigens in autoimmune disease.

Autoantigens Self-antigens to which the immune response may direct antibodies against in autoimmune disease.

Autograft Cells or tissue transplanted from one site to another within an individual.

Autoimmune hemolytic anemia (AIHA) A relatively uncommon disorder in which IgG or IgM antibodies bind to the surface of red blood cells. This binding activates classical complement and the membrane attack complex causing red blood cells to lyse.

Autoimmune Polyendocrinopathy-Candidiasis-Ectodermal Dystrophy (APECED) An autoimmune disorder in which AIRE (autoimmune regulator) is found to be mutated, and results in destruction of endocrine tissue and chronic candidiasis.

Autoimmunity Immune reaction to self-antigens.

Autologous transplantation Transplantation procedure in which stem cells are collected from a patient prior to a conditioning regimen and then reinfused after therapy.

B cell Lymphocyte derived from the common lymphoid progenitor and completes its development in the bone marrow. B cells express receptors in the form of membrane-bound immunoglobulins and secrete antibodies upon activation.

β_2-adrenergic receptor A cell membrane spanning receptor that is activated by binding epinephrine and induces smooth muscle relaxation.

β_2-agonist A type of drug class that binds β_2-adrenergic receptors on smooth muscle cells and induces their relaxation.

Bacille Calmette-Guerin (BCG) vaccine A tuberculosis vaccine that was developed from a live attenuated strain of *Mycobacterium bovis* and first administered to humans in 1921 to induce protection against tuberculosis. Currently, it is used to vaccinate infants against tuberculosis in many countries. It is also used as an immunostimulant in the treatment of superficial carcinoma of the bladder.

BAFF/BLyS B cell activating factor/B lymphocyte stimulator. B cell-derived cytokine in the TNF ligand family that induces cell growth, proliferation, survival and differentiation.

Basophils Least common granulocytic white blood cell that stains with basic dyes. It is involved in anti-parasitic responses, but is pathological in allergy and other diseases.

BCL6 B-cell lymphoma 6 protein, a transcription factor required for T_{FH} cell differentiation.

BCR B cell receptor. Membrane-bound antigen receptor expressed on the surface of B cells and structurally identical to antibodies.

Biosimilar A product that is identical to a biological product that is already on the market but is produced by another manufacturer, and has no clinically meaningful significant differences.

BiTE Bi-specific T cell Engager. Fusion protein containing antibody variable region fragments recognizing two antigens. In anti-cancer therapy, one antibody fragment recognizes CD3 on the surface of effector T cells while the other fragment recognizes a tumor-associated antigen, such as CD19 on malignant B cells.

Blood brain barrier (BBB) A semi-permeable border that separates circulating blood from the brain.

Bone marrow Primary lymphoid organ that produces blood cells through the process of hematopoiesis. It is also the organ where T and B cells are generated and where B cells complete their development and maturation.

Bone marrow stromal cells (BMSCs) Skeletal progenitor cells which invade and form along blood vessels in the bone marrow cavity.

Bone marrow transplant (BMT) Bone marrow transplant, a procedure which replaces bone marrow that has been destroyed by cancer or infection with bone marrow stem cells from a donor.

Bronchial associated lymphoid tissue (BALT) Tertiary lymphoid structures consisting of lymphoid follicles and immune cells that participate in mucosal immune responses in the respiratory tract.

Bronchial hyperresponsiveness (BHR) BHR or airway hyperresponsiveness (AHR) is the increased sensitivity of the airways to inhaled stimuli or constricting agonists. It is caused as a result of bronchoconstriction or bronchospasm due to constricting bronchioles and is a defining characteristic of asthma.

Bronchoalveolar lavage (BAL) fluid Fluid collected from the lungs of patients or experimental animals to assess the development of lung inflammation. The collected fluid is examined for the presence of inflammatory cells, cytokines, chemokines, and other mediators that contribute to airway inflammation.

Bronchoconstriction Constriction or narrowing of airways within the lungs due to tightening of the smooth muscles surrounding the bronchi and bronchioles. Induction of bronchoconstriction results in wheezing and shortness of breath.

C-reactive protein (CRP) Acute-phase reactant protein produced in the liver that becomes elevated in response to inflammation.

C3 Complement protein 3, which is cleaved into C3a and C3b during the complement cascade.

C3a Complement protein 3a, which acts as an anaphylatoxin, and is involved in the recruitment of inflammatory cells during the complement cascade.

C3b Complement protein 3b, which tags pathogens for opsonization by macrophages and other immune cells, also referred to as complement fixation.

C5 Complement protein C5, which is cleaved into C5a and C5b during the complement cascade.

C5a Complement protein C5a, which like C3a, also acts as an anaphylatoxin by binding to receptors on mast cells and basophils, and induces the recruitment of inflammatory cells during the complement cascade.

Calcineurin Inhibitors Drugs such as cyclosporine and tacrolimus, which bind calcineurin in cells, and prevent the activation of T cells by inhibiting the transcriptional activity of NFAT.

Candidate vaccine virus (CVV) A virus that has been prepared by a public health entity and is used by vaccine manufacturers to mass produce a vaccine.

Capillary leak syndrome (CLS) A condition caused by leakage of fluid from blood vessels to body tissues, resulting in swelling and weight gain, decrease in blood pressure, weakness, dizziness, and difficulty breathing.

CAR-T Chimeric antigen receptor-T cell therapy which reprograms the patient's own T cells to recognize and kill cancerous B cells.

Carcinoma Cancer of epithelial tissue including the skin or tissue lining organs such as the liver or kidney.

Carcinoma in situ (CIS) A group of abnormal cells that have not spread beyond where they originated.

CARS Compensatory anti-inflammatory response syndrome, a systemic deactivation of the immune system following a severe infection, characterized by a state of immune unresponsiveness, reduction in lymphocytes, cytokine expression and response, human leukocyte antigen on monocytes.

Cathelicidin A family of antimicrobial peptides that are stored in the lysosomes of macrophages and polymorphonuclear leukocytes. They are involved in innate immune defenses against various bacteria.

CD19 A transmembrane protein found on the surface of mature B cells and is critical for B cell signaling. CD19 is also found on cancerous B cells as well as follicular dendritic cells.

CD20 Molecule found on the surface of mature B cells that may be found in higher amounts on certain types of B cell leukemias and lymphomas. CD20 is present in all stages of B cell development except the first stage (pro-B cells) and the last (plasma cells).

CD28 Costimulatory molecule expressed on T cells that binds CD80 or CD86 on antigen-presenting cells. It is required for the activation of T cells.

CD3 T cell receptor accessory molecules that participate in signal transduction after the TCR recognizes an antigen.

CD4 T cell T cell subtype that recognizes antigen presented on MHC class II molecules.

A major subset of CD4 T cells are helper T cells, which comprise of various subsets that cooperate with and aid other cell types during immune responses.

CD40 Costimulatory molecule that promotes lymphocyte activation. On B cells, CD40 signaling is essential for antibody isotype switching and somatic hypermutation.

CD40L CD40 ligand. Costimulatory molecule expressed on activated T cells and interacts with CD40 on other cell types, including B cells. The CD40/CD40L interaction is essential for antibody isotype switching and somatic hypermutation.

CD8 T cell subtype that recognizes antigen presented on MHC class I molecules. It is also referred to as cytotoxic T cell and is involved in immunity to viruses and cancers.

CD80 and **CD86** Costimulatory molecules expressed on antigen-presenting cells that are required for the activation of naive T cells. They bind CD28 on the T cell.

CDR Complementarity determining regions, found in variable chains of TCRs and immunoglobulins where they bind to antigen and help constitute antigen diversity and specificity.

Cellular Adhesion Molecule (CAM) Membrane-bound molecules that facilitate cell-to-cell interactions and leukocyte migration during inflammatory responses.

Chemokine Secreted molecule that stimulates the migration of cells towards the site of inflammation.

Chimeric monoclonal antibody Synthetic monoclonal antibody that is engineered to have mouse variable region sequences and human constant regions.

Chronic bronchitis Chronic bronchitis, a type of COPD, refers to chronic or excessive mucus production accompanied by cough for most days of at least 3 months in a year, for at least 2 consecutive years, when other causes of cough have been ruled out.

Chronic kidney disease (CKD) Gradual loss of the kidney's ability to filter blood.

Chronic lymphocytic leukemia (CLL) Cancer of lymphocytes that progresses at a much slower rate than ALL. Most commonly affects older adults.

Chronic myeloid leukemia (CML) Cancer typically found in older adults originating in bone marrow affecting myeloid stem cells which can become red blood cells, platelets, or granulocytes. Progresses at a slower rate than AML.

Chronic obstructive pulmonary disease (COPD) Obstructive disease of the lungs that is characterized by progressive airflow limitation that increases with age. The disease is characterized by the development of either chronic bronchitis, emphysema, or overlapping symptoms of both. Inflammatory processes initiated by exposure to toxic gases such as tobacco smoke induce the development of inflammation, mucus hypersecretion, enlargement of alveolar sacs, and destruction of lung tissue over time.

Chronic rejection Occurs following transplantation when the immune system of a patient attacks donor-derived organs or tissues, resulting in a slow deterioration of the transplanted organ 1 or more years following the procedure.

Clinical latency Asymptomatic stage of HIV infection.

Clonal expansion Process by which clones of activated lymphocytes are generated after activation with specific antigens.

Clonal selection Theory explaining how the adaptive immune system is capable of mounting specific responses against antigens that have never been encountered while maintaining tolerance to self-antigens.

Commensal bacteria Bacteria that typically comprise the normal microbial flora present within an individual host and aid the host in a number of physiological processes including the digestion of food and the development of immunity.

Common lymphoid progenitor (CLP) Cell type that gives rise to T cells, B cells and NK cells during hematopoiesis.

Common variable immune deficiency (CVID) Primary immunodeficiency characterized by low antibody titers and susceptibility to infectious diseases.

Complement fixation The process of attachment of C3b or C4b to the surface of pathogens to facilitate their removal by phagocytosis.

Complement system A collection of plasma proteins that act in a cascade of enzymatic reactions to opsonize or destroy extracellular pathogens. Opsonized pathogens are targeted for phagocytosis. Complement components also induce inflammation by mediating the recruitment of inflammatory cells.

Congestive heart failure (CHF) A chronic progressive condition where the heart fails to pump an adequate amount of blood and oxygen to the body's tissues.

Conjugate vaccine Vaccine containing bacterial capsular polysaccharide joined to a protein carrier. It is used to stimulate T cell-dependent immunity to encapsulated bacteria. Helper T cells recognizing the conjugate activate B cells that subsequently make neutralizing antibodies against the polysaccharide capsule.

Constant region Structural region of an antibody, BCR or TCR that does not recognize antigen.

Corticosteroids A group of steroid hormones that are made by the adrenal cortex or made synthetically to be used as drugs. They include two main classes, the glucocorticoids and mineralocorticoids. The glucocorticoids are immunosuppressive, anti-inflammatory, and have vasoconstrictive effects.

Costimulation One of two signals required for T-cell activation after the T cell receptor has bound MHC and a peptide antigen on an antigen presenting cell. Costimulation is provided by the antigen-presenting cell to the T cell. An example of a costimulatory interaction includes the binding of CD28 on the T cell to the co-stimulatory ligands, B7-1 (CD80) and B7-2 (CD86), on the antigen-presenting cell.

COX Cyclooxygenase, an enzyme that mediates the production of prostaglandins and thromboxane from arachidonic acid.

Crohn's disease Chronic inflammatory disease that may affect any segment of the gastrointestinal tract, often characterized by transmural inflammation, fistulas, fibrosis, and patchy inflammation.

Cross match test Determines if the recipient has pre-existing antibodies against HLA (MHC class I or class II) antigens from the donor.

Cryopyrin-associated periodic syndromes (CAPS) A group of rare, inherited autoinflammatory diseases in which IL-1β is overproduced.

CTLA-4 Cytotoxic T-lymphocyte–associated antigen 4 expressed on the surface of activated CD4 and CD8 T-cells and constitutively expressed on regulatory T cells. It downregulates effector T cell responses by engaging costimulatory molecules on APCs.

CyP450/3A4 Enzyme expressed in the liver and intestine that contributes to drug metabolism.

Cysteinyl leukotrienes Family of lipid mediators that are synthesized from arachidonic acid by many immune cells including mast cells, basophils, and eosinophils. They play important roles in mediating the symptoms associated with asthma.

Cytokine Secreted molecule that plays a key role in cell to cell communication during an immune response.

Cytokine release syndrome (CRS) Most often a result of immunotherapy treatment and characterized by a rapid release of cytokines from immune cells. The most frequent signs and symptoms include fever, nausea, rash, headache, rapid heartbeat, difficulty breathing, and hypotension.

Cytotoxic T-lymphocyte (CTL) T cell that recognizes foreign antigens presented on MHC class I receptors on infected or damaged cells, and release cytotoxins to induce apoptosis.

CXCL8 (IL-8) A chemokine/cytokine that is secreted by macrophages and other cells during inflammation that induces the recruitment of neutrophils.

Deep Vein Thrombosis (DVT) When a thrombus (blood clot) forms in the veins usually within the lower extremities especially around the thigh area.

Defensins Antimicrobial peptides which penetrate and disrupt the integrity of bacterial and fungal cell membranes, as well as the envelope of enveloped viruses.

Dendritic cells (DCs) Professional antigen presenting cells that reside in the peripheral tissue, are commonly recognized by their dendrite-like projections, migrate to lymph nodes and present antigen to T cells to activate the adaptive immune response.

Diffuse large B cell lymphoma (DLBCL) An aggressive, fast-growing type of non-Hodgkin lymphoma.

Disease-modifying anti-rheumatic drugs **(DMARDs)** A class of drugs used to suppress the immune system in autoimmune diseases such as rheumatoid arthritis.

Disease-modifying therapies (DMTs) Drugs involved in the management of multiple sclerosis that aim to reduce relapses as well as slow down damage caused by MS over time.

Disseminated intravascular coagulation (DIC) Occurs when overactive consumption of clotting factors result in blood clot formation in blood vessels, occluding the vessel and decreasing tissue perfusion of the organ. Most often occurs during sepsis, shock, obstetric complications, or cancer.

Double-positive Thymocytes expressing both CD4 and CD8 coreceptors.

DTaP, Tdap A vaccine that helps build immunity to bacteria such as; diphtheria, tetanus, whooping cough (pertussis). Tdap is the booster.

Dysbiosis Reduction in intestinal microbial species diversity that may contribute to the pathogenesis of inflammatory bowel diseases.

Dyspnea Difficulty breathing.

Effector differentiation Phase of an adaptive immune response in which activated T cells or B cells acquire specialized functions for fighting infections.

EGF/EGFR Epidermal Growth Factor/EGF Receptor. An oncogene that is normally involved in cellular function, but is overexpressed in some types of cancers.

Eicosanoid Eicosanoids are a family of oxygenated derivatives of arachidonic acid or other 20-carbon polyunsaturated fatty acids. They include prostaglandins, leukotrienes, prostacyclins, and thromboxanes among others. They are involved in inflammation, the induction of fever, smooth muscle constriction, regulation of childbirth, pain, cell growth, blood pressure, and other physiological activities.

ELISA Enzyme-linked immunosorbent assay, a diagnostic procedure used to detect proteins, peptides, antibodies, hormones, and other soluble mediators in bodily fluids.

Emphysema Emphysema, a type of COPD, is defined in terms of anatomic pathology, characterized by the loss of elastic recoil due to permanent damage to alveolar sacs. This occurs due to inflammation in the small airways, which leads to destruction of alveolar walls, resulting in enlargement of the air sacs and loss of elasticity.

Endocytosis Cellular process in which foreign material is ingested into the cell. This is followed by invagination of an area of the plasma membrane which surrounds the foreign material, forming a vesicle.

Endothelial cell Epithelial cell lining the interior of blood vessels.

Eosinophilia The expansion and activation of eosinophils in the airways, blood, or other tissues during immune responses. The development of eosinophilia is an important characteristic of allergic diseases.

Eosinophils Granulocyte that stains with eosin and releases toxic substances when activated. Eosinophils participate in anti-parasitic responses, but are pathological in allergy and other diseases.

Eotaxin-1 Chemokine, also known as CCL11, that is secreted by T_H2 cells and is highly selective for the chemotaxis of eosinophils during immune responses.

Epithelial cell A type of cell that lines the surfaces of tissues and blood vessels.

Epitope The portion of an antigen that binds antibody or T cell receptors. It is also called as antigenic determinant.

Epstein-Barr Virus (EBV) DNA virus which is a member of the human herpesvirus family. It infects B cells and epithelial cells and is known to cause infectious mononucleosis. EBV is also associated with lymphoproliferative diseases such as Burkitt's lymphoma.

Erythrocyte Red blood cell.

Erythrocyte sedimentation rate (ESR) Nonspecific diagnostic test measuring the rate of erythrocyte settlement in anticoagulated blood.

Erythropoiesis-stimulating agents (ESAs) Erythropoiesis-stimulating agents.

Erythropoietin (EPO) A hormone produced by the kidneys in response to decreased oxygen in the blood to stimulate the bone marrow to produce more red blood cells.

Experimental autoimmune encephalomyelitis (EAE) An animal model of brain inflammation that mimics inflammatory demyelination of the CNS.

Extracellular matrix (ECM) A network of macromolecules including collagen, glycoproteins, and enzymes that provide a structural support to surrounding cells.

Extracellular pathogens Pathogens that establish infection outside cells in the extracellular space, on the surfaces of epithelial cells, or in the blood or lymph. They include many extracellular bacteria and fungi.

Extrinsic asthma Also referred to as atopic asthma, this type of asthma involves allergic reactions that are mediated by IgE antibodies and mast cells.

FasL Fas ligand, expressed on cytotoxic lymphocytes and induces apoptosis in target cells by activating Fas.

Fc Fragment crystallizable, the constant (or the "tail") region of an antibody which interacts with the rest of the immune system via Fc receptors.

FcεRI High affinity receptor for the IgE Fc region, expressed on mast cells, basophils and eosinophils.

FcRn Also referred to as the Brambell receptor, FcRn binds IgG and plays important roles in the transport of IgG molecules. It protects IgG from degradation in the vesicular compartments of cells and is responsible for increasing the half-life of IgG.

Forced expiratory volume (FEV) The amount of air a person can exhale during a forced breath.

FOXP3 Transcription factor required for the differentiation and maintenance of regulatory T cells.

Fully human monoclonal antibody A monoclonal antibody that is engineered to consist of both variable and constant regions of human origin. This is typically done by synthesizing the antibody in mice that are made to express human immunoglobulin genes.

G-CSF/GM-CSF Granulocyte-colony stimulating factor/granulocyte-macrophage colony-stimulating factor, glycoproteins that stimulate the bone marrow to produce granulocytes and release them into the bloodstream. GM-CSF also promotes monocytes.

GATA3 Transcription factor expressed in T_H2 cells that regulates the production of IL-4, IL-5 and IL-13.

GDP/GTP Guanosine-5′-triphosphate (GTP) is a purine nucleoside triphosphate.

GI Gastrointestinal.

GILZ Glucocorticoid-induced leucine zipper, gene induced by glucocorticoids that mediates that actions of glucocorticoids. Present in a wide variety of cell types.

GIST Gastrointestinal stromal tumor.

Glomerular filtration rate (GFR) Estimates the amount of blood that passes through the glomeruli each minute to determine how well blood is being filtered by the kidneys.

Glucocorticoid (GC) Also known as corticosteroids, or drugs that bind to the glucocorticoid receptor, regulating the expression of steroid-responsive genes including cytokines. Glucocorticoids generally decrease the levels of pro-inflammatory cytokines and increase anti-inflammatory cytokines.

Glucocorticoid receptor (GR) The receptor to which glucocorticoids bind.

Goodpasture's syndrome Autoimmune disorder characterized by autoantibodies produced against extracellular matrix, specifically the α3 chain of type IV collagen, mainly found in the basement membranes of the lungs and kidneys. Inflammation in the kidneys often results in renal impairment.

GPCRs G-protein coupled receptors, the largest family of membrane proteins, also known as seven transmembrane receptors which interact with G proteins in the plasma membrane.

Graft Versus Host Disease (GVHD) A complication that can arise after hematopoietic stem cell transplantation caused by donor lymphocytes attacking antigens in the tissues of transplant recipients.

Granulocyte White blood cells with irregularly shaped, multilobed nuclei, also referred to as polymorphonuclear leukocytes. They contain cytoplasmic granules which consist of several toxic substances. There are three types of granulocyte cells: neutrophils, basophils, and eosinophils.

Granuloma Site of chronic inflammation involved in immune defense against intracellular bacteria such as mycobacteria. Granulomas typically consist of a central area of macrophages that is fused to multinucleate giant cells. This area is surrounded by activated T cells.

Granzyme Enzyme released by cytotoxic T cells or NK cells that induces apoptosis in target cells by activating caspases.

Grave's disease An autoimmune disorder that affects thyroid function due to autoantibodies that bind to the thyroid stimulating hormone receptor.

GRE Glucocorticoid response element.

Gut-associated lymphoid tissue (GALT) Secondary lymphoid tissues associated with intestinal host defense, including Peyer's patches and mesenteric lymph nodes.

Hairy cell leukemia A slowly progressing cancer of B lymphocytes. Under the microscope these abnormal B cells appear "hairy", hence the name.

Haplotype A series of HLA genes by chromosome that are inherited together, and passed to the child from their mother or father.

Hapten Small molecule antigen that becomes recognizable to the immune system following its attachment to a larger molecule, termed a carrier protein.

Hashimoto's thyroiditis An autoimmune disorder that results in hypothyroidism or an underactive thyroid due to autoantibodies that bind to and lead to death of thyroid cells.

HDAC Histone deacetylase, a class of enzymes that removes acetyl groups from lysines in histones, allowing the histone proteins to be tightly wound around DNA. This contributes to the turning on or turning off of various genes during cellular processes.

Hemagglutinin (HA) A highly mutable glycoprotein found on the surface of influenza viruses.

Hematopoiesis The formation of blood cell types from self-renewing stem cells.

Hematopoietic stem cell transplantation (HSCT) The transplant of bone marrow-derived stem cells from a donor to a recipient to replace the hematopoietic system of the recipient. Stem cells may also be derived from umbilical cord blood or peripheral blood.

Hemolytic uremic syndrome (HUS) A condition which affects the blood cells, blood vessels, platelets, and kidneys and needs to be treated immediately.

Hepatitis B virus (HBV) A bloodborne and sexually transmitted DNA virus that replicates in the liver and can lead to chronic and fatal infections.

Hepatitis C virus (HCV) An enveloped, positive-strand RNA virus that causes inflammation of the liver, which can become chronic and for which there is no vaccine to induce prevention. It is spread through blood and bodily fluids. It is commonly characterized by fever, malaise, nausea, jaundice, right upper quadrant pain, and clay colored stools.

HepBsAg Hepatitis B surface antigen, an enveloped protein on the surface of the hepatitis B virus, detectable in the serum 4–12 weeks after infection.

HER2 Human epidermal growth factor receptor 2, member of the epidermal growth factor receptor family which can become mutated and overexpressed in some cancers.

Herpes simplex virus (HSV) A DNA virus of two main types (HSV-1 and HSV-2) characterized by sores or blisters that appear during outbreaks and disappear during periods of latency.

Hidradenitis suppurativa Inflammatory disease of the sweat glands producing painful nodules and cysts. HS commonly occurs in the axilla and inguinal area and causes long-term painful inflammation of the skin.

Histamine A compound released by cells in response to injury and in allergic and inflammatory reactions, causing contraction of smooth muscle.

Histone acetyl transferase (HAT) Enzymes that acetylate conserved lysine amino acids on histone proteins by transferring acetyl groups. They are involved in the turning on or turning off of genes by unwinding histone proteins around DNA.

HLA typing Methods used to test for the expression of certain HLA alleles prior to an organ transplant.

HMGB1 High mobility box group 1, a transcription factor and pro-inflammatory cytokine often found to be elevated in sepsis.

Hodgkin lymphoma A cancer of lymphocytes characterized by large lymph nodes and the presence of abnormal B cells called Reed-Sternberg cells.

Hormone refractory prostate cancer (HRPC) Prostate tumor that fails to respond to hormone therapy. May occur months to years after initiation of hormone therapy to shrink the tumor.

House dust mite (HDM) Mites of the genus *Dermatophagoides* whose feces are a major contributor to allergic reactions and are associated with asthma and allergic rhinitis.

Human immunodeficiency virus (HIV) An enveloped single-stranded RNA virus that depletes circulating CD4 T cells causing immunosuppression. HIV is responsible for the development of AIDS.

Human leukocyte antigen (HLA) complex The nomenclature used to refer to major histocompatibility genes in humans. It is located on the short arm of chromosome 6 and encodes for the polymorphic HLA Class I and II molecules and other proteins involved in immunity. Individual HLA genes are designated by capital letters such as HLA-A or HLA-DP. Alleles are designated by numbers such as HLA-DPB1∗0401.

Human papillomavirus (HPV) A nonenveloped double-stranded DNA virus, most common sexually transmitted infection in the United States, symptoms range from asymptomatic to high risk leading to genital warts and cancer.

Humanized monoclonal antibody Synthetic monoclonal antibody that is generated by converting antigen-specific mouse IgG antibodies into an antibody that resembles human IgG, but is engineered to still express the mouse CDR regions in the heavy and light chains.

Hybridoma Hybrid cells that are used to make large quantities of monoclonal antibodies for diagnostic or therapeutic purposes. They typically are comprised of a mouse B cell that is specific for the antigen of interest that has been fused to a myeloma cell that does not express immunoglobulin genes. The hybrid cells are immortalized and a continuous source of antibodies.

Hydroxychloroquine (HCQ) An anti-malarial agent that also has efficacy in the treatment of certain autoimmune diseases.

Hygiene Hypothesis The hygiene hypothesis is the proposition that the increase in hypersensitivities and autoimmune diseases in developed countries may be attributed to increased sanitation, lack of exposure to infections and germs during early childhood, and overuse of antibiotics in these countries.

Hyperacute rejection Occurs during organ or tissue transplantation when the recipient has pre-existing antibodies that recognize donor-derived antigens. It can occur within minutes to hours of a transplant.

Hypersensitivity Allergic or other types of immune reactions that are mediated by immune cells and antibody molecules to diverse antigenic substances. They are classified into four types based on the Gel and Coomb's classification system.

IBD Inflammatory bowel disease, term used to describe disorders that involve chronic inflammation of the digestive tract including ulcerative colitis and Crohn's disease.

ICAM Intracellular adhesion molecule. They are involved in leukocyte trafficking and homing to infected tissues and lymphoid organs.

ICOS Inducible T-cell Costimulator, an immune checkpoint protein expressed on activated T cells and required for T_{FH} cell differentiation.

IFN Interferon, signaling proteins produced by the host that interfere with viral replication and aid in the upregulation of the immune response to viruses and cancers.

IgA Antibody isotype that primarily functions to neutralize pathogens, toxins or target molecules.

IgE Antibody isotype that functions to sensitize mast cells or other cells expressing the high affinity Fc receptor for IgE. Antigen binding to IgE-coated mast cells triggers their degranulation and has a role in immediate hypersensitivity reactions.

IGF Insulin-like growth factor.

IgG Antibody isotype that facilitates neutralization, opsonization, complement activation or ADCC of pathogens, infected cells or target molecules.

IgM First antibody isotype produced by naive B cells and functions to activate complement following antigen binding.

IIV/aIIV/ccIIV Inactivated influenza vaccine/adjuvanted IIV/cell culture IIV.

IL-1Rα Cytokine produced by monocytes, macrophages, and other cells that antagonizes the functions of IL-1.

IL-1α and **IL-1β** Proinflammatory cytokine produced by macrophages and a number of other immune cells that induces vasodilation, promotes inflammation, and acts as a pyrogen.

IL-2 Autocrine T cell growth factor produced following their activation.

IL-3 Cytokine that is produced by T cells and other cells that stimulates the generation of cells of the myeloid lineage including granulocytes, mast cells, and macrophages.

IL-4 Cytokine produced by T_H2 cells, mast cells, basophils, eosinophils, ILC2 cells, NKT cells, and other cells that promotes T_H2 differentiation, B cell activation, and immunoglobulin class switching.

IL-5 Cytokine produced by T_H2 cells, mast cells, activated eosinophils and other cells that is essential for the differentiation and activation of eosinophils.

IL-6 Proinflammatory cytokine produced by endothelial cells, fibroblasts, macrophages, T cells, B cells, and other immune cells that induces the acute phase response, promotes T and B cell development, neoangeogenesis, osteoclastogenesis, and cholinergic neuronal survival among other functions.

IL-7 Cytokine produced by epithelial cells, DCs, B cells, keratinocytes, monocytes, and macrophages. Promotes megakaryocyte maturation, VDJ recombination, survival of naive T cells, proliferation of thymocytes, and development of ILCs. Also induces inflammatory mediator release from monocytes.

IL-8 Cytokine produced by monocytes, macrophages, neutrophils, lymphocytes, epithelial cells, endothelial cells, fibroblasts, hepatocytes, and several other cell types. Acts as a chemoattractant for neutrophils, T cells, NK cells, eosinophils, and basophils. Also mobilizes hematopoietic stem cells and promotes angiogenesis.

IL-9 Cytokine produced by T_H2, T_H17, and T_{regs}. Also produced by mast cells, eosinophils, and ILCs. Acts as a T cell and mast cell growth factor, inhibits T_H1 cytokines, promotes IgE, chemokine and mucus production in the bronchial epithelium.

IL-10 Immunoregulatory cytokine produced by macrophages, T cells, B cells, and other cells that suppresses inflammation through effects or antigen presenting cells, but stimulates NK cells, mast cells, and IgE synthesis in B cells.

IL-11 Cytokine produced by cells of the bone marrow, epithelial cells, endothelial cells, fibroblasts, smooth muscle cells, synoviocytes, and osteoblasts. Acts as a growth factor for erythrocyte, megakaryocyte, and myeloid progenitor cells. Can induce acute phase proteins, inhibit macrophage activity, and participate in bone remodeling by promoting osteoclasts and inhibiting osteoblast activity.

IL-12 Cytokine produced by monocytes/macrophages, neutrophils, B cells, DCs, and microglia which promotes development and maintenance of TH1 cells, activates NK cells, and supports maturation of DCs.

IL-13 Cytokine produced by TH2 cells, mast cells, eosinophils, basophils, ILC2 cells and other cells that promotes IgE class switching in B cells, mucus secretion, epithelial cell turnover, fibrosis, and smooth muscle hyperreactivity.

IL-17A Cytokine produced by Th17 cells and other T cells expressing RORγt. Stimulates the IL-17 receptor on mucosal surfaces, leading to the production of anti-microbial peptides and G-CSF.

IL-18 Cytokine produced by macrophages, DCs, epithelial cells, keratinocytes, chondrocytes, astrocytes, osteoblasts, and renal tubular epithelial cells. Enhances NK cell toxicity, induces IFN-gamma along with IL-12, and promotes T_H1 and T_H2 response depending on other cytokines present.

IL-23 Produced by phagocytes including macrophages and DCs. Stimulates production of IL-17, enhances T cell proliferation, promotes memory T cells, activates NK cells, and regulates antibody production.

IL-25 Also called IL-17E. Cytokine belonging to the IL-17 family involved in the generation of T_H2 responses to helminths and during allergic diseases. It is produced by epithelial cells, Paneth cells, T cells, dendritic cells, mast cells, basophils, and eosinophils.

IL-33 Cytokine belonging to the IL-1 superfamily that induces the production of type 2 cytokines from T_H2 cells, mast cells, basophils, eosinophils, and ILC2s. It is expressed by many cell types including mast cells, fibroblasts, epithelial cells, dendritic cells, and macrophages and binds the ST2 (IL1RL1) receptor on target cells.

ILC2 cells Group 2 or type 2 innate lymphoid cells that are derived from the common lymphoid progenitor, lack antigen-specific receptors, and produce type 2 cytokines. They play important roles in anti-parasitic responses and allergic diseases.

IMiD Immune modulatory imide drug.

Immediate hypersensitivity Also referred to as type I hypersensitivity. T_H2-mediated reaction in which B cells produce IgE antibodies against an allergen, sensitizing mast cells. Subsequent exposure to the allergen results in mast cell degranulation and swelling.

Immune complex A protein complex that is formed by the binding of antibodies to soluble antigens. They are typically cleared by phagocytes which have receptors for complement or the Fc portions of antibodies. Erythrocytes also participate in the removal of immune complexes. The unregulated deposition of immune complexes can be pathological during autoimmune diseases such as systemic lupus erythematosus or during type III hypersensitivity reactions such as serum sickness.

Immunization The process of inducing an immune response to an antigen by sensitizing or challenging an individual to the respective antigen. Sensitization is the first exposure to the antigen via any route. Challenges include booster doses given via the same route as sensitization or another route.

Immunological synapse The area of contact between immune cells during the process of their activation and function. It is typically used to refer to the area of contact between the antigen-presenting cell and the T cell during the activation or stimulation of T cells.

Immunoglobulin (Ig) The general name for the B cell receptor and antibody molecules.

Imprinting Process in which lymphocytes that are activated in mucosal lymphoid organs express chemokine receptors and integrins that cause them to migrate towards the muco-

sal surface where the antigen was originally encountered.

Inactivated vaccine A vaccine that contains whole microbes which have been deactivated with formalin or with physical heat or irradiation. Also referred to as a killed vaccine.

Induction therapy The use of immunosuppressive drugs to induce tolerance to transplanted organs in the initial days following transplantation.

Influenza An RNA virus that is easily spread and affects the respiratory tract. Leads to general malaise including chills, fever, muscle aches, cough, congestion, sneezing, fatigue, and headaches. Commonly referred to as the "flu".

Innate immunity Immunological subsystem that comprises the cells and mechanisms that provide the first line of defense from infection in a non-specific manner.

Innate lymphoid cell (ILCs) Leukocytes of lymphoid origin that do not express specific antigen receptors and contribute to innate immunity.

Interleukin (IL) Protein secreted by immune cells that regulates the proliferation, differentiation, and activation of other immune cells by activating a specific cell surface receptor. Also referred to as cytokine.

Intracellular pathogens Pathogens that can establish infections within cells. They include viruses and intracellular bacteria.

Intraepithelial lymphocyte (IEL) CD8 T cells residing within the epithelial compartment of the small intestine and possess both innate and adaptive immune properties.

Intravenous immunoglobulin (IVIG) IgG antibodies pooled from thousands of healthy donors. Can be given to patients with certain immunodeficiencies as well as autoimmunity

Intrinsic asthma Also referred to as non-atopic asthma, this type of asthma involves immune reactions to non-allergenic substances such as exercise, pollutants, gases, and other chemicals.

IPEX Immunodysregulation polyendocrinopathy enteropathy X-linked, a rare autoimmune disorder characterized by dysfunctional regulatory T cells caused by dysfunctional Foxp3.

IPV Injectable polio vaccine.

IRF Interferon regulatory factor. Transcription factors that induce the expression of genes containing interferon-stimulated elements in promoter regions.

Isograft The transplantation of tissues or cells between individuals who are identical twins.

Isotype switching Process in which antibody constant regions switch from IgM to another isotype in activated B cells. It involves the activity of the enzyme activation-induced cytidine deaminase and interactions between CD40 and CD40 ligand.

ITAM/ITIM Immunoreceptor tyrosine-based activation motif/Immunoreceptor tyrosine-based inhibitory motif, activating or inhibitory receptors of NK cells.

ITP Immune/idiopathic thrombocytopenia purpura, a disorder characterized by excessive bruising or bleeding.

JAK Janus Kinase protein tyrosine kinases are cytokine receptor subunits, responsible for initiating signaling cascades that activate enzymes required for embryonic development, tissue growth, and hematopoiesis.

John Cunningham virus (JCV) A double-stranded DNA virus that can cross the blood brain barrier and enter the CNS. It can cause a fatal infection in immunodeficient or immunosuppressed individuals.

Juvenile idiopathic arthritis (JIA) Autoinflammatory arthritis of unknown origin that occurs in children with various disease subtypes.

Kaposi sarcoma A cancer that forms in the cells lining lymph and blood vessels and often associated with a weakened immune system (AIDS patients and transplant patients taking immunosuppressive drugs. Lesions often appear as purple spots on the legs, feet, or face but can also develop in genital areas, mouth, or lymph nodes.

Keratinocyte A cell of the epidermis that produces keratin.

Lamina propria Loose connective tissue underlying mucosal epithelial surfaces in the GI, urogenital and respiratory tracts.

Langerhans Cells Dendritic cells that reside in the skin.

Late phase response The term late phase response refers to a second wave of inflammatory substances produced by mast cells several hours after initial activation *via* IgE antibodies and a specific allergen. Examples of inflammatory substances include *de novo* synthesized cytokines, chemokines, and lipid mediators such as the cysteinyl leukotrienes.

Leprosy A chronic and necrotic infection caused by *Mycobacterium leprae.*

Leukemia A broad term describing cancer of circulating cells, particularly white blood cells, but can also affect red blood cells, and platelets.

Leukocytes General term for white blood cells. They are an integral part of the body's defense system and comprise of myeloid cells, granulocytes, and lymphocytes.

Leukotriene A lipid metabolite that is synthesized by mast cells and other immune cells through the 5-lipoxygenase pathway of arachidonic acid metabolism. They are a hundred times more potent than histamine and induce vasoconstriction and smooth muscle constriction.

Leukotriene receptor antagonists (LTRAs) A class of non-steroidal drugs that inhibit the function of leukotrienes and thus inhibit inflammation.

LFA Lymphocyte function associated antigen-1, an integrin present on leukocytes.

LFTs Liver function tests, a panel of tests that illustrate the health of a patient's liver.

Live Attenuated Influenza Vaccine (LAIV) Live influenza vaccine in the form of a nasal spray.

Long-acting beta agonists (LABAs) Long acting beta agonists are a class of drugs that stimulate β_2 adrenergic receptors on smooth muscle cells and induce relaxation. They have a longer duration of action and are prescribed for moderate to severe persistent asthma and for patients with COPD. Examples of drugs include salmeterol and formoterol.

Long-acting muscarinic receptor antagonists (LAMAs) Long acting muscarinic antagonist are a class of drugs that inhibit muscarinic receptors on smooth muscle cells, thereby inducing relaxation. They have a longer duration of action and are recommended to reduce exacerbations in COPD patients. Examples of LAMAs include aclidinium and tiotropium.

LPS Lipopolysaccharide, a component of the cell wall of Gram-negative bacteria.

LTD4 receptor Also known as the cysteinyl leukotriene receptor 1, the LTD4 receptor, binds the leukotrienes LTD4 and LTE4, and is responsible for their effects. It is targeted by the drugs montelukast and zafirlukast in the treatment of asthma.

Lymph Fluid circulating through the lymphatic system derived from tissue interstitial fluid absorbed by lymph vessels.

Lymph node Secondary lymphoid organs where lymphocytes and other immune cells interact with each other and initiate adaptive immune responses.

Lymphatic vessels Vessels that absorb tissue interstitial fluid and drain into lymph nodes, carrying antigens and leukocytes. Lymphatic vessels ultimately drain into the thoracic duct and right lymphatic duct, where fluid enters the bloodstream.

Lymphocyte Cell types derived from the common lymphoid progenitor during hematopoiesis, including B cells, T cells and NK cells.

Lymphoid follicles Spherical lymphoid structures consisting of B cells and other cells that participate in B cell maturation and immunity. Two types of lymphoid follicles have been described: primary lymphoid follicles that do not contain germinal centers and secondary lymphoid follicles that contain germinal centers, and where B cells proliferate and divide. Lymphoid follicles are found in the secondary lymphoid organs such as the lymph nodes and spleen, and also as isolated structures in the mucosal epithelium of the intestines and other organs.

Lymphoid lineage Lineage comprising of all types of lymphocytes and the bone marrow cells (lymphoid progenitors) that give rise to them.

Lymphoma A solid lymphoid tumor.

M cell Microfold cell in follicle-associated epithelium of the GI tract that collects luminal antigens and delivers them to underlying secondary lymphoid tissues through transcytosis.

Macrophages Large white blood cells that are found in nearly all tissues that bear receptors for pathogens and phagocytose foreign substances. They develop from monocytes and contribute to both innate and adaptive immune responses. They assist in the activation of T cells by acting as antigen presenting cells.

MAdCAM-1 Mucosal vascular addressin cellular adhesion molecule-1. Adhesion molecule expressed on vascular endothelium in the GI tract and interacts with integrin a4b7 expressed on lymphocytes, resulting in their diapedesis into intestinal tissue.

Maintenance therapy The use of immunosuppressive drugs to maintain long-term tolerance to transplanted organs.

Major basic protein (MBP) A proteoglycan that is found in the granules of eosinophils and is toxic to helminths and other parasites. It also induces epithelial cell damage, inflammation, and bronchoconstriction during allergic responses.

Major histocompatibility complex (MHC) A large complex of mainly immune system genes that is present in all vertebrates. It encodes, among other proteins, the highly polymorphic MHC I and MHC II molecules, which present peptide antigens to CD8 and CD4 T cells respectively. They are the basis of an individual's tissue type or haplotype and are involved in tissue or graft rejection.

MAP Mean arterial pressure.

Mast cell Innate immune cell containing granules that plays a critical role during anti-parasitic responses. It is also involved in immunity to pathogens and cancers, and is pathological in allergic disease, autoimmunity, and other inflammatory disorders.

MBL Mannan-binding lectin, can bind to carbohydrates on the surfaces of pathogens, activate complement, and enhance phagocytosis.

MCD Multicentric Castleman's Disease, a rare disease involving multiple enlarged lymph nodes and characterized by nausea, fever, rash, and an enlarged liver and spleen. May be caused by human herpesvirus-8.

MCP Monocyte chemoattractant protein, a potent chemotactic factor, regulates migration and infiltration for monocytes and macrophages.

Megakaryocyte A bone-marrow derived cell responsible for the production of platelets.

Membrane attack complex (MAC) Consists of complement proteins C5b-C9 that forms on the surface of pathogens, creating a channel that disrupts the cell membrane leading to lysis and death of the pathogen.

Memory cell Long-lived T cell or B cell that has previously been activated with antigen and is capable of a rapid response following a secondary encounter with the same antigen.

Merkel cell carcinoma A rare form of malignant skin cancer.

MIC-A or MIC-B MHC class I-related chain like proteins that are expressed or released by cells during infection, malignant transformation, or other types of stress. They are involved in the activation of NK cells, γδ T cells, and other cell types.

MIP Macrophage inflammatory proteins, chemokines that attract macrophages to the site of inflammation.

Mixed lymphocyte reaction (MLR) Assay used to assess organ compatibility by coculturing lymphocytes derived from a potential organ donor and recipient and measuring cytotoxicity.

MMP Matrix metalloproteinase, an enzyme that is responsible for degradation of extracellular matrix proteins.

MMR Measles, mumps, and rubella vaccine. May also contain varicella (MMRV).

Monoclonal A clone that is derived from a single individual or cell.

Monoclonal antibody Therapeutic antibody derived from a single hybridoma cell line that recognizes a specific target.

Monocyte Large mononuclear cells found in the circulation; after entering tissues, they develop into macrophages.

Monophosphoryl lipid A (MPL) A detoxified form of lipid A, the active part of Gram-negative bacterial lipopolysaccharide endotoxin, and a Toll-like receptor 4 agonist, used as an adjuvant in vaccines.

Mtb *Mycobacterium tuberculosis*, pathogenic capsulated bacillus spread by aerosols and responsible for tuberculosis in humans.

mTOR Mammalian target of rapamycin, a kinase involved in signaling that regulates cell growth, survival, proliferation, and protein synthesis, among other cellular processes.

Mucosa-associated lymphoid tissue (MALT) Lymphoid tissue that is localized to mucosal surfaces including the GI tract, lungs and skin.

Mucosal immune system Lymphoid tissues associated with mucosal surfaces including the GI, urogenital and respiratory tracts.

Mucus cell hyperplasia Also referred to as mucus metaplasia or goblet cell hyperplasia, this refers to the increase in goblet cell numbers in the mucosal tissue during inflammation.

Mucus hypersecretion The enhanced production of mucus during immune responses.

Multiple Myeloma (MM) A cancer of plasma cells affecting many different areas of the body.

Multiple sclerosis (MS) A chronic neurodegenerative disease, resulting in delayed conduction of nerve impulses from the central nervous system to the spinal cord and the rest of the body as a result of the myelin sheath thinning or being damaged.

Myasthenia gravis (MG) An autoimmune disease producing irregular and progressive weakness and abnormal fatigability of striated muscles, exacerbated by exercise and repeated movement, commonly affecting the face, lips, tongue, neck, and throat.

Myeloid lineage Cell lineage comprising of granulocytes, monocytes, macrophages, dendritic cells, mast cells, and the bone marrow cells (myeloid progenitors) that give rise to them.

Myelosuppression A side effect of chemotherapy resulting in anemia, neutropenia, or thrombocytopenia.

Myopathy Disorder of skeletal muscles.

Naive lymphocyte Mature B cell or T cell that has not encountered its antigen.

Negative selection Process during T cell and B cell development in which the expression of a receptor that recognizes self-antigens will provide an apoptotic signal, resulting in cell death.

Neonatal onset multisystem inflammatory disease (NOMID) A condition characterized by persistent inflammation and tissue damage affecting the skin, nervous system, and joints.

Neuraminidase (NA) An enzyme found on the surface of the influenza virus, which cleaves sialic acid residues from the newly formed virion and host cell, allowing the virus to spread.

Neuromuscular junction (NMJ) The area of contact between the muscle fiber and motor neuron creating a chemical synapse.

Neutralization The process by which antibodies inactivate pathogens or other toxic substances. Neutralization prevents toxins, target molecules or viruses from attaching to host receptors or surfaces.

Neutropenia Abnormally low levels of neutrophils.

Neutrophil The most abundant white blood cell, that rapidly enters infected tissues and phagocytoses and destroys extracellular pathogens. They contain granules that stain with neutral dyes.

NFAT Nuclear factor of activated T cells, a transcription factor that is activated as a result of signaling from the T cell receptor. It is necessary for numerous immune responses and the activation of T cells.

NF-κB Nuclear factor kappa B, a transcription factor that is activated as a result of signaling through toll-like receptors and many other receptors on cells. It is required for the turning on of numerous immune system related genes including various cytokines and chemokines.

Nivolumab Monoclonal antagonist antibody against PD-1.

Natural Killer cells NK cells, innate immune cells of lymphoid origin which contribute to antiviral immunity and protection from the development of cancers.

Non-Hodgkin lymphoma (NHL) A cancer of lymphocytes that includes all lymphomas except Hodgkin type.

Non-small cell lung cancer (NSCLC) Any type of epithelial lung cancer. Accounts for 85% of all lung cancers.

NSAID Non-steroidal anti-inflammatory drugs (i.e. ibuprofen).

Obstructive Lung Disease Obstructive lung diseases are a category of respiratory diseases that are characterized by obstruction of the airways due to narrowing of the respiratory passages such as the bronchi. A primary characteristic of obstructive lung diseases is the inability to completely exhale inspired air. Examples of obstructive diseases include asthma, chronic obstructive pulmonary disease, bronchiolitis, and bronchiectasis.

Oncogene A gene which is capable of transforming a cell to become cancerous.

Opportunistic infection An infection caused by pathogens that do not cause disease under normal homeostatic conditions. These pathogens take advantage of an opportunity to colonize that is not normally available, thus these types of infections may arise in an immunocompromised individual or during a period of altered balance of microbiota.

Opsonization Process of coating pathogens with molecules such as complement or antibody to facilitate their removal by phagocytosis.

Original antigenic sin Modifications in successive immune responses to structurally related antigens such as those present on the influenza virus. Secondary immune responses to structurally related antigens are limited by the antigenic epitopes that were detected during the original exposure. As a result, primary immune responses are not made toward new antigens expressed on pathogens. Over time, this results in loss of immunity to novel antigenic strains.

Osteoclast Multinucleate bone cells, that are derived from macrophages, and break down bone tissue. They are involved in bone resorption and are critical for the maintenance, repair, and survival of bone cells.

Panel-reactive antibody test (PRA) Measures for the presence of antibodies recognizing HLA-derived antigens in a potential organ transplant recipient.

Pannus An abnormal layer of tissue found in rheumatoid arthritis that results from the inflammatory response.

Paresthesia An abnormal numbing, pricking, burning, or tingling sensation of the skin that has no apparent cause.

Passive immunization Administration of preformed antibodies from an immune individual to a nonimmune individual, providing defense against a pathogen; this does not confer long-term protection.

Pathogen-associated molecular patterns (PAMPs) Conserved nucleotides and polysaccharide motifs present on microbes that can be recognized by innate immune cells and stimulate an immune response.

Pattern recognition receptor (PRR) Innate immune receptors that recognize conserved structures on microbes including cell wall products, lipids and nucleic acids.

PCV Pneumococcal conjugate vaccine

PD-1/PD-L1 Programmed cell death protein-1/Programmed cell death protein ligand-1, immune checkpoint proteins. When bound together they regulate the immune system by suppressing the activity of T cells.

PDGF Platelet-derived growth factor, a growth factor that regulates cell division and growth particularly in blood vessel formation, as well as growth and proliferation of fibroblasts, osteoblasts, and vascular smooth muscle cells.

Pemphigus vulgaris A group of potentially life-threatening autoimmune diseases characterized by epithelial blistering affecting the cutaneous and mucosal lining.

Perforin Molecule released by cytotoxic CD8 T cells or NK cells that forms pores in the membrane of target cells.

Periodic Fever Syndromes A group of auto-inflammatory diseases characterized by cyclical fevers.

Petechiae Tiny circular red circular patches that appear on the skin as a result of bleeding under the skin.

Peyer's patch Lymphoid tissue associated with the gastrointestinal jejunum and ileum that functions as sites for lymphocyte activation against intestinal antigens.

Phagocytosis The ingestion of bacteria or other material by cells such as macrophages, dendritic cells, and neutrophils.

Phosphodiesterase (PDE) 4 Type 4 cyclic nucleotide phosphodiesterases are important enzymes that regulate the levels of intracellular cyclic adenosine monophosphate (cAMP) and its downstream effects. PDE4 breaks the phosphodiester bond in cAMP molecules, thus facilitating degradation of intracellular cAMP and affecting signaling pathways. PDE4 inhibitors such as roflumilast act by countering the action of PDE4 and enhancing cAMP concentration in smooth muscle cells.

Plaque psoriasis The most common form of psoriasis in which red, raised patches appear on the skin covered by white silvery scales or dead skin cells. They are painful and itchy and often appear on the scalp, lower back, knees, and elbows.

Plasma B cells A terminally differentiated form of a B cell that secretes antibodies.

Plasmacytoid dendritic cell (pDC) A type of cell, also referred to as interferon-producing cell, that makes thousand times more type I interferons than epithelial cells, after infection by viruses. It also participates in other types of immune responses such as psoriasis.

Plasmapheresis A process that removes potentially harmful antibodies from the plasma component of the blood.

Platelet A small colorless disk-shaped cell fragment without a nucleus involved in blood clotting.

Platelet activating factor (PAF) Mediator of platelet aggregation and degranulation, leukocyte function, and plays a role in vascular permeability. Most commonly produced by platelets, endothelial cells, neutrophils, monocytes, and macrophages.

Polymorphonuclear leukocyte See granulocyte.

Polyethylene glycol (PEG) A hydrophilic polymer, and as a drug is an osmotic laxative which can be used for constipation. In pharmaceutical usage, it can be covalently attached to drugs to shield them from the immune system and reduce their clearance, increase their hydrodynamic size to reduce their renal clearance, which increases the drug's half-life, allowing it to be dosed less frequently.

Positive selection Process during T cell and B cell development in which the expression of a functional antigen receptor provides a survival signal and allows lymphocytes to progress to the next stage of development.

Post transplantation lymphoproliferative disorder (PTLD) Conditions resulting in uncontrolled lymphocyte proliferation following a transplantation procedure and may result in lymphomas.

Post-exposure prophylaxis (PEP) The initiation of medical intervention after exposure to a pathogen in an effort to prevent infection.

PPSV Pneumococcal polysaccharide vaccine.

PRBCs Packed red blood cells that have been separated for transfusion, either for anemia or for patients who have lost large amounts of blood.

Pre-exposure prophylaxis (PrEP) The initiation of medical intervention before exposure to a pathogen in an effort to prevent infection.

Primary or Central Lymphoid Organs Organs of the body where lymphocytes develop and mature. They include the thymus and the bone marrow.

Primary immune response The adaptive immune response that is generated after a first exposure to an antigen.

Progressive multifocal leukoencephalopathy (PML) A disease of the white matter of the brain, caused by a viral infection that targets cells that make myelin.

Prostaglandin (PGD) A metabolically active lipid mediator released by mast cells and other immune cells as a result of arachidonic acid metabolism by cyclooxygenase enzymes.

Prostaglandin D2 (PGD2) A prostaglandin that is synthesized by mast cells and other immune cells and that binds the receptors PTGDR and CRT_H2. It plays important roles during immune responses mediated by T_H2 cells, mast cells, and eosinophils.

Prostatic acid phosphatase (PAP) An enzyme produced by the prostate and found to be increased in men with prostate cancer.

Provirus The integration of viral DNA into host DNA which results in expression of viral DNA in every daughter cell. Example: HIV.

Pruritis Itchiness.

Psoriatic arthritis A form of arthritis that affects some people who have the skin condition psoriasis.

PTLD Post-transplant lymphoproliferative disorder; uncontrolled B cell proliferation that can occur after transplantation as a result of immunosuppression. It can lead to the development of B cell lymphomas.

Pulmonary embolism (PE) A blot clot in the artery of the lung. Classic symptoms include desaturation, tachycardia, and shortness of breath.

Pure red cell aplasia (PRCA) A condition characterized by low levels of reticulocytes, loss of erythroblasts in the bone marrow, as well as neutralizing antibodies against EPO.

Purified protein derivative (PPD) A test used to detect if the patient has been exposed to Mycobacterium tuberculosis. Is also referred to as a Mantoux test.

Pyogenic (pus-causing) bacteria Bacteria such as Staphylococcus aureus, which induce the formation of pus.

Pyrogen A substance, either an endogenous cytokine or exogenous microbial product (such as LPS) that causes a fever.

RAG-1 Recombinase Activating Gene-1. Enzyme that forms a complex with RAG-2 and facilitates VDJ recombination in T cell receptor and B cell receptor genes.

RAG-2 Recombinase Activating Gene-2. Enzyme that forms a complex with RAG-1 and facilitates VDJ recombination in T cell receptor and B cell receptor genes.

RANK/RANKL Receptor activator of nuclear factor kappa-B/Receptor activator of nuclear factor kappa-B ligand, members of the TNF family which regulate differentiation and activation of osteoclasts thus, they play a role in bone remodeling.

RANTES *Regulated on activation, normal T cell expressed and secreted*; Chemokine, also referred to as CCL5, that is produced by T cells and is chemotactic for T cells, eosinophils, basophils, and other immune cells.

Rapamycin Anti-proliferative agent that suppresses mTOR.

RBCs/PRBCs Red blood cells/packed red blood cells.

Receptor editing Process during B cell development in which B cells that fail negative selection undergo further rearrangement of their light chain V,J gene segments.

Recombinant vaccine Vaccine which utilizes DNA technology to create an antigen that will be utilized in the vaccine.

Regulatory T cell A subset of CD4 T cells that modulates the immune system, suppresses the functions of antigen-specific activated CD4 T cells, maintains tolerance to self-antigens, and prevent autoimmune disease.

REMS Risk evaluation and mitigation strategies, a safety program that the FDA requires for certain medications with serious safety concerns.

Restrictive lung diseases Restrictive lung diseases are respiratory diseases that are characterized by the inability to fully expand the lungs after inhalation of inspired air. This may occur due to alterations in the lung parenchyma as a result of inflammation or due to damage to the chest wall, pleura, muscles, or nerves. Examples of restrictive lung diseases include interstitial lung disease, sarcoidosis, and amyotrophic lateral sclerosis (ALS).

RF Rheumatoid factor, an autoantibody found in RA that has specificity for the Fc portion of IgG antibodies.

Rh factor Rhesus factor, an inherited protein found on the surface of red blood cells.

Rheumatoid arthritis (RA) A chronic, systemic, inflammatory disease, primarily attacking the synovial membrane of peripheral joints and surrounding muscles, tendons, ligaments, and blood vessels.

RIV Recombinant influenza vaccine, a vaccine created used DNA technology.

SAA Serum amyloid A.

sAg, SAg Surface antigen, superantigen.

Sarcoma Tumor of the connective tissue.

SCIG Subcutaneous immune globulin.

Secondary immune response The adaptive immune response that is generated by a second or subsequent exposure to an antigen. Secondary immune responses are quicker and more potent. They are mediated by memory B and T lymphocytes and are also referred to as memory responses.

Secondary lymphoid organs Lymphoid organs such as the spleen and lymph nodes, where adaptive immune responses are initiated. They also include other tissues such as the mucosa-associated lymphoid tissues.

Self tolerance A process during lymphocyte development that deletes lymphocytes that react to self-antigens.

Sepsis An overwhelming immune response to infection. Systemic release of inflammatory mediators can lead to organ damage, multiple organ failure, and in some cases, death.

Severe combined immunodeficiency (SCID) Primary immunodeficiency in which individuals inherit mutations that prevent lymphocyte development. Patients with SCID are unable to develop both T and B cell responses.

Shingles Reactivation of latent herpes zoster virus which presents as a painful rash which occurs primarily on the trunk of the body.

Short acting beta agonists (SABAs) Rescue medications that initiate quick, temporary relief of asthma symptoms by relaxing bronchospasms, thus opening up the airways.

SIT [Allergen]-specific immunotherapy, also known as desensitization or hyposensitization, is a potentially disease-modifying or curative therapy to treat environmental allergies. Patients are exposed to low doses of offending allergens with the goal of shifting the immune response from one that is allergic (IgE-based) to one that is tolerant (IgG4-based) to the specific allergen.

SLAMF7 Signaling Lymphocyte Activation Molecule F7, a receptor expressed on NK cells as well as Multiple Myeloma cells.

Small cell lung cancer (SCLC) The most aggressive form of lung cancer accounting for approximately 10–15% of all lung cancers. Strongly associated with cigarette smoking. Starts in the bronchi and quickly metastasizes to other areas of the body.

SOFA Sequential organ failure assessment score, uses lab results to predict ICU mortality, particularly in cases of sepsis and septic shock. The score consists of clinical data from the respiratory, cardiovascular, hepatic, coagulation, renal and neurological systems.

Somatic hypermutation Process in which the genes encoding antibody variable regions are mutated in activated B cells, resulting in the development of variant antibodies that have a higher affinity for antigens.

Spleen Organ situated near the stomach that removes damaged or senescent red blood cells from circulation. It is a secondary lymphoid organ that is involved in the initiation of adaptive immunity to blood-borne pathogens.

STAT Signal Transducer and Activator of Transcription. Members of this family of transcription factors are phosphorylated by receptor associated kinases and then form homo- or heterodimers that translocate to the nucleus and activate various genes.

STAT6 A STAT family member that is involved in IL-4 signaling and is essential for its immunological effects.

Steven Johnson syndrome (SJS) A severe skin reaction, potentially life-threatening, that is triggered by hypersensitivity to some types of drugs. Together, with toxic epidermal necrolysis, it can lead to the blistering and peeling off of skin in the mucus membranes and multiple organ failure if not treated.

Stress proteins Proteins such as the MIC proteins that are expressed or released when cells are stressed due to infection, malignant transformation, or other means. They are involved in the activation of NK cells, γδ T cells, and other cell types.

Subunit vaccine Vaccine that contains a protein, usually the most antigenic component, which has been isolated from the pathogen.

Systemic juvenile idiopathic arthritis (SJIA) Rheumatic disease with unknown cause affecting children, usually 5 and under. Sometimes referred to as Still's disease, or Still's syndrome.

Systemic lupus erythematosus (SLE) An autoimmune disease which correlates with Hypersensitivity Type III. IgG antibodies target several surface and intracellular self-antigens forming immune complexes that get deposited in skin, kidneys, and joints resulting in inflammation.

T cell Lymphocyte derived from the common lymphoid progenitor and completes its development in the thymus. T cells express receptors that recognize peptide antigens presented on MHC class I or MHC class II molecules. They mediate cell-mediated immunity and differentiate into cytotoxic, helper, and regulatory T cell subsets.

T-bet T-box transcription factor 21 is a transcription factor encoded by the TBX21 gene that is expressed in T_H1 cells and regulates the expression of IFN-γ.

T-VEC Talimogene laherparepvec, a genetically engineered herpesvirus injected into melanoma lesions. The virus replicates in the cancer cells and causes them to lyse.

T1D Type 1 Diabetes, an autoimmune disease in which the pancreas stops producing insulin needed to regulate glucose in the body.

TCR T-cell receptor, a surface protein complex that participates in T-cell activation by recognizing foreign antigens presented by major histocompatibility complexes on APCs.

Teratogen An agent which causes defects in the developing embryo or fetus during gestation.

T_{FH} cells Follicular helper T cells, specialized T cells that provide help to B cells, and are essential for the development of memory B cells and high affinity antibodies.

TGF Transforming growth factor, a cytokine secreted by macrophages, B cells, and T cells. It functions in cell growth, cell differentiation, apoptosis and cellular homeostasis when bound to its receptor, TGFβ type II receptor.

TGF-β Anti-inflammatory cytokine that helps to resolve inflammation following an immune response. Contributes to T_H17 and T_{reg} differentiation.

T_H cells CD4 T helper cells, a type of T cell that cooperates with other types of cells and aids in their activation and function, such as inducing antibody production.

T_H1 cells A subset of helper T cells that is involved in cell-mediated responses and host defense against intracellular pathogens. It produces the cytokines IFN-γ and TNF-α which induce macrophage activation, nitric oxide production, and promote cytotoxic T lymphocyte activity. They are involved in autoimmune diseases, including rheumatoid arthritis and multiple sclerosis.

T_H17 cells A subset of activated helper T cells that promotes immunity to extracellular bacteria and fungi by inducing neutrophil activation. They are also implicated in autoimmune responses. They produce the cytokines IL-17A, IL-17F, IL-21, IL-22, IL-26, GM-CSF, macrophage inflammatory protein 3a, and TNF-α.

T_H2 cells A subset of effector helper T cells that coordinates immune responses to large extracellular pathogens such as parasites. They are also involved in humoral immunity. They produce the cytokines IL-4, IL-5, IL-9, IL-10, and IL-13. They are pathogenic in allergic diseases.

T_H22 cells A subset of helper T cells that produces IL-22 and is found in increased numbers in skin lesions of patients with atopic dermatitis and psoriasis. IL-22 produced by T_H22 cells is required for the homeostatic integrity of the skin and maintaining the balance between homeostasis and skin disease.

Thrombocytopenia Abnormally low platelet count.

Thrombopoietin (TPO) A glycoprotein hormone that stimulates the production of platelets.

Thymic stromal lymphopoietin (TSLP) A cytokine that induces the maturation of T cells by modulating dendritic cell or macrophage function.

Thymocyte Pre-T cell undergoing development in the thymus.

Thymus Primary lymphoid organ in the mediastinum that is responsible for the development and maturation of T cells.

TIM1 T cell transmembrane, immunoglobulin, and mucin gene 1, which has been linked to susceptibility to developing asthma in humans, through undefined mechanisms.

TLR Toll-like receptor, a set of proteins expressed on innate immune cells that recognize non-specific molecular patterns on microbes.

TNF Tumor necrosis factor, a pro-inflammatory cytokine, that is rapidly produced during inflammation. It is involved in the acute phase reaction. It is mainly released by macrophages, but is also produced by many other leukocytes. It promotes vasodilation, induces the expression of adhesion molecules on blood vessels, and induces a wide variety of cellular functions including immune regulation, cellular proliferation, and apoptosis.

Tolerance Immunological non-responsiveness to an antigen.

Tonsil Lymphoid tissues in the throat.

Total parental nutrition (TPN) A method of supplying all nutritional requirements to the body that bypasses the GI tract, usually through an intravenous catheter.

Toxic epidermal necrolysis (TEN) A potentially life threatening dermatologic reaction to certain medications. It involves the blistering and peeling off of the skin, exposing the raw skin. Mucus membranes are often involved. It can lead to multiple organ failure if not treated.

Toxic shock syndrome (TSS) An acute systemic illness commonly characterized by fever, hypotension, and rash secondary to infection. Historically associated with tampon use in otherwise healthy women.

Toxoid vaccine A vaccine created using the inactivated toxin from certain bacteria in order to elicit an immune response and memory immunity to the toxin.

TRH Thyrotropin-releasing hormone.

TSH/TSHR Thyroid stimulating hormone/Thyroid stimulating hormone receptor; proteins that are involved in the production of the thyroid hormones triiodothyronine and thyroxine that regulate cellular function, metabolism, and body temperature. Their activity is controlled by the pituitary gland and their dysfunction is associated with thyroid diseases.

TSI Thyroid-stimulating immunoglobulin, presence may indicate Grave's disease.

Tumor lysis syndrome (TLS) A condition that results from quick breakdown of cancer cells. Characterized by nausea, vomiting, diarrhea, lack of energy, as well as painful sores or ulcers on the skin, mouth, or lips.

Tumor-associated antigens Antigens that may be expressed on tumor cells in higher amounts than is expressed on normal cells.

Tumor-associated macrophage (TAM) A macrophage that becomes polarized within the tumor to promote its growth.

Tumor-specific antigens Antigens that are found only on tumor cells and not on normal cells.

Type I interferons Interferon molecules such as IFN-α and IFN-β that are rapidly produced by epithelial cells and plasmacytoid dendritic cells after viral infections and that serve to alert the rest of the immune system. They induce the activation of NK cells and participate in the interferon response.

Type I hypersensitivity See immediate hypersensitivity.

Type II hypersensitivity Immune reactions that are induced to antigens resulting from the interactions of small chemically reactive molecules with cell surface components. They are mediated by IgG antibodies that activate Fc-bearing phagocytes and other cells, causing tissue damage.

Type III hypersensitivity Immune reactions that are mediated by immune complexes that are formed during secondary immune responses to soluble proteins of non-human origin. The IgG-containing immune complexes cause tissue damage when they are deposited in various tissues.

Type IV hypersensitivity Immune reactions mediated by activated memory T cells to specific antigens. It is also referred to as delayed type hypersensitivity because it takes several days to be established. It is called cell-mediated immunity as opposed to hypersensitivity mediated by antibodies. An example of a type IV hypersensitivity reaction is the tuberculin test, which involves the activation of T_H1 cells to purified protein derivative from the mycobacteria that cause tuberculosis.

Ulcerative colitis (UC) A chronic inflammation of the large intestine characterized by ulcers and inflammation of the colon and rectum.

Uveitis Inflammation of the uvea, which consists of the iris, ciliary body, and choroid. If not treated quickly it can cause permanent damage to eye tissue resulting in permanent vision loss.

Vaccination The administration of antigens to an individual in order to stimulate an adaptive immune response that will protect against a certain disease.

Variable region Antigen-binding region of an antibody, BCR or TCR.

Varicella zoster virus (VZV) One of eight herpes viruses that infects humans exclusively and is highly infectious. It causes chickenpox in children and teens, and shingles in older adults.

Vasopressor A drug class that works to constrict the blood vessels, thus raising blood pressure.

VCAM Vascular cell adhesion protein, a molecule that is expressed on activated endothelial cells ad binds to $\alpha_4\beta_1$ integrin on leukocytes to mediate their adhesion (or sticking) to the endothelium.

VDJ Variable, Diversity and Joining gene segments that encode for the variable regions of T cell receptors and B cell receptors. These segments randomly associate during the recombination process to create unique and diverse antigen receptor repertoires.

VEGF Vascular endothelial growth factor is a signaling protein that helps stimulate the growth of new blood vessels.

VLPs Virus-like particles resemble a virus but lack genetic material; therefore, they are not infectious. They are composed of structural proteins which allow them to initiate an immune response making them desirable for vaccine development.

WBC White blood cells, also known as leukocytes, are derived from stem cells to fight off foreign invaders in the body including viruses, bacteria and germs. There are five different types of white blood cells; neutrophils, lymphocytes, basophils, monocytes, and eosinophils.

Xenograft The transplantation of tissues or cells from one species to another.

Xenotransplantation The transfer of cells, tissues and organs from one species into another to replace damaged or missing components.

Index

Printed in the United States
By Bookmasters